The
IMAGE
PROCESSING
Handbook
Third Edition

John C. Russ

Materials Science and Engineering Department
North Carolina State University
Raleigh, North Carolina

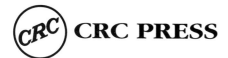 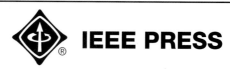

A CRC Handbook Published in Cooperation with IEEE Press

Publisher: Ron Powers
Project Editor: Carol Whitehead
Marketing Manager: Jane Stark
Cover Design: Jon Pennell
Manufacturing: Carol Slatter

Library of Congress Cataloging-in-Publication Data

Russ, John C.
    The image processing handbook / John C. Russ. -- 3rd ed.
        p.   cm.
    Includes bibliographical references and index.
    ISBN 0-8493-2532-3 (alk. paper)
    1. Image processing. I. Title
TA1637.R87 1998
    621.36'7--dc21   98-24465
                                                                      CIP

Introduction

Image processing is used for two somewhat different purposes:

a) improving the visual appearance of images to a human viewer, and

b) preparing images for measurement of the features and structures present.

The techniques that are appropriate for each of these tasks are not always the same, but there is considerable overlap. This book covers methods that are used for both purposes.

To do the best possible job, it helps to know about the uses to which the processed images will be put. For visual enhancement, this means having some familiarity with the human visual process, and an appreciation of what cues the viewer responds to in images. It also is useful to know about the printing process, since many images are processed in the context of reproduction or transmission.

The measurement of images generally requires that features be well defined, either by edges or unique (and uniform) brightness or color, texture, or some combination of these factors. The types of measurements that will be performed on entire scenes or individual features are important in determining the appropriate processing steps.

It may help to recall that image processing, like food processing or word processing, does not reduce the amount of data present but simply rearranges it. Some arrangements may be more appealing to the senses, and some may convey more meaning, but these two criteria may not be identical nor use identical methods.

This handbook presents an extensive collection of image processing tools, so that the user of computer-based systems can both understand those methods provided in packaged software, and program those additions which may be needed for particular applications. Comparisons are presented of different algorithms that may be used for similar purposes, using a selection of representative pictures from light and electron microscopes, as well as macroscopic, satellite and astronomical images.

In revising the book for this new edition, I have tried to respond to some of the comments and requests of readers and reviewers. New chapters on the measurement of images and the subsequent interpretation of the data were added in the second edition, and now there is a major new section on the important subject of surface images which includes both processing and measurement. The sections on the ever-advancing hardware for image capture and printing have been expanded and information added on the newest technologies. More examples have been added in every chapter, and the reference list expanded and brought up to date.

However, I have resisted suggestions to put "more of the math" into the book. There are excellent texts on image processing, compression, mathematical morphology, etc., that provide as much rigor and as many derivations as may be needed. Many of them are referenced here. But the thrust of this book remains teaching by example. Few people learn the principles of image processing from the equations. Just as we use images to "do science," so most of us use images to learn about many things, including imaging itself. The hope is that by seeing what various operations do to representative images, you will discover how and why to use them. Then, if you need to look up the mathematical foundations, they will be easier to understand.

The reader is encouraged to use this book in concert with a real source of images and a computer-based system, and to freely experiment with different methods to determine which are most appropriate for his or her particular needs. Selection of image processing tools to explore images when you don't know the contents beforehand is a much more difficult task than using tools to make it easier for another viewer or a measurement program to see the same things you have discovered. It places greater demand on computing speed and the interactive nature of the interface. But it particularly requires that you become a very analytical observer of images. If you can learn to see what the computer sees, you will become a better viewer and obtain the best possible images, suitable for further processing.

To facilitate this hands-on learning process, I have collaborated with my son, Chris Russ, to produce a CD-ROM that can be used as a companion to this book. The Image Processing Tool Kit contains more than 200 images, many of them the examples from this book, plus over 100 Photoshop-compatible plug-ins that implement many of the algorithms discussed here. These can be used with Adobe Photoshop® or any of the numerous programs (some of them free) that implement the Photoshop plug-in interface, on either Macintosh or Windows computers. Information about the CD-ROM is available on-line at http://members.AOL.com/ImagProcTK/.

Acknowledgments
All of the image processing and the creation of the resulting figures included in this book were performed on an Apple Macintosh®

computer. Many of the images were acquired directly from various microscopes and other sources using color or monochrome video cameras and digitized directly into the computer. Others were digitized using a digital camera (Polaroid DMC), and some were obtained using a 24-bit color scanner, often from images supplied by many coworkers and researchers. These are acknowledged wherever the origin of an image could be determined. A few examples, taken from the literature, are individually referenced.

The book was produced by directly making color-separated films with an imagesetter without intermediate hard copy, negatives or prints of the images, etc. Amongst other things, this means that the author must bear full responsibility for any errors, since no traditional typesetting was involved. (It has also forced me to learn more than I ever hoped to know about some aspects of this technology!) However, going directly from disk file to print also shortens the time needed in production and helps to keep costs down, while preserving the full quality of the images.

Special thanks are due to Chris Russ (Reindeer Games, Inc., Asheville, NC) who has helped to program many of these algorithms and contributed invaluable comments, and to Helen Adams, who has proofread many pages, endured many discussions, and provided the moral support that makes writing projects such as this possible.

John C. Russ
Raleigh, NC

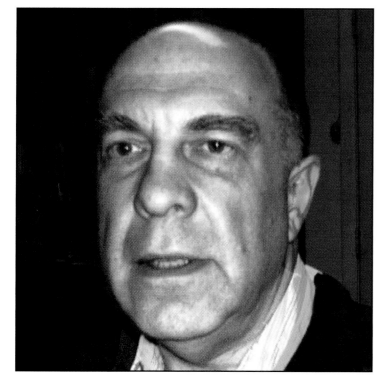

The author, in stereo.

Contents

1 Acquiring Images **1**

Human reliance on images for information *1*
Using video cameras to acquire images *7*
Electronics and bandwidth limitations *15*
High resolution imaging *25*
Color imaging *32*
Digital cameras *41*
Color spaces *47*
Color displays *56*
Image types *59*
Range imaging *61*
Multiple images *68*
Stereoscopy *72*
Imaging requirements *80*

2 Printing and Storage **87**

Printing *87*
Dots on paper *92*
Color printing *98*
Printing hardware *104*
Film recorders *110*
File storage *113*
Optical storage media *114*
Magnetic recording *118*
Databases for images *120*
Browsing and thumbnails *124*
Lossless coding *128*
Color palettes *135*
Lossy compression *136*
Other compression methods *155*
Digital movies *158*

3 Correcting Imaging Defects 161

Noisy images 162
Neighborhood averaging 166
Neighborhood ranking 174
Other neighborhood noise reduction methods . 182
Maximum entropy 189
Contrast expansion 191
Nonuniform illumination 194
Fitting a background function 196
Rank leveling 199
Color shading 205
Nonplanar views 209
Computer graphics 210
Geometrical distortion 213
Alignment 216
Morphing 222

4 Image Enhancement 227

Contrast manipulation 228
Histogram equalization 233
Laplacian 242
Derivatives 250
The Sobel and Kirsch operators 255
Rank operations 268
Texture 278
Fractal analysis 282
Implementation notes 288
Image math 290
Subtracting images 292
Multiplication and division 295

5 Processing Images in Frequency Space 305

Some necessary mathematical preliminaries .. 305
    What frequency space is all about 305
    The Fourier transform 307
    Fourier transforms of real functions 311
    Frequencies and orientations 318
Measuring images in the frequency domain ... 320
    Orientation and spacing 320
    Preferred orientation 324
    Texture and fractals 330

Filtering images 334
   Isolating periodic noise 334
   Masks and filters 341
   Selection of periodic information 348
Convolution and correlation 354
   Fundamentals of convolution 354
   Imaging system characteristics 358
   Removing motion blur and other defects 362
   Template matching and correlation 365
   Autocorrelation 367
Conclusion 370

6 Segmentation and Thresholding 371

Thresholding 371
Multiband images 374
Two-dimensional thresholds 377
Multiband thresholding 381
Thresholding from texture 386
Multiple thresholding criteria 391
Textural orientation 395
Accuracy and reproducibility 400
Including position information 403
Selective histograms 410
Boundary lines 413
Contours 416
Image representation 420
Other segmentation methods 423
The general classification problem 427

7 Processing Binary Images 431

Boolean operations 431
Combining Boolean operations 434
Masks 438
From pixels to features 440
Boolean logic with features 447
Selecting features by location 451
Double thresholding 456
Erosion and dilation 460
Opening and closing 461
Isotropy 465

Measurements using erosion and dilation 467
Extension to grey scale images 469
Coefficient and depth parameters 471
Examples of use 476
The custer 481
Skeletonization 483
Boundary lines and thickening 485
Euclidean distance map 489
Watershed segmentation 494
Ultimate eroded points 498
Fractal dimension measurement 501
Medial axis transform 501
Cluster analysis 504

8 Image Measurements 509

Brightness measurements 510
Determining location 516
Orientation 518
Neighbor relationships 519
Alignment 523
Counting features 529
Special counting procedures 532
Feature size 536
Caliper dimensions 543
Perimeter 549
Ellipse fitting 551
Describing shape 553
Fractal dimension 555
Harmonic analysis 559
Topology 562
Feature identification 566
Three-dimensional measurements 569

9 3D Image Acquisition 575

Volume imaging vs. sections 575
Basics of reconstruction 578
Algebraic reconstruction methods 585
Maximum entropy 590
Defects in reconstructed images 592
Imaging geometries 603
Three-dimensional tomography 605
High-resolution tomography 613

10 3D Image Visualization 617

Sources of 3D data 617
Serial sections 619
Optical sectioning 624
Sequential removal 627
Stereo 629
3D data sets 633
Slicing the data set 636
Arbitrary section planes 641
The use of color 645
Volumetric display 646
Stereo viewing 650
Special display hardware 654
Ray tracing 657
Reflection 662
Surfaces 667
Multiply connected surfaces 673
Image processing in 3D 679
Measurements on 3D images 683
Conclusion 686

11 Imaging Surfaces 689

Producing surfaces 689
Devices that image surfaces by
    physical contact 692
Noncontacting measurements 696
Microscopy of surfaces 700
Surface composition imaging 703
Processing of range images 706
Processing of composition maps 710
Data presentation and visualization 712
Rendering and visualization 717
Analysis of surface data 722
Profile measurements 725
The Birmingham measurement suite 729
New approaches — topographic analysis
    and fractal dimensions 737

References 747

Index 763

The
IMAGE
PROCESSING
Handbook
Third Edition

1

Acquiring Images

Human reliance on images for information

Humans are primarily visual creatures. Not all animals depend on their eyes, as we do, for 99% or more of the information received about their surroundings. Bats use high frequency sound, cats have poor vision but a rich sense of smell, snakes locate prey by heat emission, and fish have organs that sense (and in some cases generate) electrical fields. Even birds, which are highly visual, do not have our eye configuration. Their eyes are on opposite sides of their heads, providing nearly 360-degree coverage but little in the way of stereopsis, and they have four or five different color receptors (we have three, loosely described as red, green, and blue). It is difficult to imagine what the world "looks like" to such animals. Even the word "imagine" contains within it our bias towards images, as does much of our language. People with vision defects wear glasses because of their dependence on this sense. We tolerate considerable hearing loss before resorting to a hearing aid and there are, practically speaking, no prosthetic devices for the other senses.

This bias in everyday life extends to how we pursue more technical goals as well. Scientific instruments commonly produce images to communicate results to the operator, rather than generating an audible tone or emitting a smell. Space missions to other planets and Comet Halley always include cameras as major components, and we judge the success of those missions by the quality of the images returned. This suggests a few of the ways in which we have extended the range of our natural

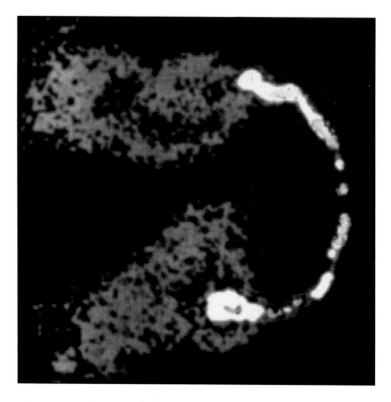

Figure 1. Radio astronomy produces images such as this view of NGC1265. These are often displayed with false colors to emphasize subtle variations in signal brightness.

vision. Simple optical devices such as microscopes and telescopes allow us to see things that are vastly smaller or larger than we could otherwise. Beyond the visible portion of the electromagnetic spectrum (a narrow range of wavelengths between about 400 and 700 nanometers) we now have sensors capable of detecting infrared and ultraviolet light, X-rays, and radio waves. **Figure 1** shows an example, an image presenting radio telescope data in the form of an image in which grey scale brightness represents radio intensity. Such devices and presentations are used to further extend our imaging capability.

Signals other than electromagnetic radiation can be used to produce images as well. Acoustic waves at low frequency produce

Figure 2. Scanning acoustic microscope image (with superimposed signal profile along one scan line) of a polished cross section through a composite. The central white feature is a fiber intersecting the surface at an angle. The arcs on either side are interference patterns which can be used to measure the fiber angle.

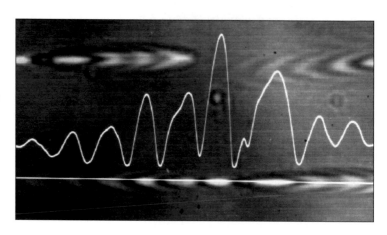

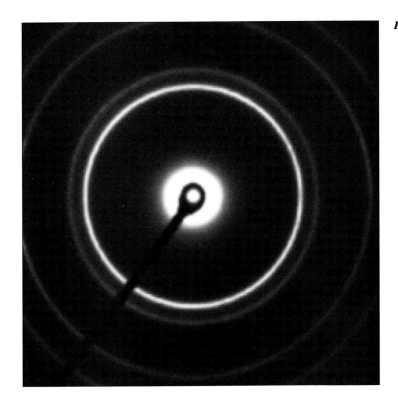

Figure 3. An electron diffraction pattern from a thin foil of gold. The ring diameters correspond to diffraction angles that identify the spacings of planes of atoms in the crystal structure.

sonar images, while at gigahertz frequencies the acoustic microscope produces images with resolution similar to that of the light microscope, but with image contrast that is produced by local variations in the attenuation and refraction of sound waves rather

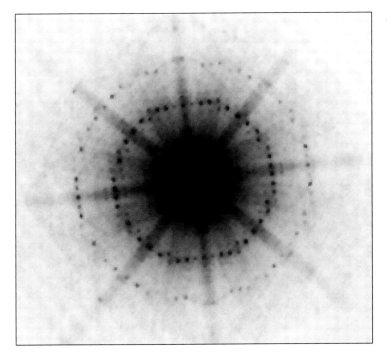

Figure 4. A convergent beam electron diffraction (CBED) pattern from an oxide microcrystal, which can be indexed and measured to provide high accuracy values for the atomic unit cell dimensions.

Figure 5. *Typical graphics used to communicate news information (Source:* USA Today).

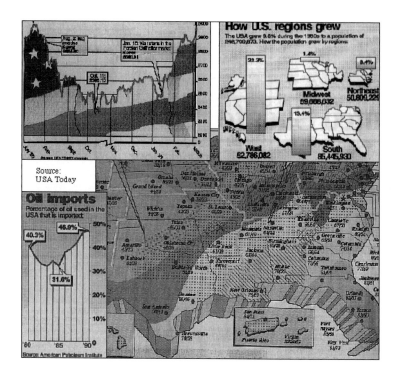

than light. **Figure 2** shows an acoustic microscope image of a composite material.

Some images such as holograms or electron diffraction patterns are recorded in terms of brightness as a function of position, but are unfamiliar to the observer. **Figures 3** and **4** show electron diffraction patterns from a transmission electron microscope, in which the atomic structure of the samples is revealed (but only to those who know how to interpret the image). Other kinds of data including weather maps with isotherms, elaborate graphs of business profit and expenses, and charts with axes representing time, family income, cholesterol level, or even more obscure parameters, have become part of our daily lives. **Figure 5** shows a few examples. The latest developments in computer interfaces and displays make extensive use of graphics, again to take advantage of the large bandwidth of the human visual pathway.

There are some important differences between human vision, the kind of information it yields from images, and the ways in which it seems to do so, compared to the use of imaging devices with computers for technical purposes. Human vision is primarily qualitative and comparative, rather than quantitative. We judge the relative size and shape of objects by mentally rotating them to the same orientation, overlapping them in our minds, and performing a direct comparison. This has been shown by tests in which the time required to recognize features as being the same or different is proportional to the degree of misorientation or intervening distance. **Figure 6** shows an example.

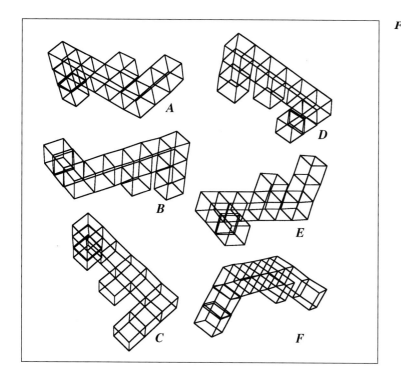

Figure 6. *Several views of a complex three-dimensional figure. Which of the representations is/are identical and which are mirror images? The time needed to decide is proportional to the misalignment, indicating that we literally "turn the objects over" in our minds to compare them.*

Humans are especially poor at judging color or brightness of features within images unless they can be exactly compared by making them adjacent. Gradual changes in brightness with position or

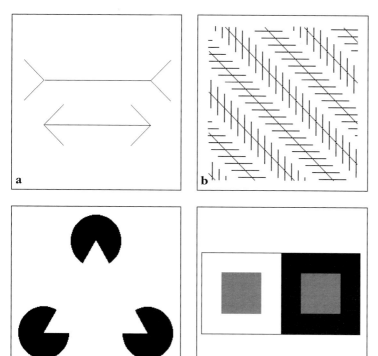

Figure 7. A few common illusions:

a) *the two horizontal lines are identical in length, but appear different because of grouping with the diagonal lines;*

b) *the diagonal lines are parallel, but the crossing lines cause them to appear to diverge due to grouping and inhibition;*

c) *the illusory triangle may appear brighter than the surrounding paper, due to grouping and completion;*

d) *the two inner squares have the same brightness, but the outer frames cause us to judge them as different due to brightness inhibition.*

Figure 8. An example of camouflage. Grouping together of many seemingly distinct features in the image and ignoring apparent similarities between others allows the eye to find the real structures present.

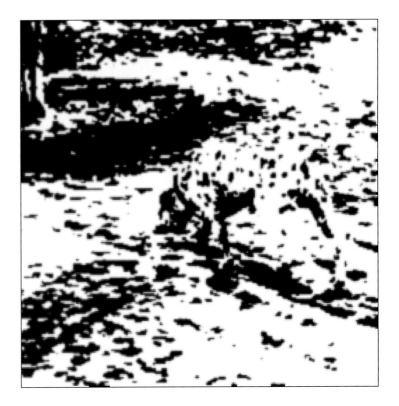

over time are generally ignored as representing variations in illumination, for which the human visual system compensates automatically. This means that only abrupt changes in brightness are easily seen. It is believed that only these discontinuities, which usually correspond to physical boundaries or other important structures in the scene being viewed, are extracted from the raw image falling on the retina and sent up to the higher-level processing centers in the cortex.

These characteristics of the visual system allow a variety of visual illusions (**Figure 7**). Some of these illusions enable researchers to study the visual system itself, and others suggest ways that computer-based systems can emulate some of the very efficient (if not always exact) ways that our eyes extract information. Gestalt theory says that this is done by dealing with the image as a whole, rather than by breaking it down to constituent parts. The idea that grouping of parts within images is done automatically by our vision system, and is central to our understanding of scenes, has been confirmed by many experiments and offers important insights into human physiology and psychology. One of the things it explains is why camouflage works (**Figure 8**). Our purpose in this book is not to study the human visual pathway, but a brief overview can help us to understand how we see things so that we become better observers. The interested reader may want to read Frisby, 1980; Marr, 1982; Rock, 1984; and Hubel, 1988. Computer-based image processing and analysis use

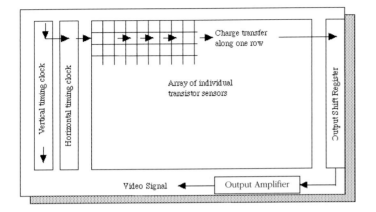

Figure 9. *Diagram of a typical CCD camera chip. The vertical timing clock selects each line of pixel detectors in turn. Then the horizontal clock shifts the contents from each detector to its neighbor, causing the line to read out sequentially into a shift register and amplifier that produces an analog voltage as a function of time.*

algorithms based on human vision methods when possible, but also employ other methods that seem not to have counterparts in human vision.

Using video cameras to acquire images

The first important difference between human vision and computer-based image analysis arises from the ways the images are acquired. The most common sensor is a standard video camera, but there are several important variations available. Solid-state cameras use a chip with an array of individual pixel (picture element) sensors. With current technology, it is possible to place arrays of more than 500,000 devices in an area of less than 1 square centimeter. Each detector functions as a photon counter, as electrons are raised to the conduction band in an isolated well. The signal is read out from each line of detectors to produce the analog voltage. **Figure 9** shows a schematic diagram of a typical device.

Several different types of circuitry are used to read the contents of the detectors, giving rise to CCD (charge coupled device), CID (charge injection device), and other designations. **Figure 10** shows an example. The most important effect of these differences is that some camera designs allow dim images to be accumulated for extended periods of time in the chip or (conversely) very short duration events to be captured in high speed imaging, and be read out nondestructively, while others can only function

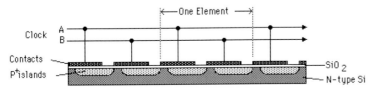

Figure 10. *Schematic diagram of the chip in a solid state camera. Each sensor records the incident illumination; the signals are read out sequentially to form the raster scan.*

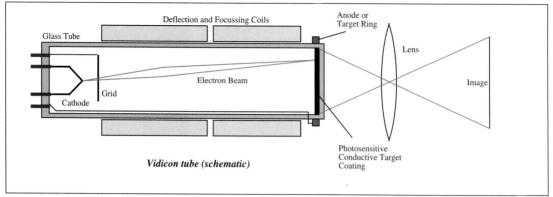

Vidicon tube (schematic)

Figure 11. *Functional diagram of a Vidicon tube. Light striking the coating changes its resistance and hence the current that flows as the electron beam scans in a raster pattern.*

Figure 12. *Response of photographic film. The "H&D" curve includes the linear response range in which the slope distinguishes high- and low-contrast films. High contrast means that a small range of exposure causes a large change in film density. Density is defined as the base-ten logarithm of the fraction of incident light that is transmitted.*

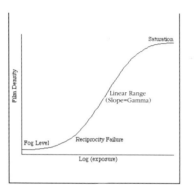

Figure 13. *Response of a light sensor. Gamma values greater or less than 1.0 expand or compress the contrast range at the dark or light end of the range.*

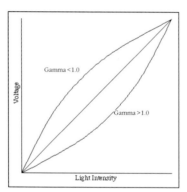

with continuous scanning. Cameras used to store the very low-intensity images encountered in astronomy, fluorescence microscopy, and some X-ray imaging devices are usually cooled to keep the electronic noise down. Integration times up to many minutes are not uncommon.

The older type of video camera uses a vacuum tube. Light passes inside the glass envelope to strike a coating whose conductivity is altered by the photons. A scanning electron beam strikes this coating, and the change in resistance is converted to the image signal. Many varieties of tube design are used, some

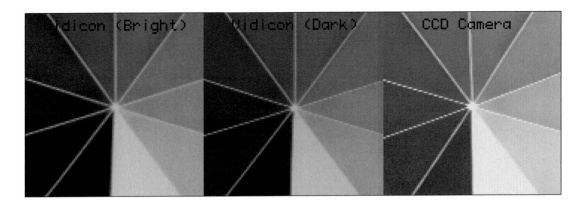

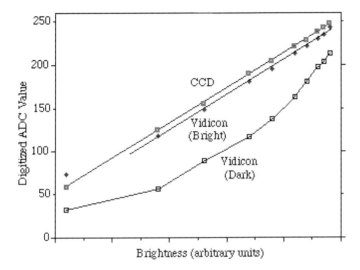

Figure 14. *Camera response curves determined by measuring an image of a series of photographic density steps as shown. The CCD camera is linear (gamma=1) while the vidicon varies with overall illumination level.*

with intermediate cathode layers or special coatings for low-light-level sensitivity. The simple vidicon shown in **Figure 11** is the least expensive and most common type, and can serve as a prototype for comparison to solid-state cameras.

Electronic cameras are similar to film in some respects. Film is characterized by a response to light exposure which (after chemical development) produces a density vs. exposure curve such as that shown in **Figure 12**. The low end of this curve represents the fog level of the film, the density that is present even without exposure. At the high end, the film saturates to a maximum optical density, for instance based on the maximum physical density of silver particles. In between, it has a linear relationship whose slope represents the contrast of the film. A high slope corresponds to a high-contrast film that exhibits a large change in optical density with a small change in exposure. Conversely, a low-contrast film has a broader latitude to record a scene with a greater range of brightnesses. A value of gamma greater or less than 1 indicates that the curve is not linear, but instead compresses either the dark or bright end of the range, as indicated in **Figure 13**.

Both solid-state and tube-type cameras are characterized by contrast and latitude, and may have values of gamma that are not equal to 1. Sometimes, special electronics circuits are used to vary gamma intentionally. Solid-state cameras are inherently linear. Some tube-type cameras are also linear, but the most common type, the vidicon, is quite nonlinear when the average illumination level is low, and becomes linear for bright scenes. **Figure 14** shows images of a grey scale wedge (as used in the photographic darkroom) obtained with a CCD camera and with a vidicon. The CCD response is linear, while that for the vidicon changes with the overall brightness level. This variability introduces some problems for image processing.

Solid-state cameras have several advantages and some drawbacks, as compared to tube-type cameras. Tube cameras may suffer from blooming, in which a bright spot is enlarged due to the spreading of light or electrons in the coating. Dissipation within the coating also makes integration of dim images impractical, while the time lag required for the coating material to respond causes "comet tails" behind moving bright spots. **Figure 15** shows examples of blooming and comet tails. These cameras may also exhibit distortion in the raster scan, producing either pincushion or barrel distortion (**Figure 16**) or more complicated effects, especially if used near instruments or wiring that generate stray magnetic fields. Keeping the two interlaced fields within each full frame in exact alignment can also be a problem.

Defocusing of the electron beam at the corners of the tube face may cause the corners and edges of the image to degrade in sharpness, while light absorbed in passing through the thicker glass near edges may cause the corners and edges to be dim.

Figure 15. *Blooming in a vidicon camera. The bright spot is of constant actual size but appears to grow larger as its brightness increases. There is also tailing on the right side (shown in the brightness profiles) due to the recovery time of the tube electronics. The fourth image at the right shows a dark comet tail when the spot is moved, due to the long recovery time of the phosphor coating.*

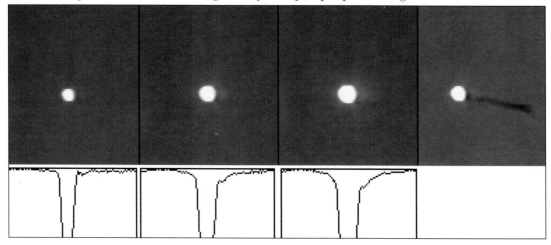

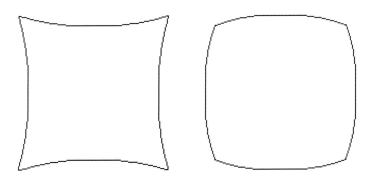

Figure 16. *Pincushion and barrel distortion. The ideal raster scan is rectilinear, but the use of magnetic deflection, and the curvature of the front face of the camera tube, may cause distortion. The variation in distance from the electron gun to the front face may also require dynamic focusing to keep edges and corners from blurring.*

Figure 17 shows an example of this vignetting. The simplest design tube cameras, such as the vidicon, have a relationship between output signal and illumination that varies as the average brightness level varies, which confuses absolute measurements of brightness or density. Tube cameras also degrade with time when installed in a vertical orientation (such as mounted to the top of a microscope), as internal contaminants settle onto the coating. They are also usually physically larger, heavier and more fragile than solid-state cameras.

On the other hand, solid state cameras rely on each of the 500,000 or more sensors being identical, which is difficult even with modern chip fabrication techniques. Variations in sensitivity show up as noise in the image. Chip cameras are also most sensitive at the red end of the visible spectrum, as shown in **Figure 18**. Many are also sensitive to infrared light that, if not eliminated in the optics, can produce an overall blur or fogging since it is unlikely to be correctly focused. For some astronomical and remote sensing applications in which extended infrared sensitivity is desired, the spectral response of the CCD can be extended even further. One way this is done is by thinning the substrate and illuminating the chip from the back side so that the light can reach the active region with less absorption in the overlying metal or silicide gate contacts. Another approach uses other semiconductors, such as In-Sb, instead of silicon.

By comparison, tube cameras can use coating materials that duplicate the spectral sensitivity of the human eye, or may be tailored to selected parts of the spectrum. However, most of these materials have a spectral response that is a function of the total brightness, so that "color shifts" may occur. This means that the same color object will appear different at different illumination levels, or the difference in brightness between two different color objects will vary at different illumination levels. These color shifts make attempts to perform colorimetry (the measurement of color, typically for quality control purposes) using video cameras extremely difficult to standardize or to keep in calibration.

Figure 17. *Darkening of edges and corners of an image of a blank grey card acquired with a vidicon, shown as originally acquired and with the contrast expanded to make the vignetting more obvious. Printing technology causes the apparent stepped or contoured variation in brightness, which is actually a smoothly varying function of position.*

The size of the chip used in cameras has been reduced from 1 inch to 2/3, 1/2 and now 1/3 inch (diagonal), in order to take advantage of improvements in reducing the size of devices in integrated circuits to obtain higher yields and reduced cost. The need to keep some space between the individual transistors for electrical isolation, and to prevent light from scattering from one to another, means that as the overall size of the chip is reduced, the fraction of coverage by active devices drops, in some cases to as little as 50%. This means that half of the light is discarded. If interline transfer devices are used (in which a row of light-shielded transistors is interposed between the rows of active ones

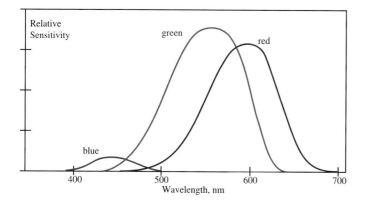

a

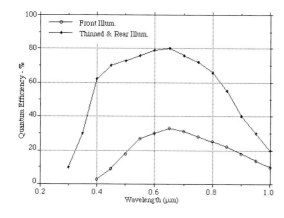
b

Figure 18. Spectral response:
a) sensitivity of the cones in the human retina; while they are commonly identified as red-, green- and blue-sensitive, each actually responds to a wide range of wavelengths;
b) response of a solid state detector for the normal case of front illumination, and rear illumination after thinning the support, showing greater red and infrared sensitivity.

to assist in readout) they also take up space and reduce efficiency. One solution is to cover the transistor array on the chip with an array of "lenslets." Each tiny lens collects light and directs it to one individual detector. There is no attempt to focus the light, just to collect it so that essentially 100% of the light falling on the chip is measured. Assuring the uniformity of the lenslet array still presents challenges to camera performance in technical applications.

The trend is clearly toward solid-state cameras, which are continually improving in resolution (number of individual sensors), uniformity, and cost. It remains to be seen whether the commercial development of high-definition television (HDTV) will result in a significant improvement of cameras, which are not the weakest link in the imaging chain used for commercial television.

Regardless of what type of camera is employed to acquire images, it is important to focus the optics correctly to capture the fine details in the image. Usually the human eye is used to perform this task. In some situations, such as automated microscopy of pathology slides or surveillance tracking of vehicles, automatic focusing

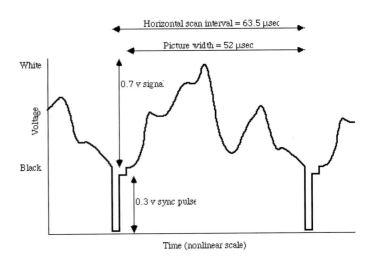

Figure 19. *Composite video signal used in US television. Each scan line duration is 63.5 μsec, of which 52 μsec contains one line of the image. The remainder contains the 5 μsec horizontal sync pulse, plus other timing and color calibration data.*

is required. This brings computer processing into the initial step of image capture. Sometimes, in the interests of speed, the processing is performed in dedicated hardware circuits attached to the camera. But in any case the algorithms are the same as might be applied in the computer, and in many cases the focusing is accomplished in software by stepping the optics through a range of settings and choosing the one that gives the "best" picture.

Several different approaches to automatic focus are used. Cameras used for macroscopic scenes may employ methods that use some distance measuring technology, e.g., using high frequency sound or infrared light, to determine the distance to the subject so that the lens position can be adjusted. In microscopy applications this is impractical and the variation in the image itself with focus adjustment must be used. Several different algorithms are used to detect the quality of image sharpness, and all are successful for the majority of images in which there is good contrast and fine detail present. Each approach selects some implementation of a high pass filter output which can be realized in various ways, using either hardware or software, but must take into account the effect of high frequency noise in the image and the optical transfer function of the optics (Green et al., 1985; Firestone et al., 1991; Boddeke et al, 1994; Santos et al., 1997).

Figure 20. *The interlaced raster scan used in standard video equipment records the even-numbered scan lines comprising one half-field in 1/60th of a second, and then scans the odd-numbered lines comprising the second half-field in the next 1/60th of a second, giving a complete frame every 30th of a second. European TV is based on 1/50th of a second, corresponding to the 50 Hz frequency of their power grid.*

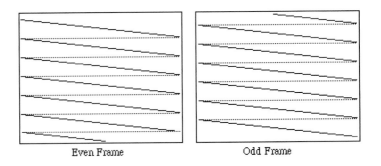

Even Frame   Odd Frame

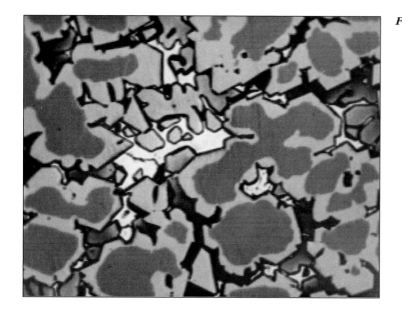

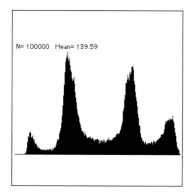

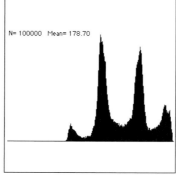

Figure 21. *A grey-scale image digitized from a metallographic microscope and its brightness histogram (white at the left, dark at the right). A bright reflection within the camera tube causes the automatic gain circuit to shift the histogram, even though the bright spot is not within the digitized area. This shifting would cause the same structure to have different grey values in successive images.*

Electronics and bandwidth limitations

Video cameras of either the solid-state or tube type produce analog voltage signals corresponding to the brightness at different points in the image. In the standard RS-170 signal convention, the voltage varies over a 0.7-volt range from minimum to maximum brightness, as shown in **Figure 19**. The scan is nominally 525 lines per full frame, with two interlaced 1/60th-second fields combining to make an entire image (**Figure 20**). Only about 480 of the scan lines are actually usable, with the remainder lost during vertical retrace. In a typical broadcast television picture, more of these lines are lost due to overscanning, leaving fewer than 400 lines in the actual viewed area. The time duration of each scan line is 62.5 μs, part of which is used for horizontal retrace. This leaves 52 μs for the image data, which must be subdivided into the horizontal spacing of discernible pixels. For PAL (European) television, these values are slightly different based on a 1/25th-second frame time and more scan lines, but the resulting resolution is not significantly different.

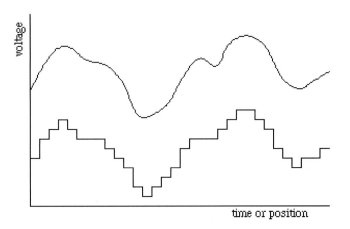

Figure 22. Digitization of an analog voltage signal such as one line in a video image (top) produces a series of numbers that represent a series of steps equal in time and rounded to integral multiples of the smallest height increment (bottom).

Broadcast television stations are given only a 4-MHz bandwidth for their signals, which must carry color and sound information as well as the brightness signal we have so far been discussing. This narrow bandwidth limits the number of separate voltage values that can be distinguished along each scan line to a maximum of 330. Even this value is reduced if the signal is degraded by the electronics or by recording using standard videotape recorders. Many consumer-quality videotape recorders reduce the effective resolution to about 200 points per line. In "freeze frame" playback, they display only one of the two interlaced fields, so that only 240 lines are resolved vertically. Using such equipment as part of an image analysis system makes choices of cameras or digitizer cards on the basis of resolution quite irrelevant.

Even the best system can be degraded in performance by such simple things as cables, connectors, or incorrect termination impedance. Another practical caution in the use of standard cameras is to avoid automatic gain or brightness compensation circuits. These can change the image contrast or linearity in response to bright or dark regions that do not even lie within the digitized portion of the image, and increase the gain and noise for a dim signal.

Figure 21 shows a micrograph with its brightness histogram. This is an important tool for image analysis, which plots the number of pixels as a function of their brightness values. The histogram is initially well spread out over the available 256 brightness levels, with peaks corresponding to each of the phases in the metal sample. When an internal reflection in the microscope causes a bright light to fall on a portion of the detector in the solid-state camera that is not part of the digitized image area, the automatic gain circuits in the camera alter the brightness-voltage relationship so that the image changes, as shown in the second histogram. This same effect occurs when a white or dark mask is used to surround images placed under a camera on

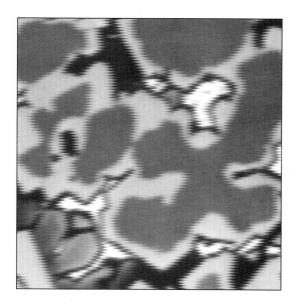

Figure 23. Example of interlace tearing when horizontal sync pulses between half-fields are inadequate to trigger the clock in the ADC correctly. Even and odd lines are systematically displaced.

a copy stand. The relationship between structure and brightness is changed, making subsequent analysis more difficult.

Issues involving color will be dealt with later, but obtaining absolute color information from video cameras is nearly impossible considering the variation in illumination color (e.g., with slight voltage changes on an incandescent bulb) and the way the color information is encoded. This is in addition to the problems of color sensitivity varying with illumination level mentioned above.

The analog voltage signal is usually digitized with an 8 bit "flash" ADC (analog-to-digital converter). This is a chip using successive approximation techniques to rapidly sample and measure the voltage in less than 100 ns, producing a number value from 0 to 255 that represents the brightness. This number is immediately stored in memory and another reading made, so that a series of brightness values is obtained along each scan line. **Figure 22** illustrates the digitization of a signal into equal steps both in time and value. Additional circuitry is needed to trigger each series of readings on the retrace events so that positions along successive lines are consistent.

Degraded signals, especially from videotape playback, can cause the even and odd fields of a full frame to be offset from each other, producing a significant degradation of the image. **Figure 23** shows the consequences of offset in the interlace correction, which can occur if the horizontal retrace signal is imprecise or difficult for the electronics to lock onto. This is a particular problem with signals played back from consumer video recorders. Digitizing several hundred points along each scan line, repeating the process for each line, and storing the values into memory

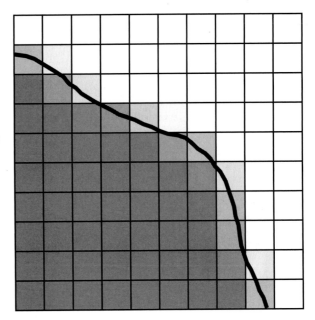

Figure 24. *Pixels have a finite area, and those straddling the boundary of a feature or region will have an intermediate brightness value resulting from averaging of the two levels. Accurate definition of the location of the boundary requires that the pixels be small and the number of grey values be large.*

while adjusting for the interlace of alternate fields produces a digitized image for further processing or analysis.

It is most desirable to have the spacing of the pixel values be the same in the horizontal and vertical directions (i.e., square pixels), as this simplifies many processing and measurement operations. Accomplishing this goal requires a well-adjusted clock to control the acquisition. Since the standard video image is not square, but has a width-to-height ratio of 4:3, the digitized image may represent only a portion of the entire field of view. Digitizing boards, also known as frame grabbers, were first designed to record 512×512 arrays of values, since the power-of-two dimension simplified design and memory addressing. Many of the newer boards acquire a 640 wide by 480 high array, which matches the image proportions while keeping the pixels square. Because of the variation in clocks between cameras and digitizers, it is common to find distortions of a few percent in pixel squareness. This can be measured, and compensated for after acquisition by resampling the pixels in the image as discussed in Chapter 3.

Of course, digitizing 640 values along a scan line that is limited by electronic bandwidth and only contains 300+ meaningfully different values produces an image with unsharp or fuzzy edges and "empty" magnification. Cameras which are capable of resolving more than 600 points along each scan line can sometimes be connected directly to the digitizing electronics to reduce this loss of horizontal resolution. Other camera designs bypass the analog transmission altogether, sending digital values to the computer, but these are generally much slower than standard video systems. They are discussed below.

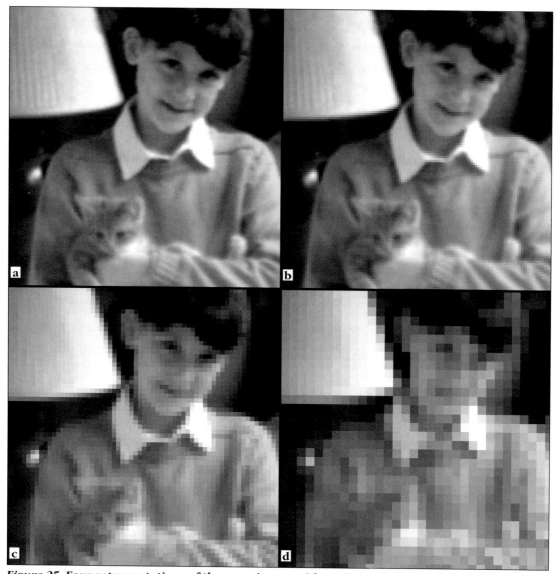

Figure 25. Four representations of the same image, with variation in the number of pixels used:
a) 256×256; *b)* 128×128; *c)* 64×64, *d)* 32×32.
In all cases, a full 256 grey values are retained. Each step in coarsening of the image is accomplished by averaging the brightness of the region covered by the larger pixels.

Since pixels have a finite area, those which straddle a boundary effectively average the brightness levels of two regions and have an intermediate brightness that depends on how the pixels lie with respect to the boundary. **Figure 24** illustrates this schematically. This means that a high lateral pixel resolution and a large number of distinguishable grey levels are needed to accurately locate boundaries. **Figure 25** shows several examples of an image with varying numbers of pixels across its width, and **Figure 26** shows the same image with varying numbers of grey levels.

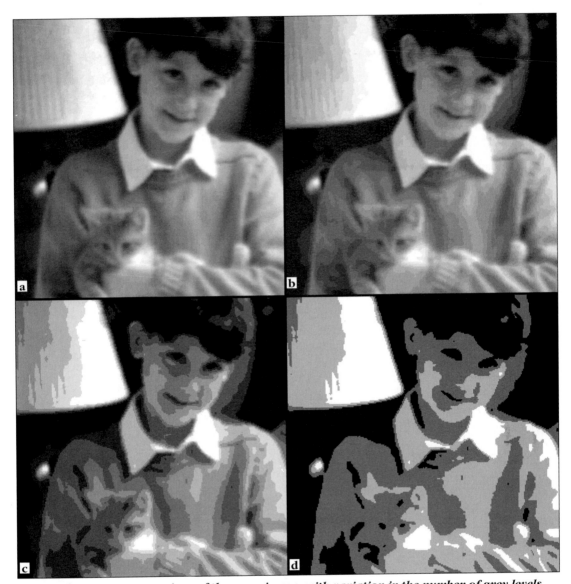

Figure 26. Four representations of the same image, with variation in the number of grey levels used: a) *32;* **b)** *16;* **c)** *8;* **d)** *4.*
In all cases, a full 256×256 array of pixels is retained. Each step in the coarsening of the image is accomplished by rounding the brightness of the original pixel value.

For the most common types of image acquisition devices, such as video cameras, the pixels represent an averaging of the signal across a finite area of the scene or specimen. However, there are other situations in which this is not so. At low magnification, for example, the scanning electron microscope beam samples a volume of the specimen much smaller than the dimension of a pixel in the image. Range imaging of the moon from the Clementine orbiter read the elevation of points a few inches in diameter using a laser rangefinder, but the points were spaced apart by 100 meters or more.

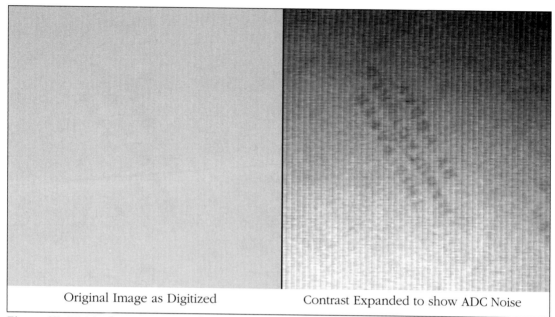

| Original Image as Digitized | Contrast Expanded to show ADC Noise |

Figure 27. *Digitized camera image of the back of a photographic print, showing the periodic noise present in the lowest few bits of the data from the electronics (especially the clock) in the analog to digital converter.*

In these cases, the interpretation of the relationship between adjacent pixels is slightly different. Instead of averaging across boundaries, the pixels sample points that are discrete and well separated. Cases of intermediate or gradually varying values from pixel to pixel are rare, and the problem instead becomes how to locate a boundary between two sampled points on either side. If there are many points along both sides of the boundary, and the boundary can be assumed to have some geometric shape (such as a straight line), fitting methods can be used to locate it to a fraction of the pixel spacing. These methods are discussed further in Chapter 8 on image measurements.

In addition to defining the number of sampled points along each scan line, and hence the resolution of the image, the design of the ADC board also controls the precision of each measurement. Inexpensive commercial flash analog-to-digital converters usually measure each voltage reading to produce an 8-bit number from 0 to 255. This range may not be used entirely for an actual image, since it may not vary from full black to white. Also, the quality of most cameras and other associated electronics rarely produces voltages that are free enough from electronic noise to justify full 8-bit digitization anyway. A typical "good" camera specification of 49 dB signal-to-noise ratio implies that only 7 bits of real information are available, and the eighth bit is random noise. But 8 bits corresponds nicely to the most common organization of computer memory into bytes, so that one byte of storage can hold the brightness value from one pixel in the image.

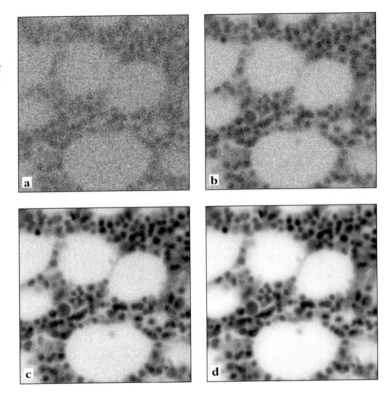

Figure 28. Averaging of a noisy (low photon-intensity) image (light microscope image of bone marrow): **a)** one frame; **b, c, d)** addition of 4, 16 and 256 frames.

Figure 27 shows an image that appears to be a uniform grey. When the contrast range is expanded we can see the faint lettering present on the back of this photographic print. Also evident is a series of vertical lines which are due to the digitizing circuitry, in this case electronic noise from the high-frequency clock used to control the time base for the digitization. Nonlinearities in the ADC, electronic noise from the camera itself, and degradation in the amplifier circuitry combine to make the lowest two bits of most standard video images useless, so that only about 64 grey levels are actually distinguishable in the data. Higher performance cameras and circuits exist, but do not generally offer "real time" speed (30 frames per second).

When this stored image is subsequently displayed from memory, the numbers are used in a digital-to-analog converter to produce voltages that control the brightness of a display, often a cathode ray tube (CRT). This process is comparatively noise-free and high resolution, since computer display technology has been developed to a high level for other purposes. A monochrome (black/grey/white) image displayed in this way, with 640×480 pixels, each of which can be set to one of 256 brightness levels (or colors using pseudo-color techniques to be discussed below), can be used with many desktop computers.

The human eye cannot distinguish all 256 different levels of brightness in this type of display, nor can they be successfully

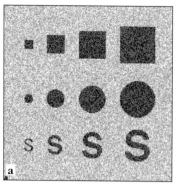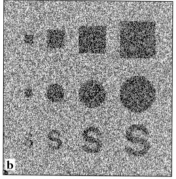

Figure 29. Features on a noisy background:
a) *signal to noise ratio 1:1;*
b) *signal to noise ratio 1:3;*
c) *signal to noise ratio 1:7;*
d) *image c after spatial smoothing.*

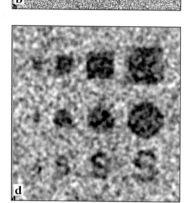

recorded photographically or printed using inexpensive technology, such as ink-jet or laser printers discussed in Chapter 2. About 30 grey levels can be visually distinguished on a CRT or photographic print, suggesting that the performance of the digitizers in this regard is more than adequate, at least for those applications where the performance of the eye was enough to begin with.

Images acquired in very dim light, or some other imaging modalities such as X-ray mapping in the scanning electron microscope (SEM), impose another limitation of the grey scale depth of the image. When the number of photons (or other particles) collected for each image pixel is low, statistical fluctuations become important. **Figure 28a** shows a fluorescence microscope image in which a single video frame illustrates extreme statistical noise, which would prevent distinguishing or measuring the structures present.

Images in which the pixel values vary even within regions that are ideally uniform in the original scene can arise either because of limited counting statistics for the photons or other signals, or due to electronic noise in the amplifiers or cabling. In either case, the variation is generally referred to as noise, and the ratio of the contrast which is actually due to structural difference to the noise level is the signal-to-noise ratio. When this is low, the features present may be invisible to the observer. **Figure 29** shows an

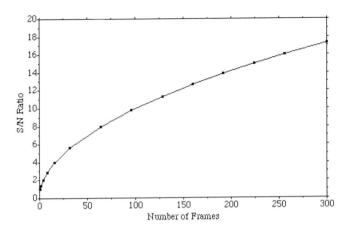

Figure 30. Signal-to-noise ratio of averaged image improves as the square root of the number of frames summed.

example in which several features of different size and shape are superimposed on a noisy background with different signal-to-noise ratios. The ability to discern the presence of the features is generally proportional to their area, and independent of shape.

In the figure, a smoothing operation is performed on the image with the poorest signal-to-noise ratio, which somewhat improves the visibility of the features. The methods available for smoothing noisy images by image processing are discussed in the chapters on spatial and frequency domain methods. However, the best approach to noisy images, when it is available, is simply to collect more signal and improve the statistics.

Adding together more video frames is shown in **Figure 28**. The improvement in quality is proportional to the square root of the number of frames (**Figure 30**). Since each frame is digitized to 8 bits, adding together up to 256 frames as shown requires a total image storage capability that is 16 bits deep. Acquiring frames and adding together the pixels at video rates generally requires specialized hardware, and performing the operation in a general-purpose computer limits the practical acquisition to only a few of the video frames per second. This limitation discards a large percentage of the photons that reach the detector. It is more efficient to use a camera capable of integrating the signal directly for the appropriate length of time, and then to read the final image to the computer. Cameras are available with this capability, and with cooled chips to reduce electronic noise during long acquisitions of many minutes. They are intended primarily for use in astronomy, where dim images are often encountered, but are equally suitable for other applications. Most uncooled camera chips will begin to show unacceptable pixel noise with integration times of more than a few seconds.

Acquiring images from a video camera is sometimes referred to as "real time" imaging, but of course this term should properly be reserved for any imaging rate that is adequate to reveal temporal changes in a particular application. For some situations, time-lapse photography may only require one frame to be taken at periods of many minutes. For others, very short exposures and high rates are needed. Special cameras that do not use video frame rates or bandwidths can achieve rates up to ten times that of a standard video camera for full frames, and even higher for small image dimensions. These cameras typically use a single line of detectors and optical deflection (e.g., a rotating mirror or prism) to cover the image.

For many applications, the repetition rate does not need to be that high. Either stroboscopic imaging or simply a fast shutter speed may be enough to stop the important motion to provide a sharp image. Electronic shutters can be used to control solid state imaging devices, instead of a mechanical shutter. Exposure times under 1/1000th of a second can easily be achieved, but of course this short exposure requires plenty of light.

High resolution imaging

The use of commercial video cameras as sources of images for technical purposes such as industrial quality control, scientific or medical research seems rather limiting. Much better cameras exist, and avoiding the use of an analog signal path for the information can reduce the degradation and improve resolution. Chips with 1000×1000, 2000×2000 and even 4000×4000 arrays of sensors are available. The cost of these cameras rises extremely rapidly, because the market is small, the yield of fabricating these devices is small, and only a few will fit on a single wafer. But they are used at present for some rather specialized imaging purposes, such as astronomical cameras. It seems unlikely that either the number of sensors will increase dramatically or the cost will drop sharply in the near future.

It is also possible to increase the "depth" of the display, or the number of grey levels that can be distinguished at each point. Whereas an 8-bit ADC gives 2^8 = 256 brightness levels, using 12 bits gives 2^{12} = 4096 levels, and 16 bits gives 2^{16} = 65,536 levels. Such great depth is needed when the brightness range of the image is extreme (as for instance in astronomy, fluorescence microsopy and some other specialized applications) in order to acquire enough signal to show detail in the dark regions of the image without the bright areas saturating so that information is lost. These depths are achievable, although they require cooling the camera to reduce electronic noise, and much slower image acquisition and digitization than the 1/30 second per full frame associated with "real time" video.

Other devices that produce data sets that are often treated as images for viewing and measurement produce data with a much greater range. For instance, a scanned stylus instrument that measures the elevation of points on a surface may have a vertical resolution of a few nanometers with a maximum vertical travel of hundreds of micrometers, for a range-to-resolution value of 10^5. This would require storing data in a format that preserved the full resolution values, and such instruments typically use 4 bytes per pixel.

In some cases with cameras having a large brightness range, the entire 12- or 16-bit depth of each pixel is stored. However, since this depth exceeds the capabilities of most CRTs to display, or of the user to see, reduction may be appropriate. If the actual brightness range of the image does not cover the entire possible range, scaling (either manual or automatic) to select just the range actually used can significantly reduce storage requirements. In other cases, especially when performing densitometry, a nonlinear conversion table is used. For densitometry, the desired density value varies as the logarithm of the brightness; this is discussed in detail in Chapter 8. A range of 256 brightness steps is not adequate to cover a typical range from 0 to greater than 2 in optical density with useful precision, because at the dark end of the range, 1 part in 256 represents a step of more than 0.1 in optical density. Using a digitization with 12 bits (1 part in 4096) solves this problem, but it is efficient to convert the resulting value with a logarithmic lookup table to store an 8-bit value (occupying a single computer byte) that is the optical density.

Lookup tables (LUTs) may be implemented either in hardware or software. They simply use the original value as an index into a stored or precalculated table, which then provides the derived value. This process is fast enough that acquisition is not affected. The context for LUTs discussed here is for image acquisition, converting a 12- or 16-bit digitized value with a nonlinear table to an 8-bit value that can be stored. LUTs are also used for displaying stored images, particularly to substitute colors for grey scale values to create pseudo-color displays. This topic is discussed in later chapters.

Many images do not have a brightness range that covers the full dynamic range of the digitizer. The result is an image whose histogram covers only a portion of the available values for storage or for display. **Figure 31** shows a histogram of such an image. The flat (empty) regions of the plot indicate brightness values at both the light and dark ends that are not used by any of the pixels in the image. Expanding the brightness scale by spreading the histogram out to the full available range, as shown in the figure, may improve the visibility of features and the perceived contrast in local structures. The same number of brightness values are missing from the image, as shown by the gaps in the histogram, but now they are spread uniformly throughout the range.

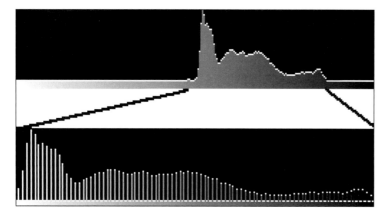

Figure 31. *Linear expansion of a histogram to cover the full range of storage and/or display.*

Other ways to stretch the histogram nonlinearly are discussed in Chapter 3.

Because the contrast range of many astronomical images is too great for photographic printing, special darkroom techniques have been developed. "Unsharp masking" (**Figure 32**) increases the ability to show local contrast by suppressing the overall brightness range of the image. The suppression is done by first printing a "mask" image, slightly out of focus, onto another negative. This negative is developed and then placed on the original to make the final print. This superposition reduces the exposure in the bright areas so that the detail can be shown. The same method can also be used in digital image processing, either by subtracting a smoothed version of the image or by using a Laplacian operator (both are discussed in Chapter 4 on spatial domain processing). When the entire depth of a 12- or 16-bit image is stored, such processing may be needed in order to display the image for viewing on a CRT.

Some perspective on camera performance levels is needed. While a standard video camera has about 300,000 sensors, and a

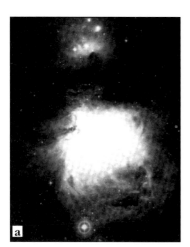
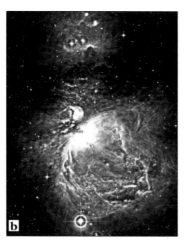

Figure 32. Unsharp masking:
a) *a telescope image of the Orion nebula originally recorded on film;*
b) *the same image using unsharp masking. An out-of-focus photographic print is made onto negative material, which is then placed on the original to reduce the exposure in bright areas when the final print is made. This process reduces the overall contrast so that local variations show. Laplacian filtering performs the same function in digital image analysis (From a Kodak darkroom manual, circa 1920).*

high performance camera may have a few million, the human eye has about $1.5 \cdot 10^8$. Furthermore, these are clustered particularly tightly in the fovea, the central area where we concentrate our attention. While it is true that only a few dozen brightness levels can be distinguished in a single field, the eye adjusts automatically to overall brightness levels covering nine orders of magnitude to select the optimal range (although color sensitivity is lost in the darkest part of this range).

Just as video cameras offer a major challenge to conventional film-based movie cameras, there is a trend in still cameras toward replacing the film with a CCD array. High-end camera models for scientific and technical applications, and used by professional photographers, can employ a filter wheel and three exposures to collect a color image. The same procedure is possible with inexpensive monochrome CCD cameras. Three images can be captured with red, green, and blue filters (e.g., Kodak Wratten filters 25=Red, 58=Green, and 47 or 47B=Blue) and then combined using software. Of course, stability of camera position, lack of motion, and constant lighting are required. Filter selection depends on the sensitivity of the camera (CCDs tend to be less blue sensitive and more red sensitive than vidicons for instance) and on lighting.

Some of these cameras use a single-line CCD instead of a two-dimensional array. This gives high resolution but requires physically scanning the line across the film plane, much like a flat-bed scanner. Most of these systems store the image digitally, converting the signal to a full color image (for instance with 8 or 10 bits each of red, green, and blue data). At the lower end, cameras intended for the consumer or desktop publishing market use a CCD similar in performance to the detector in a typical video camera. The direct video signal is often stored in an analog format, for instance on a 2-inch magnetic disk. The recording typically adheres to normal video standards, with interlaced scan lines and the same color encoding as broadcast or video tape recording. This allows the signal to be played back on standard video equipment, but it must be separately digitized if it is to be accessed by a computer.

There is a major difference between the interlace scan used in conventional television and a noninterlaced or "progressive" scan. The latter gives better quality because there are no line-to-line alignment or shift problems. Most high definition television (HDTV) proposals use progressive scan. The format requires a higher rate of repetition of frames to fool the human eye into seeing continuous motion, but it has many other advantages. These include simpler logic to read data from the camera (which may be incorporated directly on the chip), more opportunity for data compression because of redundancies between successive lines, and simpler display or storage devices. Most scientific imaging systems such as high-performance cameras, direct-scan microscopes (the scanning electron microscope or SEM, scanning tunneling microscope or STM, the atomic force microscope or AFM, etc.), flat-bed scanners, film or slide digitizers, and similar devices, use progressive rather than interlaced scan.

HDTV proposals include many more differences from conventional television than the use of progressive scan. The pixel density is much higher, with a wider aspect ratio of 16:9 (instead of the 4:3 used in NTSC television) and the pixels are square. A typical HDTV proposal presents 1920×1080 pixel images at the rate of 30 full scans per second, for a total data rate exceeding 1 gigabit per second, several hundred times as much data as current broadcast television. One consequence of this high data rate is the interest in data compression techniques, discussed in the next chapter, and the investigation of digital transmission techniques, perhaps using cable or optical fiber instead of broadcast channels. Whatever the details of the outcome in terms of consumer television, the development of HDTV hardware is likely to produce spin-off effects for computer imaging, such as high pixel density cameras with progressive scan output, high bandwidth recording devices, and superior CRT displays. For example, color cameras being designed for HDTV applications output digital rather than analog information by performing the analog-to-digital conversion within the camera, with ≥10 bits each for red, green, and blue.

An important development in present models of solid-state cameras is toward higher pixel density and lower noise, for technical applications such as astronomy and fluorescence microscopy. These cameras offer more than 8 bits of dynamic range, with capabilities up to 12, 14 or even more. With 12 bits, for instance, the dynamic range is $2^{12} = 4096$. These four thousand grey levels are still usually linearly proportional to brightness, and a logarithmic conversion corresponding to human vision reduces the dynamic range somewhat, but these cameras still have a dynamic range that compares favorably to film.

In order to achieve this performance, the chip must be cooled to reduce thermal noise. Since the solid state detector functions by storing the electrons elevated across a band gap, it is necessary to prevent the "dark current" of electrons raised across the band gap by thermal energy, and also to reduce the variation in current that occurs when the device is read out. Cooling the chip accomplishes both tasks. A camera used to record infrared (low energy) photons in an astronomical application will have a very small band gap (consequently more thermal or dark current) and may need to be cooled to liquid nitrogen or even liquid helium temperatures. But for a camera used for visible light, cooling to −40°C or less reduces the thermal noise dramatically. Such cooling can be accomplished thermoelectrically by connecting a Peltier cooler to the chip.

Care is still required to cool the chip evenly, compensate for any heating due to the electronics themselves, and so on, but a typical inexpensive cooled camera for astronomical or fluorescent microscopy applications can collect the signal for several minutes before the thermal dark current becomes significant. This collection time allows it to sum up quite faint signals, without noise. At the same time, the large dynamic range afforded by a readout with 10 or even 14 bits prevents the bright pixels from saturating. Thus, quantitative measurements of brightness over the full dynamic range become possible.

This capability has revolutionized astronomy, and comparatively inexpensive cameras have been developed for the high-end amateur market. Typically, they incorporate a Peltier cooler and digital readout directly to a computer. They are fundamentally monochrome cameras, but can be used to obtain color images by recording several images through different color filters. The least-expensive cameras may have only a small number of pixels, in order to keep costs down, while the somewhat more costly units can have resolutions up to 2000×2000, much higher than a video camera. These devices are progressive scan, and many perform the digitization on-chip, or at least within the camera, so that only digital information needs to be transmitted over wires to the computer (further reducing noise). Their principal drawback, besides a cost of $10,000 to $50,000, is the slow speed of the readout. Without a "live" image to allow easy focusing or selection of the field of view, other optical or video aids must be provided for those purposes. Some large format cameras address this problem by providing a readout at a rate of several frames per second from a reduced area of the array, or from every nth pixel.

It is also interesting to compare video technology to other kinds of image acquisition devices. The scanning electron (SEM) or scanning tunneling microscope (STM) typically use from a few hundred to about 1000 scan lines. Those that digitize the signals use 8 or sometimes 12 bits, and so are similar in image resolution and size to many camera systems. **Figure 33** shows schematically the function of an SEM. The focused beam of electrons is scanned over the sample surface in a raster pattern while various signals generated by the electrons are detected. These include secondary and backscattered electrons, characteristic X-rays, visible light, and electronic effects in the sample.

Other point-scanning microscopes, such as the STM, the confocal scanning light microscope (CSLM), and even contact profilometers, produce very different signals and information. All provide a time-varying signal that is related to spatial locations on the sample by knowing the scanning speed and parameters, which allows storing the data as an image.

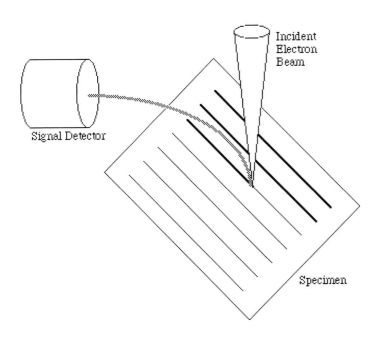

Figure 33. *The scanning electron microscope (SEM) focuses a fine beam of electrons on the specimen, producing various signals that may be used for imaging as the beam is scanned in a raster pattern.*

Significantly larger arrays of pixels are available from flat-bed scanners. These devices use a linear solid-state detector array, and can typically scan areas at least 8 inches × 10 inches, and sometimes up to four times that size. While primarily intended for the desktop publishing market, they are readily adapted to scan electrophoresis gels used for protein separation, or photographic prints or negatives. A high-quality negative can record several hundred discrete brightness levels and several thousand points per inch (both values are much better than prints). Scanners are also used for digitizing photographic negatives such as medical X-rays and 35 mm slides. Commercial scanners are used in publishing and to convert films to digital values for storage (for instance in Kodak's Photo-CD format). At the consumer level, scanners with 300 to as many as 1200 pixels per inch are common for large-area reflective originals, and 2500 to 3500 pixels per inch for 35 mm slide film. Most digitize full-color red, green, and blue (RGB) images, which are discussed below.

These devices are quite inexpensive, but rather slow, taking tens of seconds to digitize the scan area. Another characteristic problem they exhibit is pattern noise in the sensors: if all of the detectors along the row are not identical in performance a "striping" effect will appear in the image as the sensor is scanned across the picture. If the scan motion is not perfectly smooth, it can produce striping in the other direction. This latter effect is particularly troublesome with hand-held scanners that rely on the user to move them and sense the motion with a contact roller that can skip, but these devices should not be used for inputting images for measurement anyway, because of the tendency to skip or twist in motion.

By far the greatest difficulty with such scanners arises from the illumination. There is often a drop-off in intensity near the edges of the scanned field because of the short length of the light source. Even more troublesome is the warm-up time for the light source to become stable. In scanners that digitize color images in a single pass by turning lights on and off, stability and consistent color is especially hard to obtain. On the other hand, making three separate passes for red, green, and blue often causes registration difficulties. Even for monochrome scanning, it may take several repeated scans before the light source and other electronics become stable enough for consistent measurements.

Color imaging

Most real-world images are not monochrome, of course, but full color. The light microscope produces color images, and many tissue specimen preparation techniques make use of color to identify structure or localize chemical activity in novel ways. Even for inorganic materials, the use of polarized light or surface oxidation produces color images to delineate structure. The SEM would seem to be a strictly monochromatic imaging tool, but color may be introduced based on X-ray energy or backscattered electron energy. **Figure 34** shows individual grey scale images from the electron and X-ray signals from a mineral sample imaged in the SEM. The secondary electron image shows the general topography of the sample surface, and the X-ray maps show the variation in composition of the sample for each of four elements (Si, Fe, Cu, Ag). There are more individual images than the three red, green, and blue display planes, and no obvious "correct" choice for assigning colors to elements. **Figure 35** shows a few possibilities, but it is important to keep in mind that no single color image can show all of the elements at once. Assigning several of these arbitrarily, e.g., to the red, green, and blue planes of a display, may aid the user in judging the alignment of regions and areas containing two or more elements. Colored X-ray maps are now fairly common with the SEM, but other uses of color such as energy loss in the transmission electron microscope (TEM) are still experimental.

Similar use of color is potentially useful with other kinds of microscopes, although in many cases these possibilities have not been exploited in commercial instruments. This is also true for macroscopic imaging tools. A simple example is the use of color to show altitude in air traffic control displays. This use of color increases the bandwidth for communicating multidimensional information to the user, but the effective use of these methods

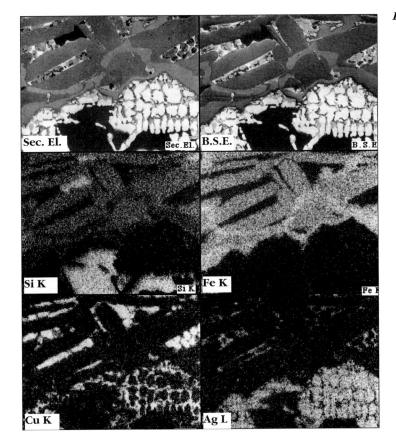

Figure 34. Scanning electron microscope images of a mineral. The secondary and backscattered electron images delineate the various structures, and the silicon, iron, copper and silver X-ray images show which structures contain those elements (image courtesy of Amray Corp., Bedford, MA).

will require some education of users, and would benefit from some standardization.

The use of color to encode richly multidimensional information must be distinguished from the very common use of false-color or pseudo-color to substitute colors for brightness in a monochrome image. Pseudo-color is used because of the limitation mentioned before in our visual ability to distinguish subtle differences in brightness. Although we can only distinguish about 30 shades of grey in a monochrome image, we can distinguish hundreds of different colors. Also, it is easier to describe a particular feature of interest as "the dark blue one" rather than "the medium grey one."

The use of color scales as a substitute for brightness values lets us show and see small changes locally, and identify the same brightness values globally in an image. This should be a great benefit, since these are among the goals for imaging discussed below. Pseudo-color has been used particularly for many of the images returned from space probes. It would be interesting to know how many people think that the rings around Saturn really are brightly colored, or that Comet Halley really is surrounded by a rainbow-colored halo! The danger in the use of pseudo-color is

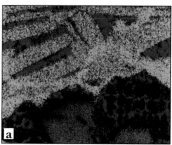 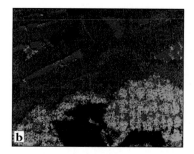 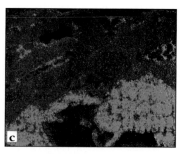

Figure 35. Color composites made from SEM electron and X-ray images in Figure 34:
a) *Red=Silicon, Green=Iron, Blue=Copper;*
b) *Red=Iron, Green=Silver, Blue=Copper;*
c) *Cyan=Silicon, Magenta=Silver, Yellow=Copper, Black=Electrons.*

that it can obscure the real contents of an image. The colors force us to concentrate on the details of the image, and to lose the gestalt information. Examples of image processing in this book will use pseudo-color selectively to illustrate some of the processing effects and the changes in pixel values that are produced, but usually pseudo-color distracts the human eye from seeing the real contents of the enhanced image.

Pseudo-color displays as used in this context simply substitute a color from a stored or precalculated table for each discrete stored brightness value. As shown in **Figure 36**, this should be distinguished from some other uses of color displays to identify structures or indicate feature properties. These also rely on the use of color to communicate rich information to the viewer, but require considerable processing and measurement of the image before this information becomes available.

Color can be used to encode elevation of surfaces (see Chapters 8 and 11). In scientific visualization it is used for velocity, density, composition, and many less-obvious properties. These uses generally have little to do with the properties of the image and simply take advantage of the human ability to distinguish more colors than grey scale values.

Most computer-based imaging systems make it easy to substitute various LUTs of colors for the brightness values in a stored image. These work in the same way as input lookup tables, described before. The stored grey scale value is used to select a set of red, green, and blue brightnesses in the LUT that are the voltages sent to the display tube. Many systems also provide utilities for creating tables of these colors, but there are few guidelines to assist in constructing useful ones. All we can do here is advise caution. One approach is to systematically and gradually vary color along a path through color space. Examples (**Figure 37**) are a rainbow spectrum of colors or a progression from brown through red and yellow to white and then blue, the so-called heat scale. This gradual variation can help to organize the different parts of the scene. Another approach is to rapidly shift colors, for instance by varying the hue sinusoidally. This enhances gradients and makes it easy to see local variations, but may completely hide the overall contents of some images (**Figure 38**).

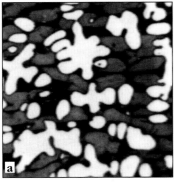

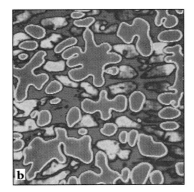

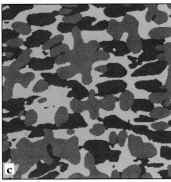

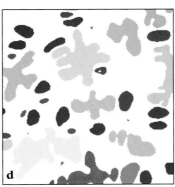

Figure 36. Uses for pseudo-color displays:

a) Portion of a grey-scale microscope image of a polished metallographic specimen with three phases having different average brightnesses;

b) Image **a** with pseudo-color palette or LUT which replaces grey values with colors. Note the misleading colors along boundaries between light and dark phases);

c) Image **a** with colors assigned to phases. This requires segmentation of the image by thresholding and other logic to assign each pixel to a phase based on grey-scale brightness and neighboring pixel classification;

d) Lightest features from image **a** with colors assigned based on feature size. This requires the steps to create image **c**, plus collection of all touching pixels into a feature and the measurement of that feature.

Some image sources may use color to encode a variety of different kinds of information, such as the intensity and polarization of radio waves in astronomy. However, by far the most common type of color image is that produced by recording the intensity at three different wavelengths of visible light. Video deserves consideration as a suitable medium for this type of image, since standard broadcast television uses color effectively. The NTSC color encoding scheme used in the U.S. was developed as a compatible add-on to existing monochrome television broadcasts. It adds

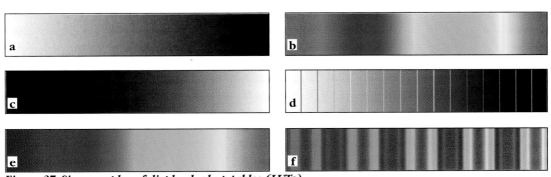

Figure 37. Six examples of display lookup tables (LUTs).

a) Monochrome (grey-scale);

b) Spectrum or rainbow (linear variation of hue, maximum saturation and intensity);

c) Heat scale;

d) Monochrome with contour lines (rainbow colors substituted every 16th value);

e) Linear variation of hue, saturation and intensity;

f) Sinusoidal variation of hue with linear variation of saturation and intensity.

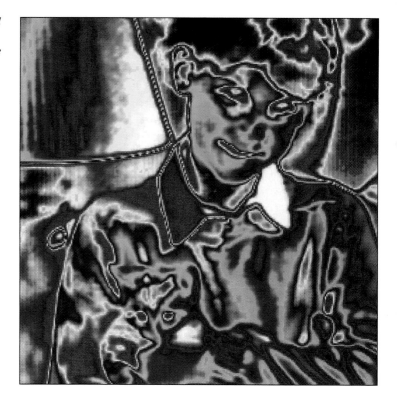

Figure 38. The same image used in Figures 25 and 26 with a pseudo-color display LUT. The gestalt contents of the image are obscured.

the color information within the same, already narrow bandwidth limitation. The result is that the color has even less lateral resolution than the brightness information.

This limitation is acceptable for television pictures, since the viewer tolerates colors that are less sharply bounded and uses the edges of features defined by the brightness component of the image where they do not exactly correspond. The same tolerance has been used effectively by painters, and may be familiar to parents whose young children have not yet learned to color "inside the lines." **Figure 39** shows an example in which the bleeding of color across boundaries or variations within regions is not confusing to the eye.

The poor spatial sharpness of NTSC color is matched by its poor consistency in representing the actual color values (a common joke is that NTSC means "Never The Same Color" instead of "National Television Systems Committee"). Videotape recordings of color images are even less useful for analysis than monochrome ones. But the limitations imposed by the broadcast channel do not necessarily mean that the cameras and other components may not be useful. An improvement in the sharpness of the color information in these images is afforded by Super-VHS or S-video recording equipment, also called component video, in which the brightness or luminance and color or chrominance information are transmitted and recorded separately, as discussed below.

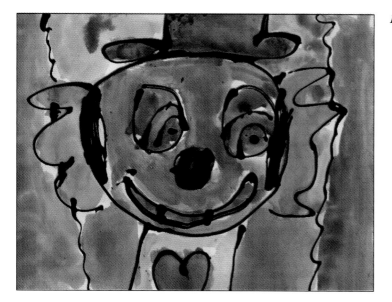

Figure 39. *A child's painting of a clown. Notice that the colors are unrealistic but their relative intensities are correct, and that the painted areas are not exactly bounded by the lines. The dark lines nevertheless give dimensions and shape to the features, and we are not confused by the colors which extend beyond their regions.*

The least-expensive color cameras, developed in response to consumer demand, are solid state. The chips are identical to those used in monochrome cameras, except that some of the sensors are made sensitive only to red, green, and blue light. This may be done either by adjusting the electrical band gap in the semiconductor, or more commonly by simply applying a filter coating to absorb the complementary colors. The detection of the red, green, and blue primary colors allows the camera electronics to produce the encoded color signal. This particular encoding scheme (YIQ) is discussed below, along with others.

In a single-chip color camera an array of red, green and blue filters is used to control the light reaching the individual transistors (**Figure 40**). Notice that twice as many transistors are used to measure green as compared to red or blue, which compensates for the greater sensitivity of human vision to that portion of the spectrum. Interpolation is used between transistors for each color, but in effect a 2×2 block of transistors is required to measure the color information for a pixel, which reduces the overall resolution of the camera. Some cameras use a different filter arrangement consisting of color stripes, which further reduces horizontal resolution. For still images, some cameras shift either the pixel array or the incoming light to acquire four images so that the color-filtered transistors can sample all of the information present in the image, but of course this cannot be done for continuous video imaging.

In so-called 3-chip cameras (**Figure 41**), a dichroic prism beam splitter separates the incoming light into red, green and blue wavelength components which are then each imaged by a high resolution monochrome CCD chip. The electrical signals are later

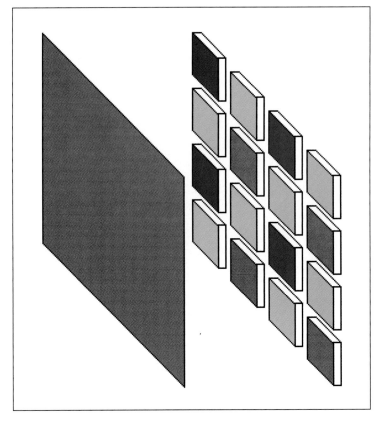

Figure 40. *Filters used in a typical CCD single chip color camera. An infrared cutoff filter removes long wavelength light, and individual red, green, and blue filters correspond to each transistor.*

recombined to produce the color video signal. This provides much higher lateral resolution since the individual color signals are measured using the full resolution of the transistors on each chip. These cameras are, of course, more expensive.

Some color cameras intended for technical purposes bring out the red, green, and blue signals separately so that they can be individually digitized. Recording the image in computer memory then simply involves treating each signal as a monochrome one,

Figure 41. *Function of a beam splitter to separate RGB images in a 3-chip camera.*

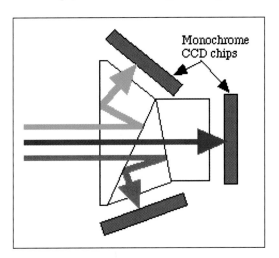

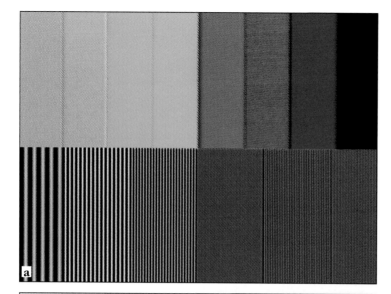

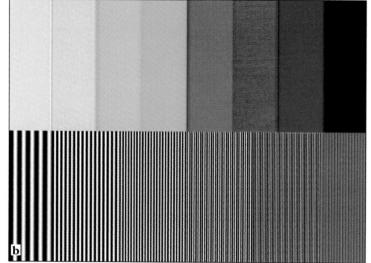

Figure 42. Comparison of
a) *composite and*
b) *component video signals from a signal generator, digitized using the same interface board. Note the differences in resolution of the black and white stripes and the boundaries between different colors.*

converting it to a set of numbers, and storing it in memory. If the signals have first been combined, the encoding scheme used is likely to be YIQ or YUV (defined below), which are closely related to the NTSC broadcasting scheme.

However, much better fidelity in the image can be preserved by not mixing together the color and brightness information. Instead of the composite signal carried on a single wire, some cameras and recorders separate the chrominance (color) and luminance (brightness) signals onto separate wires. This so-called component, Y-C or S-video format is used for high-end consumer camcorders (Hi-8 and S-VHS formats). Many computer interfaces accept this format, which gives significant improvement in the quality of digitized images, as shown in **Figure 42**.

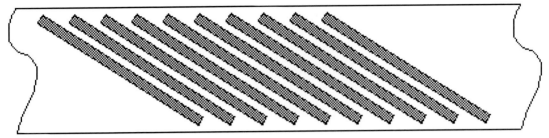

Figure 43. *In digital video, each video frame is recorded digitally in 10 tracks on the metal-coated tape (12 tracks for the larger PAL format). Each track contains video, audio, and timing information.*

As mentioned above, the newest video format uses a wide screen instead of the current standard 4:3 proportions, the window width to height ratio will be 16:9. This "landscape" format more closely approximates that used in movie film, which will make it easier to broadcast entertainment. Cameras, recorders and other equipment will become available that support this format, and of course they will be used in scientific applications as well. This is not a desirable change from the standpoint of technical measurements, which would prefer to have a square image that would make the most use of available data from the various kinds of image sources (microscopes, etc.). On the other hand, some of the other changes associated with high definition television (HDTV) will be welcome. These include progressive scan rather than interlace, which will eliminate line offsets and jitter in merging the two fields or half-frames that make up a conventional interlaced scan image, square pixels, and possibly a signal to noise ratio that would justify more than 6 or 7 bits of digitization (perhaps up to 10, or one part in 1024).

The other development in video that is important is digital video (DV) recording. Like analog video tape recorders, digital video writes each scan line onto the tape at an angle using a moving head that rotates as the tape moves past it (**Figure 43**). However, the signal is encoded as a series of digital bits that offers several advantages. Just as CD technology replaced analog audio tapes, the digital video signal is not subject to loss of fidelity as images are transmitted or copies are made. More important, the high frequency information that is discarded in analog recording because of the 4 MHz upper frequency limit imposed by conventional broadcast TV is preserved in DV. Digital video records up to 13.5 MHz for the luminance (brightness) information, and up to one-fourth that for the chrominance (color) information. This produces much sharper edge delineation in the color portion of the image, and greatly improves the usefulness of the resulting images. The digital video signal is fully preserved on the tape recording, unlike conventional analog recorders which impose a further bandwidth reduction on the data.

The result is that DV images really do have about 500×500 pixel resolution and nearly 8 bits of contrast, and can be read into the computer without a separate digitizer board since they are already digital in format. The IEEE 1394 standard protocol for digital video (also known as firewire) establishes a standard serial interface convention that is becoming available on consumer-priced cameras and decks, and is being supported by computer manufacturers as well. Inexpensive interface boards are available, and it seems likely that the interface will be built into the basic circuitry of personal computers within a short time (Sony already offers this). Most of these digital cameras can be controlled by the computer to select individual frames for transfer. They can also be used to record single frames annotated with date and time, turning the digital video tape cartridge into a tiny but high fidelity storage format for hundreds of single images.

Digital cameras

Another current development is the digital still-frame cameras that are being brought to the consumer market by practically every traditional maker of film cameras and photographic supplies. Many of these are unsuitable for technical applications because of limitations in the optics (fixed focus lenses with geometric distortions), and limited resolution (although even a low end 320×240 pixel camera chip is as good as conventional analog video recording). Some cameras try to interpolate between the transistors on the chip, or capture several images with tiny geometrical shifts, to create images that have more pixels than the camera chip can really deliver. In most cases this produces artefacts in the image that are serious impediments to quantitative measurement.

But it is the use of image compression that creates the most important problem. In an effort to pack many images into the smallest possible memory, JPEG and other forms of image compression are used. As discussed elsewhere, these are lossy techniques that discard information from the image. The discarded data is selected to minimally impact the human interpretation of common images — snapshots of the kids and the dog — but the effect on quantitative image analysis can be severe. Edges are broken up and shifted, color and density values are altered, and fine details can be eliminated or moved.

Some of the higher end cameras offer storage or transfer to the computer without any lossy compression, and this is much preferred for technical applications. At this writing, cameras from Polaroid, Kodak and a few other manufacturers offer excellent performance in the mid-price range (a few thousand dollars). The Polaroid DMC can be directly mounted onto a microscope, telescope or any optics that accept a C-mount. Somewhat more costly (up to ten thousand dollars) camera backs from Kodak, Nikon, Canon and others allow capture of high quality images with standard interchangeable lenses and other camera accessories (although they do not capture the same area as a standard

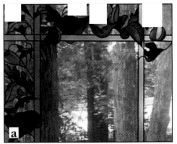 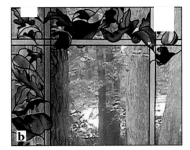 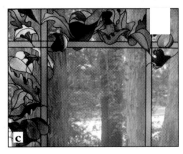

Figure 44. Images of the same scene (see text) recorded using:

a) *a 3-chip video camera (Sony) and analog to digital converter;*

b) *a high-end consumer digital camera (Sony Mavica MVC-7), and*

c) *a research-grade digital camera (Polaroid DMC).*

35mm camera back and so the effective focal length of the lenses is changed).

Figure 44 compares images of the same scene using three different cameras. The subject is a difficult view through a stained glass window, with a dark interior and bright daytime exterior. This produces a very high contrast range, regions that are saturated in color and others with low saturation, subtle differences and fine detail. The first image is video from a 3-chip color camera (Sony) acquired using a high quality analog-to-digital converter producing a 640×480 pixel image and averaging eight frames. The second image was acquired with a high end consumer digital camera (Sony Mavica), also as a 640×480 pixel image, using the highest quality compression setting (least compression). The third image was acquired with a research-grade digital camera (Polaroid DMC) as a 1600×1200 pixel image.

The colors in the original are represented with greater fidelity in the third image. In addition to color shifts, the first two images have brightness values that are clipped to maximum and minimum values, and the video image does not produce 256 distinct values of red, green and blue so that the image has missing values within the range. The consumer digital camera apparently applies a hi-pass or sharpening filter that exaggerates contrast at edges producing dark and light borders. There are other artefacts present in the first two images as well: scan line noise in the video image and square blocks resulting from the JPEG compression in the consumer digital camera image. Enlarging the image to see fine details makes apparent the far higher resolution

Figure 45. *Enlarged regions of the images in the preceding figure, showing the greater resolution and fidelity in the DMC image.*

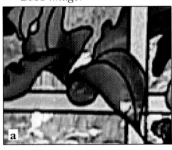 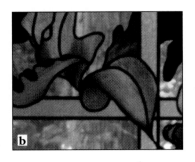 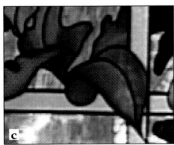

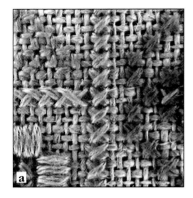
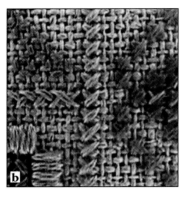
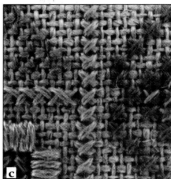

Figure 46. Images of stitchery using the same three cameras as in Figures 44 and 45.

of the research grade digital image. In **Figure 45** a region is expanded to show fine details in each of the images. The research grade digital camera image renders these with greater fidelity in both the high brightness and high saturation regions.

The research grade digital camera offers the same advantages for recording of images in microscope and other technical applications. **Figure 46** shows three images obtained with the same three cameras using a low power microscope to view an antique cross-stitch specimen. Identification of individual characteristics (and occasional errors) in the formation of the stitches and tension on the threads is of interest to cultural anthropologists to identify individual handiwork. This requires a low enough magnification to see the overall pattern, while identification of the threads and dyes used requires a high enough resolution to see individual fibers. **Figure 47** shows an enlargement of one small region of the three images. The differences in resolution and color fidelity between these images is another demonstration of the importance of using a high quality camera.

A few words of caution may be useful. The slower readout from digital cameras makes focusing more difficult: the camera produces a grey scale preview image that updates a few times a second. This is fine for selecting fields of view, but for convenient focusing it is important to adjust the optics so that the camera is

Figure 47. Enlargement of a portion of the images in the preceding figure.

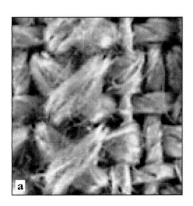
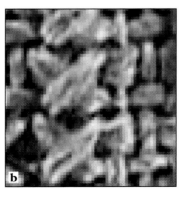
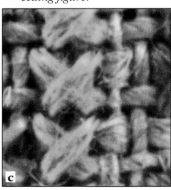

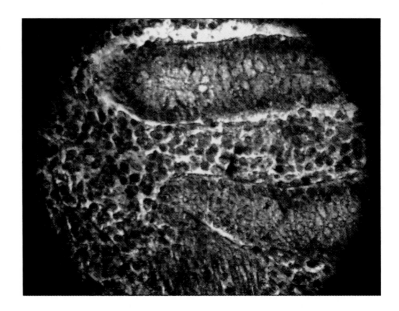

Figure 48. View of a biological thin section using a video conferencing camera placed on the eyepiece of a bench microscope.

truly parfocal with the eyepiece image. Some digital cameras do not have a useful preview image but instead rely on a viewfinder that is of little practical use. Also the area of the image sensing chip is smaller than film but larger than many video cameras so that standard transfer optics may not provide complete coverage; clipping or vignetting can result. Exposure times of a second or more produce significant pixel noise (visible as red, green, and blue color spots in the image) unless the chip is cooled to reduce thermal electron noise.

The dramatic reductions in price and improvements in capabilities of digital cameras brought about as a result of consumer demand offers some intriguing possibilities for technical image processing and analysis. For instance, a digital camera intended for video conferencing is available at this writing which delivers 64 grey levels or 32 levels of red, green and blue with 320×240 pixel resolution (about as good as many examples of digitized video!) at about 10 frames per second via a simple serial or parallel interface to the computer. No digitizer or separate power supply is required, and the digitization is built into the camera chip requiring no hardware to be added to the computer. This camera is available for about $60 with grey scale output or about $150 with color (and both the performance and cost will probably be bettered by new models in the time it takes to get this into print).

This camera is actually useful for some technical purposes, such as capturing an image for videoconferencing. The illustration in **Figure 48** was obtained by placing the camera directly onto the eyepiece of a microscope (it could have been attached there with duct tape). The automatic gain control in the software was turned off as the black area around the image confused the automatic

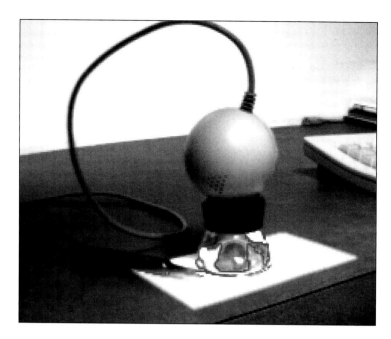

Figure 49. *Using the same camera as in Figure 48 with a loupe to record an image for forensic examination.*

adjustment. **Figure 49** shows another example of the use of the same camera. Placing it on an 8X loupe allows direct capture of images when (as in this forensic case) it was essential to collect images and nothing else except the camera and a laptop computer was available. The biggest flaws with this setup were the difficulty in controlling the specimen illumination and the distortion caused by the very wide angle view from the optics.

Consumer digital cameras are widely available in the price range from $200 to under $1000. These usually have fixed focus, fairly wide angle optics with limited macro (closeup) capability. It is not easy to remove the optics to replace them with something better. Many cameras in the class offer a preview image on an LCD display, and have a serial interface to the computer to transfer stored images, and in some cases to control capture. Most will store dozens of images within the camera, and some use removable memory cards or floppy disks that allow unlimited storage. The typical resolution is often stated as 640×480 but this is just the number of pixels stored and does not reflect the actual resolution capability. Most cameras use single chip arrays with about 350,000 transistors, some used for red, green, and blue respectively, so it seems safe to estimate the actual resolution as about 400×300. This is still quite comparable to typical consumer video cameras and would actually be quite useful and respectable for many purposes.

The critical flaw (besides the optical limitations) is that these cameras use compression to squeeze lots of images into their limited memory, and have no way to turn that compression off. As will be discussed later, this compression is a lossy process designed to preserve those aspects of images that seem important to people when looking at familiar scenes and objects. Compression can be as great as 100:1 (99% of the data in the image is discarded) without losing the ability to recognize and enjoy the contents of such pictures. But the data discarded in lossy compression destroys much of the utility of the images for quantitative purposes. Edges are shifted, and either blurred or (more typically) have their contrast increased, color and brightness values change, and so on. The use of any kind of lossy compression for images of unfamiliar objects is also dubious because it isn't possible to know what is unimportant and can be safely discarded. Avoiding any kind of compression for images destined for analysis is a good idea.

Cameras intended for technical applications have no compression, employ flexible optics, and provide high resolution. All of these cameras produce large data files, which quickly fill up storage (a topic discussed later). There are three basic types:

a) Cameras using a monochrome chip (perhaps cooled to reduce thermal noise and allow 12 or more bits of grey scale information) with at least a million transistors, and a slow (i.e., not real time) readout which can make it difficult to focus and adjust. This is often compensated by allowing more rapid (several updates per second) readout of a small area. Such cameras can capture color images by using a filter wheel to capture three sequential images if required. Typical cost of these cameras is $20K or more (Photometrix is a typical example of this class of camera. Diagnostic Instruments also makes a cooled camera with a color CCD array and a built-in filter wheel). The cameras are expensive because they are not made or marketed in consumer quantities, but they provide outstanding performance if you need it.

b) Cameras using a scanning linear array, one very high resolution set of sensors filtered for red, green and blue which are scanned across the film plane of the camera and read the data directly to the computer. These provide excellent resolution, as good as 35 mm color film, but take several minutes to scan the entire area so they are only suitable for static images. The typical cost is $5–10K (Leaf/Scitex is a typical example of this class of camera).

c) Cameras using megapixel RGB chips which read out more slowly than video cameras to achieve much better dynamic range and noise characteristics (examples are the Kodak DCS 400 series and Polaroid PDC and DMC, which cost $5–10K). These are a good compromise for most applications because they have direct high speed SCSI interfaces to the computer and/or lots of on-board storage for images, which can be quite large, and use no compression. Some can quickly read out a small area for focus and adjustment. There are also 3-chip versions of this type of camera, but they are considerably more expensive and require fairly intense lighting, so that the area of application is usually restricted to studio photography.

Prices will no doubt continue to drop in all categories due to competitive pressure and the demand of a large and growing marketplace, and fueled by the ever present decline in the cost of components.

Color spaces

Conversion from RGB (the brightness of the individual red, green, and blue signals at defined wavelengths) to YIQ/YUV and to the other color encoding schemes is straightforward and loses no information. Y, the "luminance" signal, is just the brightness of a panchromatic monochrome image that would be displayed by a black-and-white television receiver. It combines the red, green, and blue signals in proportion to the human eye's sensitivity to them. The I and Q (U and V) components of the color signal are chosen for compatibility with the hardware used in broadcasting; the I signal is essentially red minus cyan, while Q is magenta minus green. The relationship between YIQ and RGB is shown in **Table 1**. An inverse conversion from the encoded YIQ signal to RGB simply requires inverting the matrix of values.

Table 1. Interconversion of RGB and YIQ color scales

Y	=	0.299 R	+	0.587 G	+	0.114 B		R	=	1.000 Y	+	0.956 I	+	0.621 Q
I	=	0.596 R	−	0.274 G	−	0.322 B		G	=	1.000 Y	−	0.272 I	−	0.647 Q
Q	=	0.211 R	−	0.523 G	+	0.312 B		B	=	1.000 Y	−	1.106 I	+	1.703 Q

RGB (and the complementary CMY subtractive primary colors used for printing) and YIQ are both hardware-oriented schemes. RGB comes from the way camera sensors and display phosphors work, while YIQ or YUV stem from broadcast considerations. **Figure 50** shows the "space" defined by RGB signals: it is a Cartesian cubic space, since the red, green, and blue signals are independent and can be added to produce any color within the cube. There are other encoding schemes that are more useful for image processing, since they are more closely related to human perception.

The oldest of these is the CIE (Commission Internationale de L'Éclairage) chromaticity diagram. This is a two-dimensional plot defining color, shown in **Figure 51**. The third axis is the luminance, which corresponds to the panchromatic brightness which, like the Y value in YUV, would produce a monochrome (grey scale) image. The other two primaries, called x and y are always positive (unlike the U and V values) and combine to define any color that we can see.

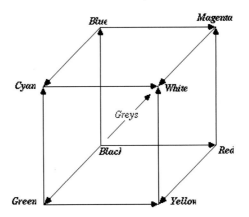

Figure 50. RGB Color Space, showing the additive progression from Black to White. Combining Red and Green produces Yellow, Green plus Blue produces Cyan, and Blue plus Red produces Yellow. Greys lie along the cube diagonal. Cyan, Yellow and Magenta are subtractive primaries used in printing, which if subtracted from White leave Red, Blue and Green, respectively.

Instruments for color measurement utilize the CIE primaries, which define the dominant wavelength and purity of any color. Mixing any two colors corresponds to selecting a new point in the diagram along a straight line between the two original colors. This means that a triangle on the CIE diagram with its corners at the red, green, and blue locations of emission phosphors used in a cathode ray tube (CRT) defines all of the colors that the tube can display. Some colors cannot be created by mixing these three phosphor colors, shown by the fact that they lie outside the triangle. The range of possible colors for any display or other output device is the gamut; hardcopy printers generally have a much smaller gamut than display tubes. The edge of the bounded region in the diagram corresponds to pure colors, and is marked with the wavelength in nanometers.

Complementary colors are shown in the CIE diagram by drawing a line through the central point, which corresponds to white

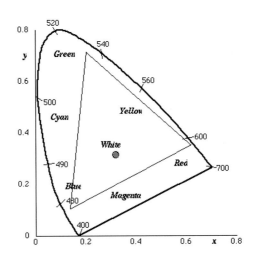

Figure 51. The CIE chromaticity diagram. The dark outline contains visible colors, which are fully saturated along the edge. Numbers give the wavelength of light in nanometers. The inscribed triangle shows the colors that typical color CRTs can produce by mixing of red, green and blue.

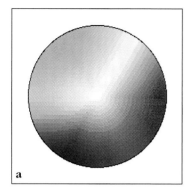

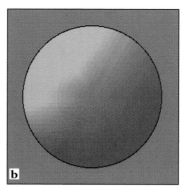

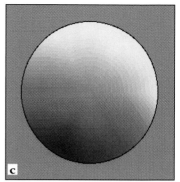

Figure 52. The U and V axes in YUV color representation used in video transmission:

a) the familiar color wheel;

b) U components of the colors, corresponding approximately to green minus magenta;

c) V components of the colors, corresponding approximately to blue minus yellow.

light. Thus, a line from green passes through white to magenta. One of the drawbacks of the CIE diagram is that it does not indicate the variation in color that can be discerned by eye. Sometimes this is shown by plotting a series of ellipses on the diagram. These are much larger in the green area, where small changes are poorly perceived, than elsewhere. In terms of the familiar color wheel representation shown in **Figure 52**, the U and V axes correspond approximately to green-magenta and blue-yellow axes.

The CIE diagram provides a tool for color definition, but corresponds neither to the operation of hardware nor directly to human vision. An approach that does is embodied in the HSV (hue, saturation, and value), HSI (hue, saturation, and intensity) and HLS (hue, lightness, and saturation) systems. These are closely related to each other and to the artist's concept of tint, shade and tone. In this system, hue is the color as described by wavelength, for instance the distinction between red and yellow. Saturation is the amount of the color that is present, for instance the distinction between red and pink. The third axis (called lightness, intensity or value) is the amount of light, the distinction between a dark red and light red or between dark grey and light grey.

The space in which these three values is plotted can be shown as a circular or hexagonal cone or double cone, all of which can be stretched to correspond. It is useful to imagine the space as a double cone, in which the axis of the cone is the grey scale progression from black to white, distance from the central axis is the saturation, and the direction is the hue. **Figure 53** shows this concept schematically. The relationship between RGB and HSI is shown in **Table 2**.

Table 2. Conversion from RGB color coordinates to HSI coordinates

---

H = $[\pi/2 - \arctan\{(2 \cdot R - G - B)/\sqrt{3} \cdot (G - B)\} + \pi; G < B] / 2\pi$
I = $(R + G + B) / 3$
S = $1 - [\min(R,G,B) / I]$

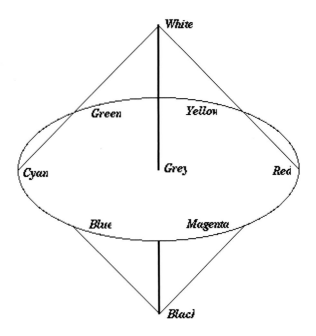

Figure 53. *Bi-conic representation of Hue-Saturation-Intensity Space. Greys lie along the central axis. Distance from the axis gives the Saturation, while direction specifies the Hue.*

This space has many advantages for image processing. For instance, if the algorithms discussed in Chapter 3 such as spatial smoothing or median filtering are used to reduce noise in an image, applying them to the RGB signals separately will cause color shifts in the result, but applying them to the HSI components will not. **Figure 54** shows an example of processing to sharpen an image with a high-pass filter. Also, the use of hue (in particular) for distinguishing features in the process called segmentation (Chapter 6) often corresponds to human perception and ignores shading effects. On the other hand, because the HSI components do not correspond to the way that most hardware works (either for acquisition or display), it requires a significant amount of computation or custom hardware to convert RGB-encoded images to HSI and back.

The HSI and HSL spaces are useful for image processing because they separate the color information in ways that correspond to the human visual system's response, and also because the axes correspond to many physical characteristics of specimens. One example of this is the staining of biological tissue. To a useful approximation, hue represents the stain color, saturation represents the amount of stain, and intensity represents the specimen density. But these spaces are awkward ones mathematically: not only does the hue value cycle through the angles from 0 to 360 degrees and then wrap around, but the conical spaces mean that increasing the intensity or luminance can alter the saturation. A geometrically simpler space that is close enough to the HSI approach for most applications and easier to deal with mathematically is the spherical L·a·b model. L as usual is the grey scale

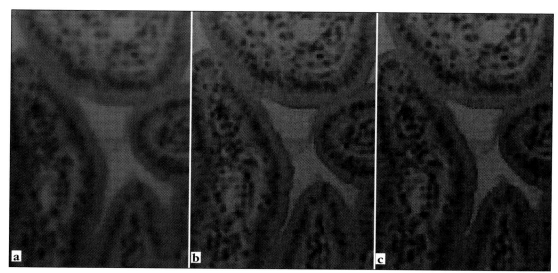

Figure 54. Portion of the color image described in Figure 58, expanded to show individual pixels:

a) *original image;*

b) *filtered to sharpen the image using the red, green and blue planes; note the appearance of false colors near boundaries;*

c) *filtered to sharpen the image by processing the hue, saturation and intensity components.*

axis, or luminance, while **a** and **b** are two orthogonal axes that together define the color and saturation (**Figure 55**). The **a** axis runs from red (+**a**) to green (–**a**) and the **b** axis from yellow (+**b**) to blue (–**b**). Notice that the hues do not have the same angular distribution in this space as in the usual color wheel. These axes offer a practical compromise between the simplicity of the RGB space that corresponds to hardware and the more physiologically based spaces such as CIE and HSI which are used in many color management systems, spectrophotometers and colorimeters.

Hardware for digitizing color images accepts either direct RGB signals from the camera, or the Y-C component signals, or a composite signal (e.g., NTSC) and uses electronic filters to separate the individual components and extract the red, green, and blue

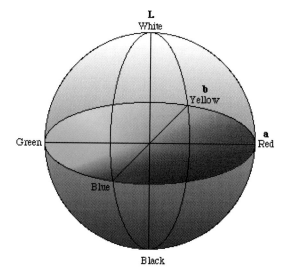

Figure 55. The L·a·b color space.

signals. As for the monochrome case discussed above, these signals are then digitized to produce values, usually 8-bit ones ranging from 0 to 255 each for R, G, and B. This takes 3 bytes of storage per pixel, so a 640×480 pixel image would require nearly 1 megabyte of storage space in the computer. With most cameras and electronics, the signals do not contain quite this much information, and the lowest 2 or more bits are noise. Consequently, some systems keep only 5 bits each for R, G, and B, which can be fit into two bytes. This reduction is often adequate for desktop publishing work, but when packed this way, the color information is hard to get at for any processing or analysis operations.

Color images are typically digitized as 24 bit RGB, meaning that 8 bits or 256 (linear) levels of brightness for red, green, and blue are stored. This is more than enough to allow display on video or computer screens, or for printing purposes, but depending on the dynamic range of the data may not be enough to adequately measure small variations within the image. Since photographic film can capture large dynamic ranges, some scanners intended for transparency or film scanning provide greater range — as much as 12 bits (4096 linear levels) for R, B and B. These 36 bit images are generally reduced to an "optimum" 8 bits when the image is stored. One of the problems with the dynamic range of color or grey scale storage is that the brightness values are linear, whereas the film (and for that matter human vision) are fundamentally logarithmic, so that in the dark regions of an image the smallest brightness step that can be stored is quite large and may result in visual artefacts or poor measurement precision for density values.

Further reduction of color images to 256 colors using a lookup table in which the best 256 colors to match the contents of the image is commonly used for computer images, in order to reduce the file size. The lookup table itself requires only 3 · 256 bytes to specify the R, G, B values for the 256 colors, which are written to the display hardware. Only a single byte per pixel is needed to select from this palette of colors. The most common technique for selecting the optimum palette is the Heckbert or median cut algorithm, which subdivides color space based on the actual RGB values of the pixels in the original image. For visual purposes such a reduction often provides a displayed image that is satisfactory, but for image analysis purposes this should be avoided.

In many situations, although color images are acquired, the "absolute" color information is not useful for image analysis. Instead, it is the relative differences in color from one region to another that can be used to distinguish the structures and features present. In such cases, it may not be necessary to store the entire color image. Various kinds of color separations are available. Calculation of the RGB components (or the complementary

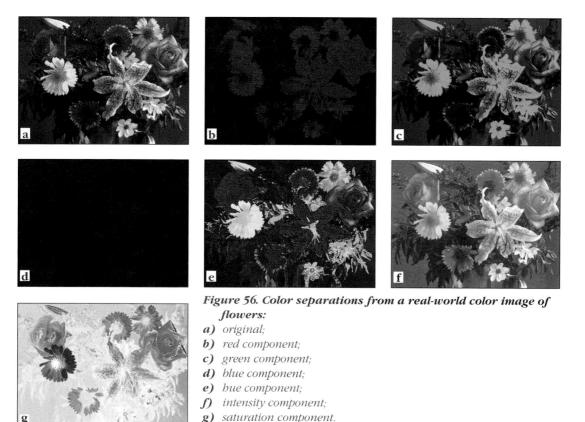

Figure 56. Color separations from a real-world color image of flowers:

a) *original;*
b) *red component;*
c) *green component;*
d) *blue component;*
e) *hue component;*
f) *intensity component;*
g) *saturation component.*

CMY values) is commonly used in desktop publishing, but as we have seen is not often useful for image analysis. Separating the image into hue, saturation, and intensity components can also be performed. **Figures 56** and **57** show two examples, one a real-world image of flowers, and the second a microscope image of stained biological tissue. Note that some structures are much more evident in one separation than another (e.g., the pink spots on the white lily petals are not visible in the red image, but are much more evident in the green or saturation images). Also, note that for the stained tissue, the hue image shows where the stains are and the saturation image shows how much of the stain is present. This distinction is also evident in the stained tissue sample shown in **Figure 58**.

It is possible to compute the amount of any particular "color" (hue) in the image. This calculation is equivalent to the physical insertion of a transmission filter in front of a monochrome camera. The filter can be selected to absorb a complementary color (for instance, a blue filter will darken yellow regions by absorbing the yellow light) and transmit light of the same color, so that the resulting image contrast can be based on the color distribution in the image. Photographers have long used yellow filters to darken the blue sky and produce monochrome images with dramatic

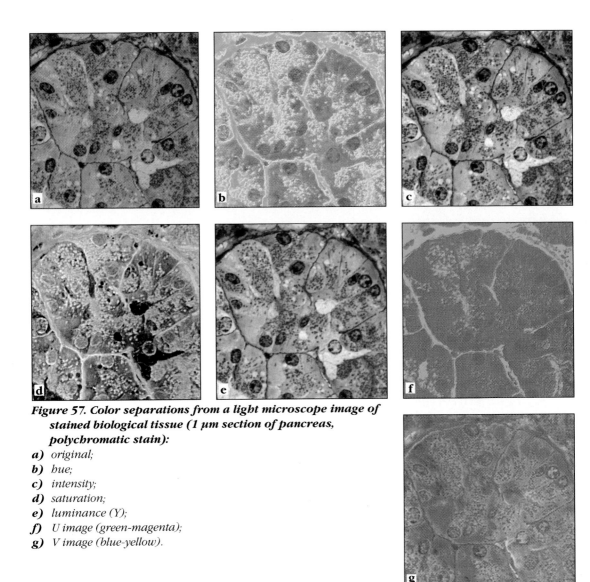

Figure 57. Color separations from a light microscope image of stained biological tissue (1 µm section of pancreas, polychromatic stain):

a) *original;*

b) *hue;*

c) *intensity;*

d) *saturation;*

e) *luminance (Y);*

f) *U image (green-magenta);*

g) *V image (blue-yellow).*

contrast for clouds, for example. The same color filtering can be used to convert color images to monochrome (grey scale). **Figures 59** and **60** show examples in which the computer is used to apply the filter. This method offers greater flexibility than physical filters, since the desired wavelength can be specified, and a drawer full of physical filters (some very difficult to make) is not needed.

Reducing a color image to grey scale is useful in many situations and can be accomplished in many ways in addition to the obvious methods of selecting an R, G, B or H, S, I image plane, or applying a selected color filter. If obtaining the maximum grey scale contrast between structures present in the image is desired

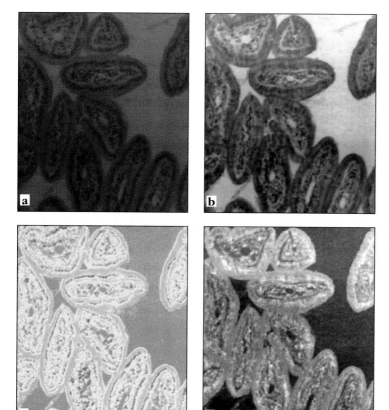

to facilitate grey scale image thresholding and measurement, then a unique function can be calculated for each image that fits a line through the points representing all of the pixels' color coordinates in color space. This least-square-fit line gives the greatest separation of the various pixel color values and the position of each pixel's coordinates as projected onto the line can be used as a grey scale value that gives the optimum contrast (Russ, 1995e). **Figure 61** shows an example.

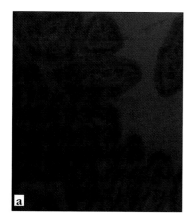
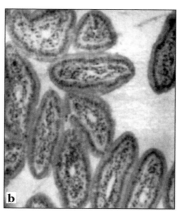

Figure 59. Filtering of the image in Figure 58:
a) application of a 480 nm filter to the original color image;
*b) monochrome intensity from image **c**.*

Figure 60. Cast aluminum alloy containing 7.4% Ca, 0.8%Si, 0.2%Ti, showing two intermetallic phases (Al_4Ca in blue, $CaSi_2$ in reddish violet); (original image from H-E. Bühler, H. P. Hougardy (1980) Atlas of Interference Layer Metallography, *Deutsche Gesellschaft für Metallkunde, Oberursel)*:

a) original color image;
b) the panchromatic intensity component of image *a* showing inability to distinguish two of the phases;
c) application of a 590 nm filter;
d) monochrome intensity from image *c* ;
e) the hue component of image *a* .

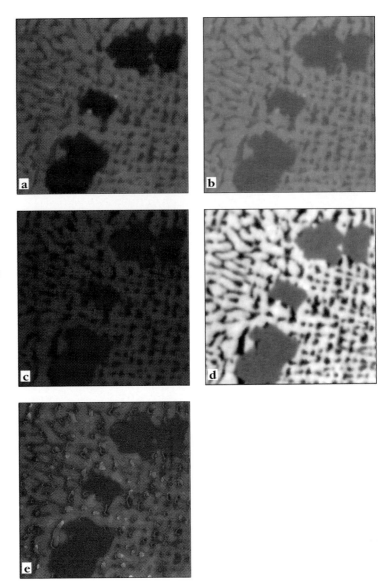

Color displays

Of course, color is also important as a vehicle for communicating to the computer user. Most computers use color monitors that have much higher resolution than a television set but operate on essentially the same principle. Smaller phosphor dots, a higher frequency scan, and a single progressive scan (rather than inter-lace) produce much greater sharpness and color purity.

Besides color video monitors, other kinds of displays may be used with desktop computers. For example, many notebook computers use a liquid crystal display (LCD). The passive type of LCD display has much poorer saturation and is also slower than the somewhat more costly active-matrix type that uses a separate

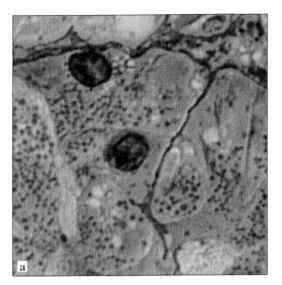

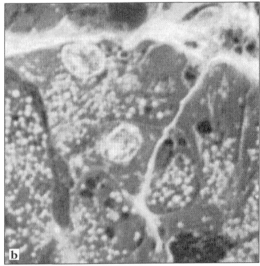

Figure 61. Color image of *(a)* stained biological tissue and *(b)* the optimal grey scale image produced by fitting a line through the pixel color coordinates.

transistor to control each pixel (or actually, each of the RGB cells that together make up a pixel in a color display). However, even the best active-matrix color LCDs are inferior to most CRTs because of their lower brightness and narrower viewing angle. They also have an inferior brightness and contrast range for each color, which reduces the number of distinct colors that can be displayed.

These same display devices may be connected to a computer and placed on an overhead projector to show images on a screen. While very convenient, and acceptable for presentations in a small room, they are inferior to dedicated projection devices. These may either use a very bright (and color corrected) light source with a small LCD panel and appropriate optics, or three separate CRTs with red, green, and blue filters. In the latter case, the resolution is potentially higher because the individual CRTs have continuous phosphor coatings. However, careful alignment of the optics is needed to keep the three images in registration; readjustment is needed every time the equipment is moved or even as it heats up. Getting enough brightness for viewing large images in rooms with imperfect light control is also a challenge.

A new class of displays uses the digital light modulation principle developed by Texas Instruments. An array of tiny mirrors produced by photolithography on silicon wafers (the same technology used to create electronic devices) is used to reflect light from the illumination source through appropriate optics to a viewing screen. The mirrors can be flipped from the "on" to the "off" position in nanoseconds. Moving each mirror back and forth rapidly to control the fraction of the time that it is in the "on" position controls the brightness of each pixel. Separate arrays for red, green, and blue light, or a single array with a rapidly rotating color filter wheel, produce full color images. The contrast and intensity of these displays is much higher than LCD panels can provide, since no light is lost to absorption. These devices are already being used in high-end projection and display systems and will probably become price competitive for consumer displays in the future.

Other kinds of flat-panel computer displays, including electroluminescence and plasma (gas discharge), are fundamentally monochrome. Arrays of red, green, and blue LEDs could in principle be arranged to make a flat-panel display, but the difficulty of generating blue light with these devices and the prohibitive cost of such devices has so far prevented their common use. Arrays of colored light bulbs are used to show images in some sports stadia.

It takes combinations of three color phosphors (RGB) to produce the range of colors displayed on the CRT. The brightness of each phosphor is controlled by modulating the intensity of the electron beam in the CRT that strikes each phosphor. Using a separate electron gun for each color and arranging the colored dots as triads is the most common method for achieving this control. To prevent stray electrons from striking the adjacent phosphor dot, a shadow mask of metal with holes for each triad of dots can be used. Each of the three electron beams passes through the same hole in the shadow mask and strikes the corresponding dot. The shadow mask increases the sharpness and contrast of the image, but reduces the total intensity of light that can be generated by the CRT.

A simpler design that increases the brightness applies the phosphor colors to the CRT in vertical stripes. It uses either a slotted pattern in the shadow mask or no mask at all. The simplicity of the Sony Trinitron design makes a tube with lower cost, no curvature of the glass in the vertical direction, high display brightness, and fewer alignment problems. However, the vertical extent of the phosphor and of the electron beam tends to blur edges in the vertical direction on the screen. While this design has become fairly common for home television, most high-performance computer CRTs use triads of phosphor dots because of the greater sharpness it affords the image, particularly for lines and edges.

Image types

In traditional images with which we are visually experienced, the brightness of a point is a function of the brightness and location of the light source combined with the orientation and nature of the surface being viewed. These "surface" or "real-world" images are actually rather difficult to interpret using computer algorithms, because of their three-dimensional nature, and the fact that some surfaces may obscure others. Even for relatively flat scenes in which precedence is not a problem and the light source is well controlled, the combination of effects of surface orientation and the color, texture, and other variables make it difficult to quantitatively interpret these parameters independently. Only in the case of a carefully prepared flat and polished surface (as in the typical metallographic microscope) can interpretation of contrast as delineating phases, inclusions, grains or other structures be successful.

A second class of images that commonly arises in microscopy shows the intensity of light (or other radiation) that has come through the sample. These transmission images start with a uniform light source, usually of known intensity and color. The absorption of the light at each point is a measure of the density of the specimen along that path. For some kinds of transmission images, such as those formed with electrons and X-rays, diffraction effects due to the coherent scattering of the radiation by atomic or molecular structures in the sample may also be present. These often complicate analysis, because diffraction is strongly dependent on the exact orientation of the crystalline lattice or other periodic microstructure.

To illustrate the complications that factors other than simple density can cause, **Figure 62** shows a transmission electron microscope (TEM) image of a thin cobalt foil. The evident structure is the magnetic domains in this ferromagnetic material. In each striped domain, the electron spins on the atoms have spontaneously aligned. There is no change in the atomic structure, sample density, or thickness, although the image certainly can fool the eye into thinking such variations may be present.

Likewise, **Figure 63** shows an image of a colloidal gold particle on an amorphous carbon film viewed in a high-resolution TEM. The so-called atomic resolution shows a pattern of dark spots on the substrate that appear more-or-less random, while in the gold

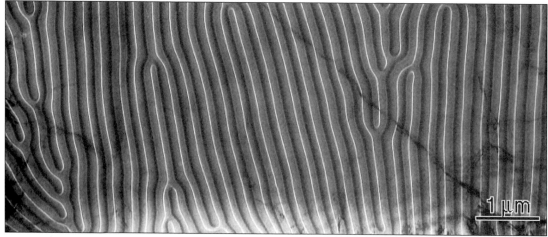

Figure 62. TEM image of a thin metal foil of cobalt. The striped pattern reveals ferromagnetic domains, in which the electron spins of the atoms are aligned in one of two possible directions. (Courtesy Hitachi Scientific Instruments)

particle they are regularly arranged. The arrangement is a result of the crystalline structure of the particle, and the spots are related to the atom positions. However, the spots are not simply the atoms; the relationship between the structure and the image is very complex and depends strongly on the microscope parameters and on the amount of defocus in the lens. Calculating the expected image contrast from a predicted structure is possible, and can be done routinely for simple structures. The inverse calculation (structure from image) is more interesting, but can only be accomplished by iteration.

Figure 63. TEM image of colloidal gold particle on an amorphous carbon substrate, used to show extremely high microscope resolution. (Courtesy Hitachi Scientific Instruments)

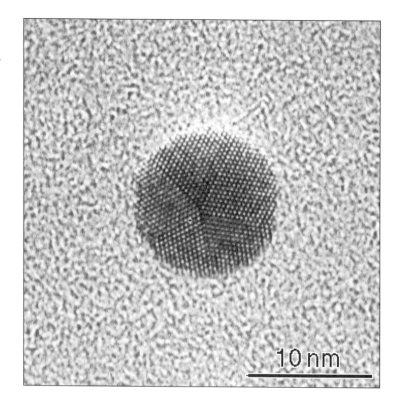

In another subclass of transmission images, some colors (or energies) of radiation may be selectively absorbed by the sample according to its chemical composition or the presence of selective stains and dyes. Sometimes, these dyes also emit light of a different color themselves, which can be imaged to localize particular structures. In principle, this is very similar to the so-called "X-ray maps" made with the scanning electron microscope (SEM), in which electrons excite the atoms of the sample to emit their characteristic X-rays. These are imaged using the time-base of the raster scan of the microscope to form a spatial image of the distribution of each selected element, since the wavelengths of the X-rays from each atom are unique. In many of these emission images, density variations, changes in the thickness of the specimen, or the presence of other elements can cause at least minor difficulties in interpreting the pixel brightness in terms of concentration or amount of the selected target element or compound.

A third class of images uses the pixel brightness to record distances. For example, an atomic force microscope image of a surface shows the elevation of each point on the surface, represented as a grey-scale (or pseudo-color) value. Range images are produced by raster-scan microscopes such as the scanning tunneling (STM) and atomic force (AFM) microscopes, or by physical scanning with a profilometer stylus. They are also produced by interferometric light microscopes, and at larger scales by laser ranging, synthetic aperture radar, side-scan sonar, and other techniques. Additional methods that present an image in which pixel brightness values represent range information obtained indirectly by other means include stereoscopy, shape-from-shading, and motion blur.

Range imaging

Most of the measurement tools available for very flat surfaces provide a single-valued elevation reading at each point in an x, y raster or grid. Chapter 11 discusses the processing and measurement of surface range images in detail. This set of data is blind to any undercuts that may be present. Just as radar and sonar have wavelengths in the range of centimeters to meters (and thus are useful for measurements of large objects such as geologic landforms), so a much shorter measuring scale is needed for high precision, or very flat surfaces. Attempts to use SEM, conventional light microscopy, or confocal scanning light microscopy (CSLM) either on the original surfaces or on vertical sections cut through them, have been only partially satisfactory. The lateral resolution of the SEM is very good, but its depth resolution is not. Stereo pair measurements are both difficult to perform and time consuming to convert to an elevation map or range image of the surface, and the resulting depth resolution is still much poorer than the lateral resolution.

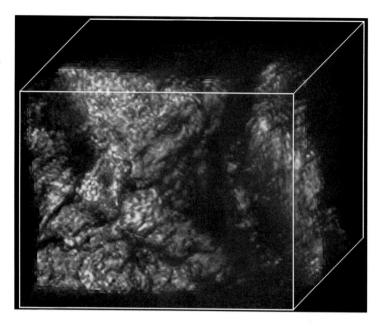

Figure 64. Reconstructed 3D image of a brittle fracture surface in a ceramic, imaged with a confocal scanning light microscope.

Conventional light microscopy has a lateral resolution of better than one micrometer, but the depth of field is neither great enough to view an entire rough surface nor shallow enough to isolate points along one iso-elevation contour line. The CSLM improves the lateral resolution slightly and greatly reduces the depth of field while at the same time rejecting scattered light from out-of-focus locations. The result is an instrument that can image an entire rough surface by moving the sample vertically and keeping only the brightest light value at each location, or can produce a range image by keeping track of the sample's vertical motion when the brightest reflected light value is obtained for each point in the image. It is the latter mode that is most interesting for surface measurement purposes. The resolution is better than one micrometer in all directions.

Figure 64 shows a reconstructed view of the surface of a fracture in a brittle ceramic. It is formed from 26 planes, separated by 1 μm in the z direction, each of which records a pixel only if that location is brighter than any other plane. The perspective view can be rotated to present a very realistic image of the surface. However, plotting the same information in the form of a range image (in which each pixel brightness corresponds to the plane in which the brightest reflection was recorded) is more useful for measurement. **Figure 65** shows this presentation of the same surface along with an elevation profile along an arbitrary line across the surface.

This method is interesting for many macroscopically rough samples, such as fractures and some deposited coatings, but it is not adequate for the really flat surfaces that are currently being produced in many applications. The surface irregularities on a

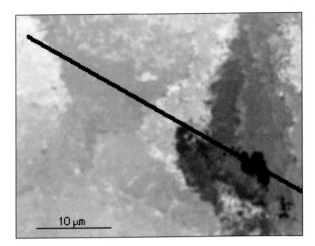

10 μm

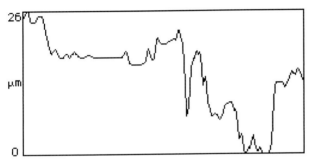

typical polished silicon wafer or precision-machined mirror surface are typically of the order of nanometers.

Three principal methods have been applied to such surfaces. Historically, the profilometer provided a tool that could accurately measure vertical elevation with a resolution approaching a nanometer. Although it has been widely used, the profilometer has two serious disadvantages for many surface applications. The first is that it determines elevations only along a single profile. While the analysis of such elevation profiles is straightforward, their relevance to complex surfaces that may have anisotropic properties is questionable. The second limitation is the large tip size, which makes it impossible to follow steep slopes or steps accurately.

This leaves the interferometric light microscope and the AFM as the methods of choice for studying very flat surfaces. Both are somewhat novel instruments. One is a modern implementation of the principles of light interference discovered a century ago, while the other is a technology invented and rapidly commercialized only within the past decade.

The interferometric light microscope (see the review by Robinson et al., 1991) reflects light from the sample surface as one leg

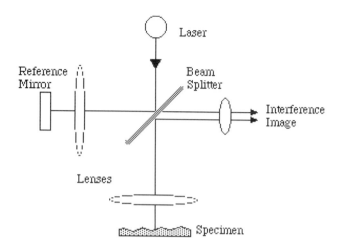

Figure 66. *Schematic diagram of an interference microscope.*

Laser

Reference Mirror

Beam Splitter

Interference Image

Lenses

Specimen

in a classic interferometer, which is then combined with light from a reference leg. **Figure 66** shows a schematic diagram. The usual principles of phase-sensitive interference occur so that changes in path length (due to different elevations of points on the surface) produce changes in the intensity of the light. This image is then digitized using an appropriate CCD detector array and analog-to-digital conversion, so that a brightness value (and from it a derived elevation value) is recorded for each point on the surface. Although the wavelength of light used is typically about 630 nm, phase differences between the two legs of the interferometer of one-thousandth of the wavelength produce a change in intensity so that the vertical resolution is a few angstroms. The lateral resolution, however, is still of the order of one micrometer, limited by the wavelength of the light used and the design of the optics.

The interferometric light microscope suffers if the surface has very high slopes and a highly specular finish, since no light will be reflected back to the detector. Such points become drop-outs in the final image. For visual purposes, it is satisfactory to fill in such missing points with a median or smoothing filter (Chapter 3), but of course this may bias subsequent measurements.

The vertical resolution of the interferometric microscope is very high, approaching atomic dimensions. Although the lateral resolution is much lower, it should be quite suitable for many purposes. The absolute height difference between widely separated points is not measured precisely, because the overall surface alignment and the shape or "figure" of the part is not known. It is common to deal with the problems of alignment and shape by fitting a function to the data. Determining a best-fit plane or other low-order polynomial function by least squares fitting to all of the elevation data and then subtracting it is called "detrending" the data or "form removal." It is then possible to display the magnitude of deviations of points from this surface. However,

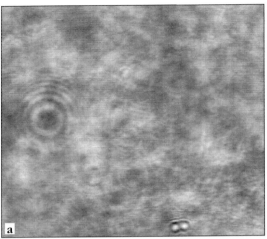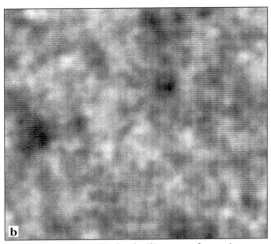

Figure 67. Comparison of interferometric range images on a flat polished silicon wafer using **a)** *Fizeau and* **b)** *Mirau optics.*

the absolute difference between points that are widely separated is affected by the detrending plane, and the ability to distinguish small differences between points that are far apart is reduced.

Figure 67 shows a very flat surface (produced by polishing a silicon wafer) imaged in a commercial interferometric light microscope (Zygo) using both Fizeau and Mirau sets of optics. The field of view is the same in both images, and the total vertical range of elevations is only about 2 nm. The two bright white spots toward the bottom of the image are probably due to dirt somewhere in the optics. These artefacts are much less pronounced with the Mirau optics. In addition, the ringing (oscillation or ripple pattern) around features that can be seen in the Fizeau image is not present with the Mirau optics. These characteristics are usually interpreted as indicating that the Mirau optics are superior for the measurement of very flat surfaces. On the other hand, the Mirau image seems to have less lateral resolution (it appears to be "smoothed"). A pattern of horizontal lines can be discerned that may come from the alignment of the diffuser plate with the raster scan pattern of the camera.

The AFM is in essence a profilometer that scans a complete raster over the sample surface, but with a very small tip (see the review by Wickramasinghe, 1989). The standard profilometer tip cannot follow very small or very steep-sided irregularities on the surface because of its dimensions, which are of the order of μm. The AFM tip can be much smaller and sharper, although it is still not usually fine enough to handle the abrupt steps (or even undercuts) present in microelectronic circuits and some other surfaces. The tip can be operated in either an attractive or repulsive mode of interaction between the electrons around the atom(s) in the tip and those in the surface. Usually, repulsive mode (in which the tip is pressed against the surface) does a somewhat better job

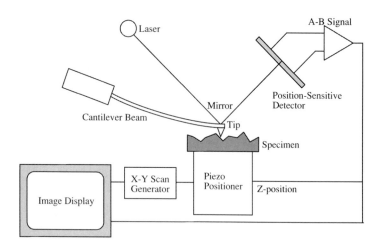

of following small irregularities, but it may also cause deformation of the surface and the displacement of atoms.

There are other modalities of interaction for these scanned-tip microscopes. The STM was the original, but it can only be used for conductive specimens and is strongly sensitive to surface electronic states, surface contamination, and oxidation. Lateral force and other modes of operation developed within the last few years offer the ability to characterize many aspects of surface composition and properties, but the straightforward AFM mode is most often used to determine surface geometry, and presents quite enough complexities for understanding.

As indicated in the schematic diagram of **Figure 68**, the usual mode of operation for the AFM is to move the sample in x, y, and z. The x, y scan covers the region of interest, while the z motion brings the tip back to the same null position as judged by the reflection of a laser beam. The necessary motion is recorded in a computer to produce the resulting image. Modifications that move the tip instead of the sample, or use a linear-array light sensor to measure the deflection of the tip rather than wait for the specimen to be moved in z, do not change the basic principle. The motion is usually accomplished with piezoelectric elements whose dimensions can be sensitively adjusted by varying the applied voltage. However, there is a time lag or creep associated with these motions that appears in the modulation transfer function (MTF) of the microscope as a loss of sensitivity at the largest or smallest dimensions (lowest and highest frequencies). Locating the x, y coordinates of the tip interferometrically instead of based on the piezo driver voltages can overcome some of these problems.

Although the AFM has in principle a lateral resolution of a few Angstroms, as well as vertical sensitivity in this range, it is not

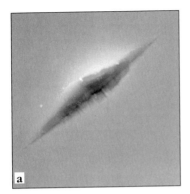
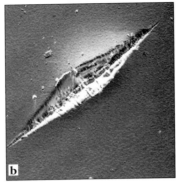
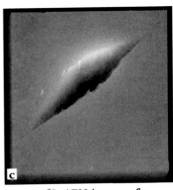

Figure 69. AFM image of a Knoop hardness indentation, shown as
a) range,
b) rendered and
c) isometric presentations.

always possible to realize that performance. For one thing, the adjustment of scan speeds and amplifier time constants for the visually best picture may eliminate some of the fine-scale roughness and thus bias subsequent analysis. Conversely, it may introduce additional noise from electrical or mechanical sources. Special care must also be taken to eliminate vibration.

Most of the attention to the performance of the AFM, STM, and related instruments has been concerned with the high-resolution limit (Denley, 1990a; Denley, 1990b; Grigg et al., 1992). This is generally set by the shape of the tip, which is not easy to characterize. Many authors (Reiss et al., 1990; Pancorbo et al., 1991; Aguilar et al., 1992) have suggested that it may be possible to deconvolve the tip shape and improve the image sharpness in exactly the same way that it is done for other imaging systems. This type of deconvolution is discussed in Chapters 4 and 11.

Figure 69 shows a sample of polished silicon (traditional roughness values indicate 0.2–0.3 nm magnitude, near the nominal vertical resolution limit for interferometry and STM) with a hardness indentation. One limitation of the STM can be seen by generating a rendered or isotropic display of the indentation, which shows that the left side of the indentation appears to be smoother than the right. This difference is an artefact of the scanning, since the tip response dynamics are different when following a surface down (where it may lag behind the actual surface and fail to record deviations) or up (where contact forces it to follow irregularities). In addition, the measured depth of the indentation is much less than the actual depth, because the tip cannot follow the deepest part of the indentation and because the calibration of the AFM in the vertical direction is less precise than in the x, y directions.

Tools for surface characterization are available with sufficient lateral and vertical resolution for application to a variety of surface range measurements. The interferometer is more convenient to use than the AFM, operates over a wide range of magnifications,

Figure 70. *Scanning tunneling microscope (STM) image. The specimen actually is flat-surfaced silicon, with apparent relief showing altered electron levels in a 2 µm wide region with implanted phosphorus. (Image courtesy of J. Labrasca, North Carolina State University, and R. Chapman, Microelectronics Center of North Carolina)*

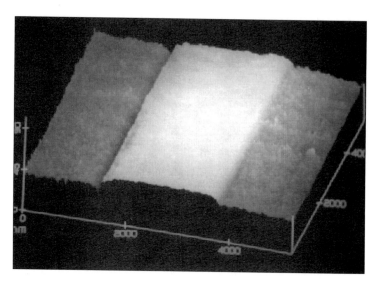

and accepts large samples. It also introduces less directional anisotropy due to the instrument characteristics. The AFM, on the other hand, has higher lateral resolution which may be required for the metrology of very fine features, now becoming commonplace in integrated circuit fabrication and nanotechnology.

It is important to keep in mind that the signal produced by many microscopes is only indirectly related to the surface elevation. In some cases, it may represent quite different characteristics of the sample such as compositional variations or electronic properties. In **Figure 70**, the apparent step in surface elevation provides an example. The surface is actually flat, but the electronic properties of the sample (a junction in a microelectronic device) produce the variation in signal.

Multiple images

For many applications, a single image is not enough. Multiple images may constitute a series of views of the same area, using different wavelengths of light or other signals. Examples include the images produced by satellites, such as the various visible and infrared wavelengths recorded by the Landsat Thematic Mapper (TM), and images from the SEM in which as many as a dozen different elements may be represented by their X-ray intensities. These images may each require processing; for example, X-ray maps are usually very noisy. They are then often combined either by using ratios, such as the ratio of different wavelengths used to identify crops in TM images, or Boolean logic, such as locating regions that contain iron and sulfur in an SEM image of a mineral. **Figure 71** shows an example in which two satellite color photographs of the same region, one covering the usual visual range of wavelengths and one extending into the near infrared, are combined by constructing the ratio of infrared to

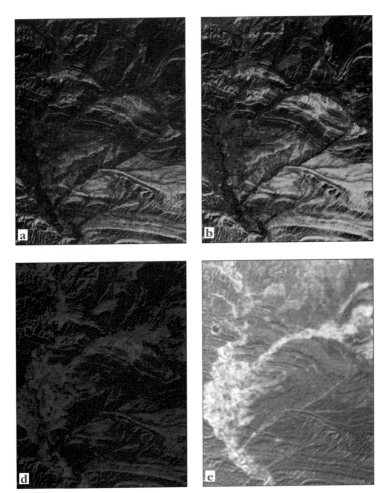

Figure 71. Landsat Thematic Mapper images in visual and infrared color *(20 km region at Thermopolis, Wyoming, original image from F. F. Sabins (1987)* Remote Sensing: Principles and Interpretation, *W. H. Freeman, New York):*

a) *visible light;*
b) *infrared light;*
c) *result of filtering the visible image at 520 nm;*
d) *filtering the infrared image at 1100 nm;*
e) *the ratio of the green (visible) to red (IR) filtered intensities.*

green intensity. Combinations reduce, but only slightly, the amount of data to be stored.

Another multiple image situation is a time sequence. This could be a series of satellite images used to track the motion of weather systems or a series of microscope images used to track the motion of cells or beating of cilia. In all of these cases, the need is usually to identify and locate the same features in each of the images, even though there may be some gradual changes in feature appearance from one image to the next. If the images can be reduced to data on the location of only a small number of features, then the storage requirements are greatly reduced.

A technique known as motion flow works at a lower level. With this approach, matching of pixel patterns by a correlation method is used to create a vector field showing the motion between successive images. This method is particularly used in machine vision and robotics work, in which the successive images are very closely spaced in time. Simplifying the vector field can again result in modest amounts of data, and these are usually processed

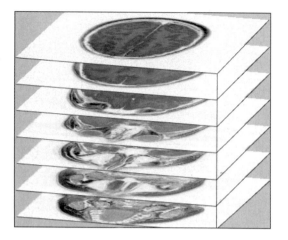

Figure 72. Multiple planes of pixels fill three-dimensional space. Voxels (volume elements) are ideally cubic for processing and measurement of 3D images.

in real time so that storage is not an issue. The principal requirement is that the local texture information needed for matching be present. Hence, the images must be low in noise and each image should contain simple and distinctive surfaces with consistent illumination. The matching is performed using cross-correlation matching, in either the spatial or frequency domain.

A set of images can also produce three-dimensional information. These are usually a series of parallel slice images through a solid object (**Figure 72**). Medical imaging methods such as tomography and magnetic resonance images can produce this sort of data. So can some seismic imaging techniques. Even more common are various serial section methods used in microscopy. The classic method for producing such a series of images is to microtome a series of sections from the original sample, image each separately in the light or electron microscope, and then align the images afterwards.

Optical sectioning, especially with the CSLM, which has a very shallow depth of field and can collect images from deep in partially transparent specimens, eliminates the problems of alignment. **Figure 73** shows several focal section planes from a CSLM. Some imaging methods, such as the SIMS (Secondary Ion Mass Spectrometer), produce a series of images in depth by physically eroding the sample, which also preserves alignment. **Figure 74** shows an example of SIMS images. Sequential polishing of harder samples such as metals also produces new surfaces for imaging, but it is generally difficult to control the depth to space them uniformly.

The ideal situation for three-dimensional interpretation of structure calls for the lateral resolution of serial section image planes to be equal to the spacing between the planes. This produces cubic "voxels" (volume elements), which have the same advantages for processing and measurement in three dimensions that square pixels have in two. However, it is usually the case that the

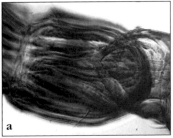 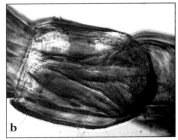 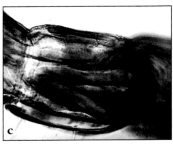

Figure 73. Serial section images formed by transmission confocal scanning laser microscopy (CSLM). These are selected views from a series of sections through the leg joint of a head louse, with section thickness less than 0.5 μm.

planes are spaced apart by much more than their lateral resolution, and special attention is given to interpolating between the planes. In the case of the SIMS, the situation is reversed and the plane spacing (as little as a few atom dimensions) is much less than the lateral resolution in each plane (typically about 1 μm).

There are techniques that directly produce cubic voxel images, such as three-dimensional tomography. In one case, a series of projection images, generally using X-rays or electrons, are obtained as the sample is rotated to different orientations, and then mathematical reconstruction calculates the density of each voxel. The resulting large, three-dimensional image arrays may be stored as a series of planar slices. When a three-dimensional data set is used, a variety of processing and display modes are

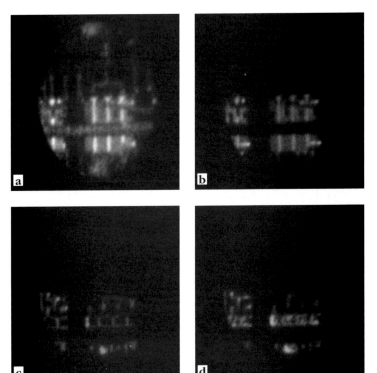

Figure 74. SIMS (Secondary Ion Mass Spectrometer) images of boron implanted in a microelectronic device. The images are selected from a sequence of 29 images covering a total of about 1 μm in depth. Each image is produced by physically removing layers of atoms from the surface, which erodes the sample progressively to reveal structures at greater depth.

Figure 75. Examples of three-dimensional data sets formed by a series of planar images:

a) *A sintered ceramic imaged by X-ray tomography (CAT), with a characteristic dimension of a few μm; the dark regions are voids. The poorer resolution in the vertical direction is due to the spacing of the image planes, which is greater than the lateral pixel resolution within each plane.*

b) *A human head imaged by magnetic resonance (MRI), with characteristic dimension of cm. The section planes can be positioned arbitrarily and moved to reveal the internal structure.*

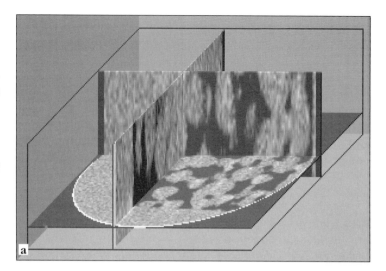

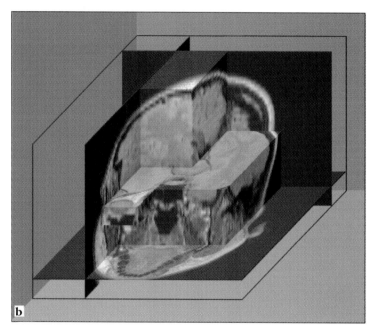

available. These are discussed in more detail in Chapter 10. **Figure 75** shows an example of sectioning through a series of magnetic resonance images (MRI) in the *x*, *y*, and *z* planes.

Stereoscopy

Three-dimensional information can also be obtained from two images of the same scene, taken from slightly different viewpoints. Human stereoscopy gives us depth perception, although we also get important data from relative size, precedence, perspective, and other cues. Like other aspects of human vision, stereoscopy is primarily comparative, with the change of vergence angle of

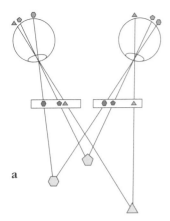

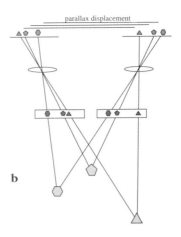

parallax displacement

a

b

Figure 76. Stereoscopic depth perception:
a) *The relative distance to each feature identified in both the left and right eye views is given by differences in the vergence angles by which the eyes must rotate inwards to bring each feature to the central fovea in each eye. This is accomplished one feature at a time. Viewing stereo pair images provides the same visual cues to the eyes and produces the same interpretation.*
b) *Measurement of images to obtain actual distances uses the different parallax displacements of the features in two images. The distance between the two view points must be known. Identifying the same feature in both images is the greatest difficulty for automated analysis.*

the eyes as we shift attention from one feature to another indicating to the brain which is closer. **Figure 76** shows schematically the principle of stereo fusion, in which the images from each eye are compared to locate the same feature in each view. The eye muscles rotate the eye to bring this feature to the fovea, and the muscles provide the vergence information to the brain. Notice that this implies that stereoscopy is only applied to one feature in the field of view at a time, and not to the entire scene. From the amount of vergence motion needed, the relative distance of the object is ascertained. Since only comparative measurements are made, only the direction or relative amount of motion required to fuse the images of each object is required.

Not all animals use this method. The owl, for instance, has eyes that are not movable in their sockets. Instead, the fovea has an elongated shape along a line that is not vertical, but angled toward the owl's feet. The owl tilts his head to accomplish fusion (bringing the feature of interest to the fovea) and judges the relative distance by the angle required.

Although the human visual system makes only comparative use of the parallax, or vergence, of images of an object, it is straightforward to use the relative displacement of two objects in the field of view to calculate their relative distance, or of the angle of vergence of one object to calculate its distance from the viewer. This is routinely done at scales ranging from aerial photography and map-making to scanning electron microscopy.

Measurement of range information from two views is quite straightforward in principle. The lateral position of objects in these two views is different depending on their distance. From these parallax displacements, the distance can be computed by a process called stereoscopy. However, computer fusion of images is a difficult task that requires locating matching points in the images. Brute-force correlation methods that try to match many points based on local texture are fundamentally similar to the motion flow approach. This produces many false matches, but these are assumed to be removed by subsequent noise filtering. The alternate approach is to locate selected points in the images that are "interesting" based on their representing important boundaries or feature edges, which can then be matched more confidently. However, the areas between the matched points are then assumed to be simple planes.

However fusion is accomplished, the displacement of the points in the two images, or parallax, gives the range. This method is used for surface elevation mapping, ranging from satellite or aerial pictures used to produce topographic maps (in which the two images are taken a short time apart as the satellite or airplane position changes) to scanning electron microscope metrology of semiconductor chips (in which the two images are produced by tilting the sample). **Figure 77** shows an example of a stereo pair from an SEM; **Figure 78** shows two aerial photographs and a complete topographic map drawn from them.

The utility of a stereoscopic view of the world to communicate depth information resulted in the use of stereo cameras to produce "stereopticon" slides for viewing, which was very popular more than 50 years ago. Stereo movies (requiring the viewer to wear polarized glasses) have enjoyed brief vogues from time to time. Publication of stereo-pair views to illustrate scientific papers is now relatively common. The most common formats are two side-by-side images about 7.5 cm apart (the distance between human eyes), which an experienced viewer can see without optical aids by looking straight ahead and allowing the brain to fuse the two images, and the use of different colors for each image. Overprinting the same image in red and green (or red and blue) allows the viewer with colored glasses to see the correct image in each eye, and again the brain can sort out the depth information (**Figure 79**). Some SEMs display true stereo views of surfaces using this method. Of course, this only works for grey scale images. Computer displays using polarized light and glasses are also used to display three-dimensional data, usually synthesized from calculations or simulations rather than direct imaging.

There are several different measurement geometries (Boyde, 1973). In all cases, the same scene is viewed from two different locations and the distance between those locations is precisely known. Sometimes this is accomplished by moving the viewpoint, for instance the airplane carrying the camera. In aerial photography, the plane's speed and direction are known and the time of each picture is recorded with it to give the distance traveled.

In **Figure 80**, S is the shift distance (either the distance the plane has traveled or the distance the SEM stage was translated) and

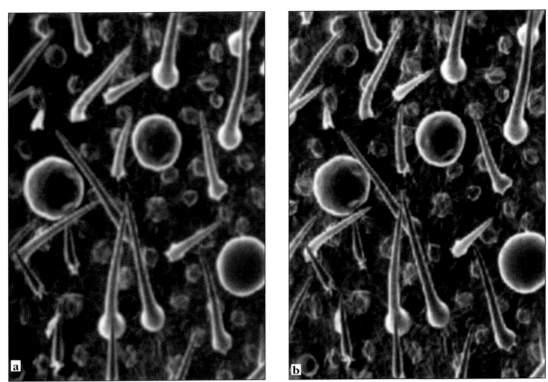

Figure 77. *Stereo pair images from the scanning electron microscope (SEM). The specimen is the surface of a leaf; the two images were obtained by tilting the beam incident on the specimen by 8° to produce two points of view.*

Figure 78. *Stereo pair images from aerial photography, and the topographic map showing iso-elevation contour lines derived from the parallax in the images. The scene is a portion of the Wind River in Wyoming (from Sabins, 1987)*

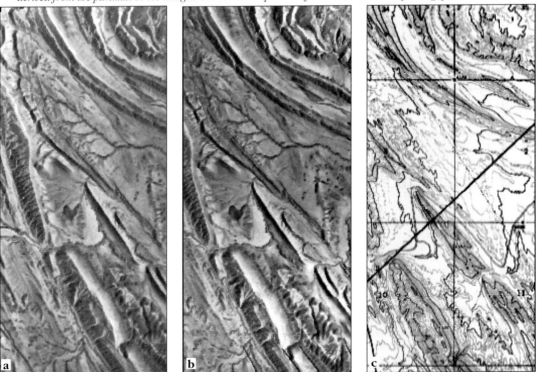

Figure 79. *Red/Cyan stereo image (Japanese lantern in the author's back yard). This image was captured directly into the computer using a digital camera, shifted to take each grey scale picture sequentially, and then superimposing them as different color planes. To view the image, use glasses with a red filter in front of the left eye, and either a green or blue filter in front of the right eye. (See also the example in the Introduction).*

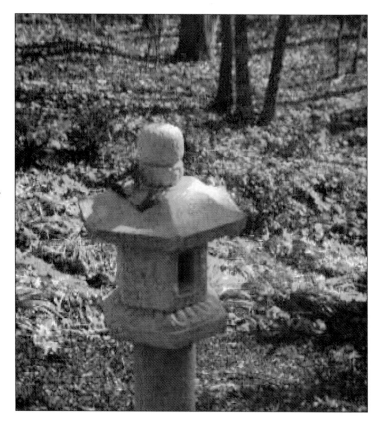

WD is the working distance or altitude. The parallax $(d_1 - d_2)$ from the distances between two points as they appear in the two different images (measured in a direction parallel to the shift) is proportional to the elevation difference between the two points.

$$h = WD \cdot (d_1 - d_2) / S$$

If the vertical relief of the surface being measured is a significant fraction of WD, then foreshortening of lateral distances as a function of elevation will also be present in the images. The x and y coordinates of points in the images can be corrected with the following equations. This means that rubber-sheeting to correct the foreshortening is needed to allow fitting or "tiling" together a mosaic of pictures into a seamless whole.

$$X' = X \cdot (WD - h) / WD$$
$$Y' = Y \cdot (WD - h) / WD$$

Much greater displacement between the two eyepoints can be achieved if the two views are not in parallel directions, but are instead directed inwards toward the same central point in each scene. This is rarely done in aerial photography, because it is impractical when trying to cover a large region with a mosaic of pictures and is not usually necessary to obtain sufficient parallax

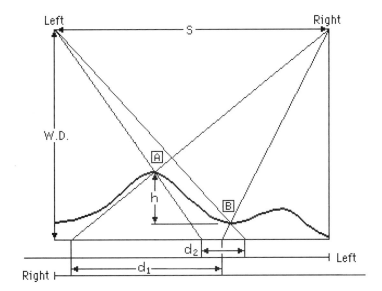

Figure 80: *Geometry used to measure the vertical height difference between objects viewed in two different images obtained by shifting the sample or viewpoint.*

for measurement. However, when examining samples in the SEM, it is very easy to accomplish this by tilting the sample between two views. In **Figure 81**, the two images represent two views obtained by tilting the specimen about a vertical axis. The points A and B are separated by a horizontal distance d_1 or d_2 that is different in the two images. From this parallax value and the known tilt angle δ applied between the two images, the height difference h and the angle θ of a line joining the points (usually a surface defined by the points) can be calculated (Boyde, 1973) as:

$$\theta = \tan^{-1}\{(\cos \delta - d_2/d_1)/\sin \delta\}$$
$$h_1 = (d_1 \cdot \cos \delta - d_2)/\sin \delta$$

Notice that the angle θ is independent of the magnification, since the distances enter as a ratio.

When two angled views of the same region of the surface are available, the relative displacement or parallax of features can be made quite large relative to their lateral magnification. This makes it possible to measure relatively small amounts of surface relief. Angles of 5 to 10 degrees are commonly used; for very flat surfaces, tilt angles in excess of 20 degrees can sometimes be useful. When large angles are used with rough surfaces, the images contain shadow areas where features are not visible in both images and fusion becomes very difficult. Also, when the parallax becomes too great in a pair of images, it can be difficult for the human observer to fuse the two images visually if this step is used in the measurement operation.

Many of the measurements made with stereo-pair photographs from both SEM and aerial photography are made using extensive

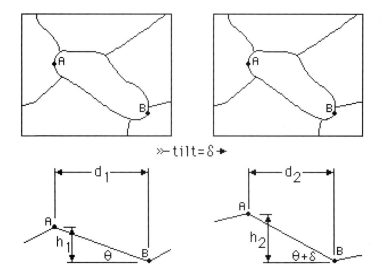

Figure 81: *Stereo pair images used to measure the vertical height difference between points, viewed in two different images obtained by tilting the sample.*

human interaction. The algorithms that have been developed for automatic fusion are relatively complex, requiring many of the image processing operations that will be described in later chapters to make possible the identification of the same features in each image. For the moment, it is enough to understand the principle that identifying the same points in left and right images, and measuring the parallax, gives the elevation. With data for many different pairs of points, it is possible to construct a complete map of the surface. The elevation data can then be presented in a variety of formats, including a range image encoding elevation as the brightness or color of each pixel in the array. Other display modes, such as contour maps, isometric views, or shaded renderings can be generated to assist the viewer in interpreting these images, which are not common to our everyday experience. The range image data are in a suitable form for many types of image processing and for the measurement of the surface area or the volume above or below the surface.

The majority of elevation maps of the earth's surface being made today are determined by the stereoscopic measurement of images, either taken from aerial photography or satellite remote imaging. Of course, two-thirds of the earth is covered by water and cannot be measured this way. Portions of the sea bottom have been mapped stereoscopically by side-scanned sonar. The technology is very similar to that used for the radar mapping of Venus, except that sonar uses sound waves (which can propagate through water) and radar uses high-frequency (millimeter length) electromagnetic radiation that can penetrate the opaque clouds covering Venus.

The synthetic aperture radar (SAR) used by the Magellan probe to map Venus does not directly give elevation data to produce a range image. The principle of SAR is not new, nor restricted to satellites and space probes. Aerial mapping of desert regions has been used to penetrate through the dry sand and map the under-lying land to find ancient watercourses, for instance. The princi-ple of SAR is that the moving satellite (or other platform) emits a series of short pulses directed downwards and to one side of the track along which it is moving. Direction parallel to the track is called the azimuth and the direction perpendicular to it is called the range (not to be confused with the range image that encodes the elevation information). The name "synthetic aperture" refers to the fact that the moving antenna effectively acts as a much larger antenna (equal in size to the distance the antenna moves during the pulse) that can more accurately resolve directions in azimuth.

The radar records the intensity of the returning pulse, the travel time, and the Doppler shift. The intensity is a measure of the sur-face characteristics, although the radar (or sonar) reflectivity is not always easy to interpret in terms of the surface structure and is not directly related to the albedo (or reflectivity) for visible light. The travel time for the pulse gives the range. For a per-fectly flat surface, there would be an arc of locations on the sur-face that would have the same range from the antenna. Because of the motion of the satellite or airplane, each point along this arc would produce a different Doppler shift in the signal frequency. Measuring the Doppler shift of each returned pulse provides res-olution along the arc. Each point on the ground contributes to the return pulse with a unique range and Doppler shift, which allows a range map of the ground to be reconstructed.

However, since the surface is not flat, there are multiple possible combinations of location and elevation that could produce the same return signal. Combining the measurements from several overlapping sweeps (for Magellan, several sequential orbits) allows the elevation data to be refined. The database for Venus resolves points on the ground with about 120-meter spacing and has elevation data with resolutions that vary from 120 to 300 meters (depending on where along the track, and how far from the center of the track, they were located). For each point, the elevation and the reflectivity are stored (**Figure 82**). In many of the published renderings of these data, the elevation values are used to construct the surface shape and the reflectivity values are used to color the surface (**Figure 83**). Of course, the colors do not reflect the actual visual appearance of the surface.

Synthetic aperture ranging with either radar or sonar is not the only way these signals can be used to construct a range map. Directing a beam straight down and measuring the echo, or return time, gives the range at a single point. Many such mea-surements can be used to construct a map or image. The simple "fish-finder" type of sonar can be used to construct a map of a

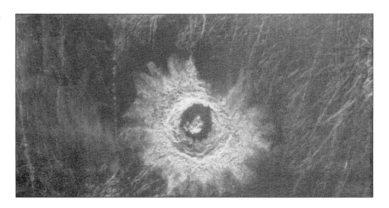

Figure 82. Range image of Venus obtained from synthetic aperture radar. (Courtesy JPL)

lake bottom in this way, if the boat is steered back and forth in a raster pattern to cover the whole surface. Other signals can be used, as well. The Clementine mission to the moon used a laser beam from the orbiting space craft in a similar fashion. By pulsing the laser and waiting for the echo, points were measured every few hundred meters across the entire lunar surface with a vertical resolution of about 40 meters.

Imaging requirements

Given the diversity of image types and sources described above, there are several general criteria we can prescribe for images intended for computer processing and analysis. The first is the need for global uniformity. The same type of feature should look the same wherever it appears in the image. This implies that brightness and color values should be the same and, consequently,

Figure 83. Rendered surface of Venus from SAR data (Courtesy JPL).

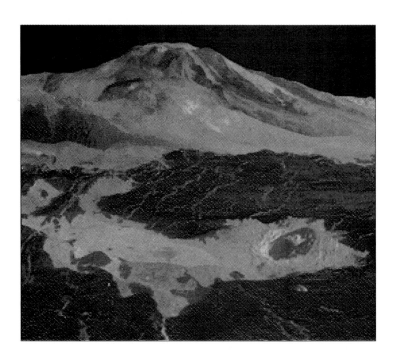

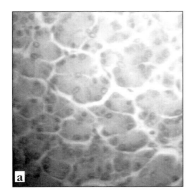

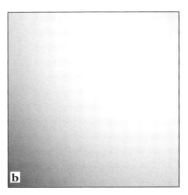

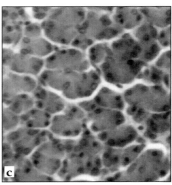

Figure 84. *A microscope image obtained with nonuniform illumination (due to a misaligned condenser). The "background" image was collected under the same conditions, with no sample present (by moving to an adjacent region on the slide). Subtracting the background image and expanding the contrast of the difference produces a "leveled" image with uniform brightness values for similar structures.*

that illumination must be uniform and stable for images acquired at different times. When surfaces are nonplanar, such as the earth as viewed from a satellite or a fracture surface in the microscope, corrections for the changing local orientation may be possible, but this usually requires extensive calculation and/or prior knowledge of the surface and source of illumination.

Figure 84 shows an example of a microscope image with nonuniform illumination. Storing a "background" image with no specimen present (by moving to a clear space on the slide) allows this nonuniformity to be leveled. The background image is either subtracted from or divided into the original (depending on whether the camera has a linear or logarithmic response). This type of leveling is discussed in Chapter 2 on correcting image defects, along with other ways to obtain the background image when it cannot be acquired directly.

The requirement for uniformity limits the kinds of surfaces that are normally imaged. Planar surfaces, or at least simple and known ones, are much easier to deal with than complex surfaces. Simply connected surfaces are much easier to interpret than ones with arches and loops that hide some of the structure. Features that have precedence problems, in which some features hide entirely or in part behind others, present difficulties for interpretation or measurement. Illumination that casts strong shadows, especially to one side, is also undesirable in most cases. The exception occurs when well-spaced features cast shadows that do not interfere with each other. The shadow lengths can be used with the known geometry to calculate feature heights. **Figure 85** shows an example in aerial photography. One form of sample preparation for the TEM deposits a thin film of metal or carbon from a point source, which also leaves shadow areas behind particles or other protrusions that can be used in the same way (**Figure 86**).

In addition to global uniformity, we generally want local sensitivity to variations. This means that edges and boundaries must be well delineated and accurately located. The resolution of the

Figure 85. *Aerial photograph in which length of shadows and knowledge of the sun position permit calculation of the heights of trees and the height of the piles of logs in the lumberyard, from which the amount of wood can be estimated.*

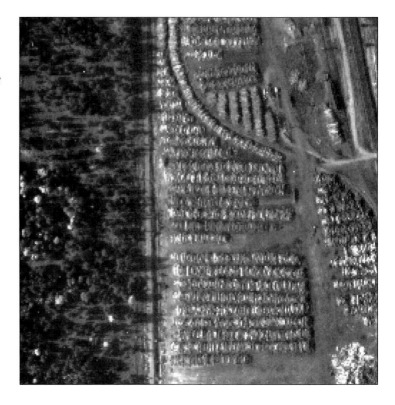

camera sensor was discussed above. Generally, anything that degrades high frequencies in the signal chain will disturb the subsequent ability to identify feature boundaries or locate edges for measurement. On the other hand, such simple problems as dust on the optics can introduce local variations that may be mistaken for image features, causing serious errors.

Figure 86. *Electron microscope image showing shadowed particles delineating the gap junctions between cells, revealed by freeze-fracturing the tissue.*

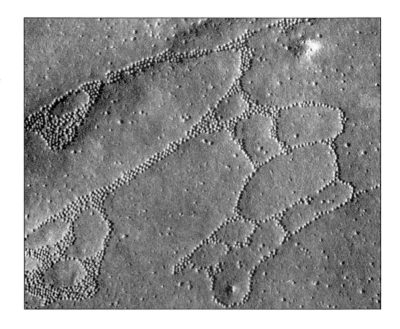

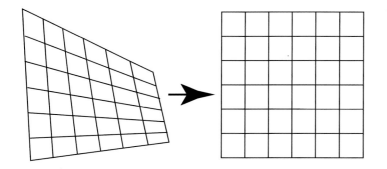

Figure 87. Geometric distortion occurs when a surface is viewed from a position away from the surface normal. Correcting this distortion to obtain a rectilinear image which can be properly processed and measured, or fitted together with adjoining images, requires knowing the viewing geometry and/or including some known fiducial marks in the scene which can be used to determine it.

Measurement of dimensions requires that the geometry of the imaging system be well known. Knowing the magnification of a microscope or the altitude of a satellite is usually straightforward. Calibrating the lateral scale can be accomplished either by knowledge of the optics or by using an image of a known scale or standard. When the viewing geometry is more complicated, either because the surface is not planar or the viewing angle is not perpendicular, measurement is more difficult and requires determination of the geometry first.

Figure 87 shows the simplest kind of distortion when a planar surface is viewed at an angle. Different portions of the image have different magnification scales, which makes subsequent analysis difficult. It also prevents combining multiple images of a complex surface into a mosaic. This problem is evident in two applications at very different scales. Satellite images of the surface of planets are assembled into mosaics covering large areas only with elaborate image warping to bring the edges into registration. This type of warping is discussed in Chapter 3. SEM images of rough surfaces are more difficult to assemble in this way, because the overall specimen geometry is not so well known, and the required computer processing is more difficult to justify.

Measuring brightness information, such as density or color values, requires a very stable illumination source and sensor. Color measurements are easily affected by changes in the color temperature of an incandescent bulb due to minor voltage fluctuations or as the bulb warms up or ages. Fluorescent lighting, especially when used in light boxes with X-ray films or densitometry gels, may be unstable or may introduce interference in solid-state cameras due to the high-frequency flickering of the fluorescent tube. Bright specular reflections may cause saturation, blooming, or shifts in the camera gain.

It will help to bear in mind what the purpose is when digitizing an image into a computer. Some of the possibilities are listed below, and these place different restrictions and demands on the hardware and software used. Subsequent chapters discuss these topics in greater detail.

Storing and filing of images becomes more attractive as massive storage devices (such as optical disks) drop in price or where multiple master copies of images may be needed in more than one location. In many cases, this application also involves hardcopy printing of the stored images and transmission of images to other locations. If further processing or measurement is not required, then compression of the images is worthwhile. The advantage of electronic storage is that the images do not degrade with time and can be accessed by appropriate filing and cross-indexing routines. On the other hand, film storage is far cheaper and offers much higher storage density and higher image resolution.

Enhancement of images for visual examination requires a large number of pixels and adequate pixel depth so that the image can be acquired with enough information to perform the filtering or other operations with fidelity and then display the result with enough detail for the viewer. Uniformity of illumination and control of geometry are not of great importance. When large images are used, and especially for some of the more time-consuming processing operations, or when interactive experimentation with many different operations is intended, this application may benefit from very fast computers or specialized hardware.

Measurement of dimensions and density values can often be performed with modest image resolution if the magnification or illumination can be adjusted beforehand to make the best use of the image sensor. Processing may be required before measurement (for instance, derivatives are often used to delineate edges for measurement) but this can usually be handled completely in software. The most important constraints are tight control over the imaging geometry and the uniformity and constancy of illumination.

Quality control applications usually do not involve absolute measurements so much as watching for variations. In many cases, this is handled simply by subtracting a reference image from each acquired image, point by point, to detect gross changes. This can be done with analog electronics at real-time speeds. Preventing variation due to accidental changes in the position of camera or targets, or in illumination, is a central concern.

Structural research in either two or three dimensions usually starts with image measurement and has the same requirements as noted above, plus the ability to subject the measurement values to appropriate stereological and statistical analysis. Interpretation of images in terms of structure is different for images of planar cross sections or projections (**Figure 88**). The latter are familiar to human vision, while the former are not. However, section images, such as the one in **Figure 89**, contain rich information for measurement in three dimensions that can be revealed by statistical analysis. Projection images, such as the one in **Figure 90**, present greater difficulties for interpretation.

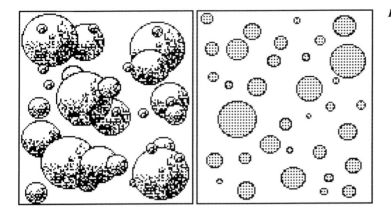

Figure 88. Projection images, such as the spheres shown at left, are familiar, showing the external surfaces of features. However, some features are partially or entirely obscured and it is not possible to determine the number or size distribution. Cross section images, as shown at right, are unfamiliar and do not show the maximum extent of features, but statistically it is possible to predict the size distribution and number of the spheres.

Three-dimensional imaging utilizes large data sets, and in most cases the alignment of two-dimensional images is of critical importance. Some three-dimensional structural parameters can be inferred from two-dimensional images. Others, principally topological information, can only be determined from the full three-dimensional data set. Processing and measurement operations in three dimensions place extreme demands on computer storage and speed. Displays of three-dimensional information in ways interpretable by, if not familiar to, human users are improving, but need further development of algorithms. They also place considerable demands on processor and display speed.

Pattern recognition is generally considered to be the high-end task for computer-based image analysis. It ranges in complexity from locating and recognizing isolated objects belonging to a few well-established classes to much more open-ended problems. Examples of the former are locating objects for robotic manipulation or recognizing targets in surveillance photos. An example of the latter is medical diagnosis, in which much of the important information comes from sources other than the image itself. Fuzzy logic, expert systems, and neural nets are all being applied to these tasks with some success. Extracting the correct

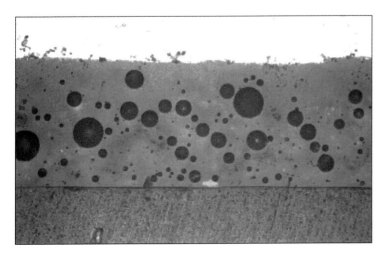

Figure 89. Light microscope image of section through a colored enamel coating applied to steel (Courtesy V. Benes, Research Inst. for Metals, Panenské Brezany, Czechoslovakia). The spherical bubbles arise during the firing of the enamel. They are sectioned to show circles with diameters which are smaller than the maximum diameter of the spheres, but since the shape of the bubbles is known, it is possible to infer the number and size distribution of the spheres from the data measured on the circles.

Figure 90. *Transmission electron microscope image of latex spheres in a thick, transparent section. Some of the spheres are partially hidden by others. If the section thickness is known, the size distribution and volume fraction occupied by the spheres can be estimated. However, some small features may be entirely obscured and cannot be determined.*

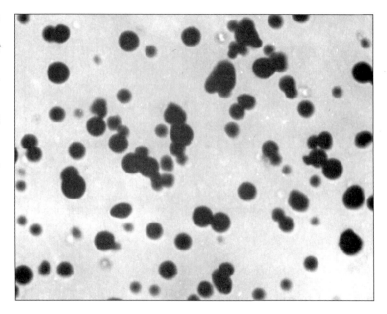

information from the image to feed the decision-making process is more complicated than simple processing or measurement, because the best algorithms for a specific application must themselves be determined as part of the logic process.

These tasks all require the computer-based image processing and analysis system, and by inference the image acquisition hardware, to duplicate some operations of the human visual system. In many cases they do so in ways that copy the algorithms we believe are used in vision, but in others quite different approaches are used. While no computer-based image system can come close to duplicating the overall performance of human vision in its flexibility or speed, there are specific tasks at which the computer surpasses any human. It can detect many more imaging signals than just visible light; is unaffected by outside influences, fatigue or distraction; performs absolute measurements rather than relative comparisons; can transform images into other spaces that are beyond normal human experience (e.g., Fourier or Hough space) to extract hidden data; and can apply statistical techniques to see through the chaotic and noisy data that may be present to identify underlying trends and similarities.

These attributes have made computer-based image analysis an important tool in many diverse fields. The image scale may vary from the microscopic to the astronomical, with substantially the same operations used. For the use of images at these scales, see especially Inoue and Spring (1997) and Sabins (1987). Familiarity with computer methods also makes most users better observers of images, able to interpret unusual imaging modes (such as cross sections) that are not encountered in normal scenes, and conscious of both the gestalt and details of images and their visual response to them.

2
Printing and Storage

reating hardcopy representations of images, for example to use as illustrations in reports, is important to many users of image processing equipment. It may also be important to store the images so that they can be retrieved later, for instance to compare with new ones or to transmit to another worker. Both of these activities are necessary because it is usually not possible to reduce an image to a compact verbal description or a series of measurements that will communicate to someone else what we see or believe to be important in the image. In fact, it is often difficult to draw someone else's attention to the particular details or general structure that may be present in an image that we may feel are the significant characteristics present, based on our examination of that image and many more. Faced with the inability to find descriptive words or numbers, we resort to passing a representation of the image on, perhaps with some annotation. Arlo Guthrie describes this procedure well in his song "Alice's Restaurant" as "twenty-seven 8 by 10 color glossy pictures with circles and arrows and a paragraph on the back of each one."

Printing

This book is printed in color, using high-end printing technology not normally available to a single image processing user. But many everyday jobs can be handled quite well using comparatively inexpensive machines; the quality, speed, and cost of both monochrome and color printers are improving rapidly. A typical monochrome (black on white) laser printer costs about a thou-

Figure 1. *Portion of a 1960s era teletype printout of a Christmas calendar poster.*

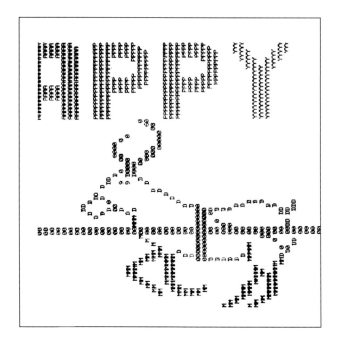

sand dollars and has become a common accessory to desktop computer systems. These printers are designed primarily to print text, and simple graphics such as line drawings. Most can, however, be used to print images as well. We have come a very long way since computer graphics consisted of printing Snoopy Christmas posters using Xs and Os to represent different grey levels (**Figure 1**). In this chapter we will examine the technology for printing images that can be used in desktop computer-based image processing systems.

For this purpose it does not matter whether or not the printers use a high level page description language such as PostScript®, which is used to produce smooth characters and lines at the maximum printer resolution, so long as they allow the computer to transmit to the printer an array of individual pixel brightness values. Most printers that can create any graphics output in addition to simply printing text can be controlled in this way. This means that "daisy wheel" or other formed-character printers (now virtually obsolete) are not useful for imaging. That is how the Snoopy posters were made, by creatively arranging to overprint groups of characters to produce different levels of darkness. But dot-matrix printers using inked ribbons, ink jet printers, thermal printers, and other devices that form their output as an array of dots on paper *can* be used to print images. The quality of the result is primarily a function of the size and spacing of the dots.

A basic level of confusion that often arises in interpreting the specifications of a printer in terms of image quality has to do with "dots per inch" or dpi. For any of the printers mentioned above, but particularly for laser printers, the specification of dpi

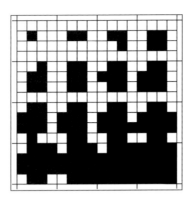

Figure 2. *Halftone grey scale produced with a 4×4 dot cell. Printing dots in all, some or none of the locations can generate 17 different grey values.*

resolution is the number of tiny black dots (or whatever color ink is used) that the printer can deposit on paper. Usually, it is the same in both the line and page directions on the paper, although some printers have different dpi resolution in the two directions. Normally, the dots are used to form characters and lines. A low number of dpi will cause the characters to look rough and the lines to appear stair-stepped or "aliased." Resolution approaching 200 dpi with dot-matrix and thermal printers and 300 to 600 dpi or more for laser printers is now very common. It is capable of producing quite acceptable output for text and line drawings used in reports and correspondence.

However, the dots placed on the paper by these printers are black, and do not have an adjustable grey scale needed to print images. To create a grey scale for images, it is necessary to use groups of these dots, a technique generally known as halftoning that has been used since early teletype transmission of images. It is commonly used in newspapers, magazines, and books (including this one), and as we will see can be used for color as well as monochrome images. The differences in halftone quality between (for instance) a newspaper and a book lie fundamentally in the number of dots per inch that can be placed on the paper and the way they are organized to produce a grey scale result.

The basis of halftoning lies in the grouping of the individual black dots produced by the printer. A group of (for instance) 16 dots in a 4×4 array may be called a halftone cell. Within the cell, some or all of the dots may actually be printed. Where no dot is printed, the white paper shows through. If the cell is reasonably small, the observer will not see the individual dots but will instead visually average the amount of dark ink and light paper, to form a grey scale. In this example, shown in **Figure 2**, there are 17 possible levels of grey ranging from solid black (all dots printed) to solid white (no dots printed).

In a 300 dpi printer, the individual black dots can be placed on the paper with a spacing of 1/300th of an inch in each direction. Grouping these into 4×4 halftone cells would produce $300 \div 4 = 75$ cells per inch. This is close to the resolution of pixels on a typical

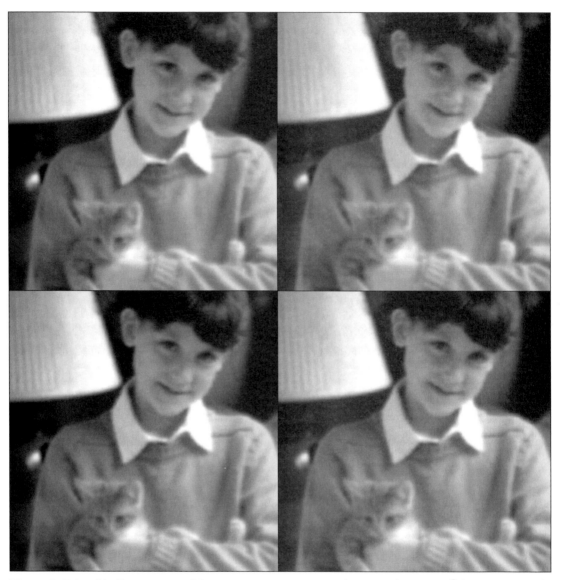

Figure 3. *Printed halftone images of the same image using a 300 dot per inch Postscript® laser printer, with halftone grids of 32, 50, 75 and 100 cells per inch. Increasing the number of cells improves the lateral resolution at the expense of the number of grey levels which can be shown, which in this example are 82, 37, 17 and 10, respectively.*

video display used with an image-processing computer. If each pixel corresponds to a halftone cell, then an image can be printed with about the same dimension as it appears on the screen. Each halftone cell uses one of its 17 possible grey levels to represent the grey scale of the pixel.

Of course, since the original image might typically have 256 grey levels, this seems like a rather poor representation of the brightness information. However, that is not the only nor even the most serious limitation. Instant prints from Polaroid® film show only about the same number of distinct grey levels (the film is quite a bit better than the print) and are considered quite useful for many scientific as well as casual purposes (for instance, the recording of scanning electron microscope images).

One problem with the halftoning method illustrated above is that the dots and cells are large enough to be visually distinguished by the observer. In a magazine or book, the size of the cells is smaller. The cell size is usually described as a halftone screen or grid: the spacing of the screen in number of lines per inch corresponds to the number of cells per inch discussed above. A screen with well over 100 lines per inch (often 115 or 133 lines per inch) is used to produce high quality printed illustrations. Even in a newspaper illustration, a screen of at least 95 lines per inch is typically used. **Figure 3** shows several examples of halftone output from a 300 dpi laser printer, in which the number of halftone cells is varied to trade off grey scale vs. lateral resolution. The output from the current generation of desktop laser printers is adequate for some reports.

Not only are more lines per inch of resolution desired to preserve the sharpness of features in the image, at the same time more grey levels must be represented by these more finely spaced cells. That means that the printer (or imagesetter, as these higher-quality devices are generally called) must be capable of placing a much larger number of very much smaller dots. A grey scale of 65 levels can be formed with an 8×8 array of dots in a cell. With a 125-line screen, this would correspond to 8×125=1000 dpi. This is about the starting point for typeset quality used to print images for commercial purposes. Color (introduced below) imposes additional restrictions that require even higher resolution.

An additional difficulty with the halftoning method outlined above arises from the dots themselves. Each of the various printing methods produces dots in a different way. Dot-matrix printers use small pins to press an inked ribbon against the paper. Ink-jet printers produce a stream of fine ink drops, some of which are electrostatically deflected away from the paper. The drops that strike the paper produce dots. Some of these printers deposit the ink in a liquid form that penetrates into the paper making slightly fuzzy dots, while in others the ink has solidified and adheres to the paper without penetration. Thermal printers use a pin to pass an electrical current through the coating on a paper. One common kind of paper is coated with a white oxide of zinc that is reduced by the current to deposit a dark spot of metal at the location; other thermal papers are based on the chemistry of silver. Laser printers work essentially like a xerographic copier. The light from the laser (or in some versions from a photodiode) falls on a selenium-coated drum and by the photoelectric effect produces a localized electrostatic charge. This in turn picks up carbon particles (the toner or "ink"), which are then transferred to the paper and subsequently heated to remain permanently.

Figure 4. *A 6×6 dot halftone that can produce 37 grey levels. The use of approximately round dots large enough to touch diagonally causes them to overlap and produce darker cells than ideal.*

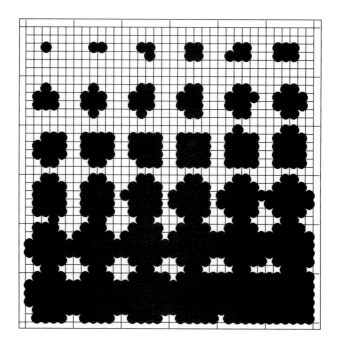

Dots on paper

All of these technologies are limited by the ability to make a small, dark spot on the paper. The size of the carbon particles used as the toner in standard copier or laser printer cartridges is adequate for 300 dpi printing, but special finely ground toner is needed for higher resolutions, which are now becoming common at 600 dpi and even higher values. The limitation in making higher resolution laser printers is not primarily in the additional memory needed in the printer, nor by the need to focus the light to a smaller spot on the drum, but in the toner particle size. Some systems disperse the toner using liquid carriers to improve the control of toner placement.

Similar restrictions limit the other printing methods. The difficulty of depositing a small but dark ink spot by the impact of a pin onto a ribbon, or the fuzziness of the dot written by thermal printing, have prevented those techniques from advancing to higher resolutions. Ink-jet printers can generate small drops and hence deposit small dots, but the inks tend to spread on the paper. Indeed, the roughness of the paper surface, and the need for special coatings to prevent the inks from soaking into the paper fibers or spreading across the surface or the toner particles from falling off, become critical issues. It is not enough to purchase a high quality printer; the use of special paper with a proper surface finish for the particular printer is needed to achieve the quality of image printing that the printer technology makes available (Lee & Winslow, 1993).

Because the dots produced by printers are generally imperfect and rough-edged, it is hard to control them so that the grey scale produced by the array of dots within the cell is uniform. Most dots are larger than their spacing so that solid black areas can be printed. This is good for printing text characters, which are intended to be solid black. However, it means that the dots overlap some of the white areas in the cell, which darkens the halftone grey scale. **Figure 4** shows this for the case of a 6×6 dot halftone cell. At the dark end of the scale, adjacent grey levels may be indistinguishable, while at the light end the difference between the first few levels may be very great.

For the case of a 4×4 dot cell illustrated above using a 300 dpi printer, 17 nominal grey levels, and 75 lines (or cells) per inch, the darkening or "gain" of the grey scale will produce images of marginal quality. If the printer resolution is much higher so that finer halftone cells with more steps can be created, it is possible to correct for this tendency to darken the images by constructing a mapping that translates the pixel grey value to a printed grey value that compensates for this effect. These "gamma" curves are applied within the software so that more-or-less equal steps of brightness can be printed on the page.

However, the human eye does not respond linearly to grey scale, but logarithmically. This means that to produce a printed image in which the visual impression of brightness varies linearly with pixel value, a further adjustment of the gamma curve is needed (as shown in **Figure 5**) to compress the dark values even more and expand the light ones. Because of these limitations, a printing scale with 65 grey values defined by an 8×8 dot halftone cell may be able to show only about half that many shades in the actual printed image.

Halftone grids in a typesetter or imagesetter are not limited by the size or perfection of the dots. Instead of coarse toner particles or contact with an inked ribbon, typesetters use light to expose a photographic emulsion, which is then developed to produce either a film or a print. The size of the silver grains in the film emulsion is far smaller than the effective dot size and the dots can be controlled in both size and shape with great precision. There is still a need for a gamma curve to compensate for the nonlinear response of human vision, however.

If the variation of brightness across an image is gradual and the total number of grey levels is small, it is possible to generate a visual effect known as banding or posterization. This is illustrated in **Figure 6**. The step from one brightness level to the next appears as a contour line in the printed image and is visually recognized as a feature in the picture, when in fact it is purely an artefact of the printing process. Banding can be avoided by increasing the number of grey levels used, or in some cases by modifying the way in which the dots within the halftone cell are used to generate the grey scale. Generally, the rule for the maximum number of grey shades available is $1+(dpi/lpi)^2$, where *dpi* is the printer resolution in dots per inch (e.g., 300 for a typical

Figure 5. A linear grey scale bar

(a) *and the use of a gamma compensation curve*

(b) *to make the visual appearance of the values appear more regular* **(c)**.

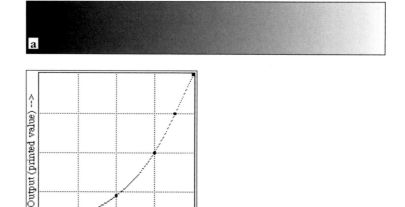

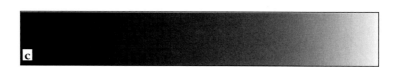

laser printer) and *lpi* is the lines per inch of the halftone screen (e.g., 75 lines per inch for the example discussed above). This assumes that all of the grey levels can actually be used, subject to the darkening ("dot gain") and gamma effects mentioned above.

In the examples shown in **Figures 2** and **3**, an arrangement of dots was used that produced more-or-less round regions of black within a white frame. With a larger dot array in each cell, an even more regular circular pattern can be constructed. The round dot pattern is one of the more commonly used arrangements; however, many others are possible, including lines and crosses (**Figure 7**). Each of these produces some visual artefacts. For instance, the diamond pattern used by most Postscript printers as an approximation to round dots causes dot densities less than 50% black to appear quite different from ones that are 50% or more black. The reason for this is that at the 50% point the dots touch from one cell to the next so that the eye perceives a sudden transition from dark dots on a white background to the reverse, even if the individual dots are not visually evident. Of course, all such artefacts degrade the representation of the original grey scale image.

Figure 6. *The same grey scale bar from Figure 5a showing banding when printed with only 32 grey steps.*

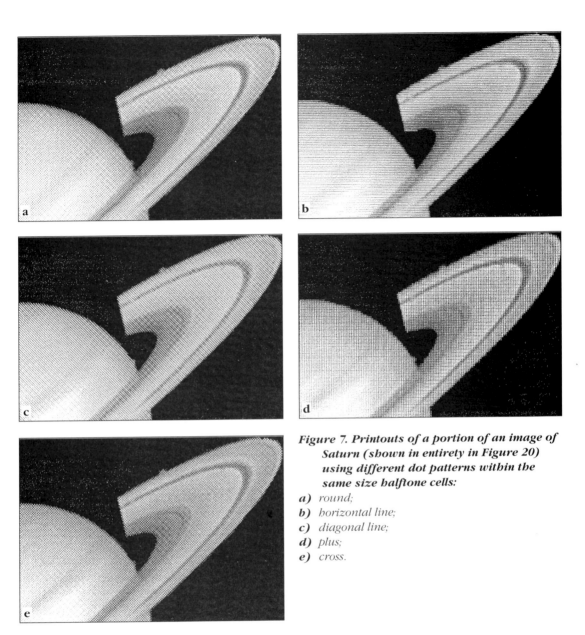

Figure 7. Printouts of a portion of an image of Saturn (shown in entirety in Figure 20) using different dot patterns within the same size halftone cells:

a) *round;*
b) *horizontal line;*
c) *diagonal line;*
d) *plus;*
e) *cross.*

If the dots within each halftone cell are randomly distributed, fewer visual artefacts are likely. However, this requires additional computer processing within the printer and is not a commonly available feature. Other printers use programs that analyze the neighbor cells (pixels). If cells on one side are dark and on the other side are light, the program may use a pattern of dots that is shifted toward the dark neighbors to produce a smoother edge. This works quite well for generating smooth boundaries for printed text characters and minimizing jagged edges on lines, but it is not clear that it is a benefit for grey scale image printing.

Figure 8. Two different dither patterns for the "girl" image (shown in Figure 19):

a) *random dots;*
b) *patterned dots.*

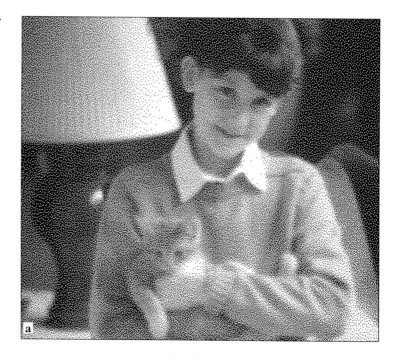

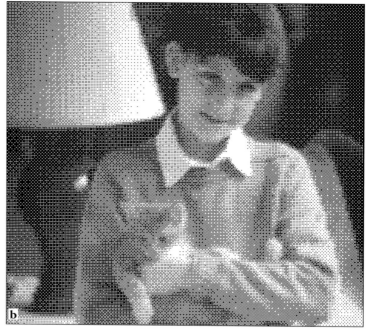

Printers of modest dpi resolution have difficulty producing halftone cells that are small and still represent many grey levels; visually distracting patterns may appear in those images if regular patterns of dots are used within the cells. Hence, another approach used with these printers is to use "dithering" to represent the image. In a simple random dither, each possible position where the printer can place a black dot corresponds to a point in the image whose grey scale value is examined. If the point is very dark, there is a high probability that the dot should be printed (and vice versa). A random number is generated and compared to the grey scale; if the number is below the grey scale value for that point (both properly scaled), then the dot is printed on the page.

As shown in **Figure 8**, dithering can produce a coarse but viewable representation of an image. In fact, there are many different types of dithering patterns that are used, some of them random or pseudo-random and others with various patterned arrangements of the dots. Usually, the particular dither pattern used is determined either by the printer itself or the interface software provided for it. There is a rich literature on the design of dither patterns, but the user of the image analysis system is not likely to have much control or choice of them. Dithered images are generally good at showing gradually varying brightness gradients, since human vision responds to an average dot density or spacing. But sharp edges will be blurred, broken up, or displaced because there is no continuous line or boundary printed, and it is difficult to compare the brightness of regions within the image. Dithered printing is usually considered to be a "low-end" method for producing crude hard copy and not suitable for use in reports or publications.

In spite of the limitations discussed above, monochrome image printing using a halftoning method and a printer with 300–600 dpi capability is adequate for many kinds of image processing applications. The resulting images are suitable in quality for reports and may even be used in some publications. For higher quality work, photographic recording as discussed below can be used with comparative simplicity by displaying the image on a high-quality monochrome monitor and using a camera. This can be a conventional one mounted on a tripod in a darkened room, or a dedicated camera rigidly attached to its own monitor. In either case, the images are recorded on film for subsequent processing.

This process may seem like a step backwards, especially when the image may have started out on film in the first place before it was digitized into the computer. But since facilities for handling photographic images, duplicating them, and making halftone screens photographically for printing are well developed, fully understood, and comparatively inexpensive, this is often the most effective solution. Forcing a "high tech" solution in which images are directly merged into a report within the computer may not be worthwhile in terms of time or cost if only a small number of copies are needed. Mounting photographs on a few pages or inserting them as separate pages is still a quite suitable presentation method. No doubt as printing technology continues to advance, the balance will shift toward direct printing from the computer.

Figure 9. The CIE color diagram discussed in Chapter 1:

a) *the linear combination of colors in CIE space;*

b) *RGB colors produced by the phosphors in a cathode ray tube;*

c) *CMY colors produced by printing inks.*

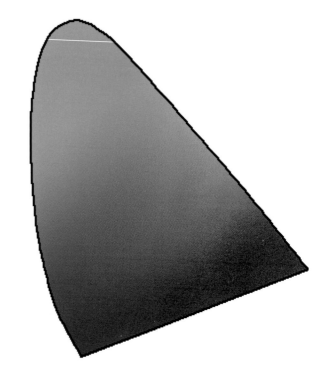

a

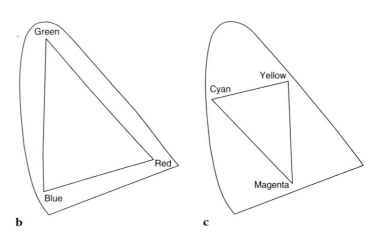

b   c

Color printing

Printing color images is much more complicated and difficult. The usual method, which you can see by looking at the color images in this book or in a magazine, is to create halftones for each of several different color inks and superimpose them to produce the printed color image. There are many complexities in this process, however. The following section discusses those that are important for most dedicated or desktop color printers.

Displaying a color image on a computer monitor or television set is accomplished by illuminating red, green, and blue phos-

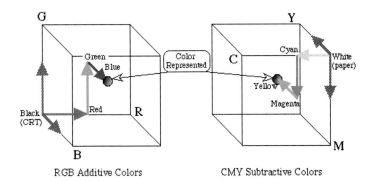

Figure 10. Comparison of RGB (additive) and CMY (subtractive) color spaces. The additive color space adds red, green and blue emissive colors to a black background, while subtractive color space removes cyan, magenta and yellow colors from a white background.

phors with the electron beam in the cathode ray tube (CRT). There are exceptions, of course, the most important being the flat-panel liquid crystal (LCD) displays used for overhead projectors and some notebook computers. There are also large-screen displays (such as used at sporting events) that consist of arrays of discrete lights. Each of these methods generate the colors in different ways, but it is still the visual mixing together of red, green, and blue that produces the full range of colors that can be shown.

This range is called the "gamut" of the device. In a display that emits red, green, and blue light (RGB), it is possible to generate a very large fraction of the total range of colors that the human eye can see. **Figure 9** shows the CIE color diagram that was introduced in Chapter 1, adding the typical color gamut for an RGB display superimposed on the CIE diagram. Notice that one of the features of the CIE diagram is that colors add along straight lines, so the three phosphor colors define the corners of a triangle that enclose all of the possible color combinations. The missing colors that cannot be generated using these particular phosphors include points near the outside of the diagram, which are the most saturated colors.

The concept of the color gamut applies equally well to other color display and recording devices. However, the gamut is not always as simple in shape as the triangle shown on the CIE diagram. For one thing, printing uses subtractive rather than additive color. In terms of the color cube (also introduced in Chapter 1 and shown again in **Figure 10**) the blank paper starts off as white and the addition of cyan, magenta, and yellow inks removes the complementary colors (red, green, and blue respectively) from the reflected light to produce the possible range of colors. It is common to call these colors CMY to distinguish them from the additive RGB colors.

Notice that on the CIE color diagram, a triangle formed by three points at cyan, magenta and yellow would omit a large portion of the color space (as shown in **Figure 9**), producing a small gamut of mostly rather unsaturated colors. This is in fact one of

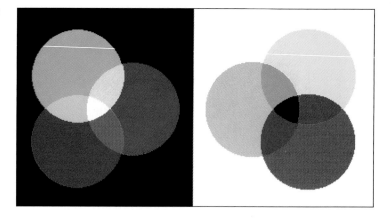

Figure 11. Combinations of RGB additive colors on a black background, and CMY subtractive colors on a white background.

the important problems with color printing, which has difficulty producing strong, vibrant colors.

The CIE diagram does not show another limitation of CMY printing. The theory of subtractive printing, summarized in **Figure 11**, suggests that the mixture of all three colors will produce black (just as with additive RGB color, the summation of all three colors produces white). However, actual printing with CMY inks generally cannot produce a very good black, but instead gives a muddy greyish brown because of impurities in the inks, reflection of light from the surface of the ink (so that it does not pass through all of the ink layers to be absorbed), and difficulty in getting complete coverage of the white paper.

The most common solution is to add a separate, black ink to the printing process. This reduces the need for large amounts of the colored inks, reduces the thickness of ink buildup on the page, and reduces cost. But from the standpoint of image quality, the most important factor is that it allows dark colors to be printed without appearing muddy. The four-color cyan-magenta-yellow-black system (CMYK) uses four halftone screens, one for each ink. However, while converting from RGB colors (or CIE, HSI, or any other equivalent color space coordinate system) to CMY (often called process color) is straightforward, converting to CMYK is not. Rules to calculate how much black to put into various color representations depend far more on visual response to colors, the kind of paper to be printed, the illumination the print will be viewed with, and even the contents of the images.

Algorithms for converting from CMY to CMYK involve specifying levels of undercolor removal (UCR) and grey component replacement (GCR) which are essentially arbitrary, are little documented, and vary considerably from one software program to another (Agfa, 1992). The general approach is to use the value of whichever of the three components (CMY) is darkest to determine an amount of black to be added. For instance, for a color containing 80% cyan, 50% magenta, and 30% yellow, the 30%

value would be taken as an index into a built-in calibration curve. This might indicate that a 15% value for the black ink should be chosen for grey component replacement. Then, the amount of the principal color (in this example cyan), or, according to some algorithms, the amounts of all of the colors, would be reduced (grey component replacement). It is difficult to design algorithms for these substitutions that do not cause color shifts. Also, the substitutions do not work equally well for printing with different combinations of ink, paper finish, etc.

The gamut limitation of CMY and CMYK printers is also being addressed by designing printers with more than three colored inks; some with as many as eight are not available. These allow more saturated colors to be printed, but the algorithms for selecting the combinations of inks and the order in which they are printed (since they usually overlap on the page) are highly specific and not generally documented.

The result of these limitations is that color prints are generally not as vivid or saturated as the image appeared on the CRT. In addition, the colors depend critically on the paper finish and viewing conditions. Changing the room light will slightly alter the visual appearance of colors on an RGB monitor, but because the monitor is generating its own illumination this is a secondary effect. Since a print is viewed by reflected light, changing the amount of light or the color temperature of room light with a print can completely alter the appearance of the image. The color temperatures (a handy way of describing the spectrum of intensity vs. color) of incandescent bulbs, fluorescent bulbs, direct sunlight, or open sky are all quite different.

Human vision can be tricked by combinations of illumination and shadow, inks or other colored coatings, surface finish (smooth, or textured in various ways), and even the presence of other adjacent colors in the field of view to change the way we judge colors in an image. These other colors may even lie outside the image itself; consider how a colored mat can change the appearance of an art print. When "true" color prints of an image are required, it is necessary to perform extensive calibrations of a specific printer and monitor so that acceptable fidelity is obtained. This is of great concern in advertising; if you purchase clothing from a mail order catalog, you expect the colors of the cloth to match the printed photograph, which is no easy task.

For most (but certainly not all) applications of image processing, the purpose of printing in color is to distinguish the variously colored regions present; some inaccuracy in the fidelity of the colors is acceptable. If exact color matching is not necessary in a particular application then the task becomes much easier, although you will still need to be concerned about the color gamut of the printer, the consistency of colors (to allow comparison of different images or regions), and of course the resolution of the printer. The color gamut is important because colors of

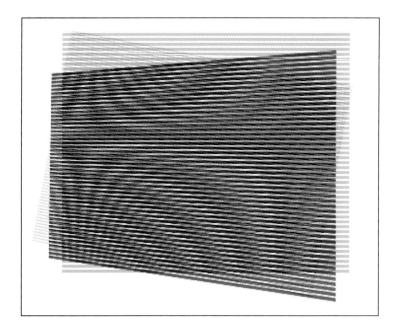

Figure 12. *Moiré pattern produced by overlaying arrays of color dots.*

increasing saturation in the original image, which can be distinguished on the video display, may become similar in the print image if the saturation exceeds the range of the printer.

Producing CMYK halftones (so-called color separations) and superimposing them to produce color prints sounds simple enough, but it harbors many problems that commercial printers

Figure 13. *Ideal screen angles for CMYK color printing place the halftone screens at angles of 45° (Black), 75° (Magenta), 90° (Yellow), and 105° (Cyan).*

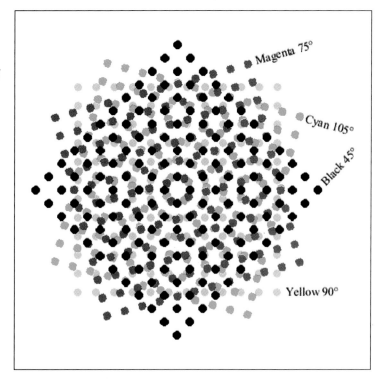

must deal with routinely. One is how to superimpose the halftone screens so that they do not produce visual moiré patterns in the image. **Figure 12** shows an example of a moiré effect produced by different color patterns. The lines that appear are an artefact of the spacing of the individual patterns. Traditional offset printing defines "ideal" screen angles for the four CMYK screens as 45, 70, 90 and 105 degrees respectively, as shown in **Figure 13**. This aligns the colored dots to form small rosettes that together make up the color. Note that some of the dots may be superimposed on each other. Since some inks are partially transparent, this can produce various color biases depending on the order of printing.

In most printing, the colors are not so much superimposed on each other as printed adjacent to each other. This is another reason that high-resolution halftone screens and very small printing dots must be used. Superimposing 300 dpi arrays would overlay one ink on top of another, producing a very dark and muddy result. With some kinds of ink and paper, it might also result in physical mixing of the inks and unexpected smearing of the image. Generally, when four halftone grids or color separations are used, the dpi of the printer must be doubled for each color to get an equivalent printing resolution as equivalent monochrome printing. In other words, each pixel now requires four interleaved halftone cells, one for each color. Since the dot size for each of the four colors is only one fourth of the area, printing a solid expanse of one color is not possible, which further reduces the maximum saturation that can be achieved and hence the gamut of the printer.

Most desktop printers cannot provide control over the screen angles, and some printers simply use a zero angle for all four screens due to the way the printing mechanism works (for instance, a typical color ink-jet printer). Some page description languages (e.g., PostScript Level 2) include provision for such control, but only high-end typesetters and imagesetters generally respond to those commands.

All of the problems present in printing monochrome or grey scale images, such as banding, posterization, limited numbers of grey levels, and so forth, are also present in producing the color separations. In addition, color printing introduces the additional problems of screen angles and moiré patterns. Finally, alignment and registration of the colors must be considered, since in general they are printed one at a time and the paper must be handled in several passes. Some alternative printing methods exist that deposit multiple colors in a single pass, but these have their own problems of allowing inks to dry without mixing.

The printing and registration of colors presents one additional (and somewhat unexpected) problem in some cases. Consider a region of a uniform color that is a mixture of two or more of the primary printed colors and is adjacent to a region of a different color, as shown schematically in **Figure 14**. At the boundary, the

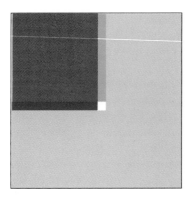

Figure 14. Enlarged schematic diagram illustrating the need for trapping. Printing the red color requires both yellow and magenta inks. Since the halftone pattern used for each is offset slightly, the boundary between the red and cyan areas will have narrow lines that appear either green (yellow + cyan) or blue (magenta + cyan) depending on which dot pattern extends past the other.

colors must change abruptly from one color to the other. However, the two color screens are not aligned dot for dot, and along the boundary there will be cases in which one of the two left-side color dots may be present close to one of the two right-side color dots. This can give rise to false color lines along boundaries. In graphic arts, such artefacts are usually avoided by trapping to remove the colors at the boundaries in a particular order, or covering up the boundary with a black line. Obviously, such tricks are not available in printing real images where every pixel may be different.

Printing hardware

The discussion so far of converting the image to CMY or CMYK values and superimposing them as separate halftone screens on the printed page has ignored the physical ways that such color printing is performed. Most color printers are still somewhat costly for a dedicated desktop image processing system, but may be available via network connections within an organization. There is a considerable variation in the quality, cost, and performance of different types of printers. Some of the more common currently available methods include ink jet, thermal wax, dye sublimation, and color laser printers. This section will offer some comparisons and introduce newer technology as well.

The currently available crop of color printers has been developed primarily with an eye toward a market that only peripherally involves scientific image processing. Most of the images people want to print are graphics generated within the computer, rather than natural images. And most of the printing is done for reports, desktop publishing, and other generally nontechnical purposes. However, the much larger market represented by those applications is lucrative enough to have generated intense competition between companies and technologies, with the result that performance and price have improved (and will likely continue to improve) dramatically.

The dominant technologies at the present time, more or less in order of cost, are ink jet, thermal wax, color laser, and dye

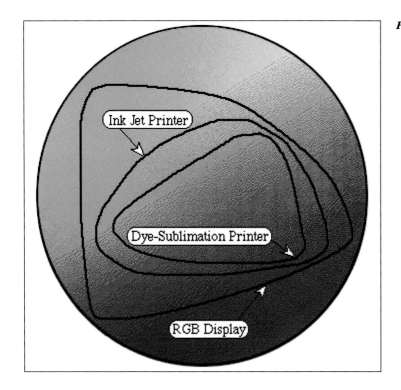

Figure 15. *Color gamuts for different output devices are frequently shown on a color wheel. In this space the boundaries are not straight lines (as in the CIE diagram). The gamut for an RGB display is greater than for printers. The printer gamuts are also affected by paper surfaces.*

sublimation. Ink-jet printers cost less than hundreds of dollars, while thermal-wax machines typically cost about a thousand and laser or dye sublimation printers are several thousand and up. These prices do not include the cost of consumables needed to print the image, which can run to several dollars per page.

Even with the relatively inexpensive ink-jet printers, the type of paper used is very important. Printers may be advertised as using "plain paper," but quality prints require coated paper to provide a flatter surface and to prevent the ink from being absorbed into the fibers and spreading out to form splotches. Furthermore, the liquid ink-jet prints take some time to dry and can be easily smudged, while the solid ink jets (which are melted just before spraying onto the paper and dry quickly) have a very textured and dull finish on the page. Even after drying, most inks can be smeared by other liquids and the solid inks can be cracked by bending the paper.

Dry inks, because they are not absorbed into the paper, are generally brighter and produce somewhat more saturated colors and a greater color gamut than liquid inks. But ink-jet printers do not produce a very broad gamut of colors anyway (**Figure 15**), because the individual inks do not completely cover the paper and so produce only medium levels of saturation. Rather than producing a true halftone screen in which the dots are grouped to produce many different levels for each color, ink-jet printers may dither the image by overprinting the various color dots just as a monochrome image can be dithered (**Figure 16**).

Figure 16. *Detail of two CMYK color images printed with halftone and dither patterns.*

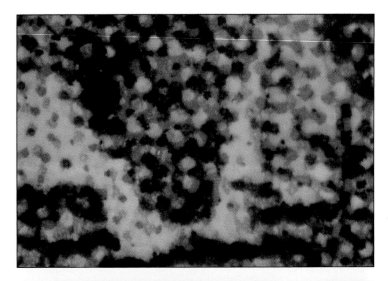

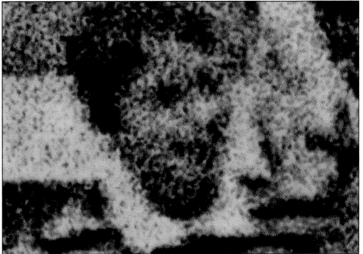

The relatively few intensity levels available produce banding problems, and at the same time the resolution is not very high. A 300 dpi color ink-jet printer that has four colors (CMYK) produces only 75 dpi of each color uniquely without overprinting (each dot is either on or off). Grouping these into 3×3 cells to allow only 10 shades of each color would reduce the overall image resolution to the rough equivalent of 25 lpi. This is not fine enough to trick the eye into seeing a continuous image, and fine details are lost.

Thermal-wax printers need paper with a very smooth finish so that the wax-based inks can adhere. They work well on overhead transparencies, which are fine for producing business graphics presentations, but are not usually an acceptable medium for image-processing output. Thermal-wax output produces a very glossy image with vivid colors. The colors are deposited from a roll of plastic film coated with wax-based pigments (CMY or CMYK). Each ink panel is as large as the page to be printed, and one panel of each color is used per page, even if very little of the color is required. By comparison, ink-jet and color laser printers use only as much ink or toner as is actually deposited on the paper. The print head in a thermal-wax printer contains heating elements that melt the wax and transfer the color to the paper. This process is repeated for each color, which may cause alignment problems. As for the ink-jet printers, the dots are too large and the resulting number of shades for each color too small, and the resolution too poor, to show details well in images.

Color laser printers work by separating the image into three CMY (or sometimes four CMYK) colors and using each to control the illumination of a separate charged drum that picks up the corresponding color toner and deposits it on the paper. One major problem with these printers is the difficulty of keeping everything in alignment, so that the paper doesn't shrink or shift as it goes from one drum through a heater to bake the toner and on to the next drum. The use of a relatively thick paper with a smooth finish helps. In addition, the order in which the toners must be applied is critical, because with most models presently available the dots are not really laid down as a set of halftone screens at different angles (as discussed above). Instead, they tend to overlay each other so that the lighter ones must be on the bottom and the darker on top. This makes it difficult to achieve good color saturation or accurate color blending. The gamut is small and the image may appear muddy. However, printing is fast and multiple copies can be made efficiently.

Dye-sublimation (or dye-diffusion) printers require special coated paper (or transparency material). The inks or dyes are transferred one at a time from a master color sheet or ribbon to the paper, with a typical resolution of about 300 dpi. A portion of the color ribbon as large as the paper is consumed in making each print, even if only a small amount of the color is needed. However, it is possible to control the amount of dye that is transferred from the ribbon to each dot by heating the print head to sublime or vaporize varying amounts of dye. A control to one part in 256 is typical, although the use of a corrective gamma function for each color to balance the colors so that the print appears similar to the screen image (so-called "color-matching") may reduce the effective dynamic range for each color to about 1 part in 100. Still, that means that about 1 million (100^3) different color combinations can be deposited at each point in the recorded image. Dye-sublimation printers do not use a halftone or dither pattern. The dyes diffuse into the polyester coating on the paper and blend to produce continuous color scales.

The lack of any halftone or dither pattern and the blending and spreading of the color dyes within the coating (instead of lying on the surface as inks do) produces an image that is very smooth and pleasing in its appearance. It is sometimes claimed that these printers are "near photographic" in output quality, but in several important respects that is not true. The saturation is somewhat less than a good photographic print, so that the color gamut is lower, and the 300 dpi resolution of the better machines, compounded by the spreading of the dye in the coating, produces much poorer sharpness than a photographic print (which can easily resolve several thousand dots per inch). This spreading is somewhat worse along the direction of paper movement than across it, which can cause some distortion in images or make some edges less sharp than others. On the dye-sublimation print, large areas of uniform or gradually varying color will appear quite smooth because there is no dither or halftone to break them up, but edges and lines will appear fuzzy.

In addition to these technical limitations, the relatively high cost of dye-sublimation printers and of their materials has limited their use as dedicated printers for individual imaging systems. At the same time, their rather slow speed (since each print requires three or four separate passes with a different color ribbon or a ribbon with alternating color panels) has made them of limited use on networks or for making multiple copies. Still, they have been the preferred choice for making direct hardcopy printouts of images. They are even finding use in commercial outlets, where consumers can insert their slides or color negatives into a machine (from Kodak), select the image and mask it if desired, and then directly print out a hard copy to take home. The glossy finish of the coated paper probably causes many customers to think they have a traditional photographic print.

The involvement of companies like Kodak, Canon, Sharp, and Polaroid in this market suggests that photography, copiers, and color printers are converging and overlapping in a way that is likely to revolutionize all three. (It is no coincidence that these same companies are offering digital cameras as well as traditional film cameras.) A new technology recently announced by Polaroid appears to offer a challenge both to dye-sublimation printing and to photographic recording. It offers the same advantage of continuous color intensity over a large dynamic range, but with the high resolution usually associated with photographic prints (and without some of the disadvantages).

The basis for this new "Sunspot" technology is a new thermal medium designed to be exposed by high-powered (500 mW) semiconductor diode lasers emitting in the near infrared (wavelengths between 750 and 950 nm.). The recording medium consists of three imaging layers laid down as coatings, either on a transparent or white substrate. Each layer is addressed by a laser emitting at a different infrared wavelength and each provides an image in one of the three (CMY) subtractive colors. The active layers exhibit negligible absorption or scattering of visible light and thus appear virtually transparent. Moreover, the only step required to form a stable image is the laser exposure itself. There is no need for pre- or post-processing and no waste materials (chemicals, paper strips, etc.) as encountered with conventional or "instant" photographic materials. The material can also be handled in full normal light before and after imaging.

Sunspot uses a mechanism quite unlike conventional thermal systems. Typically, such conventional printers use heat to drive a colored material from one place to another (as in thermal transfer printing) or to mix together reactive components (the mechanism of most direct thermal media). In Sunspot, however, color is generated from colorless "dye-precursor" molecules by a thermally induced chemical reaction within the molecules themselves (in chemical parlance, an "intramolecular" reaction). The kinetics of this reaction are designed so that negligible thermal coloration occurs in storage at or near room temperature for a period of years, but substantial reaction occurs in a microsecond or so at the elevated temperatures attained during laser exposure.

Together with the dye precursor, the only other components in each imaging layer are an infrared absorber and a polymeric binder in which the dye precursor and absorber are dispersed. The function of the infrared absorber is to convert the infrared radiation supplied by the laser into heat. The constraints upon the absorbers are severe: they must have a minimum fluorescence yield and be thermally stable under imaging conditions, and have a high absorbance in the near infrared but negligible absorption in the visible region of the spectrum. High infrared absorption is necessary to make the laser exposure efficient, but since the absorbers remain in the system after exposure, their visible light absorption must be low enough not to interfere with the final quality or long-term stability of the image.

In addition, in order to produce color images, the three layers with dye precursors corresponding to C, M, and Y must each have an infrared absorber with a narrow absorption bandwidth in the 750–950 nm range to allow each layer to be individually addressed by the energy from one laser without crosstalk or filtering. The resolution of the medium is limited only by the size of the addressing laser, which can readily produce dot sizes of a few micrometers. Resolution is easily competitive with photographic recording and much higher than the other conventional printing methods discussed here. Speed of writing is constrained by the kinetics of the thermal coloration reaction and the requirements of room-temperature stability, requiring addressing energies of about 1 joule/cm^2 for each color. Recording times of about 2 minutes per image are typical. The optical density of each color layer can range from nearly transparent (about 0.1) to extremely dense (in excess of 3.0), giving extraordinary dynamic range and color saturation without crosstalk between colors. Depending on the substrate, it can be used for either transparencies (e.g., 35 mm slides) or prints, with the cost of consumables competitive with other color printing methods. However, the printer's cost is somewhat higher than the dye-sublimation and color laser printers.

Of course, the traditional high-end printing method is a type-setter or imagesetter such as used to produce this book. This is also a photographic method, using halftone screens with well over a thousand dpi at accurate screen angles, which are subsequently used for offset printing of each of the separated CMY or CMYK colors. Such a method is obviously impractical for routine use on single images, but may be suitable for preparing a report requiring many copies. In such cases, the fact that most typesetters use the same PostScript language as many of the dedicated printers allows a less-expensive printer to be used to create proofs, with the final output made when everything has been corrected. Most of the current crop of printers, even many of the least-expensive ink-jets, offer PostScript compatible controllers. This is not really necessary for printing images, which consist in their most basic form of a very large array of color or brightness values, but it does provide a consistent printer interface that allows programs to send their image data to any of several printers without requiring internal changes or user adjustments.

Film recorders

We have seen that in many cases, especially for color images, printing directly from the computer to paper is expensive and difficult, and the quality limited. But the image looks good on the computer screen and it is tempting just to photograph it from there to create slides or prints using conventional film methods. Certainly, this is convenient. I have hundreds of slides that I use regularly in lectures that were produced in exactly this way. I keep a 35 mm camera loaded with slide film on a tripod near my desk. When there is something on the screen that might be useful as a slide, I just move the camera into position and with a permanent exposure setting of f8 at 1/2 second (for ASA 100 slide film), snap the picture. You do need to make sure that there are no reflections of windows or room lights on the monitor. When the roll is finished, I send it off and get back a box of quite useful slides. I've done this enough times to know that there is no need even to bracket the exposures. The exposure setting of f8 is about optimal for lens sharpness and gives plenty of depth of field for the slight curvature of the computer monitor, while 1/2 second is long enough to capture enough full raster scans so that no visible line shows where one scan began or ended.

While these pictures are fine for lecture slides, they are not useful for many other purposes. It is always obvious that they are photographs of the computer screen and not the actual images that have been captured or processed. This is due partly to the fact that they usually include the menu bars, cursor, and other open windows on the screen. But certainly it would be possible to eliminate those, and in fact some image-processing programs have a "photo mode" that displays just the image with the rest of the screen dark.

Unfortunately, there are other clues that reveal how such an image is recorded. It is difficult to align the camera so that it is exactly perpendicular to the center of the screen. This misalignment produces a distortion of the image. In addition, the curvature of the screen causes a pincushion distortion of the image that is hard to overcome. Special cameras intended for recording images from computer monitors have hoods to shield against stray light and align the camera lens, and may incorporate corrective optics to correct some of the distortions and minimize these problems. Still, other more serious difficulties remain.

Most color displays use an array of red, green, and blue phosphors arranged as triads of round dots. The electron beams are focused onto the phosphors and further restricted by an aperture screen (shadow mask) that prevents the electrons from straying from one dot to another. Varying the intensity of the electron beam controls the relative brightness of the phosphors and the resulting color that is perceived by the human observer, who blends the individual dots together. Modern computer displays have color triads with a spacing of about 0.25 mm. Human vision does not resolve these at normal viewing distances so that the colors are visually blended.

The other approach to monitor design, used in the Sony Trinitron, has a single electron gun, no shadow mask and the color phosphor arranged in vertical stripes. This design provides brighter images, since more of the screen is covered with phosphor and there is no shadow mask. On the other hand, the colors are less pure and lines or edges less sharp depending on their orientation. The Trinitron tube face is curved only in the horizontal direction rather than in both directions, which may reduce distortion of the photographed image.

With either of these monitor designs, the image is made up of a regular pattern of color dots that the film records, perhaps with some systematic distortion due to the screen curvature and camera position. This pattern is not visible when a slide is projected to illustrate a talk. But there is a temptation to use these films to prepare prints for publication, which reveals their major flaw. When the prints are subsequently converted to halftones, the array of dots photographed from the screen will interact with the screen of the halftone to produce a moiré pattern that can be quite objectionable (**Figure 17**).

Film has high resolution, good color saturation and dynamic range, and inexpensive processing, which make it an excellent recording medium. But photographing the color monitor is not the right way to record the image. Dedicated film recorders solve

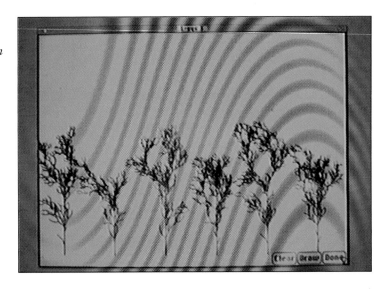

Figure 17. *Color moiré pattern produced by slight misalignments and distortion of the dot patterns when digitizing a 35mm slide photographed from the computer display.*

the problems mentioned above by using a monochrome CRT with a continuous phosphor and a very flat face. The continuous phosphor gives a very high resolution with no structure to cause moiré patterns, while the flat face eliminates distortions. With only a single electron beam, sharp focus and uniform intensity can be maintained from center to edges much better than with "television" displays; the fixed optics also provide sharp focus across the image with no vignetting or distortion.

A motorized filter wheel containing red, green, and blue filters is placed between the CRT and the camera. Software is used to separate the image into red, green, and blue components and these are displayed one at a time on the CRT with the appropriate filter in place. The filter densities are adjusted to balance the film sensitivity and the camera exposure is usually fixed for simplicity. All three color components are recorded on the same frame of the film. With most recorders, the entire process is automatic, including film transport and compensation for different film speeds and sensitivities (for instance, slide or print film).

The only drawbacks are the exposure time of several seconds and the delay until the film is developed, and of course the cost of the entire unit. The cost varies as a function of resolution (from 2000 dots horizontally up to as much as 16,000 dots), and the flexibility to handle different sizes and types of film. High-end recorders are used to expose movie film frame by frame to produce movies containing "virtual reality" and rendered computer images (e.g., *Jurassic Park*), or to restore old classics by removing dirt and making color corrections (e.g., *Snow White*). Recorders that are price-competitive with color printers can be used for routine production of 35mm slides. Nevertheless, the use of such recorders has not become widespread, and there still seems to be a preference for printing images directly onto paper.

File storage

When working on a computer-based image-analysis system, images can be saved as disk files. There seems to be no reason to consider these files as being any different from other disk files, which may contain text, drawings, or even programs. In one sense this is true: files contain a collection of bytes that can represent any of those things as well as images. But from a practical point of view, there are several reasons for treating image files as distinct, because they may require somewhat different storage considerations:

1. Image files are usually large. In terms of computer storage, the old adage that a picture is worth one thousand words is clearly a vast understatement. A single video frame (640×480 pixels) in monochrome occupies about 300 kilobytes (KB), while one in full color requires about 1 megabyte (MB). A series of images forming a time sequence, or a three-dimensional array of voxel data (which can be considered as a series of planes) can be far larger. A 500×500×500 voxel tomographic reconstruction requires 125 MB, or twice that if the density values for the voxels have a dynamic range that exceeds 256 levels. This means that the storage capacity used must be large, preferably open-ended by allowing some kind of removable media, and reasonably fast. It also increases the interest in storage methods that utilize compression to reduce file size.

2. Imaging usually requires saving a large number of files. This reinforces the requirement for large amounts of fast storage, but it also means that access to the stored images will be needed. Constructing a database that can access images in a variety of ways, including showing the user small thumbnail representations, using keywords, and other indexing tools, is an important need that has been recognized by many software producers. Automatically extracting classification data from the image to assist in searching is a more difficult problem.

3. Data management in the era of computers has not yet fully exploited the possibilities of coping with relatively straightforward records that contain text and numbers. The "file cabinet" metaphor is a poor and limited one. The real issue for computerized file storage is access to files and finding documents. Adding a field to a database primarily constructed to hold text entries does not make it into an imaging database. For instance, keeping a picture of each employee in a personnel file may be worthwhile, but it would hardly allow a user to locate employees by knowing what they looked like. That would require looking at every image.

One type of database that involves images works in essentially the opposite direction. A geographical information system (GIS) stores multiple images and maps. These record different kinds of information, which is keyed to locations. There may also be text records keyed to those locations. By overlaying and correlating the multiple map representations, it becomes possible to compare the locations of features on one map (e.g., roads or buildings) with those on others (types of soil or vegetation, underground aquifers, etc.). There are important issues to resolve in constructing a GIS, since the various maps and images (including aerial and satellite photos) must be aligned and registered, taking into account their different resolutions. In addition, displaying such rich multidimensional data presents challenges beyond those faced in most image databases.

There may be some other factors to consider in designing an optimum system for image storage. For instance, in medical and some other applications, it may be important to keep a record of all accesses to the image and of any processing or editing steps that may be applied. Also, some standardization of storage formats is important if images are to be shared between users or between different systems. Some users may want to archive images essentially forever but rarely access any particular image, while others may make continued and repeated accesses but be willing to discard images after a certain time (or when a project is completed). The data may be intended for access by many users, over a network, or be restricted to a single user. If a set of images is to be distributed widely as a permanent and unalterable resource, the requirements change again.

There are some beginnings of solutions to most of these problems and indications that many more will be forthcoming. The introduction of the Photo-CD format by Kodak indicates their expectation of considerable consumer usage of this type of storage. It is easy to imagine someone trying to find an old picture of "Aunt Sarah," for example. If the photo is stored as a faded print in an old shoe box, the searcher may have a rough idea of where to look in the attic for the box and then be willing to sort through the contents looking for the picture. But in the era of computer technology, it will seem natural that somehow the computer can find the picture just by being asked for it. Obviously, that is not a trivial task. But many companies are trying to respond to the challenge.

Optical storage media

Kodak's Photo-CD is an example of one kind of media that can be used for image storage. Actually, we will see below that Photo-CD also defines a storage format, not just the use of CD-ROM disks. And it is possible to store images on CDs in other formats as well. Projects as diverse as archaeological digs and remote sensing (satellite imagery) have found it convenient and inexpensive to distribute collections of images on CDs as a reference resource. The CD-ROM (CD meaning Compact Disk) is just a plastic platter with reflective dots imprinted onto it, physically

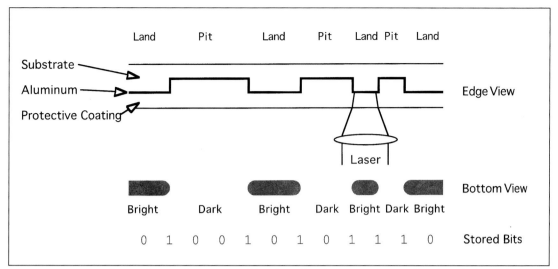

Figure 18. *Storage format for CD data. Pits and lands in the aluminum layer reflect laser light, with the pits scattering the light and producing a darker reflection. Transitions from bright to dark indicate ones and places where no transition occurs indicate zeroes.*

identical to audio CDs. The format of the dots, which mark changes from 1s to 0s rather than the actual bit values, is interesting (**Figure 18**), as is the technology used to read the disks, but not really important to the user.

The reflective dots in a "standard" CD are physically imprinted in a pressing operation and covered by a hard plastic that is quite resistant to damage. This technique lends itself to creating many copies of a disk inexpensively. Current prices for making duplicates from a master are just a few dollars per copy even in small quantities of a hundred or so, and drop to well under a dollar in larger volumes. Distributing a library of images in this way makes sense.

Data on CDs are written on one single continuous spiral track, in blocks of 2048 bytes (plus the block address and some error detection sums). Most drives that write CDs (either the standard glass masters, or the CD-R recordable disks) write the entire track at one time, which requires the data to be continuously supplied to the write head as the disk spins. The CD format is much more difficult to use as a random-access device for either writing or reading than a conventional disk with its multiple circular tracks and fixed sectors, which make locating particular blocks of data much easier.

Pressing CDs from a master creates pits in the plastic substrate that are coated with aluminum and then sealed with a protective plastic layer. The plastic layer not only prevents physical damage, but also prevents oxidation of the aluminum that would reduce its reflectivity. In a CD-R (recordable) disk, the writing is done by a laser whose light is absorbed in a dye layer. The dye decomposes and is deposited on the metal layer (gold rather than aluminum), darkens it, and produces the same pattern of reflective and dark regions that the physical lands and pits do in the CD-ROM.

CD-R disks can also be used as "write-once" storage devices for archiving files. CD-R drives cost hundreds of dollars and can be connected to a computer just like any other disk drive (for instance, using a standard SCSI or Small Computer Systems Interface). Files are written to a blank disk (which costs less than $3) as mentioned above. The writing process is not very fast; with a 4X drive it takes 15 minutes to write a full disk. But that disk provides storage of more than 600 megabytes. After it has been written, the CD-R disk can be read in exactly the same drive as a pressed CD-ROM, or used as a master to duplicate the less expensive pressed disks in quantity.

One of the limitations of the technique is that in most cases, this writing operation must be performed in a single session. All of the files to be placed on the disk must be available on the host computer and written at the same time, so that the disk directory can be created for subsequent reading. In creating the Photo-CD format, Kodak introduced the idea of multiple directories (or multiple sessions) so that a disk could be taken in to the photo finisher to add more images (e.g., another roll of film) to an existing disk. However, not all drives that can read CDs are able to access the additional directories.

At present, the most practical use of CDs would be to produce entire disks of images for distribution. The images would be archival in nature, and users would not be able to modify them on the original disk. Reading from CD-ROM drives is generally rather slow. Even the newer drives that operate at 12 times or more the speed of the platter from that used for audio disks have reading speeds an order of magnitude less than a standard magnetic hard disk used in the computer. However, for accessing archival images that speed may be quite acceptable.

Higher density CD formats such as used in the new Digital Video Disks will offer an order of magnitude more storage on the same size disk, but as yet there are few user-writable drives or media.

Optical disk storage offers more possibilities than CD-ROM, of course. Optical removable disks offering both permanent archival storage (so-called write-once read-many or WORM drives) or conventional read-write access are available for computers. The former may be useful in situations (medical imaging is certainly the most oft-cited example) in which images must be stored permanently. Such drives are also used for financial records and other applications in which assurances are needed that data cannot be tampered with, either intentionally or accidentally. With WORM drives, the data cannot be altered or erased. When changes are made to an image and it is saved again, it is actually written into another file on the disk and the original remains for comparison.

The principal difference as far as the user is concerned between optical WORM drives and CD-ROM is that the WORM drives are intended for incremental writing, so that files can be added to the disk as desired, rather than the entire disk being written at one time. There are other differences between them, of course. The CD-ROM uses a single spiral track instead of a series of concentric circles; the latter offers faster random access to files. CD drives vary the rotational speed of the disk so that the linear velocity of the bits past the head is constant, while most conventional disk drives keep the speed constant and vary the recording density across the disk surface. The storage format for the bits is different, too. But these differences are important primarily to the hardware and software designers who create them, and not to the user who properly treats any storage device as a tool. Storage capacities of about 1000 megabytes (1 gigabyte) per disk platter are available, and of course since the disks are removable, a single drive can be used to provide essentially unlimited storage.

Read-write optical disks using removable media are becoming rather common, with storage capacities from 256 megabytes up to several gigabytes. Reading is accomplished optically by reading the change in reflectivity of laser light, while writing requires both a magnetic field and a laser to be applied to create a structural change in the coating that changes the reflectivity. There is also interest in the so-called phase change method, in which the recording material in the disk is heated by the laser to write. Heating to a high temperature for a very short time causes the material to melt and then quickly solidify in an amorphous state that has low reflectivity. Heating the same spot to a lower temperature (below the melting point) allows the atoms to arrange themselves into a crystalline lattice with a high reflectivity. The reflectivity of each spot is read by the same laser at a much lower power setting. These changes are reversible, so the disks can be rewritten. Consequently, while drives now offer reading speeds close to those of typical magnetic hard disks, the writing speeds for these drives tend to be two or three times slower. This is still often fast enough for routine use.

The optical disks have the advantage of near-archival storage and immunity to stray magnetic fields. Stories abound of magnetic disks erased or corrupted by stray magnetic fields generated by airport security devices, or by the ringing bell in a desk telephone, but these fields cannot affect the magneto-optical read-write disks. Even the 256 megabyte size (3.5 inches in diameter, and small enough to put into a shirt pocket or mail in an envelope), offers enough storage for many imaging uses. This book was written and the text and images saved on such a drive. The disk was sent to the publisher, who used it to typeset the pages and produce the separated halftone images using an imagesetter. I have carried such disks literally around the world with no worries about data loss. They are far more robust than magnetic recording on removable hard disk cartridges or floppy disk media.

Magnetic recording

The most common type of hard disk used in computers is still based on magnetic storage. The disk platter (of glass or metal) is coated with a thin layer of magnetic material much like that used in audio tapes. Reading and writing are done using a magnetic head that "flies" just above the disk surface, riding on a cushion of air pressure produced by the spinning disk surface. There are exceptions to this method: Bernoulli drives use a flexible polymer substrate more like simple floppy disks, with the magnetic head in physical contact with the disk coating. Such differences can affect the long-term durability of the media, the reading and writing speed, the physical density of storage, and the amount of information that can be written onto a single disk. But again, from the user's point of view the details of the design technology are secondary considerations.

Removable magnetic storage disks with capacities of about 100 megabytes are commonly available and competitive in price and performance with read-write optical disks (e.g., the popular "Zip" disk). Emphasis has been placed here on the removable type of storage, because any conventional hard disk, even one with a gigabyte or more of storage, will sooner or later fill up with images (usually sooner). Any system that is intended for serious image analysis work is going to require some form of removable and hence unlimited storage.

The speed of access of a conventional hard disk is somewhat faster than the removable types, and quite a bit faster than slow methods like CD-ROM. This speed makes it attractive to copy files onto a hard disk for access, and to write them to the removable media only when work is temporarily complete. With that approach, the hard disk serves as a short-term storage location for work in progress, but the removable media are still used to store images for long-term purposes. The hard disk is also the place where the computer operating system, and all of the various programs including those used for image analysis, are stored.

No mention has been made of floppy disks because of their inability to hold large amounts of data. Typical diskette sizes range from about 1.4 to 20 megabytes of storage. Actually, the 20 megabyte value is not very common, as these "floptical" drives require special media with registration marks for each track, so that optical sensors in the drive's head assembly can position the magnetic head accurately enough to read and write the very high density information.

The smaller sizes most common in dedicated desktop computers can usually only hold one or a few images, and sometimes not even that. A single color image obtained from a color scanner with 600 dpi resolution (a widely available level of performance), taken from an original 8×10 inch photograph, would require about 81 megabytes of storage. Such files are not conveniently stored on floppy disks. Even a typical video image, requiring about 900 kilobytes, takes up most of one floppy disk. That may be acceptable for sending one image to a colleague but is hardly useful for storage of many images, even ignoring the rather slow reading and writing speeds of these drives.

Tape drives are even slower. A single 4 mm tape, the same type of cassette used for digital audio recording, can hold several gigabytes of files, with a drive costing a few hundred dollars. But because access to any particular location on the tape requires rewinding and searching, these devices are really only useful for backing up a random access hard disk. Saving a collection of images on a tape for archival storage might make sense, however, as it is less expensive than any other form of digital storage. Instead of using these tapes and drives simply to back up a large disk drive, it is possible with existing software to treat the tape as though it is a large (and rather slow) disk, for accessing files randomly. This requires loading a directory into memory identifying where each file is on the tape, which takes memory space. Also, the reading times are not suitable if the files must be accessed very often. But such a medium could be used as a large and inexpensive data storage medium over a network.

Generally, tapes are less robust than disks because they are subject to stretching even in normal use and can easily be damaged by mishandling. Likewise, magnetic storage is generally less "archival" than optical storage because stray fields or high temperatures can cause accidental erasure. The CD-ROM has the best claim to be archival, but this claim applies to the pressed disks and not the CD-R recordable disks.

If your purpose is archival storage of images, then regardless of what medium you select, you should prepare to invest in extra drives and interfaces. It is not likely that any of the current media will be readable by common storage devices within 5–10 years, so you will need to keep your own spare parts and working systems. And even then it may be difficult to transfer the images to the next generation of computers through different interfaces and networks. If you doubt this, consider the storage media in common use 5–10 years ago (8 inch floppy disks, punched cards, DECtape, etc.), none of which can be read with any ease today.

Another cost of archival storage is maintaining backup copies at some remote site, with appropriate security and fire protection, and having a routine method of storing regular backups there. It is really not enough simply to back up your hard disk to a tape every Friday and drop the tape off in your safety deposit box on the way home, if your data are really worth keeping for many years. This is certainly the case for remote sensing tapes (a good example, by the way, of the changing face of storage — most of the early tapes can be read only on a handful of carefully preserved drives), medical records, and so on. For many kinds of records, photographic film is still the method of choice; it offers decades of storage, takes very little space, and can be accessed with standard equipment.

But for most people, the purpose of storing large numbers of images (certainly hundreds, perhaps thousands, probably not tens of thousands) is not so much for archival preservation as for access. The ability to find a previous image, to compare it to a current one, and to find and measure similarities and differences, is an obvious need in many imaging tasks. Choosing a storage technology is not the really difficult part of filling this need. A selection between any of the technologies mentioned above can be based on the tradeoffs among cost, frequency (and speed) of access, and the size of the storage required. The technical challenge lies in finding a particular image after it has been stored.

Databases for images

Saving a large number of images raises the question of how to locate and retrieve any particular image. If the storage uses removable media, the problem is compounded. These problems exist for any large database, for instance one containing personnel or sales records. But some unique problems are involved in searching for images. Database management programs are being introduced with some features intended specifically for images, but much remains to be done in this area.

Most database management routines offer the ability to search for entries based on some logical combination of criteria based on keywords or the contents of search fields. For images, it might be useful to search, for example, for images recorded between October 1 and 15, from a video camera attached to a microscope, using transmitted light through a 500 nm color filter, obtained from slide #12345 corresponding to patient ABCDE, etc. It might also be nice to find the images that contain a particular type of feature, for example satellite images of lakes in a certain range of sizes, whose infrared signature indicates that they have a heavy crop of algae.

The first of these tasks can be handled by many existing database searching routines, provided that the classification data have been entered into the appropriate fields for each image. The second task calls for much more intensive computer processing to extract the desired information from each image. It requires close coupling of the image analysis software with the database management routine. Such a system can be implemented for a specific application, but general and flexible solutions are not yet available.

Searching through multiple fields or lists of keywords is typically specified by using Boolean logic, for instance that the creation date must lie before a certain value AND that either one OR another particular keyword must be present, but that the image must NOT be in color. These types of searches are similar to those used in other kinds of database managers. A potentially more useful type of search would use fuzzy logic. For instance looking for features that were "round" and "yellow" does not specify just what criterion is used to judge roundness, nor what range of numeric values are required, nor what combination of color components or range of hue values is sufficiently yellow.

Sometimes described as "query by image content" (QBIC), this approach seeks to include color, texture, and shape of image objects and regions (Niblack et al., 1993). Depending on the field of use, quite different criteria may be important for searching. For instance in a medical application the user might want to find "other images that contain a tumor with a texture like this one" (which implies the concept of the object named *tumor*, as well as the description of the texture), while in surveillance the target might be "other images that contain objects of similar shape to this airplane." Key issues for such a search include derivation and computation of the attributes of images and objects that provide useful query functionality, and retrieval methods based on similarity as opposed to exact match. Queries may be initiated with one or a few example images ("Query by Example"), perhaps with subsequent refinement.

Implementing a search for the example of "round" and "yellow" features would require first measuring a representative sample of features in the images in the database to obtain measures for roundness (perhaps the ratio of shortest to longest dimension, but other shape criteria are discussed in a later chapter) and hue. Histograms of frequency vs. value for these parameters would then allow conversion of the adjectives to numbers. For instance, "round" might be taken to mean objects falling within the uppermost 10–20% of the range of actual values, and "yellow" the range of hue values bracketing true yellow and enclosing a similar fraction of the observations.

An even more powerful approach to resolving fuzzy criteria into numeric values ranks all of the observations according to dimension, hue or some other objective criterion and then uses the rank numbers to decide how well a particular object conforms to the adjective used. If a feature was ranked 10th in roundness and 27th in yellowness out of a few hundred features, it would be considered round and yellow. On the other hand, if it was ranked 79th in one or the other attribute, it would not be. Both of these methods ultimately use numeric values, but judge the results in terms of the actual range of observations encountered in the particular type of application. And they do not use traditional "parametric" statistics that try to characterize a population by mean and standard deviation, or other narrow descriptors.

Fuzzy logic offers some powerful tools for classification without requiring the user to decide on numerical limits. However, although fuzzy logic has been enthusiastically applied to control circuits and consumer products, its use in database searching is still rather limited. That, combined with the time needed to measure large numbers of representative images to give meaning to the users' definition within a particular context, seems to have delayed the use of this approach in image database management. Consequently, most searching is done using specific values (e.g., a creation date after September 1, 1997, rather than "recent") and Boolean matching with user-specified criteria.

Typically, it is up to the user to establish the criteria that may be interesting for future searches before the database is established and the images are stored away. If the proper fields have not been set up, there is no place to save the values. It is impossible to overstate the importance of designing the proper search fields and lists of keywords ahead of time, and the difficulty of adding more fields retrospectively. There are no simple guidelines for setting up fields, since each imaging application has unique requirements. Establishing dozens or even hundreds of search fields with large numbers of keywords is a minimum requirement for any image database management routine.

Of course, it is still necessary to fill the search fields with appropriate values and keywords when the image is saved. Some of the fields may be filled automatically, with things like date and time, operator name, perhaps some instrument parameters such as magnification or wavelength, location (this could either be latitude and longitude, or coordinates on a microscope slide), and so forth. Even patient or sample ID numbers can in principle be logged in automatically; some laboratories are using bar code labeling and readers to automate this function. Doing this at the time the image is acquired and saved is not too burdensome, but obviously supplying such information retrospectively for a set of images is difficult and error-prone.

But the really interesting keywords and descriptors require the human observer to fill in the fields. Recognition and identification of the contents of the image, selection of important characteristics or features and ignoring the others, and then choosing the most useful keywords or values to enter in the database is highly dependent on the level of operator skill and familiarity, both with the images and with the program.

Not surprisingly, the entries can vary greatly. Different operators, or the same operator on different days, may produce different classifications. One method that is often helpful in constraining operators' choice of keywords is setting up a glossary of words that the operator can select from a menu, as opposed to free-format entry of descriptive text. The same glossary is later used in selecting logical combinations of search terms.

Values for measurement parameters that are included in the database can usually be obtained from an image analysis program. In later chapters on image measurement, we will see that automatic counting of features, measurement of their sizes, location, densities, and so forth, can be performed by computer software. But in general this requires a human to determine what it is in the image that should be measured. These programs may or may not be able to pass values directly to the database; in many practical situations manual retyping of the values into the database is required, offering further opportunities for errors to creep in.

Even in cases in which the target is pretty well known, such as examining blood smear slides, or scanning the surface of metal for cracks containing a fluorescent dye, there is enough variation in sample preparation, illumination conditions, etc., to require a modest amount of human oversight to prevent errors. And often in those cases the images themselves do not need to be saved, only the numeric measurement results. Saving entire images in a database is most common when the images are **not** all nearly the same, but vary enough to be difficult to describe by a few numbers or keywords.

A very different type of database uses the image as the organizing principle, rather than words or numbers. Numerical or text data in the database is keyed to locations on the images. This approach, mentioned above, is generally called a Geographical Information System (GIS) and is used particularly when the images are basically maps. Imagine a situation in which a number of aerial and satellite photographs of the same region have been acquired. Some of the images may show visible light information, but perhaps with different resolutions or at different times of day or seasons of the year. Other images may show the region in infrared bands or consist of range images showing elevation. There may also be maps showing roads and buildings, land use patterns, and the locations of particular kinds of objects (fire hydrants, electrical transformers). Tied to all of this may be other kinds of data including mail addresses, telephone numbers, the names of people, for example. Other kinds of information may include temperatures, traffic patterns, crop yields, mineral resources, and so forth.

Organizing this information by location is not a simple task. For one thing, the various images and maps must somehow be brought into registration so that they can be superimposed. The resolution and scales are typically different, and the "depth" of the information is quite variable as well (and certainly consists of much more than a grey scale value for each pixel). Finding ways to access and present this data so that comparisons between quite disparate kinds of information can be made presents real challenges. Even searching the database is less straightforward than might be imagined.

For instance, selecting coordinates (e.g., latitude and longitude) and then asking for various kinds of information at that location is comparatively straightforward. There are presently computerized maps (distributed on CD) that can be accessed by a laptop computer connected to a GPS (Global Positioning System) receiver. This is a tiny receiver that picks up timing signals from the network of GPS satellites to figure out location anywhere on the earth with an accuracy of tens of meters. That can obviously be used to bring up the right portion of the map. But if you are driving a car using such a system to navigate, your question may be "show me the routes to follow to the nearest gas station, or hospital, or to avoid the 5:00 P. M. traffic jam and reach the main highway." Clearly, these questions require access to additional information on streets, traffic lights and timing, and many other things. And that same database can also be accessed by entering a telephone number or zip code. This is essentially current technology; the promise is for much richer databases and more flexible ways to access and display the information.

Browsing and thumbnails

This chapter started out with the idea that saving images so that they can later be compared to other images is necessary precisely because there is no compact way to describe all of the contents of the image, nor to predict just what characteristics or features of the image may be important later. That suggests that using brief descriptors in a database may not provide a tool to locate particular images later. Consequently, most image databases also provide a way for the user to see the image, or at least a low-resolution "thumbnail" representation of it, in addition to whatever logical search criteria are employed.

Some approaches to image databases write the full image and one or more reduced resolution copies of the image onto the disk so that they can be quickly loaded when needed. This may include, in addition to the full original copy of the image, a very small version to use as a display thumbnail for browsing, a version with a resolution and color gamut appropriate for the system printer, and perhaps others. Since most of the auxiliary versions of the image are much smaller in storage requirements than the original, keeping the lower resolution copies does not significantly increase the total space required, and it can greatly speed up the process of accessing the images. Kodak's Photo-CD is an example of a storage format that maintains multiple resolution versions of each image. In some cases it is practical to use a lossy compression technique to save the lower resolution versions of the images, to further reduce their storage requirements.

The reason for thumbnails, or some kind of reduced size representation of the images in the database, is that allowing the user to "browse" through the images by showing many of them on the screen at the same time is often an essential part of the strategy of looking for a particular image. The difficulties noted above with keywords and multiple data fields mean that they can rarely be used in a Boolean search to find one particular or unique image. At best, they may isolate a small percentage of the stored images, which can then be presented to the user to make a visual selection.

Browsing through images is very different from the search strategies that are used for most other kinds of data. It is common on most computer systems, either as part of the system software itself, or as basic utility routines, or as part of applications, to incorporate intelligent search capabilities that can locate files based not only on the values of data fields (e.g., a creation date for the file) or keywords, but also by examining the actual contents of the files. For instance, the word processor being used to write this chapter can search through all of the files on my hard disk for any document containing the phrases "image" and "database" in close proximity to each other, and then show me those files by name and with the phrases displayed in context.

But that approach is possible because the files are stored as text. There may be special formatting characters present (and indeed, it is possible to search for those as well: "find documents containing the word 'large' in italics") but the bulk of the file content is a straightforward ASCII representation of the letters that make up the words and phrases. Searching strategies for text, including ignoring capitalization or requiring an exact match, and allowing for "wild card" characters (e.g., "find documents containing the phrase 'fluorescen# dye'" would find both fluorescent and fluorescence), are widely used. Much effort has gone into the development of efficient search algorithms for locating matches.

A relatively new development in text searches uses natural language rules to interpret the text. This search technique distinguishes among nouns, verbs, and adjectives to extract some meaning from the text. That, combined with the use of a thesaurus and dictionary so that words can be substituted, allows specifying target text by entering a few topical sentences, and then having the search engine look for and rank matches.

How can this technique be used for images? Certainly there is no way to simply match a specific series of bytes. The image data are typically stored on disk as a sequence of pixel values. For many monochrome images, storage requires one byte per pixel, and the values from 0 to 255 represent the grey scale of the data. For images that have greater dynamic range, two bytes per pixel may be needed; some computers store the high byte and then the low byte, and some the reverse. For color, at least three bytes per pixel are needed. These may be stored with all three values in some fixed order for each pixel, or the entire row (or even the entire image) may be stored separately for the red, green, and blue values (or other color space representation).

There are dozens of different storage formats for images, some of which will be discussed below. Few image database management routines support more than a handful of formats, expecting that most users will select a format according to specific needs, or as used by a few particular programs. When images must be imported from some "foreign" format, it is usually possible to translate them using a dedicated program. This is particularly needed when different dedicated computers and programs acquire images from various instruments, and then transmit them to a single database for later analysis.

There are a few relatively "standard" formats such as TIFF files that are used on several different computer platforms, while others may be unique to a particular type of computer (e.g., PICT on the Macintosh, BMP on the PC) or even proprietary to a particular program (e.g., the PSD format used by Adobe Photoshop®). In the latter case, the widespread use of the program can make the format a kind of standard in its own right. Some of these "standards" (TIFF is an excellent example) have so many different options that many programs do not implement all of them. The result is that a TIFF file written by one program may not be correctly read by another program that uses a different subset of the 100 or so options.

Some storage formats include various kinds of header information that describes formats, color tables and other important data more or less equivalent to the formatting of a text document. Some compress the original data in various ways, and some of the methods do so in a "lossless" manner that allows the image to be reconstructed exactly, while others accept some losses and approximate some pixel values in order to reduce the storage requirement.

For instance, the Macintosh PICT format is a lossless method that represents a line of pixels with the same value by listing the value once, and then the number of times it is repeated. For computer graphics, animation, and rendered drawings from drafting programs, this "run-length encoding" method is very efficient. It is also used to transmit faxes over telephone lines. But it does not offer much compression for typical real-world images because groups of pixels are not usually uniform.

The Amiga HAM format records only the change in value from one pixel to the next, not the actual pixel values. This format can represent an image that would normally require more than one byte per pixel (e.g., color images) quite compactly, provided there are no sudden changes in the image that require more than one byte to describe. This is a lossy method that leads to some distortion of edges and boundaries. It also makes it impossible to skip through an image to display every nth pixel as a thumbnail, or to show just a portion of the image. But the same basic idea, of recording changes rather than absolute values, is employed in sound recording on audio CDs, and gives excellent fidelity.

If compression of the data is present, the computer must read the entire image file and reconstruct the image in memory before anything can be done with it. But even if the data can be scanned directly within the disk file, how can it be searched to locate a particular image based on the contents? There is not generally a specific sequence of pixel values along one line of the image (most images are stored in a raster format, as a series of lines) that is the target. There is not even usually a specific two-dimensional pattern of pixel values. Features in images are more irregular than that, and may occur in unexpected locations, sizes and orientations.

Statistical averages of the image, as may be summarized in its brightness histogram, most predominant color, etc., may sometimes be useful, but they are rarely computed while searching for a particular image in the database. Instead, if such parameters are considered important, they are determined beforehand, when the image is stored, and written into specific fields so that they can be searched using standard logical tests.

There is one approach to data matching that is sometimes applied to this kind of searching. Cross-correlation of a target image with each image in a database is a way to look for images that are similar to the target, in a very particular sense. The use of cross-correlation is discussed and illustrated in Chapter 5, because it is usually implemented using Fourier transforms. These can be speeded up by using dedicated hardware, but even so it can be quite time consuming to search through a large database for a best match.

One application of this approach is matching surveillance photos to identify targets of possible military interest. For example, cross-correlation of an aerial image of an airport against a database of images of airplanes, each type viewed in many different orientations, will match the type of airplanes and their locations in the image. For more diverse images, or ones containing features that are more variable in their shape, contrast or color, this method is less suitable.

When images are stored in a database that extends over several physical disks, particularly when removable media are used, many of the images may not be accessible or on-line when the search is made. The usual solution to this problem is to keep the descriptive keywords and other search fields, plus at least a thumbnail representation of the image, in a file with the main program. This allows rapid searching to find a subset of the images that may be examined visually by the user. Since the program has the location of each image stored in its file, it can then request the user to insert the particular disks to load the actual images. Even with this approach, the search file can be quite large when hundreds or thousands of images are included in the database. The search file can itself require a large (and fast) disk for storage.

On the other hand, there are reasons why the search fields, keywords, thumbnails and other ancillary information should be stored with the image rather than in a central data file. Such storage makes the file containing the image self-contained, so that it can be copied with all its information intact. It is also possible to maintain a record of who has accessed the image and when, or to keep a detailed record of whatever changes have been made to an image. Such information may be very important in reconstructing the history of processing an image.

Image database programs may also be required to limit access to images, for instance with passwords. A central "file server" may allow one group of users to read images from the files, another group to add images to the database, and a third group to process or modify images. Since images are large, moving them across local area networks from a central location to many workstations is a far from trivial consideration. This is particularly a concern in medical imaging and remote sensing applications, where a large number of images are to be accessed by a moderate number of users.

Finally, the question for any image searching routine is just how it is to be used. Finding one or several images according to some criteria is usually not the end result but the beginning. How can the image(s) now be loaded into whatever program is to be used for processing or measurement? Some database management programs can act as a filter that is used by any program opening a file. This is convenient for loading images but may not lend itself to adding images to the database. Other management programs can simply locate the images and copy them onto a local disk (and perhaps convert their format or decompress them), so that the user may more easily open them into the desired application.

Lossless coding

There has already been some mention above of image compression. This is desired for storage or transmission in order to reduce the rather large size of most image files, and is quite an active area of study. We will not review all of the techniques for compression described in the literature, since most of them are not implemented in standard software packages available for dedicated image processing. Most of the methods fall into just a few categories, and representative examples of each will be discussed below.

There are two criteria by which image compression methods can be judged. One is the time needed to accomplish the compression and decompression. This is particularly important when images are being compressed for "real time" transmission, as in video conferencing, or perhaps when searching through a large database to locate particular images. The second criterion is the

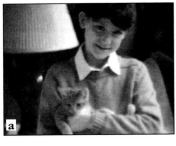

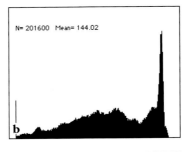

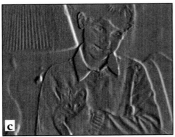

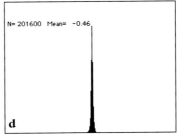

Figure 19. *Example image ("girl") with its histogram, and the results of compression by calculating differences between each pixel and its left hand neighbor. The original image has a broad range of pixel brightness values. The histograms of the original and compressed image show that the latter has most values near zero. Contrast of the displayed compression image has been expanded to show pixel differences.*

degree of preservation of the image. It is this latter area of concern that will be discussed primarily here.

The first and most important distinction between compression methods is as lossless and lossy techniques. A lossless method is one that allows exact reconstruction of all of the individual pixel values, while a lossy method does not. Lossless methods, often referred to as image coding rather than compression, have been around for some time, with much of the original development being directed toward the transmission of images from the space probes. The communication bandwidth with these low power transmitters did not allow sending many images from the remote cameras unless some method was used to reduce the number of bits per pixel.

A simple, early approach was to send just the difference between each pixel and the previous one (sometimes called "delta compression"). Since most areas of the image had little change, this reduced the average magnitude of the numbers, so that instead of requiring (for instance) 8 bits per pixel, fewer bits were needed. This is another way of saying that images are highly correlated. A histogram of the differences between adjacent pixels has a peak near zero and few large values, as shown in **Figures 19** and **20** for images that have different histograms of pixel brightness values.

Further approaches to compression used algorithms that examined several preceding pixels, predicted the next value based on some kind of fitting algorithm, and then just stored the difference from that. Advances on those methods use pixels on preceding lines as well, for further improvement in the predicted value and hence reduction in the difference values (Daut et al., 1993). Obviously, a method that looks at preceding lines is suitable for so-called progressive scan imaging rather than an interlaced scan as

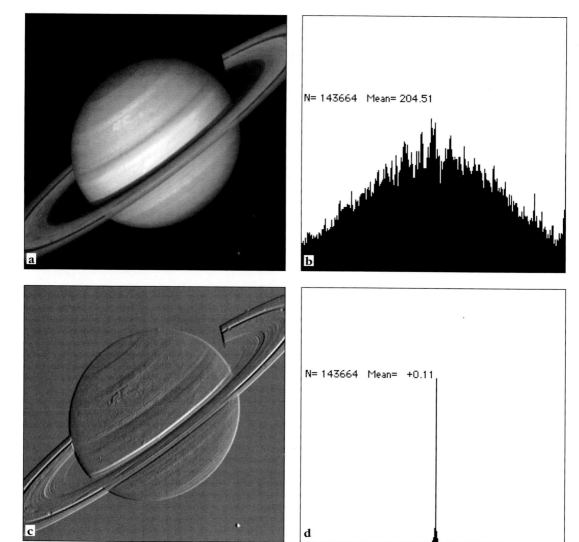

Figure 20. *Example image ("Saturn") with its histogram, and the results of compression by calculating differences between each pixel and its left hand neighbor. The original image contains many black pixels. The histograms of the original and compressed image show that the latter has most values near zero. Contrast of the displayed compression image has been expanded to show pixel differences.*

used in broadcast television. Most of these compression algorithms were originally designed and utilized with live image sources. If the image has already been stored in memory, then the full array of pixels is available.

An additional refinement codes the differences between a pixel and either its predicted value or its predecessor even more efficiently. For instance, in recording each wavelength band in Landsat images a 4 bit number is used for most differences, with two values of the 16 possible numbers reserved as flags indicating that a (rare) larger difference value follows, either positive or negative. An average of about 4.3 bits per pixel is needed to store the images, instead of the full 8 bits.

If further optimization is made to allow variable length codes to be used to represent differences, storage requirements can be further reduced to about 3.5 bits per pixel for the Landsat data. One of the most widely used variable-length coding schemes is Huffman coding. This uses the frequency with which different grey values occur in the image in order to assign a code to each value. Shorter codes are used for the more frequently occurring values, and vice versa. This can be done either for the original grey values, or for the pixel difference values. Huffman coding is also used for other types of data, including text files. Because some letters are used more than others in English, it is possible to assign shorter codes to some letters (in English, the most frequently used letter is E, followed by TAOINSHRDLU…). Morse code for letters represents an example of such a variable length coding for letters (not an optimal one).

As a simple example of the use of Huffman codes for images, consider an image in which the pixels (or the difference values) can have one of 8 brightness values. This would require 3 bits per pixel ($2^3=8$) for conventional representation. From a histogram of the image, the frequency of occurrence of each value can be determined and as an example might show the following results (**Table 1**), in which the various brightness values have been ranked in order of frequency. Huffman coding provides a straightforward way to assign codes from this frequency table, and the code values for this example are shown. Note that each code is unique and no sequence of codes can be mistaken for any other value, which is a characteristic of this type of coding.

Table 1. Example of Huffman codes assigned to brightness values

Brightness Value	Frequency	Huffman Code
4	0.45	1
5	0.21	01
3	0.12	0011
6	0.09	0010
2	0.06	0001
7	0.04	00001
1	0.02	000000
0	0.01	000001

Notice that the most commonly found pixel brightness value requires only a single bit, but some of the less common values require 5 or 6 bits, more than the three that a simple representation would need. Multiplying the frequency of occurrence of each value times the length of the code gives an overall average of

$$0.45 \cdot 1 + 0.21 \cdot 2 + 0.12 \cdot 4 + 0.09 \cdot 4 + 0.06 \cdot 4 + 0.04 \cdot 5 + 0.02 \cdot 6 + 0.01 \cdot 6$$
$$= 2.33 \text{ bits/pixel}$$

Using software to perform coding and decoding takes some time, particularly for the more "exotic" methods, but this is more than

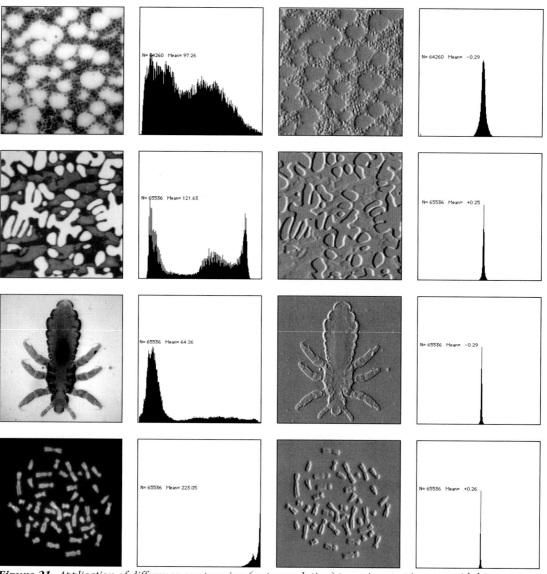

Figure 21. *Application of difference compression (autocorrelation) to various test images, with histograms of pixel values. The entropy values are listed in Table 2.*

made up in the decreased transmission time or storage requirements. This is true of all of the coding and compression methods discussed here, and is the justification for their use. Information theory sets a lower limit to the size to which an image (or any other file of data) can be reduced, based on the distribution of actual values present. If, for example, an image consists of 256 possible grey levels whose actual frequencies of occurrence (taken from a brightness histogram of the image) are p_1, p_2, ..., p_{256}, then the entropy of the image is

$$H = -\sum_{k=1}^{256} p_k \cdot \log_2 p_k$$

(1

Information theory establishes this as a theoretical limit to the number of bits per pixel needed to represent the image, and provides a performance criterion for actual coding methods. If this calculation is applied to the same example with eight grey levels as used above to illustrate Huffman coding, it calculates H=2.28 bits per pixel as a minimum. Huffman coding is not optimal except in the unique case in which the frequencies of occurrence of the various values to be represented are exactly integral powers of 1/2 (1/4, 1/8, ...). But this example indicates that it does offer a useful degree of compression with modest computational needs. Other coding techniques are available that can approach the theoretical limit, but simple methods like Huffman coding are often good enough to be widely used.

Table 2. Entropy values (bits per pixel) for representative grey scale images shown in Figures 19, 20 and 21

Image	H (original)	H (difference-coded)
girl	7.538	3.059
Saturn	4.114	2.019
bone marrow	7.780	4.690
dendrites	7.415	4.262
bug	6.929	3.151
chromosomes	5.836	2.968

Table 2 lists the entropy values for a few typical images, which are shown in **Figure 21** along with their original brightness histograms and the autocorrelation histograms of values between horizontally adjacent pixels. Some of these images have large peaks in their original histograms that indicate there are many pixels with similar brightness values. This affects both the entropy value and as discussed above the generation of an optimal Huffman code. Notice the reduction in information density (H) as the visual appearance of images becomes simpler and larger areas of uniform brightness are present. Calculating the H values for the difference coding of these images reveals a considerable reduction as shown in the table, averaging about a factor of 2 in additional compression.

The entropy definition can be expanded to cover neighbor pairs by summing the joint probabilities of all pairs of two (or more) grey values for neighbors in the same way. This would apply if a coding scheme was used for pairs or larger combinations of pixels, which in theory could compress the image even further.

While it is unusual to apply coding methods to all possible pairs of grey values present, a related coding scheme can be used with images just as it is with text files. This approach scans through the file once looking for any repeating patterns of byte values. In a text file, the letter patterns present in English (or any other human language) are far from random. Some sequences of letters such as "ing" "tion" "the" and so forth occur quite often, and can be replaced by a single character. In particular cases, common words or even entire phrases may occur often enough to allow such representation.

A dictionary of such terms can be constructed for each document, with segments selected by size and frequency to obtain maximum compression. Then the dictionary itself and the coded document must be stored or transmitted, but for a large document the combination requires less space than the original. Compression of typical text documents to 40–50% of their original size is commonly achieved in this way. For small documents, using a standard dictionary based on other samples of the language may be more economical than constructing a unique dictionary for each file. Dictionary-based methods, known as a "Lempel-Ziv" technique (or one of its variants, such as Lempel-Ziv-Welch, LZW), is commonly used to compress text to reduce file sizes on small computers.

Applying the same compression algorithm to images, treating the sequence of bytes just as though they represented ASCII characters is not so successful (Storer, 1992). There are few exactly repeating patterns in most images; even small amounts of random noise cause changes in the pixel values. These noise fluctuations may not be important, and in fact it is easy to argue that much of this "noise" arises in the camera, electronics and digitization and is not part of the scene itself. But our goal in coding the image is to preserve everything so that it can be reconstructed exactly, and there is no *a priori* reason to discard small fluctuations, or even to identify the pixel values as containing such noise. Deciding that some fluctuations in pixel values represent noise while others represent information is very difficult. Because of these fluctuations, whatever their source, few repeating patterns are found, and the compressed image is typically at most 10% smaller than the original.

A close cousin of these coding methods is run-length encoding. This was mentioned before as being used in some of the standard file formats, such as the Macintosh PICT format and the compressed TIFF format used on Mac, PC and quite a few other computer platforms. Run-length encoding (RLE) looks for any row of pixel brightness values that repeats exactly, and replaces it with the value and the number of pixels. For natural grey scale images, such rows do not occur very often and little compression is achieved. However, for computer graphics, drawings and animation images, this method can achieve very high compression ratios.

Run-length encoding is particularly appropriate for binary (black and white) images. Fax machines use RLE to send images of pages containing text or anything else via telephone lines. Thresholding is often used as discussed in a subsequent chapter to reduce images to black and white representations of features and background. Such binary images can be efficiently represented by run-length encoding, and in addition the encoded image is directly useful for performing measurements on images.

Most of the "standard" image formats used in desktop computers and workstations are lossless representations of images. Some simply record all of the pixel values in some regular order, perhaps with header information that gives the dimensions of the image in pixels, the colors represented by the various values, or other similar information. Some use modest coding schemes such as run-length encoding to speed up the reading and writing process and reduce file size. Some, like TIFF or HDF, are actually a collection of possible formats that may or may nor include coding and compression, and have within the header a flag that specifies the rest of the format in the particular file.

Fortunately, program users rarely need to know the details of the format in use. Either the images have been stored by the same program that will later read them back in, or several programs share one of the more-or-less standard formats, or there is a translation facility from one format to another within the programs or provided by a separate program. Quite a few such translation programs have been developed specifically to cope with the problems of translating image files from one computer platform to another.

Color palettes

As part of the storage format for images, many systems try to reduce the number of colors represented within each image. One reason that color images occupy so much storage space is that three color components, usually RGB, are stored for each pixel. In most cases, these occupy one byte each, giving 256 possible values for each component. In a few cases, reduction to 32 grey levels ($2^5=32$) is used to allow reducing the storage requirements to 2 bytes, but the visual artefacts in these images due to the magnitude of the changes between colors on smoothly varying surfaces may be distracting. In some other cases, more than 8 bits per color component are used, sometimes as many as the 12 bits ($2^{12}=4096$) which are generally considered to be required to capture all of the dynamic range of color slide film, and this of course represents a further increase in storage requirements.

Some images can be reduced for storage, depending on their ultimate use, by constructing a unique color coding table. This allows each pixel to have a stored value from 0 to 255 and occupy one byte, while the stored value represents an entry in a table of 256 possible colors to be used to display that image. This method may seem to reduce the amount of information in the image drastically, but it corresponds nicely to the way that many computer screens actually work. Instead of a 24-bit display with 8 bits (256 intensity values) for R, G and B, many low cost displays use an 8-bit display memory in which each of the possible 256 pixel values is used to select one of 16 million colors (2^{24}). The palette of colors corresponding to each pixel value is stored with the image (it occupies only 768 bytes), and written to the hardware of the display to control the signals that are output to the cathode ray tube (CRT) or other device. This is sometimes called a Lookup Table (LUT) since each pixel value is used to "look up" the corresponding display color. Manipulation of the same LUT to produce pseudocolor displays was described in Chapter 1.

If the LUT or palette of color values is properly selected, it can produce quite acceptable display quality. Since the selection of which 256 colors are to be used to show an entire image (typically containing from 1/4 million to 1 million pixels) is critical to the success of this method, various algorithms have been devised to meet the need. The color triplet can be considered (as discussed in Chapter 1) as a vector in a three-dimensional space, which may be RGB, HSI, etc. The process of selecting the best palette for the image consists of examining the points in this space that represent the colors of all the pixels in the image, and then finding the clusters of points in a consistent way to allow breaking the space up into boxes. Each box of points of similar color is then represented by a single color in the palette. This process is usually called vector quantization, and there are several iterative algorithms that search for optimal results and are all rather computer intensive (Heckbert, 1982; Braudaway, 1987; Gentile et al., 1990).

A new technique (Balasubramanian et al., 1994) seems to offer improvements in both quality and speed. It uses the YCC (broadcast video, also called YIQ and YUV) space with the Y (luminance, or brightness) axis given more precision than the two chrominance signals (yellow-blue and red-green), because human vision is more sensitive to changes in brightness than in color. This is the same argument used for reducing the bandwidth used to transmit the color information in television. The scaling of the values is also nonlinear, corresponding to the response of the display CRT to changes in signal intensity. In other words, the goal of the color palette compression is to reproduce the image so that visual observation of the image on a television screen will not show objectionable artefacts such as color banding. And for that goal these methods work well. But if any further quantitative use of the image is intended, the loss of true color information may create obstacles. It may even produce difficulties for printing the images, since the gamut of colors available and the response of the color intensities is different than for CRT displays.

Lossy compression

Much higher compression ratios can often be achieved for images if some loss of the exact pixel values can be tolerated. Again, there is a rich literature discussing the relative merits of different approaches. For instance, the encoding of differences between neighboring pixels can be made lossy and gain more compression simply by placing an upper limit on the values. Since most differences are small, compression can represent the small differences exactly but only allow a maximum change of ±7 grey levels. This restriction would reduce the number of bits per pixel from 8 to 4, without any other coding tricks. Larger differences, if they occur, would be spread out over several pixels. Of course, this might distort important edges or boundaries.

Two approaches have become common enough to be implemented in many desktop computers and are fairly representative of the others. There are a variety of "transform" methods that are similar in principle to the JPEG (Joint Photographers Expert Group) standard now widely used, and a proprietary fractal compression method has also shown great promise. Each will be discussed in some detail and examples shown.

The JPEG compaction scheme has several parts. First, the image is transformed from RGB to a video-based encoding scheme in which the grey scale image (the luminance) and the color information (the chrominance) are separated. Each of these is compacted separately, since for visual purposes it is possible to lose more of the color information than grey scale. This is because the eye uses the grey scale edges to indicate boundaries, and allows color to bleed across boundaries without confusion. The particular tradeoff used in most video methods reduces the precision of the color information to half that used for the brightness values.

Next, square subregions in the image are processed with a discrete cosine transform. This is similar to the FFT discussed in Chapter 4, except that the terms in the expansion are real valued (the FFT uses complex numbers). For a spatial image $f(x,y)$ the two-dimensional transform $F(u,v)$ is given by

$$F(u,v) = \frac{4\,c(u,v)}{N^2} \sum_{x=0}^{N-1} \sum_{y=0}^{N-1} f(x,y)\,\cos\frac{(2x+1)\pi u}{2N}\cos\frac{(2y+1)\pi v}{2N} \qquad (2$$

where N is the width of the image, the range for u and v is from 0 to $N-1$, and the function $c(u,v)=1$ except when u or v is 0, and is then equal to 0.5. The magnitude of these terms drops very rapidly as u and v increase, and the compression is achieved by keeping only some of them, starting from 0 and working up. The fewer terms that are kept, the greater the compression (and the greater the loss of high frequency information). This may be done separately for different areas within the image, so that the amount of color or detail preservation is varied according to the actual image contents.

Finally, additional compression is achieved by truncating the precision of the terms, and then using a coding scheme that looks for repeated characters and stores them only once with the number of repeats. From all of these operations, compression ratios in excess of 100:1 are possible, although much lower ratios of the order of 10:1 are more typical (and still very useful). **Figures 36 to 39** will show examples of images that have been compressed. There is some detectable loss of detail and sharpness which would be objectionable for measurement purposes but is not visually distracting. Depending on whether hardware or software is used to perform the transform (and its inverse, which is required to retrieve the image for display), the time required to perform the compression and decompression can vary up to tens of seconds.

The proprietary Kodak Photo-CD algorithm is also a transform method, and shares the same advantages and drawbacks as the JPEG method. Because it is intended to work from traditional photographic materials, which have a wide latitude, Photo-CD makes some provision for the extended range that may be present in such images. Whereas JPEG separates the image first into HSI components, as discussed in Chapter 1, Photo-CD uses a modification of the YCC format used for broadcast television, which has one luminance (Y) and two chrominance (C_1 and C_2 or U and V) components (one the red-green balance and the other the yellow-blue balance). However, they cover an extended range in which $Y' = 1.36 \cdot Y$, and the modified C' components are related to RGB by

$$R = Y' + C_2'$$
$$G = Y' - 0.194 \cdot C_1' - 0.509 \cdot C_2' \qquad (3$$
$$B = Y' + C_1'$$

When each of these is mapped to a 256 level (one byte) value, a nonlinear relationship is used as shown in **Figure 22**. In addition to mapping the film density to the output of a typical CRT display for viewing of the stored image, this method allows recording information beyond the nominal 100% white, which gives visually important highlights to reflections and other features that can be recorded by film, but not by most CCD cameras. However, these differences do not alter the basic similarity of approach, fidelity and efficiency which Photo-CD shares with JPEG.

For sequences of images, an additional compression based on similarity between successive frames has been proposed. The MPEG (Moving Pictures Experts Group) standard is intended for use with high definition television (HDTV), in order to compress the images enough to permit transmission within the narrow bandwidth used by present television stations. MPEG adds several additional steps to reduce the amount of data that must be transmitted. It looks for blocks of similar pixels in successive images, even if they have moved slightly. Only an average of 2 frames per second are normally sent in their entirety. The rest are either encoded as differences from preceding frames, or as interpolations between frames. This approach allows overall compression to approach 200:1 with "acceptable" visual appearance.

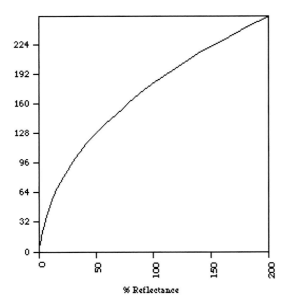

224

192

160

128

96

64

32

0

% Reflectance

Figure 22. Nonlinear encoding of brightness and extended luminance range used in Kodak's Photo-CD format.

A typical HDTV proposal presents 1920×1080 pixel images at the rate of 30 per second, for a total data rate exceeding 1 gigabit per second. The images use progressive scan (not interlaced), square pixels, and a wider image aspect ratio of 16:9 instead of the 4:3 used in NTSC video (and most computer display screens). A typical broadcast TV station has a bandwidth that is 250 times too small. Without examining the debate over HDTV, whose standards are still evolving, we can consider if and how application of these methods may be useful for technical images.

It is important to remember that the criterion for these compression methods is the visual acceptance of the reconstructed image, as it is displayed on a television screen. For instance, the MPEG standard, like present broadcast television, encodes the chrominance (color) information with half the precision as it does the luminance (brightness) information. This is because tests indicate that human vision of images displayed on a CRT is more tolerant of variations in color than in brightness. The use of images for technical purposes, or even their presentation in other forms such as printed hardcopy viewed by reflected light, may not be so forgiving.

Judging the quality of compressed and restored images is not a simple matter. Calculating the rms differences between the original pixel values and the reconstructed values is often used, but does not provide a measure that agrees very well with human judgment, nor with the needs of image measurement and analysis. Human vision responds differently to the same absolute variation between pixels depending on whether they lie in light or dark areas of the image. The same difference is usually more objectionable in the dark areas, because of the logarithmic response of human vision. Differences are also judged as more important in regions that are smooth, or strongly and regularly patterned, than in areas that are perceived as random. Displacing an edge or boundary because of pixel differences is usually considered more detrimental than a similar brightness change in the interior of a feature.

Ranking of image quality by humans is often employed to compare different methods, but even with careful comparisons the results are dependent on lighting conditions, the context of the image and others that have been seen recently, and fatigue. It was the result of extensive human comparisons that led to the selection of the JPEG standard that is now widely implemented. The JPEG method is one of many that rely on first transforming the image from the familiar spatial domain to another one that separates the information present according to a set of basis functions.

The most familiar of these transforms is the Fourier approach discussed in more detail in Chapter 5. Basically, the Fourier transform decomposes the image into a summation of sinusoidal variations in brightness, with every possible frequency and orientation, and adjusts their magnitudes and phases to match the original image. If a complete set of these functions is used, it can exactly and completely reconstruct the original image. So using the transform by itself is not a lossy method. But if the complete set of functions is used, the numbers required to specify the magnitude and phase take up just as much storage space as the original image. In fact, usually they take up more because the magnitude and phase values are real numbers, and the original pixel values are likely to have been integers that require less storage space.

The virtue of transforming the image into another space is that it collects the information together in a different way. The Fourier method separates the information present according to frequency and orientation. If very low frequency variations, such as shading in the image, are not important, they can be eliminated in the transform just by setting the magnitude of the corresponding sine functions to zero. If a particular frequency and orientation corresponds to electronic noise or a camera defect, it can be similarly eliminated.

There are of course many other sets of basis functions besides the sine functions used in the Fourier approach. Some provide a more efficient representation of the image, in which more of the terms are very small, while some are simply easier to compute. One of the popular newer methods is the wavelet transform, which offers some computational advantages and can even be obtained optically with lenses and masks (McAulay et al., 1993), or electronically with a filter bank. The wavelet transform provides a progressive or "pyramidal" encoding of the image at various scales, which is more flexible than conventional windowed approaches like the FFT. The wavelets comprise a normalized set of orthogonal functions on which the image is projected

(Chui, 1992). Each individual wavelet can be represented as a summation of Fourier terms, so the difference is primarily one of implementation. However, the wavelet basis functions each have a different extent in the spatial image, and so their use for compression avoids the "blockiness" or "quilting" sometimes seen in JPEG compression, where the image is subdivided into 8×8 pixel blocks before performing a discrete cosine transform.

Applications of this comparatively new approach to a wide variety of time- and space-dependent signals are taking advantage of its efficiency and compactness. But in principle, all of these transforms take up just as much space as the original, and are loss-free. Lossy compression of the image is accomplished by examining the magnitudes of the various terms in the transform, and eliminating those that are very small. This can reduce the amount of space required, but also produces loss in the quality of the reconstructed image.

But the idea is that the loss of particular terms from the transform may not be visible or at least objectionable to a human viewer, because the information each term represented was spread throughout the entire image and may have contributed little to any particular feature. This is not always the case. The selection of terms with a small amplitude often means the elimination of high frequency information from the image, and this may be important to define edges and boundaries in particular. Nevertheless, such compression techniques have been widely used and developed.

Figure 23 illustrates wavelet compression. At a compression ratio of about 20:1, the image is visually similar in quality to the original, at least as printed. However, when the original image is subtracted from the one that has been compressed, it becomes apparent that the compression process has altered details. When the compression ratio is increased to 60:1, the appearance of artefacts throughout the image is quite apparent. All of the lossy methods of compression introduce some alterations into images, particularly at boundaries. We will examine them in more detail in the balance of this chapter.

Compression using lossy methods is often suitable for images to be used in particular applications such as printing in which the printing device itself may set an upper limit to the frequencies that can be reproduced. It has already been suggested above that one use of compression may be to store multiple copies of an image in a database, each with appropriate quality for a specific purpose such as printing or viewing as a thumbnail for searching and recognition. It is also important to determine just how much loss of quality is produced by varying degrees of image compression, so that artefacts capable of altering the analysis of reconstructed images are avoided.

The JPEG technique is fairly representative of many of these transform-based compression methods, and uses a discrete

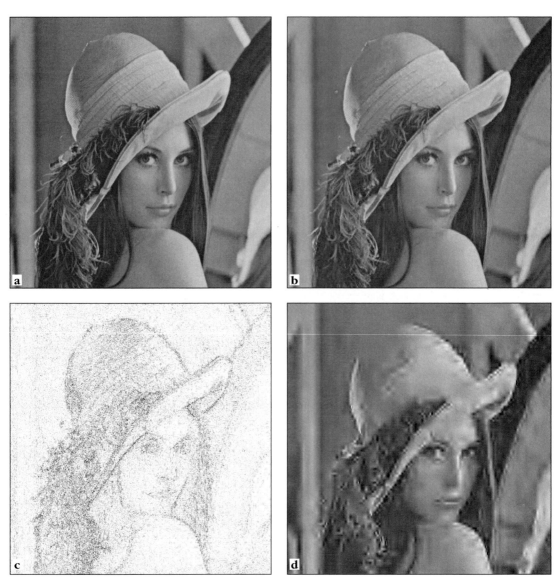

Figure 23. Example of wavelet compression:

a) original image;
b) compressed by 20:1;
c) difference between *a* and *b*;
d) compressed by 60:1.

cosine transform (DCT) that is quite similar to the Fourier transform method. Also, it is now widely implemented on small computers, either in hardware or software. Consequently, the following comparisons use this method. Broadly similar results would be expected for methods using any of the other transforms, followed by thresholding to remove terms with small magnitudes.

The JPEG standard is a collaborative effort of the CCITT (International Telegraph and Telephone Consultative Committee) and the ISO (International Standards Organization), and actually comprises a variety of methods, of which the most widely implemented to date is based on a discrete cosine transform. The methods are not explicitly intended for computer storage; it deals with a stream of bytes as might be encountered in image transmission. However, implementations for compressing images for file storage have become widely available both in hardware and software implementations.

The methods include both a compression and a decompression routine, which for the DCT are quite symmetric. Some other compression methods, more suitable for storage of moving pictures on media such as CD-ROM, are asymmetric and take much longer to achieve the compression that is needed for decompression during playback. There is nothing in the JPEG standard that deals with sequential images, but a separate standard (MPEG) still in development is intended to address those applications.

The question, of course, is what consequences such compression has on the quality of images as it may be relevant to image analysis. Some of the artefacts and loss of data which do not detract from visual examination of the images, or their printed appearance, may be objectionable when the images are to be measured. Changes in the sharpness or location of edges, the contrast across boundaries, or the absolute brightness of regions might have serious effects on image analysis procedures. General warnings are often given on these points, but few detailed evaluations have been published. The examples which follow will serve as a more explicit caution on the use of image compression, and illustrate the specific defects that compression can introduce.

A test image (**Figure 24**) was created to evaluate the effects of compression (and subsequent decompression) on image quality. The image consists of features and lines whose boundaries are sharply defined. However, the same image was repeated with different overall contrast between the light and dark regions to study the effect of brightness differences on quality. The lines and edges are mostly vertical because the DCT method used in the JPEG procedure is symmetrical with respect to vertical and horizontal directions. However, the circle was included to show any effects which might vary in intermediate directions, and corners are present to verify that they are well preserved.

This is a more complicated test pattern than the typical sets of resolution lines used to measure the modulation transfer function (MTF) of an optical system. Such a test pattern can be used to determine the smallest line spacing that is resolved, as a function of contrast, and so define the system resolution or MTF. However, it is not easy to predict from this information the influence of the optical system on corner definition, boundary sharpness, and preservation of brightness values. Since all of these are of interest in image analysis, a test pattern that might directly show these effects was used.

The actual image subjected to compression and decompression is shown in **Figure 25**. It consists of five identical panels with

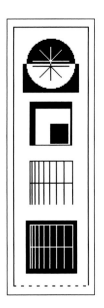

Figure 24. *Test pattern image used for compression tests.*

the same features present but with different contrast. In the left-most panel, the brightness values of the two regions are 0 and 255. In the remaining panels, the contrast is reduced to 64, 16, 4 and 1 grey level value, respectively. In the normal printing of these images, the lower values of contrast may be hidden so that they appear as solid grey panels. However, the actual stored pixel brightness values are listed for comparison in subsequent tables.

The use of a grey scale rather than a color test image does not affect the results, since the compression of a color image is performed by separately encoding three image planes, either the red, green, and blue (RGB) components of the digitized image, or another representation such as HSI (hue, saturation, and intensity) computed from the RGB values. If RGB planes are used,

Figure 25. *Image with repetitions of the test pattern at different contrast levels.*

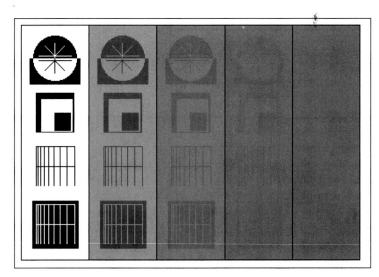

the artefacts which appear after compression and decompression (or, in fact, after any type of image processing) may modify the pixel values in ways that alter the perceived color (hue) of the final image. This visual defect can be severe, and is one reason that processing is by preference carried out in HSI space, but the presence and magnitude of the defects can be judged by the results for the individual 8 bit planes, as represented here by the single grey scale test image.

The compression and decompression of the test image were performed using both hardware and software implementations of the JPEG DCT algorithm on a Macintosh II computer. The results were indistinguishable, although the time required varied considerably (from the order of 10 seconds to essentially real time). The two routines differ in the way the user specifies the degree of compression. In both cases, a "Q" or quality value is specified that has only an indirect relationship to the ultimate file size. In general, it is not possible to specify the desired file size directly. The Q setting controls the thresholding of the various frequency terms as discussed below. The numeric values used are different in the various implementations of the technique, and in any event influence the final file size only indirectly.

Table 3. Image file sizes

Compression	File Size (Bytes)
None	100,100
PICT file	31,267
Q=5	29,207
Q=40	17,122
Q=125	12,680
Q=255	10,548

Four different degrees of compression were used, from a minimum size (maximum compression, poorest quality) up to a setting that represented the least compression that was lossy (resulted in the change of individual pixel values). The original image size of the five panels shown in **Figure 25** is 385×260≈100,000 pixels. Because this image consists of several comparatively large areas of pixels with uniform brightness, the normal run-length encoding of the image compresses it to 31,267 bytes in the Macintosh PICT format. The four JPEG compression levels, to which this can be compared, are listed in **Table 3** with the arbitrary "Q" settings used. The most extreme compression produces a file approximately 90% smaller than the original pixel array. In some examples with large color images, even larger compression ratios can be achieved but the expected quality defects would be at least as serious as those illustrated here.

The JPEG standard encompasses several compression methods, of which the discrete cosine transform is the most widely implemented. The steps in the compression algorithm are:

1. The image is separated into HSI planes and subdivided into 8×8 pixel blocks. If the image is not an exact multiple of 8 pixels in width or height, it is temporarily padded out to that size.

2. Each 8×8 pixel block is processed using the discrete cosine transform. This is closely related to the more familiar Fourier transform, except that all of the values are real instead of complex. The transform produces another 8×8 block of values for the frequency components. While the original pixel values are 1 byte = 8 bits (0...255), the transformed data are stored temporarily in 12 bits, giving 11 bits of precision plus a sign bit. Except for the possibility of round-off errors due to this finite representation, the DCT portion of the algorithm does not introduce any loss of data (i.e., the original image can be exactly reconstructed from the transform by an inverse DCT).

3. The 64 coefficients for each block are quantized to a lower precision (8 bits), and any values smaller than some threshold value which depends on the selected Q value will be arbitrarily set to zero. This is the "lossy" step in the compression. In most cases, the threshold setting for the grey scale brightness (called variously the intensity or luminance of the image) retains more terms than the setting for the color planes. This is because in the intended use of the compression method for human viewing of images, it is generally accepted that more fidelity is needed in image brightness than is needed in color. Normal television broadcasting (NTSC video) also uses a narrower bandwidth for the color (chrominance) information than it does for the brightness (luminance) signal.

4. The first of the 64 coefficients for each block is the average brightness or "DC" term. It is represented as a difference from the same term for the preceding block in the image. The blocks are listed in raster-scan order through the image.

5. The remaining 63 coefficients for each block are scanned in a zig-zag diagonal order that starts with the lowest frequencies and progresses to the highest. The nonzero terms are retained with their 8-bit precision, but after the thresholding and reduction in precision, many of the terms will now be zero. These terms are collected together and coded as the number of consecutive zero terms.

6. The entire data stream may then be further compacted by using a Huffman coding as discussed above. This step is loss-free.

The decompression or image reconstruction procedure reverses these steps to produce an image that is similar to the original image. The loss of high frequency terms results in some image defects and distortions. Since the specific terms which are thresholded to zero may be different in the various 8×8 pixel blocks in the original image, the exact nature of the defects will vary from

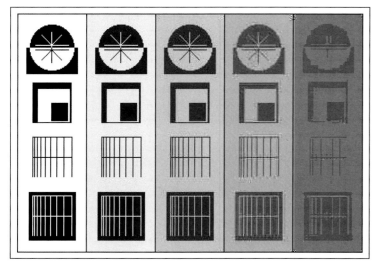

Figure 26. *Reconstruction of image after compression at Q=5 setting. Each panel has had its contrast expanded to cover the full black to white range, to show details.*

place to place. In general, sharp boundaries, edges, corners and lines require the highest frequencies to accurately reproduce, and it is these that will show the greatest degradation. An 8×8 block of pixels with a uniform grey value would be compressed to a single coefficient that would be accurately encoded, and all of the remaining coefficients would actually be zero so that no loss would occur. Small deviations from this uniform grey might or might not be preserved.

Figures 26, **27**, **28** and **29** show the test image after it has been compressed and decompressed using the algorithm described above. These images have been further processed to increase the visibility of the low contrast structures. Within each panel of the test image, the contrast has been linearly stretched to cover the full range from black to white. If applied to the original test image, this procedure would have made all panels

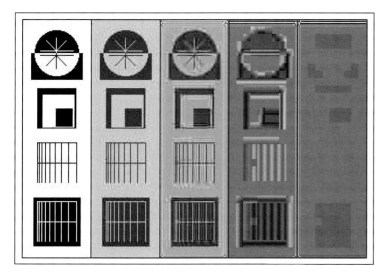

Figure 27. *Reconstruction of image after compression at Q=40 setting. Each panel has had its contrast expanded to cover the full black to white range, to show details. Many of the details have been lost from the rightmost panel (5).*

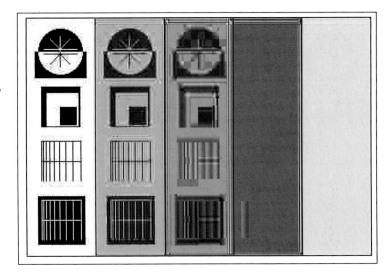

Figure 28. *Reconstruction of image after compression at Q=125 setting. Each panel has had its contrast expanded to cover the full black to white range, to show details. No details remain in the two rightmost panels (4 and 5).*

appear identical. For the reconstructed images, the presence of pixels with values brighter or darker than the original two brightness levels present causes this scaling to produce lower contrast for the features. The increased contrast allows some of the image artefacts around the feature boundaries to be visible. Several of these specific defects are described in more detail below.

As noted in the description of the algorithm, the average brightness value of each block of pixels is coded in terms of the difference from the adjacent block. This should preserve the absolute grey values for the large regions in the image. **Table 4** lists the pixel values at the center of the dark inner square in the second feature from the top of each panel, and in the light area that surrounds it. The brightness values are changed by no more than two brightness values in any of the images, even for the most extreme compression. This seems like a small change out of

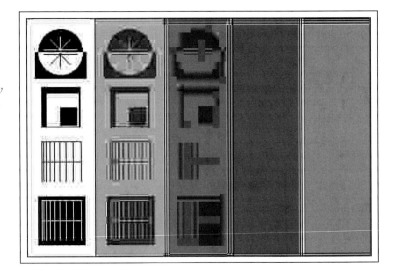

Figure 29. *Reconstruction of image after compression at Q=255 setting. Each panel has had its contrast expanded to cover the full black to white range, to show details. No details remain in the two rightmost panels (4 and 5), and many have disappeared from the center panel (3).*

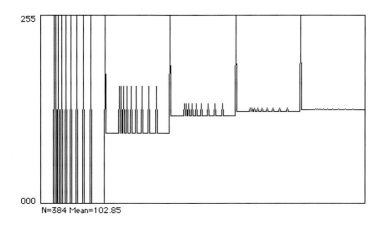

N=384 Mean=102.85

Figure 30. Brightness profile across the vertical line pattern (third feature from top) in the original test image.

the 255 brightness levels present, but unfortunately the change in the contrast levels between the two areas reaches 100% for some of the low-contrast, high-compression cases. In other words, small differences between uniform areas are reduced or wiped out entirely.

Table 4. Pixel brightness values after compression.

Image	Original	Q=5	Q=40	Q=125	Q=255
Panel 1	255-0	255-0	254-0	255-2	255-0
Panel 2	159-95	159-195	158-96	157-97	157-97
Panel 3	135-119	135-119	134-20	137-117	137-117
Panel 4	129-125	129-125	128-126	127-127	127-127
Panel 5	128-127	128-127	128-127	127-127	127-127

In addition to the change in contrast between relatively large uniform areas, the compression routine strongly affects the resolution of lines. **Figure 30** shows the brightness variation along a line profile across the pattern of dark lines in the original test pattern, and **Figures 31**, **32**, **33** and **34** show the same line for the images after compression and reconstruction. The low contrast lines disappear altogether, but in addition contrast between

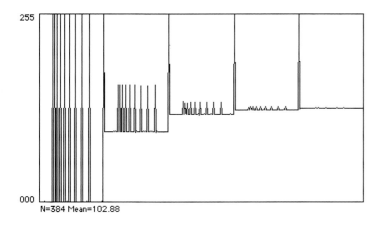

N=384 Mean=102.88

Figure 31. Brightness profile across the reconstructed image after compression at Q=5 setting. Notice that some lines in the rightmost panel are missing.

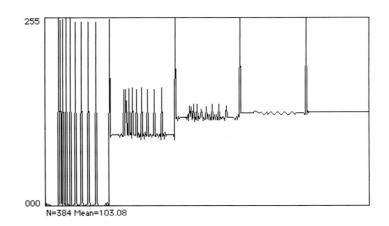

Figure 32. *Brightness profile across the reconstructed image after compression at Q=40 setting. In addition to the loss of the lines in the right panel (5), the variations in panel 4 do not correspond to the original lines, and the dark and light levels are distorted in the higher contrast panels.*

N=384 Mean=103.08

the closely spaced dark lines changes, and for some of the combinations of degree of compression and line spacing, aliasing occurs. These effects cause the individual lines to disappear, while other lines that are completely an artefact of the image processing and have different locations and spacings, appear. A similar set of artefacts appears for the light lines, which interestingly are not an exact inverse of the dark lines.

Additional artefacts appear at the corners and along the boundaries of the features. **Figure 35** shows enlargements of several of the circle and square formations. They were selected as being broadly representative of the types of defects produced by the compression. Notice that the distortions of the boundaries are not isotropic. Nor are they identical from one side to another. This is due to the way the 8×8 subdivision of the image happens to fall on the various features. Indeed, the 8×8 pixel blocks are visible in several locations in the figure, because of different average brightnesses for the reconstructed pixels. Also, some of the lines within the circle have disappeared while others have changed from being light to dark. The corners of the squares are significantly distorted, and it is clear that feature sizes and shapes

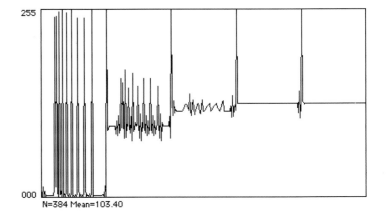

Figure 33. *Brightness profile across the reconstructed image after compression at Q=125 setting. There is no signal left in panels 4 and 5, the variations in panel 3 do not correspond to the original lines, and the dark and light levels are distorted in the higher contrast panels.*

N=384 Mean=103.40

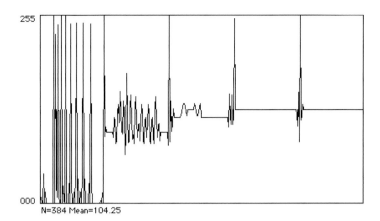

255

000

N=384 Mean=104.25

Figure 34. *Brightness profile across the reconstructed image after compression at Q=255 setting. Even in panel 2, the variations do not correspond to the original lines.*

change when image compression is used. The light and dark artefact lines that appear along boundaries result from the attempt to model a square step by a summation of cosine terms. This classic limitation of Fourier series is often described as a Gibb's phenomenon, or as "ringing."

Even at the lowest compression setting, significant artefacts are observed in this simple test image. The location and contrast of edges, especially ones with an initially low contrast, are altered. Feature shapes are changed, especially at corners, and the resolution of narrow lines is significantly reduced. For the lowest compression setting used, the file size is reduced about the same amount as run-length encoding in the standard system file format, which is a lossless compression method. At higher compression settings, the amount of image distortion increases markedly and low-contrast features disappear altogether.

In more complex images, the presence of defects of this type may be more difficult to recognize visually. However, the nature of the JPEG process which keeps the larger terms and erases the smaller ones in the discrete cosine transform of each block is likely to remove more of the small high frequency terms in

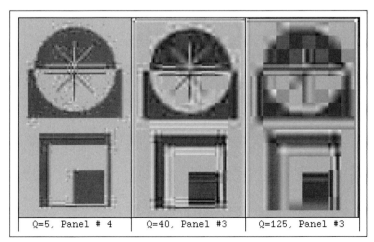

Q=5, Panel # 4   Q=40, Panel #3   Q=125, Panel #3

Figure 35. *Enlargement of several of the circle and square test features in the reconstructed images. The contrast of each has been expanded to cover the full black to white range, to show details; the original contrast values are listed in Table 4.*

Figure 36. *Image of a Debye-Scherer X-ray film before and after JPEG compression (from 136.3K to 8.1K bytes). The position and density of the vertical lines provide information about crystallographic structure. A plot of the density profile across the image shows that statistical noise in the spectrum has been removed along with some small peaks, and a new artefact peak introduced, by the compression.*

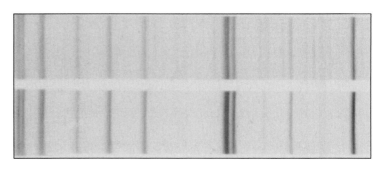

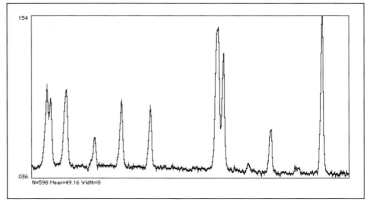

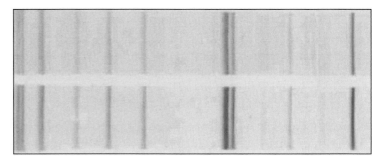

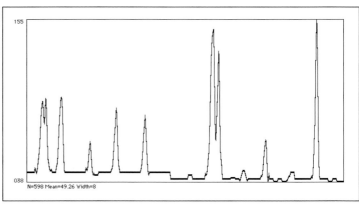

images with more detail present. This compression will produce artefacts of the same type, in at least as great a number and magnitude as those shown here.

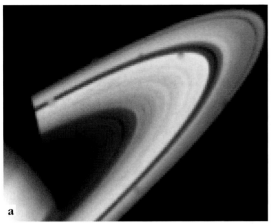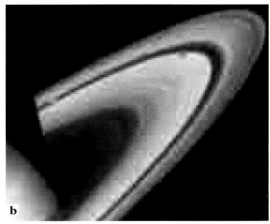

a   b

*Figure 37. Detail from the image of Saturn (Figure 20) before (**a**) and after (**b**) JPEG compression (from 63K to 10.3K bytes). Notice the alteration of pixel values along the planet's limb and in the rings, and the appearance of 8×8 pixel blocking artefacts.*

Figures 36 through **39** show examples of detail loss in several grey scale and color images, as a function of the degree of compression. For each image, the original and compressed sizes are shown. In the Debye pattern (**Figure 36**), notice that the horizontal profile of the density after compression shows that statistical fluctuations and small peaks have been eliminated, while an artefact peak has appeared. In the image of Saturn (**Figure 37**), the difference between the original and the compressed image is particularly evident along edges and in the fine detail of the rings. For the gel image (**Figure 38**), the difference between the original and the compressed image emphasizes the alteration of the grey scale vs. density calibration.

The color image of flowers (**Figure 39**) shows that even substantial compression does not necessarily degrade the visual appearance of the image as it is printed. However, as shown by the difference image and the detail images, there are changes in edge definition and color shifts along boundaries. These might be important in any subsequent use or analysis of the image.

There are several ways in which JPEG, or any other similar approach based on transforms, can be improved. One is to choose the best possible color space in which to represent the image before starting. For instance, Photo-CD uses the CIE color space while JPEG uses HSI. Second, instead of dividing the image into nonoverlapping tiles, a system using blocks that overlap in both the horizontal and vertical directions can suppress some of the artefacts that appear at block boundaries (Young & Kingsbury, 1993). Third, and perhaps most important, the thresholding of terms can be made more flexible. Different threshold values can be used for each color plane or for different colors, for different frequencies, and perhaps different directions, depending on the intended use of the image (for viewing,

Figure 38. *Image of an electrophoresis gel before and after JPEG compression (from 122.8K to 10.9K bytes). The difference image emphasizes the altered pixels, which will change the density calibration.*

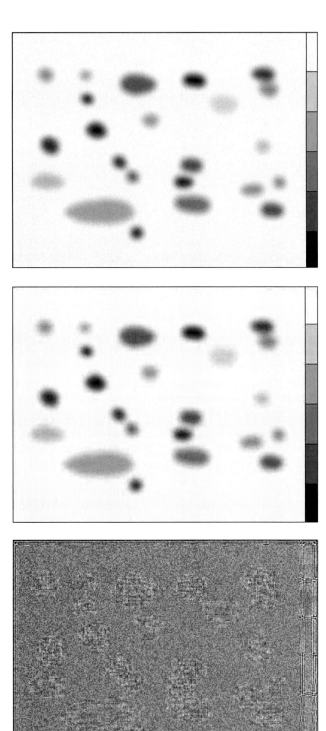

printing, etc.). These methods can improve the reconstructed image quality at a given level of compression, with no change in reconstruction time.

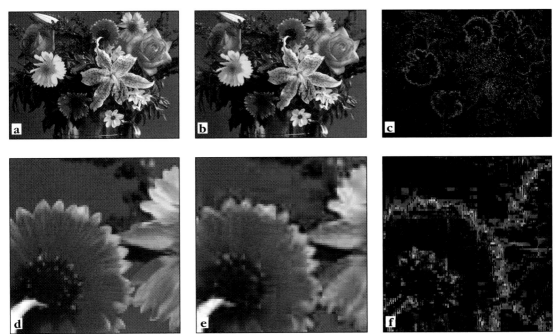

Figure 39. Image of flowers, before *(a)* and after *(b)* JPEG compression (from 523.6K to 23.5K bytes), and the difference *(c)* between the two (with contrast expanded to show details). In the enlarged details of these images *(d, e, f)* the changes in pixel values, loss of detail, alteration of contrast at boundaries and introduction of false colors can be seen.

The use of JPEG compression or indeed any "lossy" compression technique for images should be restricted to images intended for visual examination and printing, and should not be used for images intended for measurement and analysis. This is true even for relatively high "quality" settings which result in only modest compression. At high compression settings, even visual examination of images may be affected due to aliasing of edges and lines, loss of resolution, and suppression of contrast.

Another approach to achieving control over the degree of loss of fidelity is to combine lossy and lossless compression. For example, if an image or a color plane of an image has 8 bits of depth, the brightest 3 bits might be compressed with a lossless method such as differential Huffman coding, and the lowest 5 bits might be compressed using a JPEG technique (Bassiouni et al., 1993). It is also possible to imagine using different compression methods or combinations of lossy and lossless methods for the different color planes.

Other compression methods

The JPEG method is fairly representative of many transform-based techniques applied to still images. As mentioned above, transforms decompose the image into a collection of regular terms, such as the sine functions used in the Fourier approach.

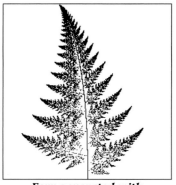
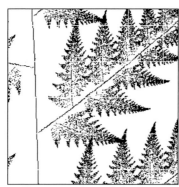
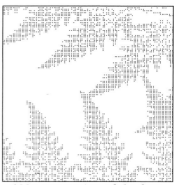

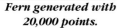
Fern generated with 20,000 points.   **5x expansion of the fern.**   **100x expansion of the fern.**

Figure 40. Image of a fern generated with the four transformation rules shown in the text. The structure remains self-similar when expanded, except for the limitation of finite numerical precision in the computer, which rounds off the values in the 100-times-expanded image.

Usually a complete set of such basis functions must be used to get a lossless or complete representation of the original image.

Barnsley (Barnsley & Hurd, 1993) has shown another way to transform an image, using what are often referred to as self-affine distortions of the image (shrinking and displacing copies of the original) as the basis functions. In principle, a complete set of these operations would give a set of parameters as large as the original image. But for many images, only a very few basis functions are required to reconstruct the original image with astonishing fidelity, providing a significant compression. The best-known example of this self-affine compression is the generation of a fern by iteratively combining smaller copies of the same basic shape.

The four rules below are able to generate a realistic image of a fern. Each rule corresponds to one rotation, displacement and shrinkage of a subelement of the structure. The rules are applied by starting at any point, selecting one of the rules (with the frequency shown by the probability values, from 1% to 84%), and then moving from the current point to the next point according to the rule. This point is plotted and the procedure iterated to produce the entire figure. The more points, the better the definition of the result. **Figure 40** shows an example. The entire fern with 20,000 points shows the self-similarity of the overall shape. As a portion of the image is blown up for examination, more points are required. Finally, the limit of magnification is set by the numerical precision of the values in the computer, as indicated in the figure.

From a mathematical point of view, the four transformations are basis functions which can be added together in proportion (the p or probability values) to produce the overall object. In Fourier analysis, the cosine terms are basis functions and the coefficients specify the amount of each to add to generate the final result. Here, the first problem is to find the correct basis functions for a given image or surface. It is expected that only a few will be needed; Barnsley has shown the ability to compress and reconstruct full-color images of arbitrary scenes with typically only a few terms. This has been used to compress full color images for storage on CD-ROM, for instance in the *Microsoft Encarta* encyclopedia.

This technique is often described by its inventors as "fractal compression" because the reconstruction can be carried out iteratively (as shown for the fern), and because it provides ever finer levels of detail. In fact, the method produces reconstructed images with detail at a much finer scale than the original used to find the basis functions. Such detail looks very impressive, since the enlarged image never shows flat or smooth areas that indicate loss of resolution. Of course, the detail may not be real. It is generated under the assumption that whatever patterns are present at large scale in the image are also present with progressively less amplitude (following a power law) at all finer scales.

Table 5. Transformations (Basis Functions) for the Fern image (Figure 40)

1 (p=0.840)	x'=+0.821·x + 0.845·y + 0.088
	y'=+0.030·x − 0.028·y − 0.176
2 (p=0.075)	x'=−0.024·x + 0.074·y + 0.470
	y'=−0.323·x − 0.356·y − 0.260
3 (p=0.075)	x'=+0.076·x + 0.204·y + 0.494
	y'=−0.257·x + 0.312·y − 0.133
4 (p=0.010)	x'=+0.000·x + 0.000·y + 0.496
	y'=+0.000·x + 0.172·y − 0.091

The same principle has been applied to the compression of photographic images with grey scale or color pixels, where it is known as the Collage Theorem. This is shown schematically in **Figure 41**, using the basis functions listed in **Table 5**. That there must be such basis functions, or rules for the self-affine distortions, and that they are in principle discoverable is known (Barnsley et al., 1986; Barnsley, 1988; Barnsley & Hurd, 1993). It has been shown that nonlinear self-affine transforms can also be used, and may be more efficient. The problem of finding the correct basis functions is, however, far from trivial. Knowing that such functions must exist gives few leads to discovering them. Each consists of a mapping (a combination of translation, scaling, rotation and warping) and a relative contribution or probability. Unlike the JPEG method, the Barnsley approach is not symmetrical. There are formal procedures for performing fractal compression (Fisher et al., 1992), although the results do not necessarily give optimal reduction in file size. The time needed to compress the image is typically much greater than that needed to reconstruct it.

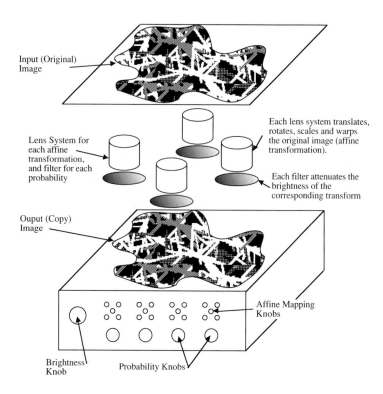

Figure 41. *Barnsley's photocopy machine (Barnsley & Hurd, 1993). His collage theorem states that there is a set of mappings and probabilities that produce an output identical to the input to any desired degree of accuracy. These geometrical transforms and probabilities constitute his image compression algorithm (U. S. Patent # 5065447). For a fractal surface image, the mappings may provide information beyond the simple fractal dimension value, which may be related to the history or properties of the surface.*

Input (Original) Image

Lens System for each affine transformation, and filter for each probability

Each lens system translates, rotates, scales and warps the original image (affine transformation).

Each filter attenuates the brightness of the corresponding transform

Ouput (Copy) Image

Affine Mapping Knobs

Brightness Knob

Probability Knobs

Digital movies

There is growing interest in using small computers to produce, edit and display digital moving pictures. Two emerging standards (or sets of standards) are Apple's Quicktime and Microsoft's Video for Windows. Both of these methods allow the use of various compression techniques, usually called CODECs (COmpressor-DECompressor). A codec is a program implementation of one of the compression algorithms such as those described above. In fact, JPEG is one of the methods provided by currently existing codecs available for both Quicktime and Video for Windows. Some of the codecs run in software only, and others use additional hardware. For JPEG, this can be either a digital signal processor chip programmed to execute the discrete cosine transform, or a dedicated chip designed specifically for the JPEG algorithm.

However, the JPEG method does not provide as much compression for digital movies as is needed to compress an entire movie onto a single CD-ROM, to broadcast HDTV images, or to allow digital video conferencing with images transmitted over relatively low bandwidth networks because it does not take into account the considerable redundancy of sequential images. In most cases, a series of images on movie film or videotape has large areas of pixels that are not changing at all with time, or are doing so in relatively smooth and continuous ways. It should be possible to compress these, and in fact quite high compression ratios can be tolerated because for such areas the needed quality of the reconstructed image is not high. Human vision tends to ignore portions of images in which nothing interesting is happening, and no changes are occurring.

The emerging MPEG (Moving Pictures Experts Group) standards follow the same approach as JPEG. They are based primarily on the need to compress images in order to transmit "consumer" video, either over low-bandwidth networks (including wire, optical fiber and broadcast channels), or using media such as CD-ROM. Of course, for more technical purposes such as tracking features in a sequence of images, or measuring density or color changes as a function of time, different requirements may place different limits on the acceptable quality of reconstruction.

Most of the moving-picture compression methods use key frames, which are compressed using the same method as a still picture. Then for every image in the sequence that follows the key frame, the differences from the previous image are determined and compressed. For these difference images, as we have seen above, the magnitude of the values is reduced. Consequently, in performing a further compression of this image by keeping only the "most important" basis functions, the number of terms eliminated can be increased significantly and much higher levels of compression achieved.

Like JPEG, MPEG consists of several options, some of which require more computation but deliver more compression. For instance, motion compensation provides a higher degree of compression because it identifies an overall translation in successive images (for instance, when the camera is slowly panned across a scene), and adjusts for that before comparing locations in one image with the previous frame. Unlike JPEG, the MPEG approach is asymmetric: it requires more computation to compress the original data than to decompress it to reconstruct the images.

One of the consequences of this approach to compression is that it is intended only to go forward in time. From a key frame and then successive differences, you can reconstruct each following image. But you cannot easily go back to reconstruct a previous image except by returning to the nearest key frame and working forward from there. In principle, one key frame at the beginning of each scene in a movie should be enough. In practice, key frames are often inserted every few seconds (for video movies reconstructed at 30 frames per second).

Other compression methods are being developed for sequential images. One is predictive vector quantization that attempts to locate boundaries in each image, track the motion of those boundaries, and use prediction to generate successive images. Sequences of 8-bit grey scale images compressed to an average data rate of less than 0.5 bits per pixel have been reported (Nicoulin et al., 1993; Wu & Gersho, 1993; Wen & Lu, 1993;

Hwang et al., 1993). Fractal compression has also been extended to deal with image sequences (Li et al., 1993).

High compression ratios for moving images are appropriate for video conferencing, where the image quality only has to show who is speaking and perhaps what they are holding. High compression is essential for consumer delivery of movies via low bandwidth transmission channels, in order to make HDTV a reality. Compression offers the convenience of enabling an entire feature-length movie to be pressed onto a single CD-ROM disk. For such consumer applications, in which the final image will be viewed on a television screen of only modest resolution, the image quality will be adequate. Tests with human television viewers have long suggested that it is the quality of the sound that is most important, and significant noise and other defects in the individual images are not objectionable.

However, for most technical applications, the types of artefacts produced by still image compression are not acceptable, and the additional ones introduced as a result of temporal compression make matters worse. The user intending to perform analysis of images from a sequence should certainly begin with no compression at all, and only accept specific compression methods if tests indicate they are acceptable for the particular purposes for which the images are to be used.

3

Correcting Imaging Defects

The first class of image processing operations considered in this chapter are those procedures applied to correct some of the defects in as-acquired images that may be present due to imperfect detectors, inadequate or nonuniform illumination, or an undesirable viewpoint. It is important to emphasize that these are corrections that are applied after the image has been digitized and stored, and therefore will be unable to deliver the highest quality result that could have been achieved by optimizing the acquisition process in the first place.

Of course, acquiring an optimum-quality image is sometimes impractical. If the camera can collect only a small number of photons in a practical time or before the scene changes, then the noise present in the image cannot be averaged out by acquiring and adding more photons or video frames, and other noise reduction means are needed. If the source of illumination cannot be controlled to be perfectly centered and normal to the viewed surface (for instance the sun), or if the surface is curved instead of planar, then the image will have nonuniform illumination that must be corrected afterwards. If the viewpoint cannot realistically be adjusted (for instance the path of a space probe or satellite), or if the surface is irregular (as in the case of a metal fracture), then some parts of the scene will be foreshortened; this must be taken into account in comparing sizes or measuring distances.

Even in typical laboratory setups such as the light microscope, keeping the instrument in ideal alignment may be very time-consuming, and achieving adequate stability to collect dim fluorescence images for a long time very difficult, so that it becomes more practical to trade off some of the ultimately achievable image quality for convenience and speed, and to utilize image processing methods to perform these corrections. When the first space probe pictures were obtained and the need for this type of correction was first appreciated, it required lengthy computations on moderate sized computers to apply them. It is now possible to implement such corrections on desktop machines in times measured in seconds, so that they can be practically applied to routine imaging needs.

Noisy images

In Chapter 1, improvement in image quality (technically, signal-to-noise ratio) by averaging a number of frames was demonstrated. The most common source of noise is counting statistics in the image detector due to a small number of incident particles (photons, electrons, etc.). This is particularly the case for X-ray images from the SEM, in which the ratio of incident electrons to detected X-rays may be from 10^5 to 10^6. In fluorescence light microscopy, the fluoresced-light photons in a narrow wavelength range from a dye or activity probe may also produce very dim images, compounded by the necessity of acquiring a series of very-short-duration images to measure activity as a function of time.

Noisy images may also occur due to instability in the light source or detector during the time required to scan or digitize an image. The pattern of this noise may be quite different from the essentially Gaussian noise due to counting statistics, but it still shows up as a variation in brightness in uniform regions of the scene. One common example is the noise in field emission SEM images due to the variation in field emission current at the tip. With a typical time constant of seconds, the electron emission may shift from one atom to another, producing a change of several percent in the beam current. The usual approach to minimize the effects of this fluctuation in the viewed image is to use scan times that are either much shorter or longer than the fluctuation time.

Similar effects can be seen in images acquired using fluorescent lighting, particularly in light boxes used to illuminate film negatives, resulting from an interference or beat between the camera and flickering of the fluorescent tube. This flickering is much greater than that of an incandescent bulb, whose thermal inertia smooths out the variation in light emission due to the alternating current. When the noise has a characteristic that is not random in time and does not exhibit "normal" statistical behavior, it is more difficult to place numeric descriptors on the amount of noise. However, many of the same techniques can be used, usually with somewhat less efficacy, to reduce the noise.

Assuming that an image represents the best quality that can practically be obtained, this section will deal with ways to suppress noise to improve the ability to visualize and demarcate for measurement the features which are present. The underlying assumptions in all of these methods are that the pixels in the image are much smaller than any of the important details, and that for most of the pixels present, most of their neighbors represent the same structure. Various averaging and comparison methods can be applied based on these assumptions.

These are very much the same assumptions as that inherent in classical image averaging, in which the assumption is that pixel readings at different times represent the same structure in the viewed scene. This directly justifies averaging (or integrating) pixel readings over time to reduce random noise. When the signal varies in other ways described above, other methods such as median filtering can be used. These methods are directly analogous to the spatial comparisons discussed here except that they utilize the time sequence of measurements at each location.

There are important differences between noise reduction by the use of frame averaging to combine many sequential readouts from a camera, and the use of a camera that can integrate the charge internally before it is read out. The latter mode is employed in astronomy, fluorescence microscopy, and other applications to very faint images, and is sometimes called "staring" mode since the camera is simply open to the incident light. The two methods might seem to be equivalent, since both add together the incoming signal over some period of time. However, it is important to understand that there are two quite different sources of noise to be considered.

In a camera used in staring mode, the electrons collected in each transistor on the CCD array include those produced by incoming photons and some from the dark current in the device itself. This current is strongly influenced by thermal noise, which can move electrons around at room temperature. Cooling the chip, either by a few tens of degrees with a Peltier cooler or by hundreds of degrees with liquid nitrogen or even liquid helium, can reduce this thermal noise. An infrared camera must be cooled more than a visible light camera, because the light photons themselves have less energy and so the production of a signal electron takes less energy, so that more dark current would be present at room temperature.

Cameras intended for staring application often specify the operating time needed to half-fill the dynamic range of the chip with dark current. For an inexpensive Peltier-cooled astronomy camera, the useful operating time may be several minutes. Collecting an image in staring mode for that length of time would raise the dark level to a medium grey, and any real signal would be superimposed on that background. Since the production of thermal electrons is a statistical process, not all pixels will have the same background level. Fluctuations in the background thus represent one type of noise in the image that may be dominant for these types of applications to very dim images.

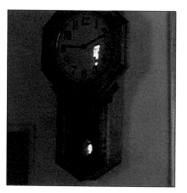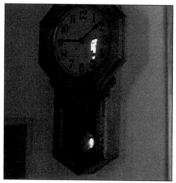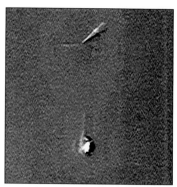

Figure 1. *Two images of the same view, acquired as sequential video frames, and the difference between them (contrast expanded to show detail).*

All cameras have some readout noise. In the typical CCD camera, the electrons from each transistor must be transferred across each line in order to be read out as a voltage to the computer. In a CCD camera, more transfers are needed to shift the electrons from one side of the image to the amplifier and so the resulting noise is greater on one side of the image than on the other. In an inter-line transfer camera, a separate row of transistors adjacent to each detector is used instead, somewhat reducing the readout noise. Of course, additional sources of noise from the other associated electronics (clock signals, wiring from the camera to the digitizer, pickup of electrical signals from the computer itself, and so forth) may degrade the signal even more. But even if those other sources of noise are minimized by careful design and proper wiring, there is an irreducible amount of noise superimposed on the signal each time the camera image is read out and digitized.

This noise is generally random, and hence is as likely to reduce as to increase the brightness of any particular pixel. **Figure 1** shows an example of two successive video frames acquired using a standard camera and dim lighting (high camera gain). The images look essentially identical except for the motion of the clock pendulum. However, subtracting one frame from the other shows the pixel noise present in the images. Averaging many frames together causes the random noise from readout to cancel while the signal continues to add up. The consequence is that frame averaging can reduce the relative magnitude of this source of noise in the image.

For a very dim image, the optimum situation is to integrate the signal within the camera chip, but without allowing any single pixel to reach saturation. Then reading the data out once will produce the minimum readout noise and the best image. For a brighter image, the optimum situation is to average together a sufficient number of frames to reduce the pixel variations due to random readout noise. This integration may be done in the frame grabber or in the computer program. The frame grabber is generally restricted by the amount of on-board memory, but can

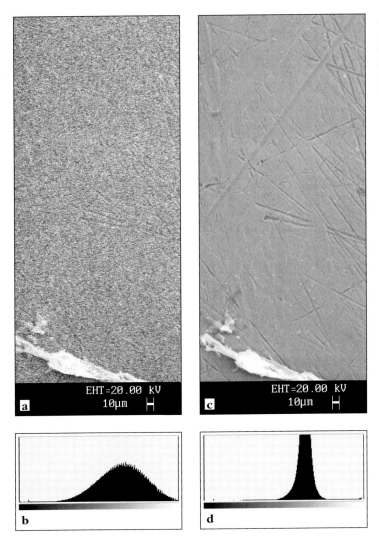

Figure 2. SEM images of a scratched metal surface:
a) 1 second scan;
b) histogram of **(a)**;
c) 20 second scan;
d) histogram of **(c)**.

often collect every frame with no loss of data. The computer program is more flexible, but the time required to add the frames together may result in discarding some of the video frames, so that the total acquisition takes longer (which may not be a problem if the image does not vary with time). Of course, in fluorescence microscopy bleaching may occur and it may be desirable to collect all of the photons as rapidly as possible, either by frame averaging, or, for a very dim image, by using staring mode if the camera is capable of this.

Figure 2 shows a comparison of two SEM images taken at different scan rates. The fast scan image collects few electrons per pixel and so has a high noise level that obscures details in the image. Slowing the scan rate down from one second to 20 seconds increases the amount of signal and reduces the noise. The histograms show that the variation of brightness within the uniform region is reduced, which is why the visibility of detail is improved (Bright et al., 1998).

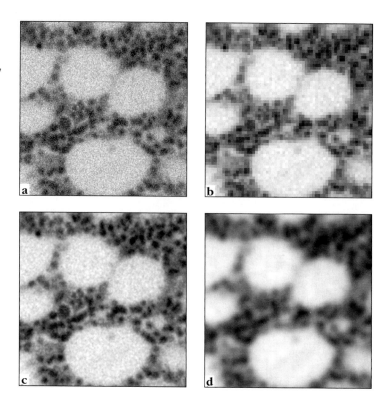

Figure 3. Smoothing by averaging:
a) *a noisy original image (fluorescence light microscopy of bone marrow);*
b) *each 4×4 block of pixels averaged;*
c) *each pixel replaced by the average of itself and its 8 neighbors in a 3×3 square block;*
d) *each pixel replaced by the average of itself and its 120 neighbors in an 11×11 square.*

Neighborhood averaging

The simplest form of spatial averaging is simply to add together the pixel brightness values in each small region of the image, divide by the number of pixels in the neighborhood, and use the resulting value to construct a new image. **Figure 3** shows that this essentially produces an image with a smaller number of pixels. The block size in **Figure 3b** is 4×4, so that sixteen pixel values are added. Since the noise in this image is random due to the counting statistics of the small number of photons, the improvement in image quality or signal-to-noise ratio is just the square root of 16, or a factor of 4. However, the image lateral resolution is seriously impacted and the small structures in the image can no longer be separately discerned.

The more common way to accomplish neighborhood averaging is to replace each pixel with the average of itself and its neighbors. This is often described as a "kernel" operation, since implementation can be generalized as the sum of the pixel values in the region multiplied by a set of integer weights.

$$P^*_{x,y} = \frac{\sum\limits_{i,j=-m}^{+m} W_{i,j} \cdot P_{x+i,\,y+j}}{\sum\limits_{ij=-m}^{+m} W_{i,j}} \tag{1}$$

Equation 1 shows the calculation performed over a square of dimension $2m + 1$, which is odd. The neighborhood sizes thus range from 3×3, upwards to 5×5, 7×7, etc. It is possible, although not common, to use nonsquare regions. The array of weights W for a simple neighbor averaging contains only 1s, and for a 3×3 region could be written as

$$
\begin{array}{ccc}
1 & 1 & 1 \\
1 & 1 & 1 \\
1 & 1 & 1
\end{array}
$$

where we understand the convention that these coefficients are to be multiplied by pixels that surround the central pixel, the total normalized by dividing by the sum of weights, and the value written to the location of the central pixel to form a new image.

As a matter of practicality, since storage space is never unlimited, it is common to write the new image back into the same memory as the original. However, when this is done it is important to use the original pixel values for the summation, and not those new ones which have already been calculated for some of the neighbors. This requires keeping a copy of a few lines of the image during the process.

Neighborhood operations including kernel multiplication are usually applied symmetrically around each pixel. This creates a problem for pixels nearer to the edge of the image than the half-width of the neighborhood. Various approaches are used to deal with this problem, including designing special asymmetrical kernels or rules along edges or in corners, assuming that the image edges are mirrors, so that each line of pixels within the image is duplicated beyond it, or assuming that the image wraps around so that the left edge and right edge, and the top and bottom edges, are continuous. In the examples shown here, an even simpler approach is used: the processing is restricted to that portion of the image where no edge conflicts arise. This leaves lines of unprocessed pixels along the edges of the images, equal in width to half the dimension of the neighborhood. None of these approaches is entirely satisfactory, and in general most processing operations sacrifice some pixels from the image edges.

Figure 3 shows the effect of smoothing using a 3×3 neighborhood average and also an 11×11 neighborhood size. The noise reduction is much greater with the larger region, but is accompanied by a significant blurring of the feature edges.

The amount of blurring can be reduced and more control exerted over the neighborhood averaging procedure by using weight values that are not 1. For example, the values

$$
\begin{array}{ccc}
1 & 2 & 1 \\
2 & 4 & 2 \\
1 & 2 & 1
\end{array}
$$

have several attractive characteristics. First, the central 4 which multiplies the original pixel contents is the largest factor, causing the central pixel to dominate the average and reducing blurring. The values of 2 for the four orthogonally touching neighbors and 1 for the four diagonally touching neighbors acknowledge the fact that the diagonal pixels are in fact farther away from the center of the neighborhood (actually by the factor $\sqrt{2}$). Finally, these weights have a total value of 16, which is a power of two and consequently very easy to divide by quickly in a computer implementation of this averaging procedure.

Similar sets of ad hoc weight values can be devised in various sizes. Integers are used to speed implementation, and storage requirements are modest. We will see in Chapter 5, in the context of processing images in frequency space, that these kernels can be analyzed quite efficiently in that domain to understand their smoothing properties. It turns out from that analysis that one of the very useful "shapes" for a weight kernel is that of a Gaussian. This is a set of integers that approximate the profile of a Gaussian function along any row, column or diagonal through the center. It is characterized by a standard deviation, expressed in terms of pixel dimensions. The size of the kernel is generally made large enough that adding another row of terms would insert negligibly small numbers, ideally zeroes into the array, but of course some zero values will be present anyway in the corners since they are farther from the central pixel.

Choosing the actual integers is something of an art, at least for the larger kernels, since the goal is to approximate the smooth analytical curve of the Gaussian. However, the total of the weights must usually be kept smaller than some practical limit to facilitate the computer arithmetic (Russ, 1995d). Several Gaussian kernels are shown below, with standard deviations that increase in geometric proportions from less than one pixel to many pixels. The standard deviation for these kernels is the radius (in pixels) containing 68% of the integrated magnitude of the coefficients, or the volume under the surface if the kernel is pictured as a 3D plot of the integer values. This is a two-dimensional generalization of the usual definition of standard deviation; for a one-dimensional Gaussian distribution, 68% of the area under the curve lies within ± one standard deviation.

Of course, the kernel size increases with the standard deviation as well. For the largest examples shown below, only the upper left quadrant of the symmetrical array is shown. Repeated application of a small kernel, or the sequential application of two or more kernels, is equivalent to the single application of a larger one, which can be constructed as the convolution of the two kernels (applying the weighting factors from one kernel to those in the other as if they were pixel values, and summing and adding to generate a new, larger array of weights).

σ=0.391 pixels (3x3)
```
 1  4  1
 4 12  4
 1  4  1
```

σ=0.625 pixels (5x5)
```
 1  2  3  2  1
 2  7 11  7  2
 3 11 17 11  3
 2  7 11  7  2
 1  2  3  2  1
```

σ=1.0 pixels (9x9)
```
 0  0  1  1  1  1  1  0  0
 0  1  2  3  3  3  2  1  0
 1  2  3  6  7  6  3  2  1
 1  3  6  9 11  9  6  3  1
 1  3  7 11 12 11  7  3  1
 1  3  6  9 11  9  6  3  1
 1  2  3  6  7  6  3  2  1
 0  1  2  3  3  3  2  1  0
 0  0  1  1  1  1  1  0  0
```

σ=1.6 pixels (11x11)
```
 1  1  1  2  2  2  2  1  1  1
 1  2  2  3  4  4  3  2  2  1
 1  2  4  5  6  7  6  5  4  2  1
 2  3  5  7  8  9  8  7  5  3  2
 2  4  6  8 10 11 10  8  6  4  2
 2  4  7  9 11 12 11  9  7  4  2
 2  4  6  8 10 11 10  8  6  4  2
 2  3  5  7  8  9  8  7  5  3  2
 1  2  4  5  6  7  6  5  4  2  1
 1  2  2  3  4  4  3  2  2  1
 1  1  1  2  2  2  2  1  1  1
```

σ=2.56 pixels (15x15)
```
 2  2  3  4  5  5  6  6  6  5  5  4  3  2  2
 2  3  4  5  7  7  8  8  8  7  7  5  4  3  2
 3  4  6  7  9 10 10 11 10 10  9  7  6  4  3
 4  5  7  9 10 12 13 13 13 12 10  9  7  5  4
 5  7  9 11 13 14 15 16 15 14 13 11  9  7  5
 5  7 10 12 14 16 17 18 17 16 14 12 10  7  5
 6  8 10 13 15 17 19 19 19 17 15 13 10  8  6
 6  8 11 13 16 18 19 20 19 18 16 13 11  8  6
 6  8 10 13 15 17 19 19 19 17 15 13 10  8  6
 5  7 10 12 14 16 17 18 17 16 14 12 10  7  5
 5  7  9 11 13 14 15 16 15 14 13 11  9  7  5
 4  5  7  9 10 12 13 13 13 12 10  9  7  5  4
 3  4  6  7  9 10 10 11 10 10  9  7  6  4  3
 2  3  4  5  7  7  8  8  8  7  7  5  4  3  2
 2  2  3  4  5  5  6  6  6  5  5  4  3  2  2
```

σ=4.096 pixels (21x21)
```
 5  6  7  8  9 10 11 12 13 13 13 13 13 12 11 10  9  8  7  6  5
 6  7  9 10 11 12 14 15 15 16 16 16 15 15 14 12 11 10  9  7  6
 7  9 10 12 13 15 16 17 18 18 19 18 18 17 16 15 13 12 10  9  7
 8 10 12 13 15 17 18 20 21 21 21 21 20 18 17 15 13 12 10  8
 9 11 13 15 17 19 21 22 23 24 24 24 23 22 21 19 17 15 13 11  9
10 12 15 17 19 21 23 25 26 27 27 27 26 25 23 21 19 17 15 12 10
11 14 16 18 21 23 25 27 28 29 29 29 28 27 25 23 21 18 16 14 11
12 15 17 20 22 25 27 29 30 31 31 31 30 29 27 25 22 20 17 15 12
13 15 18 21 23 26 28 30 32 33 33 33 32 30 28 26 23 21 18 15 13
13 16 18 21 24 27 29 31 33 34 34 34 33 31 29 27 24 21 18 16 13
13 16 19 21 24 27 29 31 33 34 34 34 33 31 29 27 24 21 19 16 13
13 16 18 21 24 27 29 31 33 34 34 34 33 31 29 27 24 21 18 16 13
13 15 18 21 23 26 28 30 32 33 33 33 32 30 28 26 23 21 18 15 13
12 15 17 20 22 25 27 29 30 31 31 31 30 29 27 25 22 20 17 15 12
11 14 16 18 21 23 25 27 28 29 29 29 28 27 25 23 21 18 16 14 11
10 12 15 17 19 21 23 25 26 27 27 27 26 25 23 21 19 17 15 12 10
 9 11 13 15 17 19 21 22 23 24 24 24 23 22 21 19 17 15 13 11  9
 8 10 12 13 15 17 18 20 21 21 21 21 20 18 17 15 13 12 10  8
 7  9 10 12 13 15 16 17 18 18 19 18 18 17 16 15 13 12 10  9  7
 6  7  9 10 11 12 14 15 15 16 16 16 15 15 14 12 11 10  9  7  6
 5  6  7  8  9 10 11 12 13 13 13 13 13 12 11 10  9  8  7  6  5
```

Figure 4 shows two of these, the 5×5 and 43×43 Gaussian kernels, plotted as an isometric view. Notice that even with the large kernel, the quantization of the weights using integers produces some distortion.

In subsequent sections on image processing, we will see other uses for these kernels in which the weights are not symmetrical

```
σ=6.536 pixels (29x29)
 7  8  9 10 10 11 12 13 13 14 14 15 15 15 15 ...
 8  9 10 11 11 12 13 14 15 15 16 16 16 17 17 ...
 9 10 11 12 13 13 14 15 16 17 17 18 18 18 18 ...
10 11 12 13 14 15 16 17 17 18 19 19 20 20 20 ...
10 11 13 14 15 16 17 18 19 20 20 21 21 21 21 ...
11 12 13 15 16 17 18 19 20 21 22 22 23 23 23 ...
12 13 14 16 17 18 19 20 21 22 23 24 24 24 24 ...
13 14 15 17 18 19 20 22 23 24 24 25 25 26 26 ...
13 15 16 17 19 20 21 23 24 25 26 26 27 27 27 ...
14 15 17 18 20 21 22 24 25 26 27 27 28 28 28 ...
14 16 17 19 20 22 23 24 26 27 28 28 29 29 29 ...
15 16 18 19 21 22 24 25 26 27 28 29 30 30 30 ...
15 16 18 20 21 23 24 25 27 28 29 30 30 30 31 ...
15 17 18 20 21 23 24 26 27 28 29 30 30 31 31 ...
15 17 18 20 21 23 24 26 27 28 29 30 31 31 31 ...
```

```
σ=10.486 pixels (43x43)
 6  6  6  7  7  7  8  8  8  9  9  9  9 10 10 10 10 10 10 10 11 11 ...
 6  6  7  7  7  8  8  8  9  9  9  9 10 10 10 10 11 11 11 11 11 11 ...
 6  7  7  7  8  8  9  9  9 10 10 10 11 11 11 11 11 12 12 12 12 12 ...
 7  7  7  8  8  9  9  9 10 10 10 11 11 11 12 12 12 12 12 12 13 ...
 7  7  8  8  9  9  9 10 10 11 11 11 12 12 12 12 13 13 13 13 13 13 ...
 7  8  8  9  9 10 10 10 11 11 12 12 12 13 13 13 13 13 14 14 14 14 ...
 8  8  9  9 10 10 11 11 12 12 13 13 13 14 14 14 14 14 14 14 ...
 8  8  9  9 10 10 11 11 12 12 13 13 13 14 14 14 15 15 15 15 15 ...
 8  9  9 10 10 11 11 12 12 13 13 14 14 14 15 15 15 15 15 16 16 16 ...
 9  9 10 10 11 11 12 12 13 13 14 14 14 15 15 15 16 16 16 16 16 ...
 9  9 10 10 11 11 12 12 13 13 14 14 15 15 15 16 16 16 16 17 17 17 ...
 9 10 10 11 11 12 12 13 13 14 14 15 15 15 16 16 16 17 17 17 17 17 ...
 9 10 11 11 12 12 13 13 14 14 15 15 16 16 17 17 17 18 18 18 ...
 9 10 11 11 12 12 13 13 14 14 15 15 16 16 17 17 17 18 18 18 18 ...
10 10 11 11 12 13 13 14 14 15 15 16 16 17 17 17 18 18 18 18 18 18 ...
10 10 11 12 12 13 13 14 15 15 16 16 17 17 17 18 18 18 18 19 19 19 ...
10 11 11 12 12 13 14 14 15 15 16 16 17 17 18 18 18 19 19 19 19 ...
10 11 11 12 13 13 14 15 15 16 16 17 17 18 18 18 19 19 19 19 19 19 ...
10 11 12 12 13 13 14 15 15 16 16 17 17 18 18 19 19 19 19 19 19 ...
10 11 12 12 13 14 14 15 15 16 17 17 18 18 19 19 19 19 19 20 20 ...
10 11 12 12 13 14 14 15 15 16 17 17 18 18 19 19 19 19 20 20 20 ...
10 11 12 12 13 14 14 15 16 16 17 17 18 18 19 19 19 19 20 20 20 ...
11 11 12 12 13 14 14 15 16 16 17 17 18 18 19 19 19 20 20 20 20 ...
11 11 12 13 13 14 14 15 16 16 17 17 18 18 19 19 19 20 20 20 20 ...
```

```
σ=16.777 pixels (55x55)
 5  5  5  5  5  5  5  6  6  6  6  6  6  6  6  7  7  7  7  7  7  7  7  7  7  7  7  7  7  7  7 ...
 5  5  5  5  5  6  6  6  6  6  6  6  6  7  7  7  7  7  7  7  7  7  7  7  7  7  7  7  7  7  7 ...
 5  5  5  5  6  6  6  6  6  6  6  6  7  7  7  7  7  7  7  7  7  7  7  7  7  7  7  7  7  7  7 ...
 5  5  5  6  6  6  6  6  6  6  7  7  7  7  7  7  7  7  7  8  8  8  8  8  8  8  8  8 ...
 5  5  6  6  6  6  6  6  6  7  7  7  7  7  7  7  7  7  8  8  8  8  8  8  8  8  8  8 ...
 5  6  6  6  6  6  6  6  7  7  7  7  7  7  7  7  8  8  8  8  8  8  8  8  8  8  8  8 ...
 5  6  6  6  6  6  6  7  7  7  7  7  7  7  7  8  8  8  8  8  8  8  8  8  8  8  8  8 ...
 6  6  6  6  6  6  7  7  7  7  7  7  7  8  8  8  8  8  8  8  8  8  8  8  8  8  8  8 ...
 6  6  6  6  6  7  7  7  7  7  7  8  8  8  8  8  8  8  8  9  9  9  9  9  9  9  9 ...
 6  6  6  6  7  7  7  7  7  7  8  8  8  8  8  8  8  8  8  9  9  9  9  9  9  9  9  9 ...
 6  6  6  7  7  7  7  7  8  8  8  8  8  8  8  9  9  9  9  9  9  9  9  9  9  9  9 ...
 6  6  6  7  7  7  7  7  8  8  8  8  8  8  8  9  9  9  9  9  9  9  9  9  9  9  9 ...
 6  6  7  7  7  7  7  8  8  8  8  8  8  8  9  9  9  9  9  9  9  9  9  9  9  9  9 ...
 6  7  7  7  7  7  8  8  8  8  8  9  9  9  9  9  9  9  9  9  9  9  9 10 10 10 ...
 6  7  7  7  7  7  8  8  8  8  8  9  9  9  9  9  9  9  9  9  9 10 10 10 10 10 10 ...
 7  7  7  7  7  8  8  8  8  8  9  9  9  9  9  9  9  9  9 10 10 10 10 10 10 10 ...
 7  7  7  7  7  8  8  8  8  8  9  9  9  9  9  9  9 10 10 10 10 10 10 10 10 10 ...
 7  7  7  7  8  8  8  8  8  9  9  9  9  9  9  9 10 10 10 10 10 10 10 10 10 10 ...
 7  7  7  7  8  8  8  8  8  9  9  9  9  9  9 10 10 10 10 10 10 10 10 10 10 10 ...
 7  7  7  7  8  8  8  8  8  9  9  9  9  9  9 10 10 10 10 10 10 10 10 10 10 10 10 ...
 7  7  7  8  8  8  8  8  9  9  9  9  9  9 10 10 10 10 10 10 10 10 10 10 10 10 ...
 7  7  7  8  8  8  8  8  9  9  9  9  9  9 10 10 10 10 10 10 10 10 10 11 11 11 11 ...
 7  7  7  8  8  8  8  9  9  9  9  9  9 10 10 10 10 10 10 10 10 10 11 11 11 11 11 ...
 7  7  7  8  8  8  8  9  9  9  9  9  9 10 10 10 10 10 10 10 10 11 11 11 11 11 11 ...
 7  7  7  8  8  8  8  8  9  9  9  9  9 10 10 10 10 10 10 10 10 11 11 11 11 11 ...
 7  7  7  8  8  8  8  8  9  9  9  9  9 10 10 10 10 10 10 10 10 11 11 11 11 11 ...
```

in magnitude or not all positive. The implementation of the kernel will remain the same, except that when negative weights are present the normalization is usually performed by division by the sum of the positive values only (because in these cases the sum of all the weights is usually zero). For the present our interest is restricted to smoothing of noise in images.

Figure 5 shows the same noisy image as **Figure 3**, along with an image of the same region using image averaging to reduce the

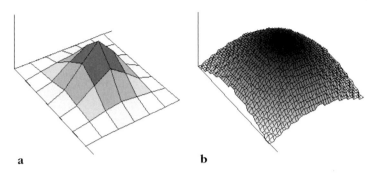

Figure 4. Isometric plots of the integers used as weight values in the Gaussian smoothing kernels:
a) *5×5, σ = 0.625 pixels;*
b) *43×43, σ = 10.486 pixels*

statistical noise, as described in Chapter 1. The figure also shows an enlargement of a portion of the image in which the individual pixels can be discerned, as an aid to judging the pixel-to-pixel noise variations in uniform regions and the sharpness of boundaries between different structures. Applying smoothing with the 5×5 kernel corresponding to a Gaussian shape with a standard deviation of 0.625 pixels produces the improvement in quality shown in **Figure 6** (for two applications of the kernel). Using a larger kernel (the 9×9 kernel with standard deviation of 1.0 pixels, applied once) produces the result shown.

This type of averaging can reduce visible noise in the image, but it also blurs edges, displaces boundaries, and reduces contrast. It can even introduce an artefact often called "pseudo-resolution"

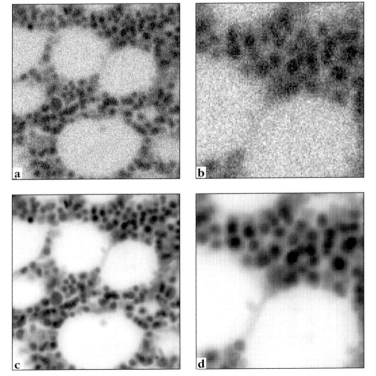

Figure 5. Test image for several neighborhood smoothing operations:
a) *original light microscope fluorescence image of bone marrow, obtained by averaging four video frames;*
b) *enlargement of a portion of image **a** to show individual pixels;*
c) *an image of the same specimen area with reduced noise obtained by averaging 256 video frames;*
d) *the same enlargement of image **c**.*

Figure 6. Neighborhood smoothing with Gaussian kernels:

a) *two applications of a 5×5 kernel with standard deviation of 0.625 pixels;*

b) *enlargement of image **a** to show pixel detail;*

c) *one application of a 9×9 kernel with standard deviation of 1.0 pixels;*

d) *the same enlargement of image **b**.*

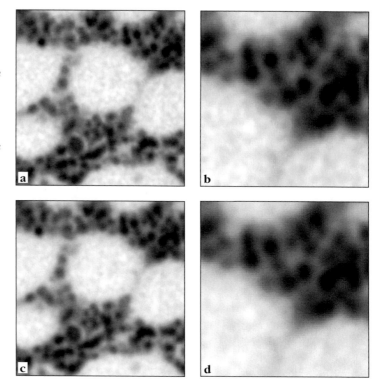

or "aliasing" when two nearby structures are averaged together in a way that creates an apparent feature between them. **Figure 7** shows an example in which the lines of the test pattern are blurred by the 11×11 averaging window causing false lines to appear between them.

Smoothing of one-dimensional signal profiles, such as X-ray diffraction patterns, spectra, or time-varying electronic signals, is often performed using a Savitsky and Golay (1964) fitting procedure. Tables of coefficients published for this purpose (and intended for efficient application in dedicated computers) are designed to be used just as the weighting coefficients discussed above, except that they operate in only one dimension. The process is equivalent to performing a least-squares fit of the data points to a polynomial. The smoothed profiles preserve the

Figure 7. *Pseudo-resolution due to smoothing. Applying an 11×11 unweighted smoothing kernel to the test pattern in image **a** produces apparent lines between the original ones, as shown in image **b**.*

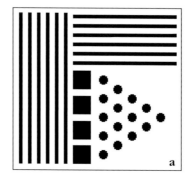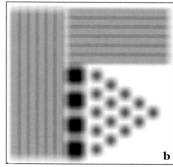

Table 1. Savitsky and Golay fitting coefficients

Quadratic polynomial fit

5	7	9	11	13	15	17	19
0	0	0	0	0	0	0	−.0602
0	0	0	0	0	0	−.065	−.0226
0	0	0	0	0	−.0706	−.0186	.0106
0	0	0	0	−.0769	−.0118	.0217	.0394
0	0	0	−.0839	0	.038	.0557	.0637
0	0	−.0909	.021	.0629	.0787	.0836	.0836
0	−.0952	.0606	.1026	.1119	.1104	.1053	.0991
−.0857	.1429	.1688	.1608	.1469	.133	.1207	.1101
.3429	.2857	.2338	.1958	.1678	.1466	.13	.1168
.4857	.3333	.2554	.2075	.1748	.1511	.1331	.119
.3429	.2857	.2338	.1958	.1678	.1466	.13	.1168
−.0857	.1429	.1688	.1608	.1469	.133	.1207	.1101
0	−.0952	.0606	.1026	.1119	.1104	.1053	.0991
0	0	−.0909	.021	.0629	.0787	.0836	.0836
0	0	0	−.0839	0	.038	.0557	.0637
0	0	0	0	−.0769	−.0118	.0217	.0394
0	0	0	0	0	−.0706	−.0186	.0106
0	0	0	0	0	0	−.065	−.0226
0	0	0	0	0	0	0	−.0602

Quartic polynomial fit

5	7	9	11	13	15	17	19
0	0	0	0	0	0	.0464	−.0343
0	0	0	0	0	.0464	−.0464	−.0565
0	0	0	0	.0452	−.0619	−.0619	−.039
0	0	0	.042	−.0814	−.0636	−.0279	.0024
0	0	.035	−.1049	−.0658	−.0036	.0322	.0545
0	.0216	−.1282	−.0233	.0452	.0813	.0988	.1063
.25	−.1299	.0699	.1399	.1604	.1624	.1572	.1494
−.5	.3247	.3147	.2797	.2468	.2192	.1965	.1777
1.5	.5671	.4172	.3333	.2785	.2395	.2103	.1875
−.5	.3247	.3147	.2797	.2468	.2192	.1965	.1777
.25	−.1299	.0699	.1399	.1604	.1624	.1572	.1494
0	.0216	−.1282	−.0233	.0452	.0813	.0988	.1063
0	0	.035	−.1049	−.0658	−.0036	.0322	.0545
0	0	0	.042	−.0814	−.0636	−.0279	.0024
0	0	0	0	.0452	−.0619	−.0619	−.039
0	0	0	0	0	.0464	−.0464	−.0565
0	0	0	0	0	0	.0464	−.0343
0	0	0	0	0	0	0	.0458

magnitude of steps while smoothing out noise. **Table 1** lists these coefficients for second (quadratic) and fourth (quartic) power polynomials, for fits extending over neighborhoods ranging from 5 to 19 points. These profiles are plotted in **Figure 8**.

This same method can be extended to two dimensions, of course (Edwards, 1982). This can be done either by first applying the coefficients in the horizontal direction and then in the vertical

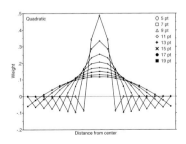
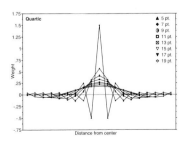

Figure 8. Savitsky and Golay linear smoothing weights for least-squares fitting to quadratic and quartic polynomials.

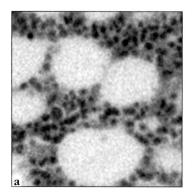 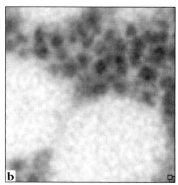

Figure 9. Smoothing with a 7-point-wide, quadratic Savitsky and Golay fit:
a) *same image as Figure 5, smoothed;*
b) *enlarged to show pixel detail.*

direction, or by constructing a full 2-D kernel. Since the points in the kernel are not all at integer distances from the center, calculation of additional weight values is needed for each specific 2D case. **Figure 9** shows the application of a 7×7 Savitsky and Golay quadratic polynomial to smooth the image from **Figure 5**.

It is interesting to compare the results of this spatial-domain smoothing to that which can be accomplished in the frequency domain. As discussed in Chapter 5, multiplication of the frequency transform by a convolution function is equivalent to application of a kernel in the spatial domain. The most common noise-filtering method is to remove high frequency information, which represents pixel-to-pixel variations associated with noise. Such removal may be done by setting an aperture on the two-dimensional transform, eliminating higher frequencies, and retransforming. **Figure 10** shows the result of applying this technique to the same image as in **Figure 5**. A circular low-pass filter with radius = 35 pixels and a 10-pixel-wide cosine edge shape (the importance of these parameters is discussed in Chapter 5) was applied. The smoothing is similar to that accomplished in the spatial domain.

Neighborhood ranking

The use of weighting kernels to average together pixels in a neighborhood is a convolution operation, which has a direct

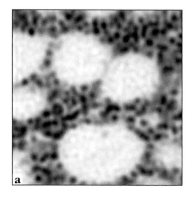 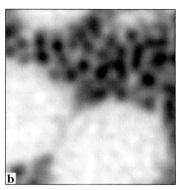

Figure 10. Smoothing in frequency space, using a circular low-pass filter with radius = 35 pixels and a 10-pixel-wide cosine edge shape:
a) *application to image in Figure 5;*
b) *enlargement to show pixel detail.*

counterpart in frequency space image processing. It is a linear operation in which no information is lost from the original image. There are other processing operations that can be performed in neighborhoods in the spatial domain that also provide noise smoothing. These are not linear and do not utilize or preserve all of the original data.

The most widely used of these methods is based on ranking of the pixels in a neighborhood according to brightness. Then, for example, the median value in this ordered list can be used as the brightness value for the central pixel. As in the case of the kernel operations, this is used to produce a new image and only the original pixel values are used in the ranking for the neighborhood around each pixel.

The median filter is an excellent rejector of certain kinds of noise, for instance "shot" noise in which individual pixels are corrupted or missing from the image. If a pixel is accidentally changed to an extreme value, it will be eliminated from the image and replaced by a "reasonable" value, the median value in the neighborhood.

Figure 11 shows an example of this type of noise. Ten percent of the pixels in the original image, selected randomly, are set to black, and another ten percent to white. This is a rather extreme amount of noise. However, a median filter is able to remove the noise and replace the bad pixels with reasonable values while causing a minimal distortion or degradation of the image. Two different neighborhoods are used: a 3×3 square containing a total of nine pixels, and a 5×5 octagonal region containing a total of 21 pixels. **Figure 12** shows several of the neighborhood regions often used for ranking. Of course, the computational effort required rises quickly with the number of values to be sorted, even using specialized methods which keep partial sets of the pixels ranked separately so that as the neighborhood is moved across the image, only a few additional pixel comparisons are needed.

Application of a median filter can also be used to reduce the type of random noise shown before in the context of averaging. **Figure 13** shows the same image as in **Figure 5**, with a 5×5 octagonal median filter applied. There are two principal advantages to the median filter as compared to multiplication by weights. First, the method does not reduce the brightness difference across steps, because the values available are only those present in the neighborhood region, not an average between those values. Second, median filtering does not shift boundaries as averaging may, depending on the relative magnitude of values present in the neighborhood. Overcoming these problems makes the median filter preferred both for visual examination and measurement of images (Huang, 1979, Yang and Huang, 1981).

The minimal degradation to edges from median filtering allows repeated application of the method. **Figure 14** shows an example

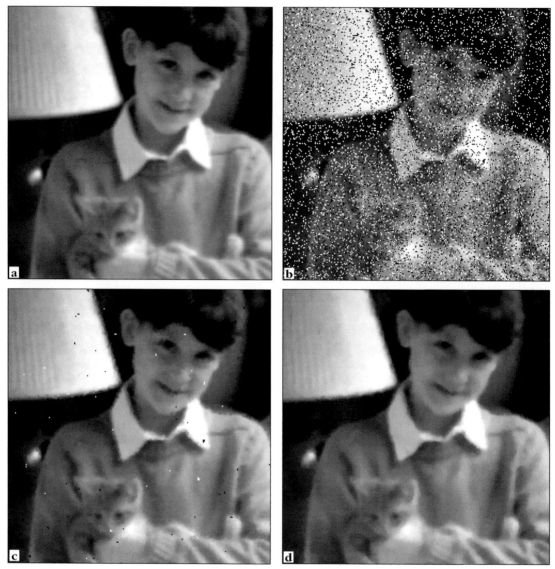

Figure 11. Removal of shot noise with a median filter:

a) *original image;*

b) *image **a** with 10% of the pixels randomly selected and set to black, and another 10% randomly selected and set to white;*

c) *application of median filtering to image **b** using a 3×3 square region;*

d) *application of median filtering to image **b** using a 5×5 octagonal region.*

in which a 5×5 octagonal median filter was applied 12 times to an image. The fine detail is erased in this process, and large regions take on the same brightness values. However, the edges remain in place and well defined. This type of leveling of brightness due to repetition of median filtering is sometimes described as contouring or posterization.

The concept of a median filter requires a ranking order for the pixels in the neighborhood, which for grey scale images is simply

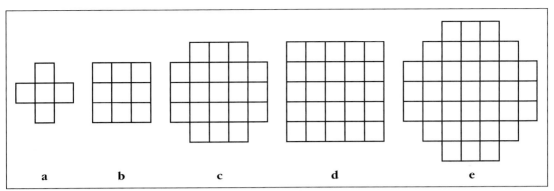

Figure 12. Neighborhood patterns used for median filtering:
a) *4 nearest-neighbor cross;* ***b)*** *3×3 square containing nine pixels;* ***c)*** *5×5 octagonal region with 21 pixels;*
   d) *5×5 square containing 25 pixels;* ***e)*** *7×7 octagonal region containing 37 pixels.*

provided by the pixel value. Color images present a challenge to this idea. A color median filter can be devised by using as the definition of the median value that pixel whose color coordinates give the smallest sum-of-squares of distances to the other pixels in the neighborhood (Astolo et al., 1990; Oistämö & Neuvo, 1990; Russ, 1995b). The choice of the color space in which these coordinate distances are measured can also present a problem. As discussed before, HSI space is generally preferred for processing to RGB space, but there is no single answer to the question of the relative scaling factors of these different spaces, or how to deal with the angular measure of hue values. **Figure 15** shows an example of a color median filter.

Sharpening of edges can be accomplished even better with a mode filter (Davies, 1988). The mode of the distribution of brightness values in each neighborhood is, by definition, the

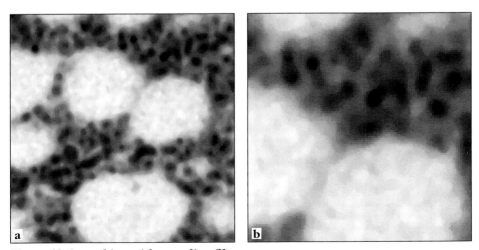

Figure 13. Smoothing with a median filter:
a) *the same image as in Figure 5 after application of a 5×5 octagonal median filter;*
b) *enlargement of image* ***a*** *to show individual pixels.*

Figure 14. Repeated application of a 5×5 octagonal median filter:
a) *original image;*
b) *after 12 applications. The fine details have been erased and textured regions leveled to a uniform shade of grey, but boundaries have not shifted.*

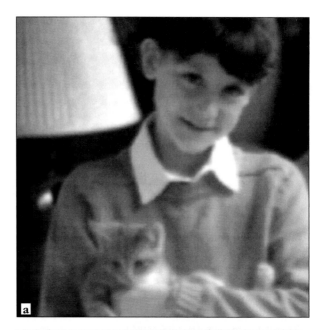

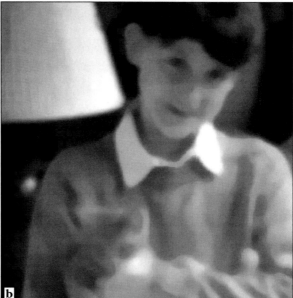

most likely value. However, for a small neighborhood, the mode is poorly defined. An approximation to this value can be obtained with a truncated median filter. For any asymmetric distribution, such as would be obtained at most locations near but not precisely straddling an edge, the mode is the highest point, and the median lies closer to the mode than the mean value. This is illustrated in **Figure 16**. The truncated median technique consists of discarding a few values from the neighborhood so that the median value of the remaining pixels is shifted toward the mode. In the example shown in **Figure 17**, this is done for

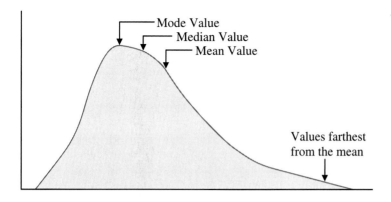

Mode Value
Median Value
Mean Value

Values farthest
from the mean

Figure 15. Schematic diagram of an asymmetric histogram distribution of brightness values, showing the relationship between the mode, median, and mean. The truncated median filter works by discarding the values in the distribution which are farthest from the mean, and then using the median of the remainder as an estimate for the mode. For a symmetrical distribution, values are discarded from both ends and the median value does not change (it is already equal to the mode).

a 3×3 neighborhood by skipping the two pixels whose brightness values are most different from the mean, ranking the remaining seven values, and assigning the median to the central pixel. This has the effect of sharpening steps, and produces posterization when it is applied repeatedly.

Another modification to the median filter is used to overcome its tendency to erase lines which are narrower than the half-width of the neighborhood, and to round corners. The so-called hybrid median, or edge-preserving median, is actually a three-step ranking operation (Nieminen et al., 1987). In a 5×5 pixel neighborhood, pixels are ranked in two different groups as shown in **Figure 18**. The median values of the 45-degree neighbors forming an "X" and the 90-degree neighbors forming a "+" (both groups include the central pixel) are compared to the central pixel and the median value of that set is then saved as the new pixel value. As shown in **Figure 19**, this method preserves lines and corners which are erased or rounded off by the conventional median, even one of smaller size which does a poorer job of eliminating noise.

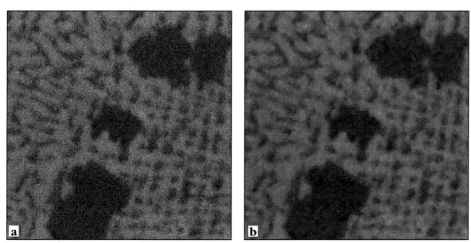

Figure 16. Application of a median filter to a noisy color image:
a) *image with noise;*
b) *median filter applied.*

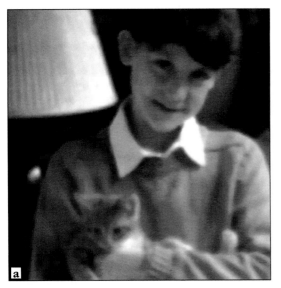

a

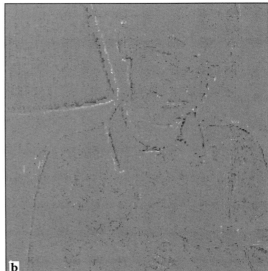

b

Figure 17. Application of the truncated median filter to posterize the image from Figure 11:

a) one application of the 3×3 truncated median;

b) difference between Figure *a* and a conventional 3×3 median filter, showing the difference in values along edges;

c) 12 applications of the truncated median filter.

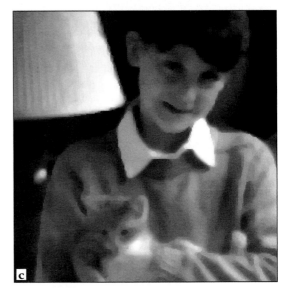

c

Figure 18. Diagram of pixels in a 5×5 neighborhood to show the groups used in the hybrid median filter. The two separately ranked groups are the vertical/horizontal lines and the diagonal lines, shown in different colors. Both groups include the central pixel. The ranked median of each group, and the central pixel, are then ranked again to select the overall median value. The white pixels are not used in the operation.

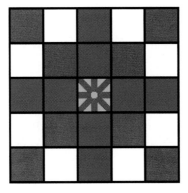

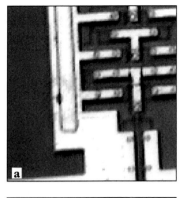

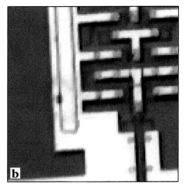

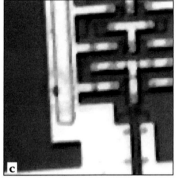

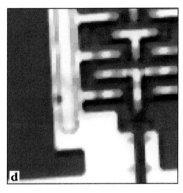

Figure 19. Application of the hybrid median filter to a light microscope image of an integrated circuit, showing the improved retention of lines and corners:

a) *original image with noise;*

b) *application of the 5×5 hybrid median filter;*

c) *application of a conventional 3×3 median, which does not remove all of the noise but still degrades corners and edges somewhat;*

d) *application of a conventional 5×5 filter, showing its effect on corners and edges.*

If the hybrid median filter is applied repeatedly, it can also produce posterization. Because the details of lines and corners are better preserved by the hybrid median than by a conventional neighborhood median, the shapes of regions are not smoothed as much, although the brightness values across steps are still sharpened and posterized, as illustrated in **Figure 20**.

The fact that the hybrid median involves three ranking operations, first within each of the two groups of pixels and then to compare those medians to the central pixel, does not impose a serious computational penalty. Each of the ranking operations is for a much smaller number of values than used in a square or octagonal region of the same size. For example, the 5 pixel wide neighborhood used in the examples contains either 25 (in the square neighborhood) or 21 pixels (in the octagonal neighborhood) which must be ranked in the traditional method. In the hybrid method, each of the two groups contains only 9 pixels, and the final comparison involves only three values. Even with the additional logic and manipulation of values, the hybrid method is at least as fast as the conventional median.

Posterizing an image, or reducing the number of grey levels so that regions become uniform in grey value and edges between regions become abrupt, falls more into the category of enhancement than correcting defects, but is included here as a side-effect of median filtering. Other methods can produce this effect. One that is related to the median is the extremum filter, which

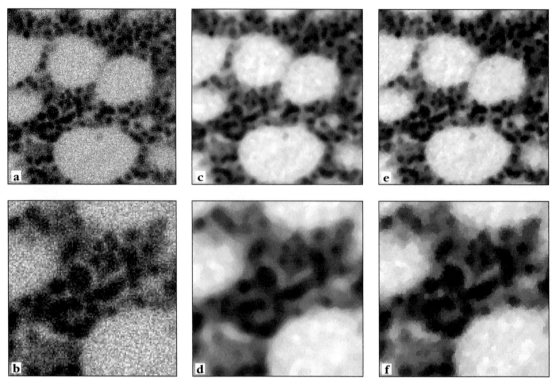

Figure 20. Repeated application of the hybrid median filter to the noisy image in Figure 3:
a) original image;
b) zoomed portion of *a* showing individual pixels;
c) repeated application of a conventional 5-pixel-wide median filter;
d) zoomed portion of *c* showing individual pixels;
e) repeated application of the hybrid 5-pixel-wide median filter;
f) zoomed portion of *e* showing individual pixels.
Notice that the brightness values are posterized and smoothed and edge contrast is sharpened, but the shapes of features and edges are not smoothed.

replaces each pixel value with either the minimum or maximum value in the neighborhood, whichever is closer to the mean value. **Figure 21** shows this operator applied to the image from **Figure 19**. This filter is not edge-preserving and may shift boundaries.

Other neighborhood noise reduction methods

A modification to the simple averaging of neighborhood values which attempts to achieve some of the advantages of the median filter is the so-called Olympic filter. The name comes from the system of scoring used in some events in the Olympic games, in which the highest and lowest scores are discarded and the remainder averaged. The same thing is done with the pixel values in the neighborhood. By discarding the extreme values, shot noise is rejected. Then the average of the remaining pixel values is used as the new brightness.

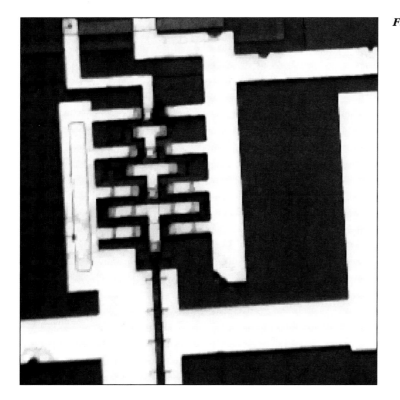

Figure 21. Posterization of the image from Figure 19, produced by applying a 3×3 extremum filter which replaces each pixel value with either the minimum or maximum value in the neighborhood, whichever is closer to the mean value.

Figure 22 shows an application of this method to the image from **Figure 3**, containing Gaussian noise (random intensity variations due to counting statistics). Because it still causes blurring of edges, is not easily adapted to weighting values that take into account the original pixel locations, and still requires sorting of the brightness values, this method is generally inferior to the others discussed and is not often used. **Figure 23** shows an application to the shot noise introduced in **Figure 11**. The performance is quite poor: the features are blurred and yet the noise is not all removed.

There are other, more complicated combinations of operations that are used for very specific types of images. For instance, synthetic aperture radar (SAR) images contain speckle noise which varies in a known way with the image brightness. To remove the

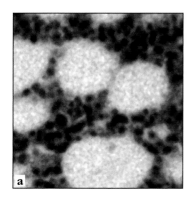
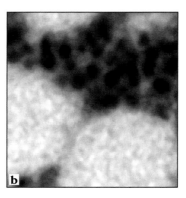

Figure 22. Application of an Olympic filter to Gaussian noise. The 4 brightest and 4 darkest pixels in each 5×5 neighborhood are ignored and the remaining 17 averaged to produce a new image:
a) *application to image in Figure 2;*
b) *enlargement to show pixel detail.*

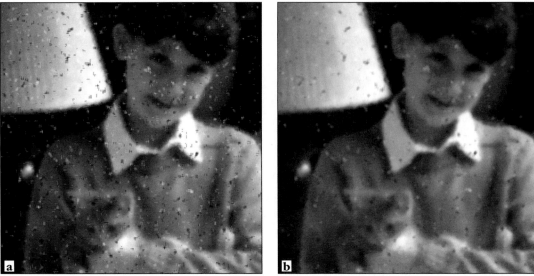

Figure 23. Application of Olympic filter to shot noise. The original image is the same as in Figure 11:
a) *the 2 brightest and 2 darkest pixels in each 3×3 neighborhood are ignored and the remaining 5 averaged;*
b) *the 4 brightest and 4 darkest pixels in each 5×5 neighborhood are ignored and the remaining 17 averaged.*

noise, the brightness of each pixel is compared to the average value of a local neighborhood. If it exceeds it by an amount calculated from the average and the standard deviation, then it is replaced by a weighted average value. Using some coefficients determined by experiment, the method is reported (Nathan & Curlander, 1990) to perform better at improving signal-to-noise than a simple median filter. This is a good example of an ad hoc processing method based on some knowledge of the characteristics of the signal and the noise in a particular situation. In general, any filtering method that chooses between several algorithms or modifies its algorithm based on the actual contents of the image or the neighborhood is called an adaptive filter (Mastin, 1985).

Another way of filtering by ranking is to use the maximum and minimum brightness rather than the median. **Figure 24** shows the results of a two-step operation. First, the brightest pixel value in each region (a 5×5 octagonal neighborhood) was used to replace the original pixel values. Then in a second transformation, the darkest pixel value in each region was selected. This type of combined operation requires two full passes through the image, and during each pass only the previous pixel brightness values are used to derive the new ones.

For reasons that will be discussed in more detail in Chapter 7, this type of operation is often described as a grey scale erosion and dilation, by analogy to the erosion and dilation steps which are performed on binary images. The sequence is also called an opening, again by analogy to operations on binary images. By adjusting the sizes of the neighborhoods (which need not be the same) used in the two separate passes, to locate the brightest and

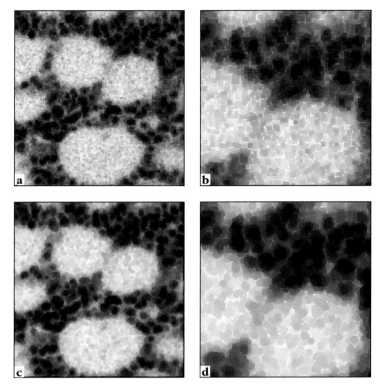

Figure 24. Grey scale opening, or erosion and dilation. Two separate ranking operations are performed on the original image from Figure 5. First each pixel value is replaced with the brightest value in the neighborhood; then using this image, each pixel value is replaced by the darkest value in the same size neighborhood:
a) application using a 3×3 square neighborhood;
b) enlargement to show pixel detail;
c) application using a 5×5 octagonal neighborhood;
d) enlarged to show pixel detail.

then the darkest values, other processing effects are obtained. These are described in Chapter 4.

A major purpose for this type of processing is to prepare an image for brightness thresholding (discussed in Chapter 6) to delineate regions for measurement. The idea is that with appropriate processing, a particular type of feature will appear with the same brightness level anywhere in the image. Then the brightness level can be used to select the pixels that make up the feature. For a noisy image, processing is needed before this assumption can be made.

Comparison of two methods for dealing with "noisy" images is shown in **Figure 25**. The image is an autoradiograph, in which silver grains in a photographic emulsion record the emission of gamma rays from a radioactive-labeled drug applied to cells. The task is to use the spotty images of the white grains (in this negative image) to mark the cells that incorporated the drug. Smoothing produces a grey scale image in which clusters of grains produce a higher brightness than in regions where grains are sparse. Thresholding this image produces outlines that mark the high brightness regions and hence the cells. However, the outlines do not necessarily delineate the cells well because of the boundary shifting produced by the smoothing.

Grey scale erosion and dilation are performed with rank operators. The example shows a grey scale closing in which each pixel is replaced by the brightest neighbor in a 9-pixel-wide circle

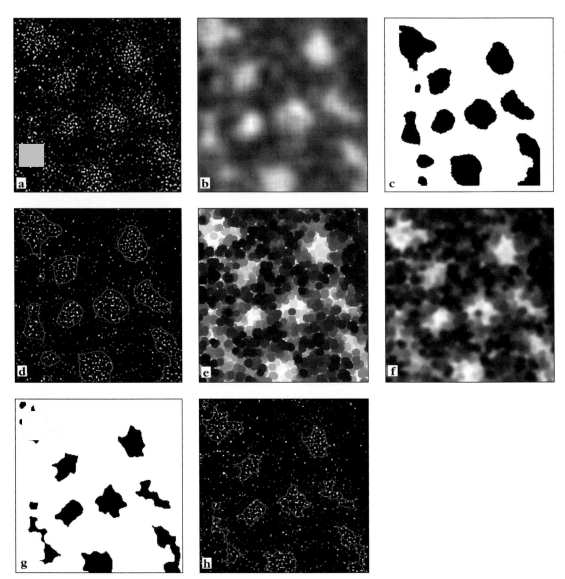

Figure 25. Delineation of cells in an autoradiograph image: a) *original;* **b)** *smoothed (Gaussian kernel, standard deviation = 4 pixels);* **c)** *brightness thresholding of* **b;** **d)** *outlines from* **c** *superimposed on the original;* **e)** *grey scale closing (erosion followed by dilation);* **f)** *smoothing (3×3 kernel) of* **e** *to blend edges;* **g)** *brightness thresholding of* **f;** **h)** *outlines from* **g** *superimposed on the original.*

(dilation of the white regions), followed by replacing each pixel with the darkest neighbor in the same size region (erosion of the white regions). A slight smoothing of the result followed by thresholding produces the region outlines shown. The erosion/dilation method does not shift boundaries, but it does impose a limitation on the size of regions and of the details of irregularities in their boundaries, as a consequence of the size of the neighborhood region used for the ranking operations.

As a method for removing noise, this technique would seem to be the antithesis of a median filter, which discards extreme values. It

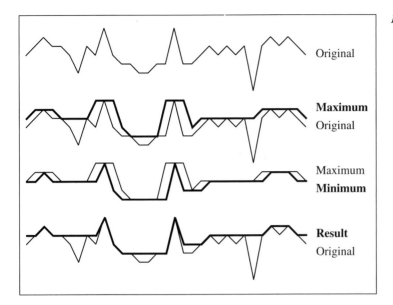

Figure 26. Schematic diagram of the operation of grey scale erosion and dilation in one dimension, showing (starting from the top): the original profile with result of first (maximum) pass, producing a new profile through brightest points; the second step in which a new profile passes through the darkest (minimum) points in the result from step 1; comparison of the final result to the original profile, showing rejection of noise and dark spikes.

may be helpful to visualize the image as a surface for which the brightness represents an elevation. **Figure 26** shows a one-dimensional representation of such a situation. In the first pass, the brightest values in each region are used to construct a new profile which follows the "tops of the trees." In the second pass, the darkest values in each region are used to bring the profile back down to those points which were large enough to survive the first one, giving a new profile that ignores the noise spikes in the original.

Profile plots sometimes offer a better tool for visualization of the reduction of noise in images than do grey scale representations. **Figure 27** shows the brightness values along the same line in several of the previous images obtained by processing **Figure 5**.

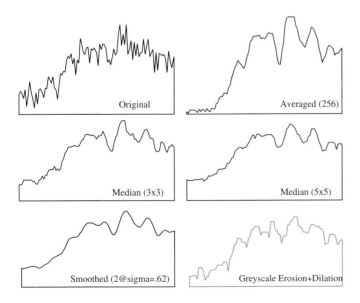

Figure 27. Profile plots on several original and smoothed images from the preceding figures, showing the variation of brightness along the same horizontal line. Except for the profile for the averaged image, all of the brightness scales are identical.

Figure 28. The "Top Hat" filter. Pixel brightness values are treated as elevations, and the filter placed at each location so that the brim rests on the surface. Any pixel that protrudes through the crown of the hat is selected either for replacement or as a feature marker. The adjustable parameters are the diameter of the brim and crown, and the height of the crown.

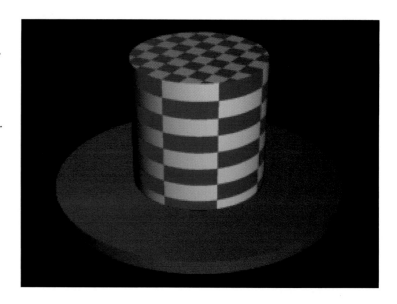

Although these are only one-dimensional traverses across a two-dimensional image and therefore cannot show all of the data that are used in the transformations based on 2D neighborhoods, the presence of the noise and its removal by various operations is evident, as is the blurring of edges.

The method shown above is closely related to a method for identifying (and removing) noise in images that is variously known as a "top hat" or "rolling ball" technique. Imagine the brightness values of the pixels to represent the elevation of a surface, as discussed above. A top hat filter consists of a flat disk that rests on the surface, and a central crown of a smaller diameter, as shown in **Figure 28**. This filter is centered on each pixel in the image, with the brim "resting" on the surface. Any pixels that "stick up" through the crown of the hat are considered to be noise, and replaced. The replacement value may be either the mean or the median value of the pixels covered by the brim of the hat. If the sense of the brightness values is reversed and darkest pixels are the target of the filter, it is usually called a rolling ball filter. The symbolism is that a sphere rolling on the surface will be unable to touch the bottom of the pit represented by the dark noise pixel.

Some systems implement the top hat/rolling ball filter directly, but many require the user to perform the operation in several steps. The rank filter is applied twice to the image, using different neighborhoods (corresponding to the diameter of the brim and crown). The resulting images are subtracted and the difference image thresholded to select pixels that represent a difference of more than the height of the crown. **Figure 29** shows an example. Those pixels that exceed this value may be replaced with the desired value.

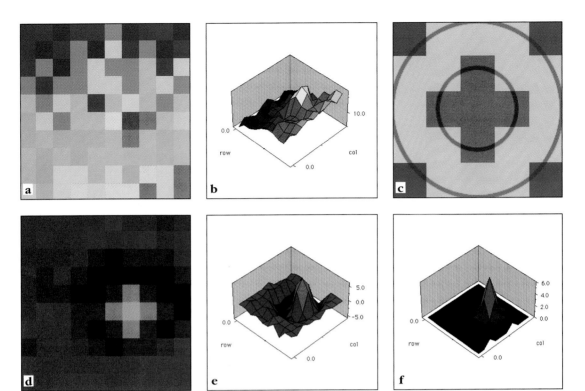

Figure 29. Example of the application of a top hat filter: a) 10×10 pixel array, color coded; *b)* the array from figure *a* shown as a surface; *c)* a top hat filter, with the ideal round shape implemented with discrete pixels; *d)* application of the top hat filter to the surface, with the resulting difference between the maximum value inside the crown and that under the brim; *e)* the array from figure *d* shown as a surface; *f)* thresholding the array to suppress negative values, leaving just a single peak.

In the next chapter we will consider the use of this same filter for a different purpose. Instead of removing extreme points as noise, the same operation can be used to find points of interest that are smaller than the crown of the hat and brighter or darker than the local neighborhood. In that case, the points that do NOT protrude through the crown are suppressed, and only those that do are kept.

Figure 30 illustrates this property of the top hat. The original image shows a cross section of muscle tissue. A top hat filter with a crown 3 pixels in diameter and a brim 7 pixels in diameter finds the small stained muscle fibers and eliminates other details from the image (**Figure 30b**). Increasing the size of the filter to a crown 9 pixels across with a brim 15 pixels across ignores the small fibers but locates the larger dark blood vessels (**Figure 30c**).

Maximum entropy

Images may contain other defects, such as blur due to motion or out-of-focus optics, in addition to noise. The "inverse filtering"

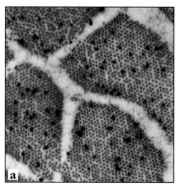 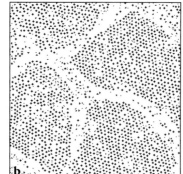 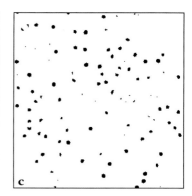

Figure 30. Stained muscle tissue:
a) *original;*
b) *application of a top hat filter with crown = 3 pixel diameter, brim = 7 pixel diameter;*
c) *application of a top hat filter with crown = 9 pixel diameter, brim = 15 pixel diameter.*

methods described in Chapter 5 are quite noise sensitive. When the noise that is present can itself be characterized, it may be possible to use a maximum entropy approach to remove the artefacts.

Maximum entropy methods represent a computer-intensive approach to removing artefacts such as noise or blur from images, based on some foreknowledge about the image contents and some assumptions about the nature of the degradation that is to be removed and the image restored (Skilling, 1986; Frieden, 1988). The conventional description of the method is to imagine an image containing N pixels, that has been formed by a total of M photons (where usually $M>>N$). The number of photons in any single pixel (i.e., the pixel's brightness value) is P_i where i is the pixel identification or location. This is usually written for convenience as a single subscript, but we understand that it really refers to a pixel at a given x,y location.

The measured image has normalized pixel brightness values $p_i=P_i/M$ that only approximate the "true" image that would be collected if there were no artefacts. The method used to approach this ideal image is to alter pixel brightness values to maximize the entropy in the image, subject to some constraints. The justification for this method is given in terms of statistical probability and Bayes' theorem, and will not be derived here. In some cases this method produces dramatic improvements in image quality.

The "entropy" of the brightness pattern is given in a formal sense by calculating the number of ways that the pattern could have been formed by rearrangement, or $S = M!/p_1! \, p_2!, \, \ldots \, p_N!$ where ! indicates factorial. For large values of M, this reduces by Stirling's approximation to the more familiar $S = - \sum p_i \log p_i$. This is the same calculation of entropy used in statistical mechanics. In the particular case of taking the log to the base 2, the entropy of the image is the number of bits per pixel needed to represent the image, according to information theory.

The entropy in the image would be maximized in an absolute sense simply by setting the brightness of each pixel to the average brightness, M/N. Clearly, this is not the "right" solution. It is the application of constraints that produce usable results. The most common constraint for images containing noise is based on a chi-squared statistic, calculated as $\chi^2 = 1/\sigma^2 \sum (p_i - p_i')^2$. In this expression the p_i values are the original pixel values and the p_i' are the altered brightness values, and σ is the standard deviation of the values. An upper limit can be set on the value of χ^2 allowed in the calculation of a new set of p_i' values to maximize the entropy. A typical (but essentially arbitrary) limit for χ^2 is N, the number of pixels in the array.

This constraint is not the only possible choice. A sum of the absolute value of differences, or some other weighting rule, could also be chosen. This is not quite enough information to produce an optimal image, and so other constraints may be added. One is that the totals of the p_i and p_i' values must be equal. Bryan and Skilling (1980) also require, for instance, that the distribution of the $p_i - p_i'$ values corresponds to the expected noise characteristics of the imaging source (e.g., a Poisson or Gaussian distribution for simple counting statistics). And, of course, we must be careful to include such seemingly "obvious" constraints as nonnegativity (no pixel can collect fewer than zero photons). Jaynes (1985) makes the point that there is practically always a significant amount of real knowledge about the image which can be used as constraints, but which is assumed to be so obvious that it is ignored.

An iterative solution for the values of p_i' produces a new image with the desired smoothness and noise characteristics which is often improved from the original image. Other formulations of the maximum entropy approach may compare one iteration of the image to the next, by calculating not the total entropy but the cross entropy, $-\sum p_i \log (p_i/q_i)$ where q_i is the previous image brightness value for the same pixel, or the modeled brightness for a theoretical image. In this formulation, the cross entropy is to be minimized. The basic principle remains the same.

Contrast expansion

Acquiring a noise-free image or processing one to reduce noise does not by itself insure that the resulting image can be viewed or interpreted well by an observer or a program. If the brightness range within the image is very small, there may not be enough contrast to assure visibility. Typical digitizers, as discussed in Chapter 1, convert the analog voltage range from the camera or other sensor to numbers from 0 to 255 (8 bits). For a common video camera, this corresponds to a total voltage range of 0.7

volts, and (depending on the camera design) to a variation in brightness covering several orders of magnitude in numbers of photons.

If the inherent range of variation in brightness of the image is much smaller than the dynamic range of the camera, subsequent electronics, and digitizer, then the actual range of numbers will be much less than the full range of 0 through 255. **Figure 31a** shows an example. The specimen is a thin section through tissue, with a blood vessel shown in cross section in a bright field microscope. Illumination in the microscope and light staining of the section produce very little total contrast. The histogram shown next to the image is a plot of the number of pixels at each of the 256 possible brightness levels. The narrow peak indicates that only a few of the levels are represented.

Visibility of the structures present can be improved by stretching the contrast so that the values of pixels are reassigned to cover the entire available range. **Figure 31b** shows this. The mapping is linear and one-to-one. This means that the darkest pixels in the original image are assigned to black, the lightest images are assigned to white, and intermediate grey values in the original image are given new values which are linearly interpolated between black and white. All of the pixels in the original image which had one particular grey value will also have only one grey value in the resulting image, but it will be a different one.

This histogram plotted with the image in the figure now shows counts of pixels for grey levels that are spread out across the available brightness scale. However, notice that most of the grey values still have no pixels in the histogram, indicating that no pixels have those values. The reassignment of grey values has increased the visual contrast for the pixels present, but has not increased the ability to discriminate subtle variations in grey scale that were not recorded in the original image. It has also magnified the brightness difference associated with noise in the original image.

Figure 31c shows the same field of view recorded to utilize the entire range of the camera and digitizer. This was actually done by averaging together several video frames. The mean brightness of various structures is similar to that shown in **Figure 31b**, after linear expansion of the contrast range. However, all of the 256 possible grey values are now present in the image, and very small variations in sample density can now be distinguished or measured in the specimen.

This is a rather extreme case. It is not always practical to adjust the illumination, camera gain, etc., to exactly fill the available pixel depth (number of grey levels that can be digitized or stored). Furthermore, increasing the brightness range too much can cause pixel values at the dark and/or light ends of the range to exceed the digitization and storage capacity and to be clipped

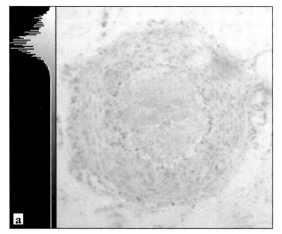

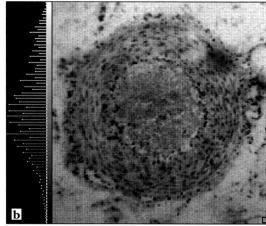

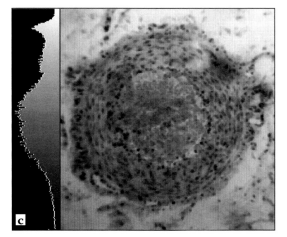

Figure 31. Contrast expansion:
a) *this light microscope image of a blood vessel has very low initial contrast, as shown by its brightness histogram;*
b) *linear expansion of the brightness range by manipulating the display shows a full range of black to white values but causes gaps in the histogram;*
c) *averaging multiple frames produces an image with more than 8 bits, which can be scaled to the full 8-bit range of the display without gaps. It also averages image noise to produce a smoother image.*

to the limiting values, which also causes loss of information. Consequently, it is common for images to be acquired that do not completely cover the available brightness range.

If these images still have enough different grey levels to reveal the important features in the specimen, then linear contrast expansion may be a useful and acceptable method to increase the viewer's visual discrimination. More important, this expansion may make it possible to more directly compare images acquired with slightly different brightness ranges by adjusting them all to the same expanded contrast scale. Of course, this only works if the brightest and darkest class of features are present in all of the images and fields of view.

Other manipulations of the pixel brightness values are also performed. Those which are one-to-one (i.e., all pixels which originally had a single grey scale value are assigned to another single value) need not be linear. An example would be one which converted brightness to density, which involves a logarithmic relationship. For color images, a transfer function can be used to correct colors for distortion due to the color temperature of the light source, or for atmospheric scattering and absorption in satellite images. These functions may be implemented with either a mathematical function or a lookup table, and for color images this is most easily done when the image is represented as hue, saturation and intensity (as opposed to red, green, blue) values for each pixel. This allows hue values to be adjusted while intensity values remain unchanged, for example. Discussion of the general use of "transfer functions," and their implementation using lookup tables, is presented in Chapter 4 on image enhancement.

Nonuniform illumination

The most straightforward strategy for image analysis uses the brightness of regions in the image as a means of identification: it is assumed that the same type of feature will have the same brightness (or color, in a color image) wherever it appears in the field of view. If this brightness is different from that of other features, or can be made so by appropriate image processing as discussed in Chapter 4, then it can be used to discriminate the features for counting, measurement or identification. Even if there are a few other types of objects that cannot be distinguished on the basis of brightness or color alone, subsequent measurements may suffice to select the ones of interest.

This approach is not without pitfalls, which are discussed further in Chapter 6 in conjunction with converting grey scale images to binary (black and white) images. And other approaches are available such as region growing or split-and-merge that do not have such stringent requirements for uniformity of illumination. But because when it can be used, simple brightness thresholding is by far the simplest and fastest method to isolate features in an image, it is important to consider the problems of shading of images.

When irregular surfaces are viewed, the amount of light scattered to the viewer or camera from each region is a function of the orientation of the surface with respect to the source of light and the viewer, even if the surface material and finish is uniform. In fact, this principle can be used to estimate the surface orientation, using a technique known as shape-from-shading. Human vision seems to apply these rules very easily and rapidly, since we are not generally confused by images of real-world objects. We will not pursue those methods here, however.

Most of the images we really want to process are essentially two-dimensional. Whether they come from light or electron microscopes, or satellite images, the variation in surface elevation is usually small compared to the lateral dimensions, giving rise to what is often called "two-and-one-half D." This is not always the case of course (consider a metal fracture surface examined in the SEM), but we will treat such problems as exceptions to the general rule and recognize that more elaborate processing may be needed.

Even surfaces of low relief need not be flat, a simple example being the curvature of the earth as viewed from a weather satellite. This will produce a shading across the field of view. So will illumination of a macroscopic or microscopic surface from one side. Even elaborate collections of lights, or ring lights, can only approximate uniform illumination of the scene.

For transmission imaging, the uniformity of the light source with a condenser lens system can be made quite good, but it is easy for these systems to get out of perfect alignment and produce shading as well. Finally, it was mentioned in Chapter 1 that lenses or the cameras themselves (especially ones with glass envelopes) may show vignetting, in which the corners of the image are darker than the center because the light is partially absorbed.

Most of these defects can be minimized by careful setup of the imaging conditions, or if they cannot be eliminated altogether, can be assumed to be constant over some period of time. This assumption allows correction by image processing. In most instances, it is possible to acquire a "background" image in which a uniform reference surface or specimen is inserted in place of the actual samples to be viewed, and the light intensity recorded. This image can then be used to "level" the subsequent images. The process is often called "background subtraction" but in many cases this is a misnomer. If the image acquisition device is logarithmic with a gamma of 1.0, then subtraction of the background image point-by-point from each acquired image is correct. If the camera or sensor is linear, then the correct procedure is to divide the acquired image by the background. For other sensor response functions, there is no simple correct arithmetic method, and the calibrated response must first be determined and applied to convert the measured signal to a linear space.

In the process of subtracting (or dividing) one image by another, some of the dynamic range of the original data will be lost. The greater the variation in background brightness, the less the remaining variation from that level can be recorded in the image and will be left after the leveling process. This loss and the inevitable increase in statistical noise that results from subtracting one signal from another argue that all practical steps should be taken first to make illumination uniform before acquiring the images, before resorting to processing methods.

Figure 84 in Chapter 1 showed an example of leveling in which the background illumination function could be acquired separately. This acquisition is most commonly done by removing the specimen from the light path, for instance a slide, and storing an image representing the variation. This image can then be used for leveling. However, in many cases it is not practical to remove the specimen, or its presence is a contributor to the brightness variation. This includes situations in which the specimen thickness varies and so the overall absorption of light is affected. Another case is that in which the surface being examined is not

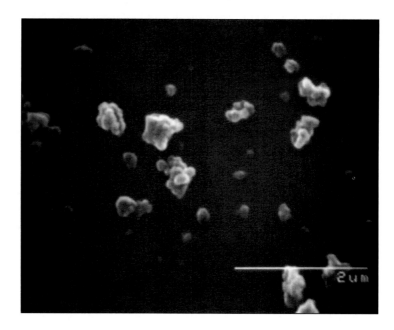

Figure 32. *SEM image of particles on a substrate showing nonuniform brightness.*

perfectly flat, which causes incident light or SEM images to show a varying background.

Figure 32 shows an example of the latter type. The SEM image shows particles on a substrate, which because of the geometry of the surface and of the SEM chamber causes a portion of the image to appear darker than the rest. The human eye is quite tolerant of this kind of gradual brightness variation, and so it is sometimes helpful to apply pseudo-color lookup tables to reveal the shading present in the image. Furthermore, moving the specimen or changing the magnification alters the pattern of light and dark, in which case it is necessary to perform the correction using the image itself. Fortunately, in many of these situations the variation of background brightness is a smooth and well behaved function of location and can be approximated by simple functions such as polynomials.

Figure 33 shows a situation in which the brightness variation can be extracted directly from the original image. By separating the red, green, and blue planes from the image it is seen that the green image contains the important detail: the blood vessels in the retina of the eye, which cannot be thresholded because of the overall brightness variation. The red image has the same variation so the ratio of the green to red levels the varying background and makes the vessels more uniform.

Fitting a background function

By selecting a number of points in the image, a list of brightness values and locations can be acquired. These can then used to perform least-squares fitting of a function $B(x,y)$ that approximates

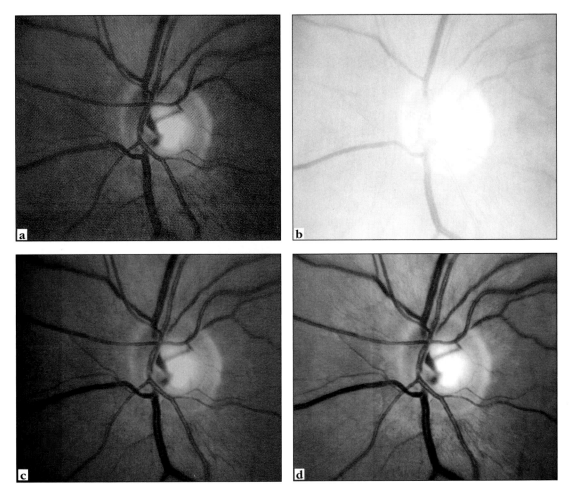

Figure 33. Image of the retina:
a) *original color image;*
b) *green image plane showing blood vessels;*
c) *red image plane showing brightness variation;*
d) *ratio of green to red showing uniform brightness.*

the background, and can be subtracted (or divided) just as a physically acquired background image would be. When the user marks these points, for instance by using a pointing device such as a mouse, trackball or light pen, it is important to select locations that should all have the same brightness and are well distributed across the image. Locating many points in one small region and few or none in other parts of the image requires the function to extrapolate the polynomial, and can introduce significant errors. For a second-order polynomial, the functional form of the fitted background is

$$B(x,y) = a_0 + a_1 \cdot x + a_2 \cdot y + a_3 \cdot x^2 + a_4 \cdot y^2 + a_5 \cdot xy \qquad (2$$

This polynomial has six fitted constants, and so in principle could be fitted with only that number of marked points. Likewise, a

Figure 34. Automatic leveling of nonuniform illumination:

a) *reflection light microscope image of ceramic specimen, with nonuniform background brightness due to a non-planar surface;*

b) *background function calculated as a polynomial fit to the brightest point in each of 81 squares (a 9×9 grid);*

c) *leveled image after subtracting* **b** *from* **a**.

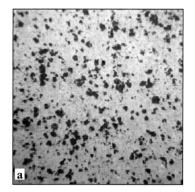

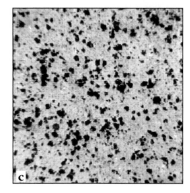

third-order polynomial would have ten coefficients. However, in order to get a good fit and diminish sensitivity to minor fluctuations in individual pixels, and to have enough points to sample the entire image area properly, it is usual to require several times this minimum number of points.

In some cases, it is practical to locate the points automatically for background fitting. Automatic leveling is easiest when there is a distinct structure or phase present that is well distributed throughout the image area and contains the darkest (or lightest) pixels present. In that case, the image can be subdivided into a grid of smaller squares or rectangles, the darkest (or lightest) pixels in each subregion located, and these points used for the fitting.

Figure 34 shows an example in which the specimen (a polished ceramic) has an overall variation in brightness due to curvature of the surface. The brightest pixels in each region of the specimen represent the matrix, and so should all be the same. Subdividing the image into a 9×9 grid and locating the brightest pixel in each square gave a total of 81 points, which were then used to calculate a second-order polynomial (six coefficients) by least-squares. The fitting routine in this case reported a fitting error (rms value) of less than 2 brightness values out of the total 0...255 range for pixels in the image.

Figure 34b shows the calculated brightness using the $B(x,y)$ function, and **Figure 34c** shows the result after subtracting the background from the original, pixel by pixel, to level the image. This leveling removes the variation in background brightness and permits setting brightness thresholds to delineate the pores for measurement, as discussed in Chapter 6.

This approach to automatic leveling can of course be applied to either a light or a dark background. By simultaneously applying it to both the lightest and darkest pixels in each region of the image, it is possible to stretch the contrast of the image as a function of location. This autocontrast method works particularly well when the image loses contrast due to nonuniform illumination or varying sample thickness. **Figure 35** shows an example.

Another approach sometimes used to remove gradual variation in overall brightness employs the frequency transforms discussed in Chapter 5. It assumes that the background variation in the image is a low-frequency signal, and can be separated in frequency space from the higher frequencies that define the features present. If this assumption is justified, and the frequencies corresponding to the background can be identified, then they can be removed by a simple filter in the frequency space representation.

Figure 36 shows an example of this approach. The brightness variation in the original image is due to off-centered illumination in the microscope. Transforming the image into frequency space with a 2D FFT (as discussed in Chapter 5), reducing the magnitude of the first four frequency components by filtering the frequency space image, and retransforming, produces the image shown in the figure.

This method is not entirely successful for this image. The edges of the image show significant variations present because the frequency transform attempts to match the left and right edges and the top and bottom edges. In addition, the brightness of dark and light regions throughout the image which have the same appearance and would be expected to properly have the same brightness show considerable local variations because the brightness variation is a function of the local details, including the actual brightness values and the shapes of the features. There are few practical situations in which leveling can be satisfactorily performed by this method.

Rank leveling

When the background variation is more irregular than can be fit to simple functions, another approach can be used. This method is especially useful when the surface is irregular, such as details on a fracture surface examined in the SEM. The assumption behind this method is that features of interest are limited in size and smaller than the scale of background variations, and that the background is everywhere either lighter than or darker than the features. Both requirements are often met in practical situations.

Figure 35. TEM image of latex particles:
a) *original, with varying contrast due to changing sample thickness;*
b) *after application of automatic contrast by fitting polynomial functions to light and dark pixel values.*

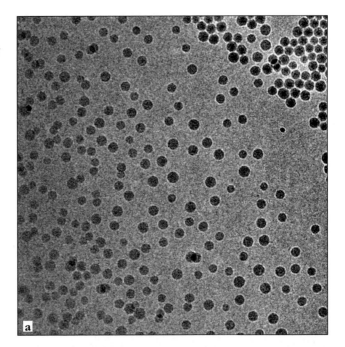

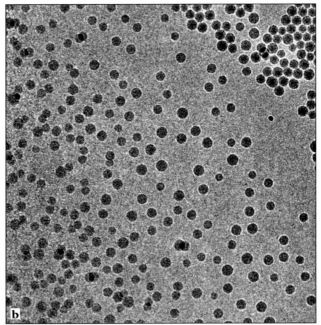

Rank neighborhood operations are discussed in detail elsewhere in this chapter, and in Chapter 4. The basic idea behind neighborhood operations is to compare each pixel to its neighbors or combine the pixel values in some small region, minimally the eight touching pixels in a 3×3 square. This operation is performed for each pixel in the image, and a new image is produced as a result. In many practical implementations, the new image replaces the original image with only a temporary requirement

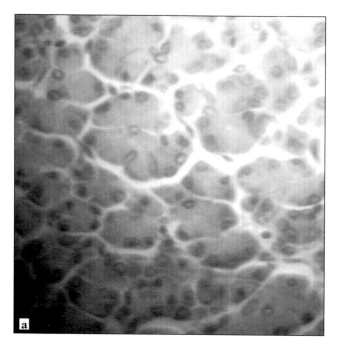

a) *original image, showing nonuniform illumination;*

b) *attempt to level the brightness by reducing the magnitude of the lowest four frequency components to zero. Notice that in addition to the variations near the edge, the brightness of similar structures is not constant throughout the image.*

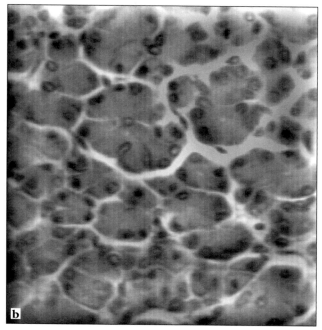

for additional storage; these implementation considerations are discussed in Chapter 4.

For our present purposes, the neighborhood comparison works as follows: for each pixel, examine the pixels in a 3×3 or other similar small region. If the background is known to be darker than the features, find the darkest pixel in each neighborhood and replace the value of the original pixel with that darker

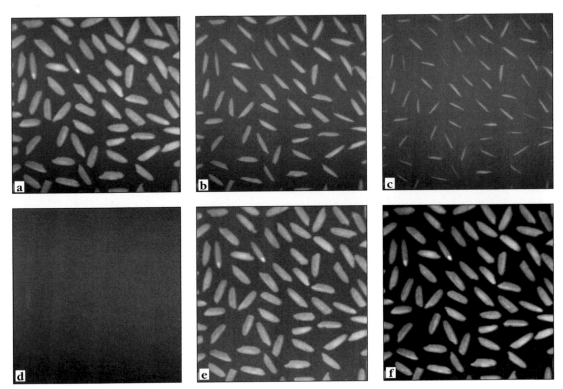

Figure 37. Constructing a background image with a rank operation:
a) *an image of rice grains with nonuniform illumination;*
b) *each pixel replaced with the darkest neighboring pixel in an octagonal 5×5 neighborhood;*
c) *another repetition of the "darkest neighbor" or grey scale erosion operation;*
d) *after four repetitions only the background remains;*
e) *result of subtracting d from a;*
f) *the leveled result with contrast expanded.*

brightness value. For the case of a background lighter than the features, the brightest pixel in the neighborhood is used instead. These operations are sometimes called grey-scale erosion and dilation, by analogy to the morphological processing discussed in Chapter 7. The result of applying this operation to the entire image is to shrink the features by the radius of the neighborhood region, and to extend the local background brightness values into the area previously covered by features.

Figure 37 illustrates this procedure for an image of rice grains on a dark and uneven background. A neighborhood is used here which consists of 21 pixels in an octagonal 5×5 pattern centered on each pixel in the image. The darkest pixel value in that region replaces the original central pixel. This operation is repeated for every pixel in the image, always using the original image pixels and not the new ones from application of the procedure to other pixels. After this procedure is complete, the rice grains are reduced in size as shown in **Figure 37b**. Repeating the operation continues to shrink the grains and to extend the background based on the local background brightness.

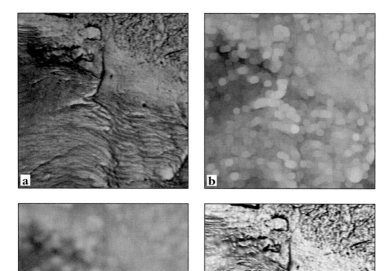

Figure 38. *Leveling an uneven fracture surface image (TEM replica):*

a) *original image shows brightness variations due to local variations in surface orientation;*

b) *two applications of a brightest rank operation using a 5×5 octagonal neighborhood around each pixel;*

c) *image **b** smoothed using a Gaussian kernel with sigma = 1.6 pixels;*

d) *subtraction of image **c** from image **a**, showing the leveled background and more visible fatigue striations.*

After four repetitions (**Figure 37d**), the rice grains have been removed. This removal is possible because the maximum width of any grain is not larger than four times the width of the 5-pixel-wide neighborhood used for the ranking. Knowing how many times to apply this operation depends upon knowing the width (smallest dimension) of the largest features present, or simply watching the progress of the operation and repeating until the features are removed. In some cases this can be judged from the disappearance of a peak from the image histogram. The background produced by this method has the large-scale variation present in the original image, and subtracting it produces a leveled image (**Figure 37f**) that clearly defines the features and allows them to be separated from the background by thresholding.

This method is particularly suitable for the quite irregular background brightness variations that occur when looking at details on fracture surfaces. **Figure 38** shows an example. The original TEM image of this fatigue fracture has facets with differing overall brightness because of their different orientations. Applying a ranking operation to select the brightest pixel in a 5-pixel-wide octagonal neighborhood produces the result shown in **Figure 38b**. This image was blurred using a Gaussian smoothing kernel with a standard deviation of 1.6 pixels (these neighborhood smoothing operations are discussed earlier in this chapter), and then subtracted from the original image to produce the result in **Figure 38d**. The

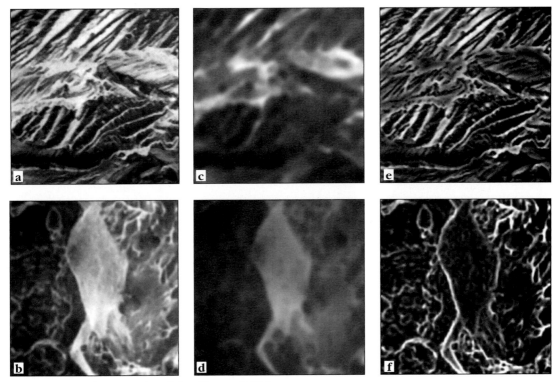

Figure 39. Application of rank leveling to SEM images:

a, b) original images of metal fractures showing local brightness variations due to surface orientation;

c, d) background image produced by two applications of a 5-pixel-wide rank filter keeping the darkest pixel in each neighborhood followed by smoothing with a Gaussian filter having a standard deviation of 1.0 pixels;

e, f) leveled result after subtraction of the background from the original.

leveled background improves the visibility of the fatigue striations on the fracture.

It is interesting in this example to note that the fatigue marks in the original image are not simply the darkest pixels in the image. Because the original image was produced by shadowing a TEM replica with carbon, each line has a white as well as a dark line. This influences the result, and the background rank leveling method provides only an approximate correction for this type of image.

Better results are often possible with SEM images in which local ridges and variations produce bright lines on a dark background. **Figure 39** shows two examples, images of fracture surfaces in metals. The background in each case was produced by two applications of the ranking operation keeping the darkest pixel in a 5 pixel wide octagonal neighborhood, followed by smoothing with a Gaussian kernel with a standard deviation of 1.0 pixels. Subtracting this background from the original makes the markings, fatigue striations in one image and brittle quasi-cleavage marks in

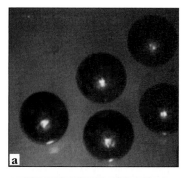

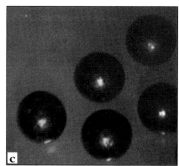

*Figure 40. **Effect of leveling on an image with limited grey scale range:***
a) *original image;*
b) *fitted polynomial background;*
c) *subtracting image **b** from **a**. The background is now uniform, but the dark features are not because the original pixels were fully black in the original image.*

the other, more visible by removing the overall variation due to surface orientation.

This method is also useful for examination of particles and other surface decorations on freeze-fractured cell walls in biological specimens, examination of surface roughness on irregular particles or pollen, and other similar problems. In some cases it can be used to enhance the visibility of dislocations in TEM images of materials, which appear as dark lines in different grains whose overall brightness varies due to lattice orientation.

However, the ability to level brightness variations by subtracting a background image, whether obtained by measurement, mathematical fitting, or image processing, is not a cost-free process. Subtraction uses up part of the dynamic range, or grey scale, of the image. **Figure 40** shows an example. The original image has a shading variation that can be fit rather well by a quadratic function, but this has a range of about half of the total 256 grey levels. After the function has been subtracted, the leveled image does not have enough remaining brightness range to show detail in the dark areas of some features. This clipping may interfere with further analysis of the image.

Color shading

Color images present significant problems for shading correction. A typical example of a situation in which this arises is aerial or satellite imagery, in which the irregularity of the ground or the curvature of the planet surface produces an overall shading. In some cases, this affects only the intensity in the image and leaves the color information unaffected. But depending on the camera response, possible texturing or specular reflection from the surface, atmospheric absorption, and other details of the imaging, it is more common to find that there are also color shifts between the areas in the image that have different illumination.

The same methods used above for grey scale images can be applied to the intensity plane from a color image, but are not usually appropriate for use with the hue and saturation planes, and they are essentially never useful for application directly to the red, green, and blue planes. When (mis)used in this way the operations produce color shifts in pixels that alter the image so that it cannot be successfully thresholded, and in most cases does not even "look" right.

Chapter 1 showed an example of another approach. While the various color planes have each been altered by the effects of geometry and other factors, to a first approximation the effect is the same across the spectrum of colors. In that case, it is appropriate to use ratios of one color plane to another to level the effects of nonuniform surface orientation or illumination. Filtering the color image in different wavelengths and then dividing one by another cancels out some of the nonuniformity and produces a leveled image in which similar features located in different areas have the same final appearance.

Figure 41 shows an example using a satellite image of the entire earth. The limb darkening around the edges of the globe is due primarily to viewing angle, and secondarily to the effects of atmospheric absorption. Histogram equalization (discussed in Chapter 4) of the individual color planes increases the contrast between features and improves the visibility of structures, but the resulting colors are not "real" and do not have any intrinsic meaning or use. Notice in particular the pink colors that appear in clouds, and the green in the oceans and along cloud edges. Separating the image into separate color planes and ratioing them reveals fine details and levels the overall contrast range. It does not produce an image of the globe in which pixels near the limb have their colors "corrected" to be similar to those in the center of the field of view.

Color correction of images is a very rich and complicated field. Generally, it requires detailed knowledge of the light source and the camera response, which must be obtained with calibration standards. Accurate colorimetry also requires extreme stability of all components. Colorimetry goes well beyond the capabilities of general purpose image processing and analysis systems, and is not considered in detail here. However, there is a more routine interest in making some adjustments to color images to permit comparisons between regions or images, or to provide some control over consistency in the printing of color images.

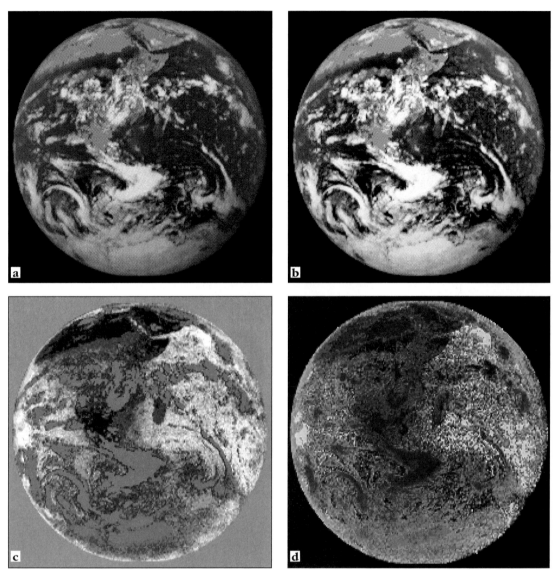

Figure 41. Satellite image of the earth:
a) *original;*
b) *with contrast increased by histogram equalization of each color plane;*
c) *ratio of the image filtered at 450 nm (blue) to that at 650 nm (orange);*
d) *ratio of the image filtered at 700 nm (red) to that at 550 (green).*

These adjustments are generally accomplished with standardization, at least of a relative kind. For instance, most printers (as discussed in Chapter 2) cannot reproduce the full gamut of colors displayed on the screen or captured by a camera. In order to calibrate the relationship between the display and the input/output devices, some systems create a test pattern that is printed on the system printer, redigitized from the printed output, and compared to the original. This comparison allows the system to construct an internal correction matrix to adjust the colors so that

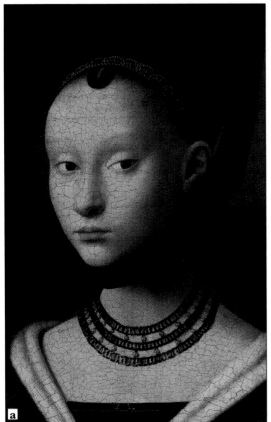
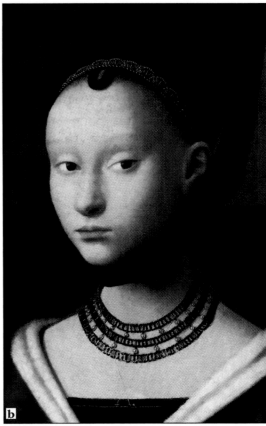

Figure 42. Portrait of a Lady, *painted in 1470 by Petrus Christus:*
  a) present appearance, showing cracks and fading of the colors;
  b) application of a median filter to fill in the dark cracks, and color compensation to adjust the colors.

the display and reproduction of colors will be more consistent. It also allows flagging those colors that cannot be printed accurately with a given printer.

Correction for a shift in colors, due for instance to a known change in lighting conditions, is also possible. Acquiring an image from a test card under each of several conditions allows the computer to build a matrix of corrections that may be expressed internally as either RGB or HSI components. These are multiplied by the incoming signal to approximately correct for the change in lighting.

One example of the use of this type of correction is to compensate for the yellowing of varnish and other coatings applied to artworks. **Figure 42** shows an example. The painting is *Portrait of a Lady*, painted in 1470 by Petrus Christus, a Flemish Renaissance painter (Gemäldegalerie der Staatlichen Museen, Berlin-Dahlem). The painting shows several defects. The two most obvious are the network of fine cracks that have formed in the paint, and the yellowing and fading of the pigments. Measurements on similar pigments freshly made and applied provide color samples that allow compensation for the color change. The application of a median filter allows filling in the cracks without blurring edges, much as the pixel noise was removed from the grey scale images shown above. The result is a restoration of the appearance of the original painting.

Nonplanar views

Computer graphics is much concerned with methods for displaying the surfaces of three-dimensional objects. Some of these methods will be used in Chapter 10 to display representations of three-dimensional structures obtained from a series of 2D image slices, or from direct 3D imaging methods such as tomography.

One particular use of computer graphics which most of us take for granted can be seen each evening on the local news program. Most TV stations in the U.S. have a weather forecast that uses satellite images from the GOES satellite. These pictures show the United States as it appears from latitude 0, longitude 108 W (the satellite is shifted to 98 W in summertime to get a better view of hurricanes developing in the south Atlantic), at a geosynchronous elevation of about 22,000 miles.

This image shows cloud patterns, and a series of images taken during the day shows movement of storms and other weather systems. In these images, the coastline, Great Lakes and a few other topographic features are evident, but may be partially obscured by clouds. Given the average citizen's geographical knowledge, that picture would not help most viewers to recognize their location. So computer graphics are used to superimpose political outlines, such as the state borders and perhaps other information such as cities, to assist the viewer. Most U.S. TV stations have heavy investments in computer graphics for advertising, news, etc., but they rarely generate these lines themselves, instead obtaining the images with the lines already present from a company which specializes in that niche market.

How are these lines generated? This is not simply a matter of overlaying a conventional map, say a Mercator's projection as used in the school classroom, over the satellite image. The curvature of the earth and the foreshortening of the image need to be taken into account. For instance, **Figure 43** shows an example of the broadcast use of these images, and **Figure 44** shows a GOES weather satellite image of North America that is clearly foreshortened at the top, and also shows noticeable curvature from west to east across the width of the country.

The coordinates, in latitude and longitude, of points on the earth's surface are used to calculate a perspective view of the roughly spherical globe as it is seen from the satellite. Since the viewpoint is constant, this is a one-time calculation, which nevertheless

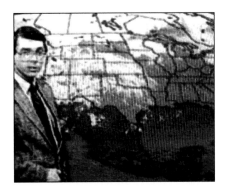

Figure 43. Television weather forecast using the GOES weather satellite image. The satellite is located on the equator and therefore shows the U.S. in a foreshortened view. There is also curvature evident from west to east. The political boundary lines are superimposed by computer graphics, as discussed in the text. (WRAL-TV, Channel 5, Raleigh, NC.)

needs to be done for a great many points to construct good outline maps for superposition. The calculation can be visualized as shown in the diagram of **Figure 45**.

The location of a point on the spherical earth (specified by its latitude and longitude) is used to determine the intersection of a view line to the satellite with a flat image plane, inserted in front of the sphere. This calculation requires only simple trigonometry as indicated in **Figure 46**. The coordinates of the points in that plane are the location of the point in the viewed image. As shown, a square on the ground is viewed as a skewed trapezoid, and if the square is large enough its sides are noticeably curved.

Computer graphics

Computer graphics is similarly used to construct perspective drawings of three-dimensional objects so that they can be viewed on the computer screen, for instance in CAD (computer-aided

Figure 44. GOES-7 image of North America with political boundary lines superimposed. The dark area just west of Baja California is the shadow of the moon, during the eclipse of 11 June, 1991. (Image courtesy National Environmental Satellite, Data and Information Service.)

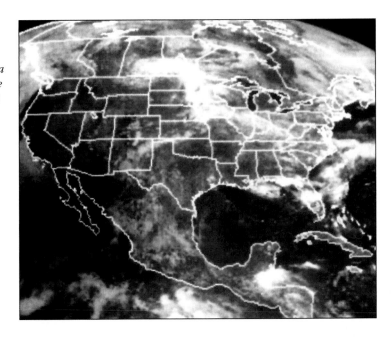

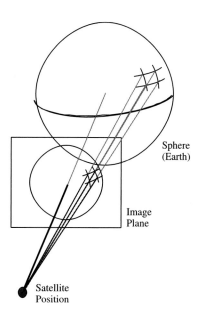

Figure 45. *Diagram of satellite imaging. As in any perspective geometry, the "flat" image is formed by projecting view lines from the three-dimensional object to the viewpoint and constructing the image from the points at which they intersect the image plane.*

Sphere (Earth)

Image Plane

Satellite Position

design) programs. The subject goes far beyond our needs here; the interested reader should refer to standard texts such as Foley & Van Dam (1984) or Hearn & Baker (1986). The display process is the same as that just described, with the addition of perspective control that allows the user to adjust the apparent distance of the camera or viewpoint so as to control the degree of foreshortening that occurs (equivalent to choosing a long or short focal length lens for a camera; the short focal length lens produces more distortion in the image).

Setting aside perspective distortion for the moment (i.e., using a telephoto lens), we can represent the translation of a point in three dimensions by matrix multiplication of its x, y, z coordinates

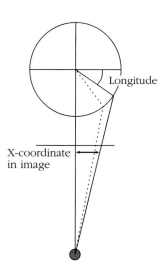

Figure 46. *Simple trigonometry can be used to calculate the location of points in the image plane from the longitude of the point on the earth, and the location of the satellite. This is the view from the North Pole; a similar view from the equator gives the y-coordinate.*

Longitude

X-coordinate in image

by a set of values that describe rotation and translation. This is simpler to examine in more detail in two dimensions, since our main interest here is with two-dimensional images. Consider a point with Cartesian X, Y coordinates and how it moves when we shift it or rotate it and the other points in the object with respect to the coordinate system.

From simple geometry we know that a translation of an object simply adds offsets to X and Y, to produce

$$X' = X + \Delta X \qquad (3$$
$$Y' = Y + \Delta Y$$

while stretching the object requires multiplicative coefficients which may not be the same

$$X' = \alpha X \qquad (4$$
$$Y' = \beta Y$$

and rotation of an object by the angle ϑ introduces an interdependence between the original X and Y coordinates of the form

$$X' = X + Y \sin \vartheta \qquad (5$$
$$Y' = Y - X \cos \vartheta$$

In general, the notation for two-dimensional translations is most commonly written using so-called homogeneous coordinates and matrix notation. The coordinates X, Y are combined in a vector along with an arbitrary constant 1 to allow the translation values to be incorporated into the matrix math, producing the result

$$[X' Y' 1] = [X \ Y \ 1] \cdot \begin{vmatrix} a & b & 0 \\ c & d & 0 \\ e & f & 1 \end{vmatrix} \qquad (6$$

which multiplies out to

$$X' = aX + cY + e \qquad (7$$
$$Y' = bX + dY + f$$

By comparing this matrix form to the examples above, we see that the e and f terms are the translational shift values. The diagonal values a and d are the stretching coefficients, while b and c are the sine and cosine terms involved in rotation. When a series of transformations is combined, including rotation, translation and stretching, a series of matrices is produced that can be multiplied together. When this happens, for instance to produce rotation about some point other than the origin, or to combine nonuniform stretching with rotation, the individual terms are combined in ways that complicate their simple interpretation. However, only the same six coefficients are needed.

If only these terms are used, we cannot produce curvature or twisting of the objects. By introducing higher order terms, more

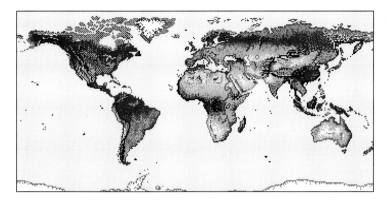

Figure 47. *The standard Mercator projection of the earth used in maps projects the points on the sphere onto a cylinder, producing distortion at high latitudes.*

complex stretching and twisting of figures is possible. This would produce a more complex equation of the form

$$X' = a_1 + a_2X + a_3Y + a_4XY + a_5X^2 + a_6Y^2 + \ldots \qquad (8$$

and a similar relationship for Y'. There is no fundamental reason to limit this polynomial expansion to any particular maximum power, except that as the complexity grows the number of coefficients needed rises (and the difficulty of obtaining them), and the mathematical precision needed to apply the transformation increases. It is unusual to have terms beyond second power, which can handle most commonly encountered cases of distortion and even approximate the curvature produced by looking at a spherical surface, at least over small ranges of angles.

Of course, some surface mappings are better handled by other functions. The standard Mercator's projection of the spherical earth onto a cylinder (**Figure 47**) sends the poles to infinity and greatly magnifies areas at high latitudes. It would require many polynomial terms to approximate it, but since the actual geometry of the mapping is known, it is easy to use the cosecant function that efficiently performs the transformation.

Geometrical distortion

Now we must examine what to do with these mathematical operations. Images are frequently obtained that are not of flat surfaces viewed normally. The example of the satellite image used above is one obvious case. So is viewing surfaces in the SEM, in which the specimen surface is often tilted to increase the contrast in the detected image. If the surface is not flat, different regions may be tilted at arbitrary angles, or continuous curvature may be present. This distortion becomes important if we want to perform any measurements of comparisons within or between images. Many airborne cameras and radars introduce a predictable distortion (which is therefore correctable) due to the use of a moving or sideways scan pattern, or by imaging a single line onto continuously moving film. In all of these cases, knowing the distortion is the key to correcting it.

This situation does not commonly arise with light microscopy because the depth of field of the optics is so low that surfaces must be flat and normal to the optical axis to remain in focus. There are other imaging technologies, however, which do frequently encounter nonideal surfaces or viewing conditions.

Making maps from aerial or satellite images is one application (Thompson, 1966). Of course, there is no perfect projection of a spherical surface onto a flat one, so various approximations and useful conventions are employed. But in each case, there is a known relationship between the coordinates on the globe and those on the map which can be expressed mathematically. But what about the image? If the viewpoint is exactly known, as for the case of the weather satellite, or can be calculated for the moment of exposure, as for the case of a space probe passing by a planet, then the same kind of mathematical relationship can be determined.

This procedure is usually impractical for aerial photographs, as the plane position is not that precisely controlled. The alternative is to locate a few reference points in the image whose locations on the globe or the map are known, and use them to determine the equations relating position in the image to location on the map. This technique is generally known as image warping or rubber sheeting, and while the equations are the same as those used in computer graphics, the techniques for determining the coefficients are quite different.

We have seen that a pair of equations calculating X', Y' coordinates for a transformed view from original coordinates X, Y may include constants, linear terms in X and Y, plus higher order terms such as XY, X^2, etc. Adding more terms of higher order makes it possible to introduce more complex distortions in the transformation. If the problem is simply one of rotation, only linear terms are needed, and a constraint on the coefficients can be introduced to preserve angles. In terms of the simple matrix shown above, this would require that the two stretching coefficients a and d must be equal. That means that only a few constants are needed, and they can be determined by locating a few known reference points and setting up simultaneous equations.

More elaborate stretching to align images with each other or with a map requires correspondingly more terms and more points. In SEM pictures of surfaces which are locally flat, but oriented at an angle to the point of view, the distortion is essentially trapezoidal as shown in **Figure 48**. The portion of the surface that is closest to the lens is magnified more than regions farther away, and distances are foreshortened in the direction of tilt. In order to measure and compare features on these surfaces, or even to properly apply image processing methods (which generally assume that the neighbor pixels in various directions are at equal distances from the center), it may be necessary to transform this

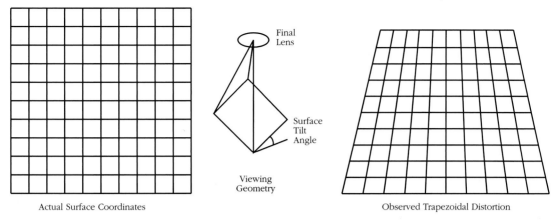

Actual Surface Coordinates   Viewing Geometry   Observed Trapezoidal Distortion

Figure 48. *Trapezoidal distortion commonly encountered in the SEM, due to observing a tilted surface with a short focal length lens.*

image to correct the distortion. Since the exact tilt angle and working distance may not be known, a method that uses only reference points within the image itself will be needed.

All that is required here is the ability to identify four points whose real X, Y coordinates on the surface are known, and whose image coordinates X', Y' can be measured. Then the following equations are written

$$X = a_1 + a_2X' + a_3Y' + a_4X'Y' \tag{9}$$

$$Y = b_1 + b_2X' + b_3Y' + b_4X'Y'$$

for each of the four sets of coordinates. This allows solving for the constants a_i and b_i. Of course, if more points are available, then they can be used to obtain a least-squares solution that minimizes the effect of the inevitable small errors in measurement of coordinates in the image.

By limiting the equation to those terms needed to accomplish the rotation and stretching involved in the trapezoidal distortion which we expect to be present, we minimize the number of points needed for the fit. More than the three terms shown above in **Equation 7** are required, because angles are not preserved in this kind of foreshortening. But using the fewest possible is preferred to a general equation involving many higher order terms, both in terms of the efficiency of the calculation (number of reference points) and the precision of the coefficients.

Likewise, if we know that the distortion in the image is that produced by viewing a globe, the appropriate sine and cosine terms can be used in the fitting equations. Of course, if we have no independent knowledge about the shape of the surface or the kind of imaging distortion, then arbitrary polynomials often represent the only practical approach.

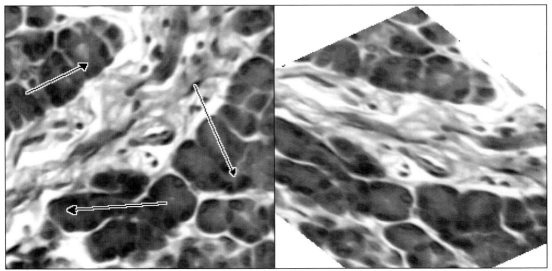

Figure 49. *An image with three displacement vectors (left), and the rotation and stretching transformation which they produce (right). Notice that portions of the original image are lost and some areas of the transformed image have no information.*

Alignment

Another very common situation is the alignment of serial section images. In this case there is usually no "ground truth" to align to, but only relative alignment between the successive slices. Either by using features within the image that can be recognized in two successive slices, or by introducing fiducial marks such as holes drilled through the specimen block before the sections are cut, this alignment can be performed. The points may be located manually by the user, or automatically by the imaging system, although the latter method works best for artificial markings such as holes, and somewhat poorly when trying to use details within the images which match only imperfectly from one section to the next. Relative alignment is discussed in more detail in Chapter 9.

Serial sections cut with a microtome from a block of embedded biological material commonly are foreshortened in the cutting direction by 5 to 15%, due to compression of the block by the knife. Then they are rotated arbitrarily before they are viewed. The result is a need for an alignment equation of the form

$$X = a_1 + a_2 X' + a_3 Y' \tag{10}$$

with only three constants (and a similar equation for Y). Hence, locating three reference points that are common to two sequential images allows one to be rotated and stretched to align with the other. **Figure 49** shows an image in which three points have been marked with vectors to indicate their movement to perform this alignment, and the resulting transformation of the image by stretching.

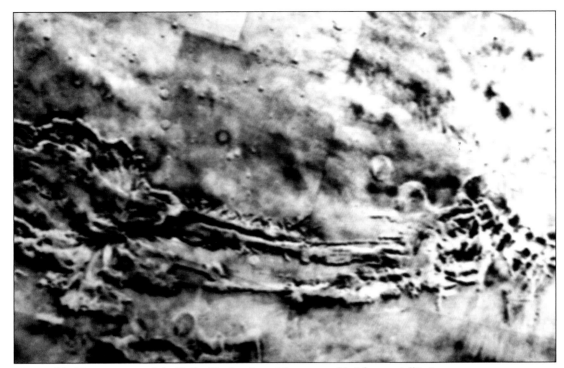

Figure 50. *Mosaic image of the Valles Marineris on Mars, assembled from satellite images.*

This kind of warping can be performed to align images with other images, as in serial section reconstruction, or to align images along their edges to permit assembling them as a mosaic (Milgram, 1975). Alignment of side-by-side sections of a mosaic is often attempted with SEM images but fails because of the trapezoidal distortion discussed above. The result is that features along the image boundaries do not quite line up, and the mosaic is imperfect. Using rubber sheeting can correct this defect.

Such correction is routinely done for satellite and space probe pictures. **Figure 50** shows an example of a mosaic image constructed from multiple images taken from orbit of the surface of Mars. Boundaries between images are visible because of brightness differences due to variations in illumination or exposure, but the features line up well across the seams. When images are being aligned, it is possible to write the equations either in terms of the coordinates in the original image as a function of the geometrically corrected one, or vice versa. In practice it is usually preferable to use the grid of x,y coordinates in the corrected image to calculate for each of the coordinates in the original image, and to perform the calculation in terms of actual pixel addresses.

Unfortunately, these calculated coordinates for the original location will only rarely be integers. This means that the location lies "between" the pixels in the original image. Several methods are used to deal with this problem. The simplest is to truncate the

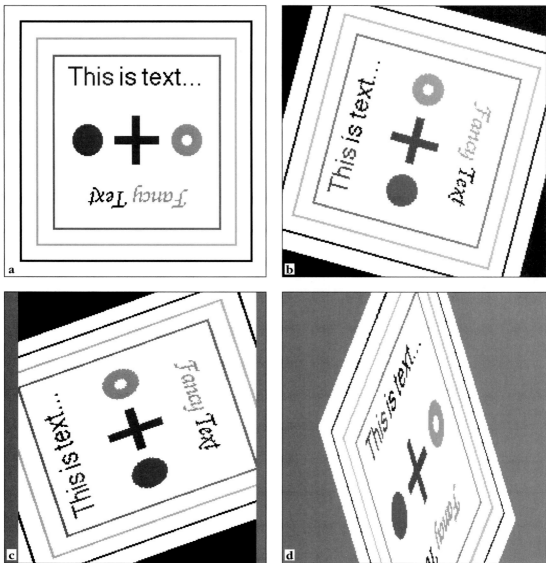

Figure 51. Rotation and stretching of a test image:
a) *original;*
b) *rotation only, no change in scale;*
c) *rotation and uniform stretching while maintaining angles;*
d) *general rotation and stretching. in which angles may vary (lines remain straight).*

calculated values so that the fractional part of the address is discarded and the pixel lying toward the origin of the coordinate system is used. Slightly better results are obtained by rounding the address values to select the nearest pixel, whose brightness is then copied to the transformed image array.

Either method introduces some error in location that can cause distortion of the transformed image. **Figure 51** shows examples using a test pattern in which the biasing of the lines and apparent variations in their width is evident.

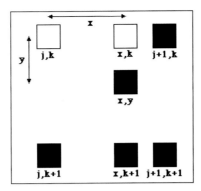

Figure 52. *Diagram of pixel interpolation. The brightness values of the neighbors are first interpolated horizontally, and then these two values are interpolated vertically, using the fractional part of the pixel addresses.*

When this distortion is unacceptable, another method may be used which requires more calculation. The brightness value for the transformed pixel may be calculated by interpolating between the four pixels surrounding the calculated address. This is called bilinear interpolation, and is calculated simply from the fractional part of the X and Y coordinates. First the interpolation is done in one direction, and then in the other, as indicated in **Figure 52**. For a location with coordinates $j+x$, $k+y$ where x and y are the fractional part of the address, the equations for the first interpolation are

$$B_{j+x,k} = (1-x) \cdot B_{j,k} + x \cdot B_{j+1,k} \tag{11}$$

$$B_{j+x,k+1} = (1-x) \cdot B_{j,k+1} + x \cdot B_{j+1,k+1}$$

and then the second interpolation, in the y direction, gives the final value

$$B_{j+x,k+y} = (1-y) \cdot B_{j+x,k} + y \cdot B_{j+x,k+1} \tag{12}$$

Weighted interpolations over larger regions are also used in some cases. One of the most popular is bicubic fitting. Whereas bilinear interpolation uses a 2×2 array of neighboring pixel values to calculate the interpolated value, the cubic method uses a 4×4 array. Using the same notation as the bilinear interpolation in equations 11 and 12, the summations now go from $k-1$ to $k+2$ and from $j-1$ to $k+2$. The intermediate values from the horizontal interpolation are

$$B_{j+x,k} = (1/6) \, (B_{j-1,k} \cdot R_1 + B_{j,k} \cdot R_2 + B_{j+1,k} \cdot R_3 + B_{j+2,k} \cdot R_4) \tag{13}$$

and the interpolation in the vertical direction is

$$B_{j+x,k+y} = (1/6) \, (B_{j+x,k-1} \cdot R_1 + B_{j+x,k} \cdot R_2 + B_{j+x,k+1} \cdot R_3 + B_{j+x,k+2} \cdot R_4) \tag{14}$$

where the weighting factors R_i are calculated from the real part (x or y respectively) of the address as

$$\begin{aligned}
R_1 &= (3+x)^3 - 4 \cdot (2+x)^3 + 6 \cdot (1+x)^3 - 4 \cdot x^3 \\
R_2 &= (2+x)^3 - 4 \cdot (1+x)^3 + 6 \cdot x^3 \\
R_3 &= (1+x)^3 - 4 \cdot x^3 \\
R_4 &= x^3
\end{aligned} \tag{15}$$

Figure 53. *Effect of rotating a one-pixel-wide black line using nearest neighbor, bilinear and bicubic interpolation.*

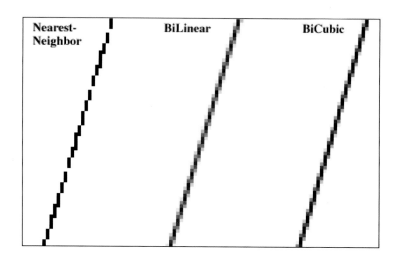

The bicubic fit is more isotropic than the bilinear method. Interpolation always has the effect of smoothing the image and removing some high frequency information, but minimizes aliasing or "stair-stepping" along lines and edges. **Figure 53** shows the results of rotating a line (originally a black vertical line one pixel wide) by seventeen degrees with no interpolation (selecting the nearest neighbor pixel value), bilinear, and bicubic interpolation. The aliasing with the nearest neighbor method is evident. Bilinear interpolation reduces the line contrast more than bicubic, and both assign grey values to adjacent pixels to smooth the appearance of the line.

The advantage of interpolation is that dimensions are altered as little as possible in the transformation, and in particular boundaries and other lines are not biased or distorted. **Figure 54** shows the same examples as **Figure 50**, with bilinear interpolation used. Careful examination of the figure shows that the lines appear straight and not "aliased" or stair-stepped, because some of the pixels along the sides of the lines have intermediate grey values resulting from the interpolation. In fact, computer graphics sometimes uses this same method to draw lines on CRT displays so that the stair-stepping inherent in drawing lines on a discrete pixel array is avoided. The technique is called anti-aliasing and produces lines whose pixels have grey values according to how close they lie to the mathematical location of the line. This fools the viewer into perceiving a smooth line.

For image warping or rubber-sheeting, interpolation has the advantage that dimensions are preserved. However, brightness values are not. With the nearest-pixel method achieved by rounding the pixel addresses, the dimensions are distorted but the brightness values are preserved. Choosing which method is appropriate to a particular imaging task depends primarily on which kind of information is more important, and secondarily

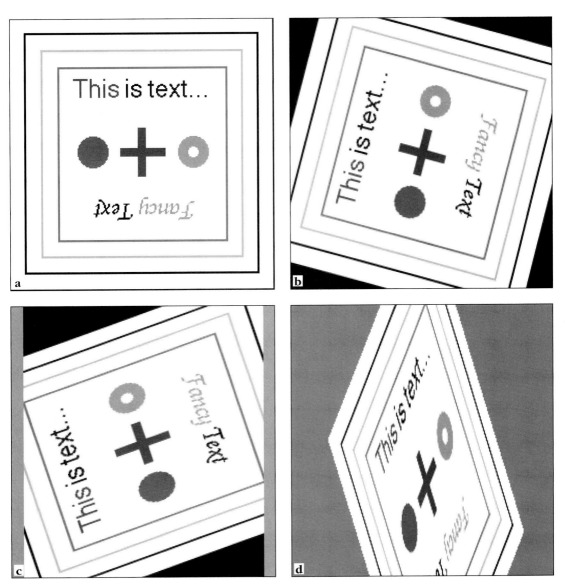

Figure 54. *Same generalized rotation and stretching as in Figure 50, but with bilinear interpolation. Note the smoothing of the lines and boundaries.*

on the additional computational effort required for the interpolation.

Figure 55 illustrates the effect of adding higher order terms to the warping equations. With quadratic terms, the trapezoidal distortion of a short focal length lens or SEM can be corrected. It is also possible to model the distortion of a spherical surface closely over modest distances. With higher order terms arbitrary distortion is possible, but this is rarely useful in an image processing situation since the reference points to determine such a distortion are not likely to be available.

Figure 55. Some additional examples of image warping:

a) *original test image;*

b) *linear warping with reversal;*

c) *quadratic warping showing trapezoidal foreshortening (no interpolation);*

d) *cubic warping in which lines are curved (approximation here is to a spherical surface);*

e) *twisting the center of the field while holding the edges fixed (also cubic warping);*

f) *arbitrary warping in which higher order and trigonometric terms are required.*

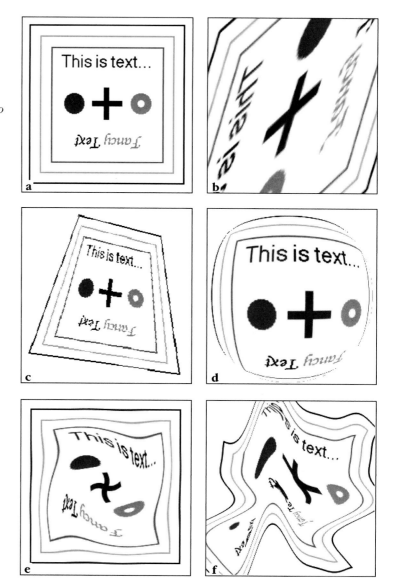

Morphing

Programs that can perform controlled warping according to mathematically defined relationships, or calculate those matrices of values from a set of identified fiducial or reference marks that apply to the entire image are generally rather specialized. But an entire class of consumer-level programs has become available for performing image morphing based on a net of user-defined control points. The points are generally placed at corresponding locations that are distinctive in the two images. For aligning two faces, for example, points at the tips of the eyes, corners of the mouth, along the hairline and chinline, and so forth are used as shown in the illustration in **Figure 56**.

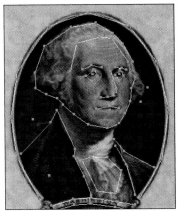
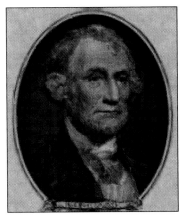
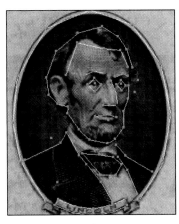

Figure 56. Transformation of George into Abe (pictures from US currency). The corresponding points marked on each end point image control the gradual distortion from one to the other. The midpoint frame is plausible as a person, and shares feature characteristics with both endpoints.

The program uses the points to form a tesselation of the first image into triangles (technically, the choice of which points to use as corners for the triangles is defined by a procedure called a Voronoi tesselation). Each triangle is uniformly stretched to fit the location of the corner points in the second image. Since the sides of the triangles are uniformly stretched, points along the edges of adjacent triangles are not displaced, although lines may be bent where they cross the boundaries. **Figure 57** shows an

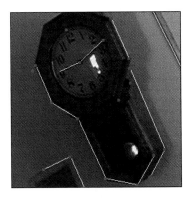
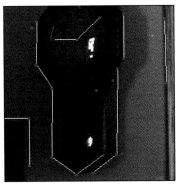

Figure 57. Alignment of two images of a clock. The control points shown on the two images allow the gradual distortion of one image to fit the second. Within the network of triangles, there are no abrupt distortions. But around the edges of the image and where pixels on one do not correspond to locations on the other, straight lines show sharp bends.

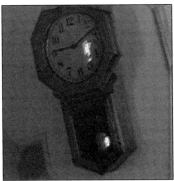

example of this effect when this procedure is used to rotate one image to match another.

With a triangular mesh and linear stretching of each triangle, lines crossing the boundaries of the triangles would be continuous, but sharply bent. Using spline or cubic equations to control the stretch gives a better appearance by making the curves smooth, but this is not a necessary indication that dimensions are preserved or that measurements can be made on such images.

The art of using these morphing programs lies primarily in using enough control points, and their careful placement. The results look quite realistic, as shown in the examples. This is especially true when a sequence of images is created with progressive motion of the control points from the original to final locations. These morphing "movies" show one image transforming gradually into the second. These effects are used routinely in creating television advertisements. It is not clear whether there are any technical applications requiring image measurement that can be satisfactorily accomplished with these programs, considering the somewhat arbitrary placement of points and distortion of dimensions and directions.

The ability to use morphing to align images of different objects and produce visually convincing images can be a powerful tool for communicating results to others. This procedure can be useful to show the similarity between two objects, but it is extraordinarily susceptible to misuse, producing apparent matching between different images that are really not the same.

Figure 58 shows an example of morphing to perform the alignment of a weather satellite image with a Mercator's projection weather map. The alignment process was carried out by locating about 30 points on each image, creating a tesselation of triangles between the points, and using them to control the distortion of one image to match the other. The original morph is a continuous movie that stretches the satellite image in some areas and directions while squeezing it in others, until it lines up with the map. An image from halfway through the process is shown in the figure. Notice that the lines are smoothly adjusted, with no sharp bends or other visual artefacts.

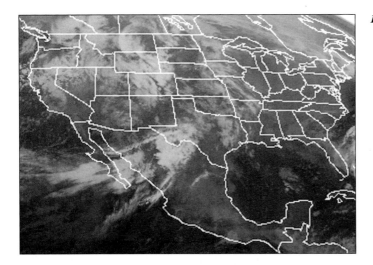

Figure 58. *Satellite image and corresponding weather map from 9:00 GMT on February 20, 1994. Morphing the satellite image to fit the Mercator projection map produces a continuous movie, the middle frame of which is shown.*

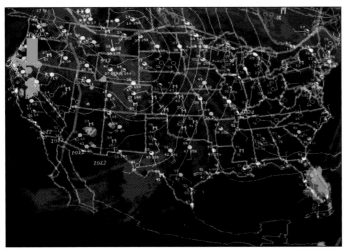

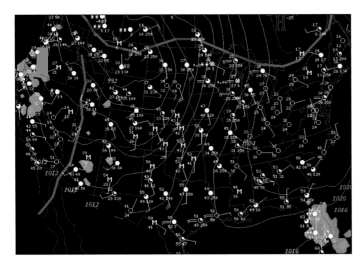

Image Enhancement

Processing in the Spatial Domain

The preceding chapter discussed methods for correcting or alleviating the principal defects in as-acquired images. There is a grey area between simply correcting these defects and going beyond to enhance the images. Enhancement is the subject of this chapter. Methods are available that increase the visibility of one portion, aspect or component of an image, though generally at the expense of others whose visibility is diminished. In this regard, image processing is a bit like word processing or food processing. It is possible to rearrange things to make a product that is more pleasing or interpretable, but the total amount of data does not change. In the case of images, this generally means that the number of bytes (or pixels) is not reduced. Most image analysis procedures attempt to extract only the "important" information from the image. An example would be to identify and count features in an image, reducing the amount of data from perhaps a million bytes to a few dozen, or even a single "Yes" or "No" answer in some quality control, medical, or forensic applications.

Image processing for purposes of enhancement can be performed in either the spatial domain (the array of pixels comprising our conventional representation of the image) or other domains, such as the Fourier domain discussed in Chapter 5. In the spatial domain, pixel values may be modified according to rules that depend on the original pixel value (local or point processes). Alternatively, pixel values may be combined with or compared to others in their immediate neighborhood in a variety of ways. Examples of each of these approaches were used in Chapter 3, to replace brightness values to expand image contrast or to smooth noise by kernel averaging or median filtering. Related techniques used in this chapter perform further enhancements.

It is worth noting here that 2D images typically consist of a very large number of pixels, from perhaps 1/4 million to several million. Even a point process that simply modifies the value of each pixel according to its previous contents requires that the computer address each pixel location. For a neighborhood process, each pixel must be addressed many times, and the processing speed slows down accordingly. Fast processors and high speed memory access (and a lot of memory) are essential requirements for this type of work. Some machines use dedicated hardware such as shift registers and array processors, or boards with dedicated memory and custom addressing circuits, or multiple processors with special programming, to permit near-real-time processing of images, when that is economically justified. As CPU speeds have increased, the need for special hardware has diminished.

Contrast manipulation

In Chapter 3, Figure 31 showed the example of expanding the contrast of a dim image by reassigning pixel brightness levels. In most systems, this can be done almost instantaneously by writing a table of values into the display hardware. This lookup table or LUT substitutes a display brightness value for each stored value and thus does not require actually modifying any of the values stored in memory for the image. Linearly expanding the contrast range by assigning the darkest pixel value to black, the brightest value to white, and each of the others to linearly interpolated shades of grey makes the best use of the display and enhances the visibility of features in the image.

It was also shown, in Chapter 1, that the same LUT approach can be used with colors by assigning a triplet of red, green, and blue values to each stored grey scale value. This pseudo-color also increases the visible difference between similar pixels; sometimes it is an aid to the user who wishes to see small or gradual changes in image brightness.

A typical computer display can show 2^8 or 256 different shades of grey, and many can produce colors with the same 2^8 brightness values for each of the red, green, and blue components to produce a total of 2^{24} or 16 million different colors. This is often described as "true color," since the gamut of colors that can be displayed is adequate to reproduce most natural scenes. It does not imply, of course, that the colors displayed are photometrically accurate or identical to the original color in the displayed scene. Indeed, that kind of accuracy is very difficult and requires special hardware and calibration.

More important, the 16 million different colors that such a system is capable of displaying, and even the 256 shades of grey, are far more than the human eye can distinguish. Under good viewing conditions, we can typically see only a few tens of different grey levels and hundreds of distinguishable colors. That means the display hardware of the image processing system is not being used very well to communicate the image information to the user. If many of the pixels in the image are quite bright, for example, they cannot be distinguished. If there are also some dark pixels present, we cannot simply expand the contrast. Instead, a more complicated relationship between stored and displayed values is needed.

In general, we can describe the manipulation terms of a transfer function relating the stored brightness value for each pixel to a displayed value. If this relationship is one-to-one, then for each stored value there will be a unique (although not necessarily visually discernible) displayed value. In some cases, it is advantageous to use transfer functions that are not one-to-one: several stored values are displayed with the same brightness value, so that other stored values can be spread further apart to increase their visual difference.

Figure 1 shows an image in which the 256 distinct pixel brightness values cannot all be discerned even on the display cathode ray tube (CRT); the printed version of the image is necessarily much worse. As discussed in Chapter 2, the number of distinct printed grey levels in a halftone image is determined by the variation in dot size of the printer. For a simple 300-dot-per-inch (dpi) laser writer, this requires a tradeoff between grey scale resolution (number of shades) and lateral resolution (number of halftone cells per inch). A typical compromise is 50 cells per inch and more than 30 grey levels, or 75 cells per inch and 17 grey levels. The imagesetter used for this book is capable of much higher resolution and more grey levels.

For comparison purposes, a good-quality photographic print can reproduce 20 to 30 grey levels (the negative can do much better). An instant print such as the Polaroid film commonly used with laboratory microscopes can show 10 to 15. However, both have much higher spatial resolution, and so the images appear sharper to the eye.

Even so, looking at the original image in **Figure 1**, the viewer cannot see the detail in the bright and dark regions of the image, even on the video screen (and certainly not on the print). Modifying the LUT can increase the visibility in one region or the other, or in both dark and bright regions, provided something else is given up in exchange. **Figure 1** shows several modifications to the original image produced simply by manipulating the transfer function and the LUT by drawing a new relationship between stored and displayed brightness. In this case, a freehand drawing was made that became the transfer function; it was adjusted purely for visual effect.

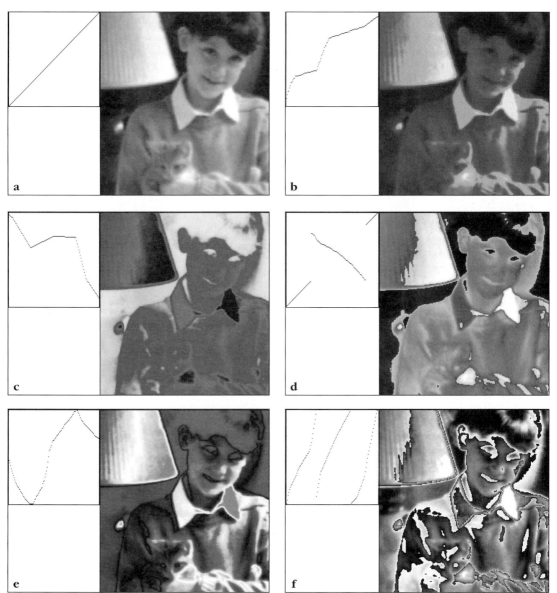

Figure 1. *An original image with a full range of brightness values and several examples of arbitrary hand-drawn display transfer functions which expand or alter the contrast in various parts of the range. The plot with each image shows the stored pixel brightness values on the horizontal axis and the displayed brightness on the vertical axis.* **Image a)** *has a transfer function that is the identity function, so that actual stored brightnesses are displayed.* **Images b)** *through* **f)** *illustrate various possibilities, including reversal and increased or decreased slope over parts of the brightness range.*

Note some of the imaging possibilities. A nonlinear relationship can expand one portion of the grey scale range while compressing another. In photographic processing and also in analog display electronics, this is called varying the gamma (the slope of the exposure-density curve). Using a computer, however, we can draw in transfer functions that are far more complicated, nonlinear, and arbitrary than can be achieved in the darkroom.

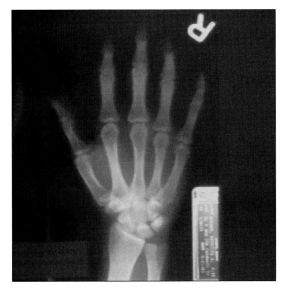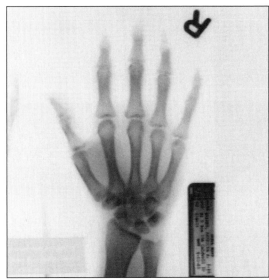

Figure 2. X-ray image of a human hand, viewed as a positive and a negative.

Reversing all of the contrast range produces the equivalent of a photographic negative, which sometimes improves the visibility of details (especially in dark regions of the original image). **Figure 2** illustrates this with an example of an X-ray image, which are commonly examined using negatives. Reversing only a portion of the brightness range produces a visually strange effect, called solarization by photographers, that can also be used to show detail in shadowed or saturated areas.

Increasing the slope of the transfer function so that it "wraps around" produces an image in which several quite different stored brightness values may have the same display brightness. If the overall organization of the image is familiar to the viewer, though, this contouring may not be too disruptive, and it can increase the visibility for small differences. However, as with the use of pseudo-color, this kind of treatment is easily overdone and may confuse rather than enhance most images.

Certainly, experimentally modifying the transfer function until the image "looks good" and best shows those features of most interest to the viewer provides an ultimately flexible (if dangerous) tool. In most cases, it is desirable to have more reproducible and meaningful transfer functions available which can be applied equally to a series of images, so that proper comparison is possible.

The most common kinds of transfer functions are shown in **Figure 3**. These are curves of displayed vs. stored brightness following simple mathematical relationships such as logarithmic or power law curves. A logarithmic or square root curve will compress the displayed brightnesses at the bright end of the scale, while expanding those at the dark end. This kind of relationship can also convert an image from a camera with a linear response

Figure 3. *Examples of display transfer functions.*

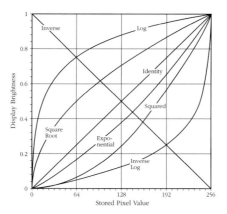

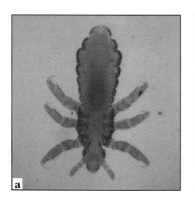
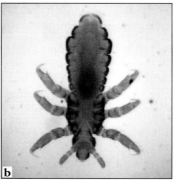
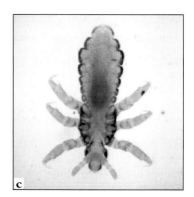

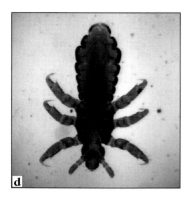
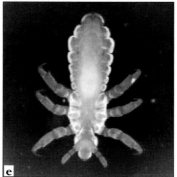
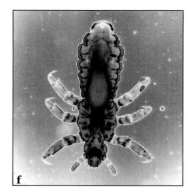

Figure 4. Manipulation of the grey scale transfer function:

a) an original, moderately low-contrast transmission light microscope image (prepared slide of a head louse);

b) expanded linear transfer function adjusted to the minimum and maximum brightness values in the image;

c) positive gamma (log) function;

d) negative gamma (log) function;

e) negative linear transfer function;

f) nonlinear transfer function (high slope linear contrast over central portion of brightness range, with negative slope or solarization for dark and bright portions).

to the more common logarithmic response. An inverse log or squared curve will do the opposite. The error-function curve compresses middle grey values and spreads the scale at both the bright and dark extremes. An inverse curve simply produces a negative image.

Any of these functions may be used in addition to contrast expansion, which stretches the original scale to the full range of the display. Curves or tables of values for these transfer functions are typically precalculated and stored, so that they can be loaded quickly to modify the display LUT. Many systems allow quite a few different tables to be kept on hand for use when an image requires it, just as a series of color LUTs may be available on disk for pseudo-color displays. **Figure 4** illustrates the use of several transfer functions to enhance the visibility of structures in an image.

Histogram equalization

In addition to precalculated and stored tables, it is sometimes advantageous to construct a transfer function for a specific image. Unlike the arbitrary hand-drawn functions shown above, however, we would like to have a specific algorithm that gives reproducible and (hopefully) optimal results. The most popular of these methods is called histogram equalization (Stark & Fitzgerald, 1996). To understand it, we must begin by understanding the image brightness histogram.

Figure 5 shows an example of an image with its histogram. The plot shows the number of pixels in the image having each of the

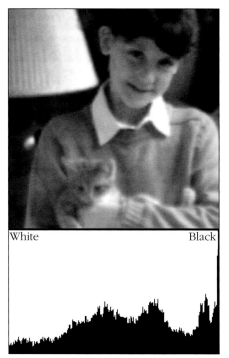

Figure 5. *An image with its brightness histogram. The plot shows the number of pixels with each of the 256 possible brightness values.*

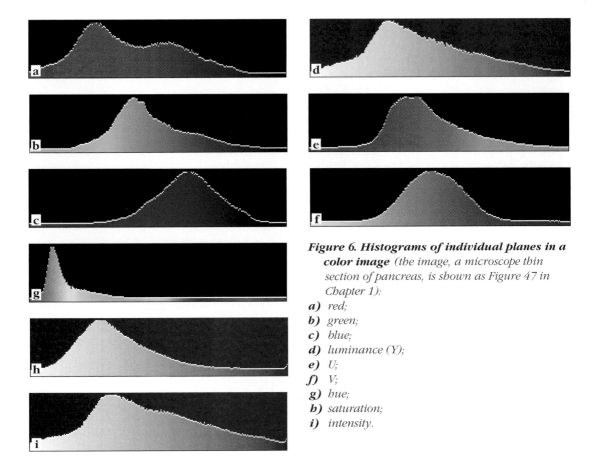

Figure 6. Histograms of individual planes in a color image *(the image, a microscope thin section of pancreas, is shown as Figure 47 in Chapter 1):*
a) *red;*
b) *green;*
c) *blue;*
d) *luminance (Y);*
e) *U;*
f) *V;*
g) *hue;*
h) *saturation;*
i) *intensity.*

256 possible values of stored brightness. Peaks in the histogram correspond to the more common brightness values, which often identify particular structures that are present. Valleys between the peaks indicate brightness values that are less common in the image. Empty regions at either end of the histogram would show that no pixels have those values, indicating that the image brightness range does not cover the full 0–255 range available.

For a color image, it is possible to show three histograms corresponding to the three color axes. As shown in **Figure 6**, this can be done equally well for RGB, HSI, or YUV color coordinates. Any of these sets of histograms are incomplete, however, in that they do not show the combinations of values that are associated in the same pixels. A three-dimensional histogram, in which points in the histogram have coordinates that correspond to the color values and show the number of pixels with each possible combination of values, is illustrated in **Figure 7**. Dark values indicate a large number of pixels with a particular combination of components. The projections of the three-dimensional histogram onto each of the two-dimensional faces of the cube are shown. This tool will be used again in Chapter 6 in the context of selecting color combinations for thresholding.

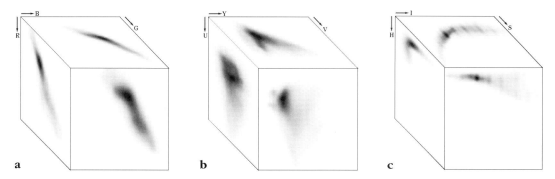

Figure 7. Three-way histograms of the same data shown in Figure 6: a) RGB; *b)* YUV; *c)* HSI.

Generally, images have unique brightness histograms. Even images of different areas of the same sample or scene, in which the various structures present have consistent brightness levels wherever they occur, will have different histograms, depending on the area fraction of each structure. Changing the overall illumination will shift the peaks in the histogram. In addition, most real images exhibit some variation in brightness within features (e.g., from the edge to the center) or in different regions.

From the standpoint of efficiently using the available grey levels on the display, some grey scale values are underutilized. It might be better to spread out the displayed grey levels in the peak areas selectively, compressing them in the valleys so that the same number of pixels in the display show each of the possible brightness levels. This is called histogram equalization. The transfer function is simply the original brightness histogram of the image, replotted as a cumulative plot as shown in **Figure 8**.

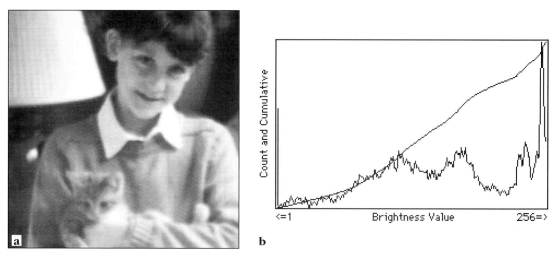

Figure 8. *The original and cumulative histogram from Figure 5. The cumulative plot (**b**) gives the transfer function for histogram equalization. The image (**a**) shows the result of applying this function.*

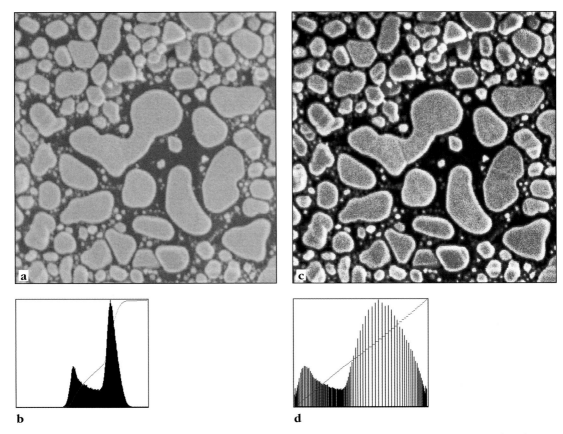

Figure 9. *An SEM image of deposited gold particles* **(a)** *with its histogram shown in conventional and cumulative form* **(b)** *. After histogram equalization* **(c)** *the cumulative histogram is a straight line* **(d)** *.*

A cumulative histogram helps to understand what histogram equalization does. **Figure 9** shows an SEM image with its original histogram shown in conventional presentation and also as a plot of the total number of pixels less than or equal to each brightness value. After equalization the latter plot is a straight line.

Histogram equalization reassigns the brightness values of pixels based on the image histogram. Individual pixels retain their brightness order (that is, they remain brighter or darker than other pixels) but the values are shifted, so that an equal number of pixels have each possible brightness value. In many cases, this spreads out the values in regions where different regions meet, showing detail in areas with a high brightness gradient.

An image having a few regions with very similar brightness values presents a histogram with peaks. The sizes of these peaks give the relative area of the different phase regions and are useful for image analysis. Performing a histogram equalization on the image spreads the peaks out, while compressing other parts of the histogram by assigning the same or very close brightness values to those pixels that are few in number and have intermediate brightnesses. This equalization makes it possible to see

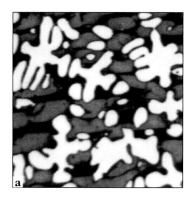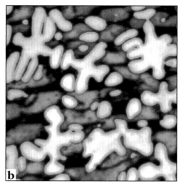

Figure 10. Metallographic light microscope image of a three-phase metal alloy. In the original image *(a)*, phase regions are characterized by fairly uniform brightness values. After histogram equalization *(b)* the shading in these regions is evident because the brightness values for the pixels have been spread apart.

minor variations within regions that appeared nearly uniform in the original image.

The process is quite simple. For each brightness level j in the original image (and its histogram), the new assigned value k is calculated as

$$k = \sum_{i=0}^{j} N_i/T \qquad (1$$

where the sum counts the number of pixels in the image (by integrating the histogram) with brightness equal to or less than j, and T is the total number of pixels (or the total area of the histogram).

Figure 10 shows an example. The original metallographic specimen has three phase regions with dark, intermediate, and light grey values. These peaks are separated in the histogram (**Figure 11**) by regions having fewer pixels with intermediate brightness values, often because they happen to fall on the boundary between lighter and darker phase regions. Histogram equalization shows the shading within the phase regions, indiscernible in the original image. It also spreads out the brightness values in the histogram, as shown.

Some pixels that originally had different values are now assigned the same value, which represents a loss of information, while other values that were once very close together have been spread out, leaving gaps in the histogram. This image of a polished metal shows well-defined peaks corresponding to different phases present. The histogram-equalized image is less satisfying in terms of showing the distinction between the phases, but much better at showing the gradation in the white phase, which was not visible in the original.

This equalization process need not be performed on an entire image. Enhancing a portion of the original image, rather than the entire area, is also useful in many situations. This is particularly true when large regions of the image correspond to different types of structures or scenes and are generally brighter or darker than the rest of the image. When portions of an image can be se-

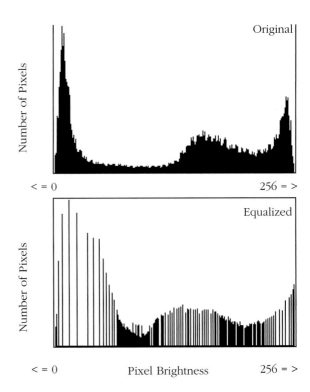

Figure 11. Brightness histograms from the images in Figure 10. The horizontal scale is brightness, from zero (white) to 255 (black). The vertical scale is the number of pixels in the image with that brightness value. The original image shows three major peaks corresponding to the three phase regions in the original specimen, with few pixels having intermediate values. After equalization, the brightness values are reassigned to cover the brightness range uniformly. This causes some pixels with initially different brightness values to be assigned the same value, and other values to be missing altogether.

lected, either manually or by some algorithm based on the variation in the brightness histogram, a selective equalization can be used to bring out local detail.

Figure 12 shows regions of the same test image used previously, with three regions separately selected and equalized. Two of these regions are arbitrary rectangular and elliptical shapes, drawn by hand. In many cases, this kind of manual selection is the most straightforward way to specify a region. The third area is the lampshade, which can be isolated from the rest of the image because locally the boundary is a sharp transition from white to black. Methods for locating boundary edges are discussed later in the chapter.

Each of the three regions shown was used to construct a brightness histogram, which was then equalized. The resulting reassigned brightness values were then substituted only for the pixels within the region. In the two dark regions (the girl's face and the region near her shoulder), equalization produces an overall brightening as well as spreading out the brightness values so that the small variations are more evident. In the bright area (the lampshade), the overall brightness is reduced; again, more variation is evident.

In all cases, the brightness values in the equalized regions show some contouring, the visible steps in brightness produced by the small number of different values present in these regions in the original image. Contouring is usually considered to be an image

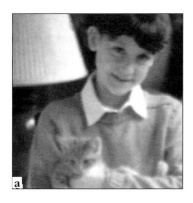 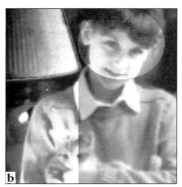

defect, since it distorts the actual smooth variation in values present in the image. When it is introduced specifically for effect, it may be called posterization (not to be confused with the use of the same term for the result of repeatedly applying a median filter, discussed in Chapter 3).

It should be noted, of course, that once a region has been selected, either manually or automatically, the contrast can be modified in any way desired: by loading a prestored LUT, calculating a histogram equalization function, or simply stretching the grey scale linearly to maximize contrast. However, when these operations are applied to only a portion of the entire image, it is not possible to manipulate only the display LUT. Since the stored grey values in other regions of the image are to be shown with their original corresponding display values, it is necessary to actually modify the contents of the stored image to alter the display. This is a very fast operation, since it is performed using a transfer function that is loaded or precalculated from the histogram and each pixel is accessed one time.

Histogram equalization of regions within an image can dramatically improve the local visibility of details, but it usually alters the relationship between brightness and structure. In most cases, it is desirable for the brightness level of pixels associated with a particular type of feature in the image to be the same, wherever in the field of view it may occur. This allows rapid classification of the features for counting or measurement. Local modification of the grey scale relationship voids this assumption, making the display brightness of features dependent on other features that happen to be nearby or in the selected region.

Histogram equalization in **Figure 12** assigns the same new grey value to each pixel having a given original grey value, everywhere in the region. The result is that regions often have very noticeable and abrupt boundaries, which may or may not follow feature boundaries in the original image. Another approach performs the equalization in a region around each pixel in the image, with the result applied separately to each individual pixel. This is normally done by specifying a neighborhood size (typically round

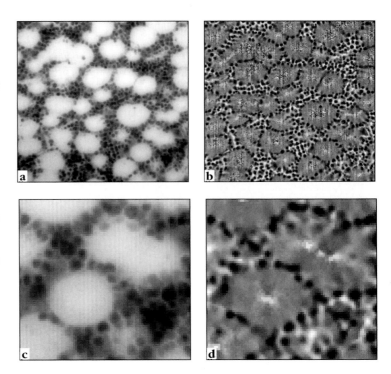

Figure 13. *Local equalization applied to every pixel in an image. This is a transmission light micrograph of bone marrow. For each pixel in the original image (a), a 9×9 neighborhood has been used to construct a histogram. Equalization of that histogram produces a new brightness value for each pixel, but this is only saved for the central pixel. The process is repeated to apply to each pixel in the original image except those too near the edge, producing the result (b). Enlargements to show individual pixels are shown in (c) and (d). The effect of this local equalization is to enhance edges and reveal detail in light and dark regions. However, in the center of uniform regions it can produce artefacts and noise.*

or square). All of the pixels in that region are counted into a histogram, but the equalization procedure is applied only to the central pixel. This process is then repeated for each pixel in the image, always using the original brightness values to construct the histogram.

Figure 13 shows an example in which the neighborhood size is a 9×9 pixel square. The process is not applied within a distance of four pixels of the edges of the image, where the region cannot be centered on a pixel. Special rules can be made for these points, if required. The calculation is quite simple in this method, since for each pixel the equalized brightness value is just the number of darker pixels in the neighborhood. For the case of a 9×9 region, the maximum number of pixels is 81, so the procedure produces an image in which the maximum number of distinct brightness values is 81, instead of the original 256.

The process of local equalization enhances contrast near edges, revealing details in both light and dark regions. However, it can be seen in the example that in the center of large, nominally uniform regions, this can produce artificial contrast variations that introduce artefacts into the image. The solution is to increase the size of the region so that it is larger than any uniform area in the image. However, this slows down the process and loses some of the ability to locally increase contrast at boundaries.

Somewhat more uniform results can be obtained with a circular region 11 pixels wide, as shown in **Figure 14**. Circular neighborhoods are generally more isotropic and produce better results

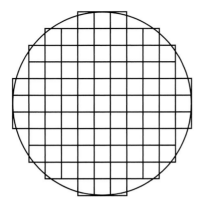

Figure 14. *Approximation to a circle 11 pixels wide contains a total of 89 pixels. Using a round neighborhood minimizes directional distortion and artefacts in the image due to local equalization.*

than square ones for all neighborhood image processing operations, but make the programming logic for pixel addressing somewhat more complicated. The 11 pixel wide circular region contains 89 pixels, including the central one. If a brightness histogram is formed from just those 89 pixels, a transfer function can be constructed that would assign a new brightness value to each pixel, but the assignment will be performed only for the one central pixel. Then the process can be repeated for the next pixel, using a slightly shifted neighborhood region of 89 pixels. Of course, it is necessary to construct a new image so that only the original values of the neighboring pixels are used to perform the equalization.

Since it is not necessary to build the entire table of substitute brightness values, an efficient way to perform this calculation is simply to count the number of pixels in the neighborhood region that are darker than or equal to the central pixel. The ratio of this number to 89 (the total number of pixels in the neighborhood), multiplied by 255 (the maximum grey value in the image, if it is a conventional 8-bit image), gives the new pixel brightness value.

Clever use of logic to add in the brightness of each new row or column of pixel values and remove the old ones as the process is repeated for each pixel in the image can make this operation moderately fast. The resulting image can have only a total of 89 different possible pixel values with this size neighborhood. Of course, larger neighborhoods can also be used with correspondingly more pixels and possible grey levels.

Figure 15 shows an example of the application of local or neighborhood equalization using the 11-pixel-wide circular region described. Notice that the gradient within each of the uniform grey or white grain areas is an artefact of the method, because the regions overlap more of the adjacent areas when they are near the edges. This method tends to highlight edges and boundaries and shows separations and detail in nearly uniform regions (note the improved separation between dark features).

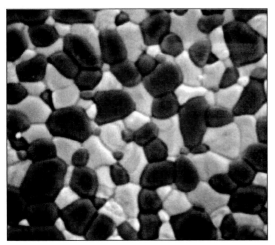
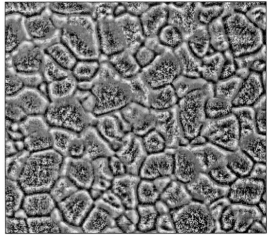

Figure 15. *Local equalization of a two-phase material (alumina-zirconia) using an 11-pixel-diameter circle. Note the increased contrast at boundaries, and the gradients within the grains producing noise artefacts within the grains.*

Local equalization is also useful for dealing with features of a consistent size that are superimposed on a varying background. **Figure 16** shows an example of a fingerprint covering some printing. The change in background brightness makes it impossible to threshold and difficult to see the important features. After local equalization the fingerprint is clear.

Laplacian

Local, or neighborhood, equalization of image contrast produces an increase in local contrast at boundaries. This has the effect of making edges easier for the viewer to see, consequently making the image appear sharper. This section will discuss several different approaches to edge enhancement that are less sensitive to overall brightness levels and feature sizes than the equalization discussed above.

The first set of operations uses neighborhoods with multiplicative kernels of integer weights identical in principle to those used in

Figure 16. *Fingerprint superimposed on printing (**a**) and revealed by local equalization (**b**).*

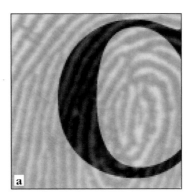
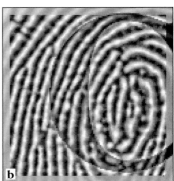

Chapter 3 for noise smoothing. In the section on smoothing, kernels were written as an array of integers. For example,

1	2	1
2	4	2
1	2	1

This 3×3 kernel is understood to mean that the central pixel brightness value is multiplied by 4, the values of the 4 touching neighbors to the sides and above and below are multiplied by 2, and the 4 diagonally touching neighbors by 1. The total value is added up and then divided by 16 (the sum of the 9 weights) to produce a new brightness value for the pixel. Other arrays of weights were also shown, some involving much larger arrays than this simple 3×3. For smoothing, all of the kernels were symmetrical about the center, and the examples shown in Chapter 3 had only positive weight values.

A very simple kernel that is still symmetrical, but does not have exclusively positive values, is the 3×3 Laplacian operator

−1	−1	−1
−1	+8	−1
−1	−1	−1

This subtracts the brightness values of each of the neighboring pixels from the central pixel. Consequently, in a region of the image that is uniform in brightness or has a uniform gradient of brightness, the result of applying this kernel is to reduce the grey level to zero. When a discontinuity is present within the neighborhood in the form of a point, line, or edge, the result of the Laplacian is a nonzero value. It may be either positive or negative, depending on where the central point lies with respect to edge, etc.

In order to display the result when both positive and negative pixel values arise, it is common to add a medium grey value (128 for the case of a single-byte-per-pixel image with grey values in the range from 0 to 255) so that the zero points are middle grey and the brighter and darker values produced by the Laplacian can be seen. Some systems plot the absolute value of the result, but this tends to produce double lines along edges that are confusing both to the viewer and to subsequent processing and measurement operations.

As the name of the Laplacian operator implies, it is an approximation to the linear second derivative of brightness B in directions x and y

$$\nabla^2 B \equiv \frac{\partial^2 B}{\partial x^2} + \frac{\partial^2 B}{\partial y^2} \qquad (2$$

which is invariant to rotation, and hence insensitive to the direction in which the discontinuity runs. This highlights the points,

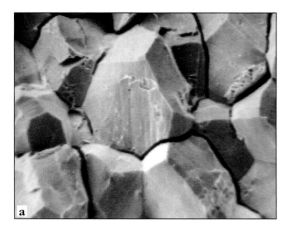

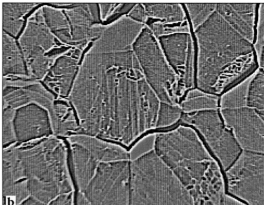

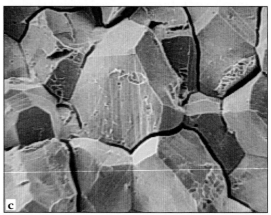

Figure 17. Enhancement of contrast at edges, lines and points using a Laplacian:
a) original SEM image of ceramic fracture;
b) application of Laplacian operator;
c) subtraction of the Laplacian from the original image.

lines, and edges in the image and suppresses uniform and smoothly varying regions, with the result shown in **Figure 17**. By itself, this Laplacian image is not very easy to interpret. Adding the Laplacian enhancement of the edges to the original image restores the overall grey scale variation which the human viewer can comfortably interpret. It also sharpens the image by locally increasing the contrast at discontinuities (**Figure 17**). This can be done simply by changing the weights in the kernel, so that it becomes

−1	−1	−1
−1	+9	−1
−1	−1	−1

This kernel is often described as a sharpening operator, because of the improved image contrast that it produces at edges. Justification for the procedure can be found in two different explanations. First, consider blur in an image to be modeled by a diffusion process, which would obey the partial differential equation

$$\frac{\partial f}{\partial t} = k\nabla^2 f \qquad (3$$

where the blur function is $f(x,y,t)$ and t is time. If this is expanded into a Taylor series around time τ, we can express the unblurred image as

$$B(x,y) = f(x,y,\tau) - \tau \frac{\partial f}{\partial t} + \frac{\tau^2}{2} \frac{\partial^2 f}{\partial t^2} - \dots$$ (4

If the higher-order terms are ignored, this is just

$$B = f - k\tau \nabla^2 f$$ (5

In other words, the unblurred image B can be restored by subtracting the Laplacian (times a constant) from the blurred image. While the modeling of image blur as a diffusion process is at best approximate and the scaling constant is unknown or arbitrary, this at least gives some plausibility to the approach.

At least equally important is the simple fact that the processed image "looks good." **Figure 18** illustrates this with an astronomical photograph of Saturn. The visibility of the fine detail in the rings and atmosphere is enhanced by processing. The human visual system itself concentrates on edges and ignores uniform regions (Marr & Hildreth, 1980; Marr, 1982; Hildreth, 1983). This capability is hard-wired into our retinas. Connected directly to

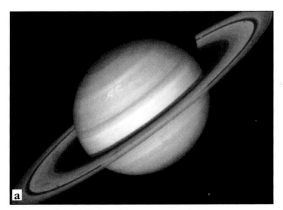

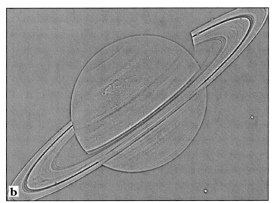

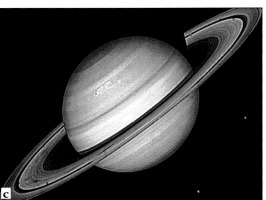

Figure 18. Application of a Laplacian operator to enhance the visibility of band structures in the rings and atmosphere of Saturn:
a) original image;
b) application of Laplacian operator (notice the haloes around the tiny moons);
c) subtraction of the Laplacian from the original image.

Figure 19. Illustration of Mach bands:

a) *uniform grey bands;*

b) *brightness profile of the bands;*

c) *application of a Laplacian to the bands in image **a**, showing increased contrast at the boundaries (this is the way the human eye perceives the uniform bands in image **a**);*

d) *brightness profile of image **c**.*

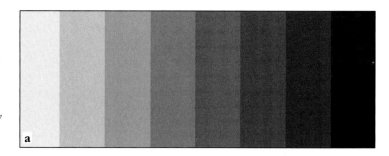

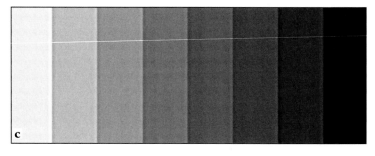

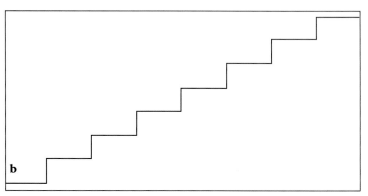

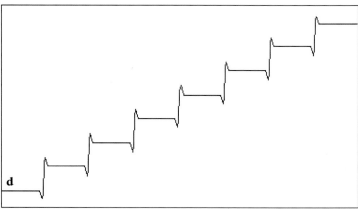

the rods and cones of the retina are two layers of processing neurons that perform an operation very similar to the Laplacian. The horizontal cells in the second layer average together the signals from several neighboring sensors in the first layer, and the bipolar cells in the third layer subtract that signal from the original sensor output. This is called local inhibition and helps us to extract boundaries and edges.

At a more practical level, consider the ability of the eye to respond to cartoons and line drawings. These are highly abstracted bits of information about the original scene, yet they are entirely recognizable and interpretable. The cartoon provides the eye with exactly the minimum information it would otherwise have to extract from the scene itself to transmit up to higher levels of processing in the brain. (Similar inhibition in the time domain, using the next two layers of retinal neurons, helps us detect motion.)

One characteristic of human vision that confirms this behavior is the presence of Mach bands, a common illusion resulting from local brightness inhibition (Mach, 1906; Cornsweet, 1970). **Figure 19** shows a series of vertical bands of uniform intensity. The human viewer does not perceive them as uniform, but sees an undershoot and overshoot on each side of the steps as shown in the plot. This increases the contrast at the step, and hence its visibility.

To see how this works using the Laplacian, we will use a one-dimensional kernel of the form

$$-1 \qquad +2 \qquad -1$$

and apply it to a series of brightness values along a line profile, across a step of moderate steepness

| 2 | 2 | 2 | 2 | 2 | 4 | 6 | 6 | 6 | 6 | 6 |

Shifting the kernel to each position, multiplying the kernel values times the brightness values, then adding, gives the result

| 0 | 0 | 0 | 0 | −2 | 0 | +2 | 0 | 0 | 0 | 0 |

which can be subtracted from the original to give

| 2 | 2 | 2 | 2 | 0 | 4 | 8 | 6 | 6 | 6 | 6 |

The undershoot and overshoot in brightness on either side of the step correspond to the Mach band effect.

Local inhibition also influences our perception of brightness and color. **Figure 20** shows the effect of the surrounding grey scale

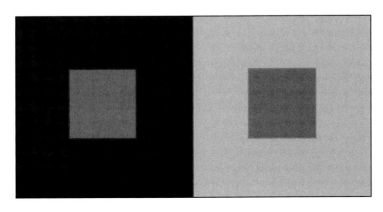

Figure 20. *Visual inhibition causes the brightness of the central grey square to appear different depending on the brightness of the surroundings.*

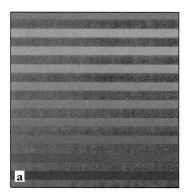

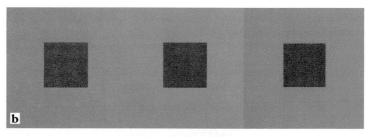

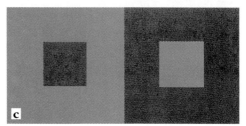

Figure 21. Inhibition in color images:

a) the red lines are constant in color and width, but appear to vary because of changes in the blue/cyan lines;

b) the central square appears to change in size and color with variations in the surroundings;

c) the color of the central square looks brighter and more saturated than the same color in the surroundings.

value on the apparent brightness and size of the central square (the two central grey squares are identical). This also happens in color. **Figure 21** illustrates several effects of local inhibition. In **Figure 21a** the reddish lines appear to change in color, brightness and thickness according to the varying colors of the intervening cyan/blue lines. In **Figure 21b**, the three identical central squares appear to vary in size, color and brightness according to the color of the surrounding square. In **Figure 21c**, the size of the two central squares appears different, and the color of the central square appears brighter and more saturated than when the same color occupies the surrounding outer patch. Similar visual illusions based on inhibition are commonly shown in many books and articles on vision and perception.

Inhibition is a process that takes place within the eye itself. Connections between the neurons within the retina suppress the output from one region according to its neighbors. Inhibition is useful for edge detection, but also affects our visual comparisons of size and orientation. **Figure 22** shows a typical result from an experiment in which the output from a single retinal ganglion in the optic nerve (shown as a time sequence across the top) is plotted as a small white target is slowly moved across the visual field. The cluster of white dots shows the location of the corresponding receptor on the retina. Notice the zone around the receptor that is very poor in white dots. Light shining on neighboring receptors inhibits the output from the central receptor. Presenting a dark spot in the visual field produces additional output from the receptor when it lies within the zone of inhibition, and suppresses output when it lies on the receptor. Selecting different ganglia will map other receptor cells, including those that surround the one shown. Each cell inhibits output from its neighbors. Other ganglia show temporal inhibition, in which output from a cell ignores the steady presence of either light or dark,

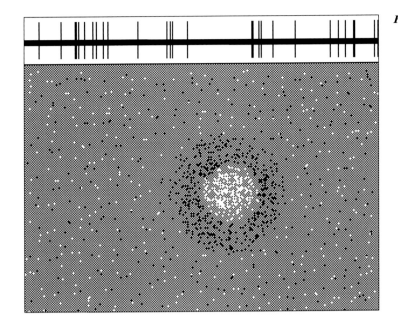

Figure 22. *Experimental results plotting the output from a single retinal ganglion in the optic nerve as targets consisting of small white or black circles are moved slowly across the visual field. The central cluster of white dots shows a positive response to the white circle, and the reduction in pulses when the white target lies in the field of a neighboring receptor. The dark target gives a complementary result.*

and responds only to changes in illumination. You can demonstrate this effect by staring at a bright red pattern and then looking away; the afterimage will appear in your eye as green.

Another way to describe the operation of the Laplacian is as a high-pass filter. In Chapter 5, image processing in the Fourier domain is discussed in terms of the high- and low-frequency components of the image brightness. A low-pass filter, such as the smoothing kernels discussed above and in Chapter 3, removes the high-frequency variability associated with noise, which can cause nearby pixels to vary in brightness. Conversely, a high-pass filter allows these high frequencies to remain (pass through the filter), while removing the low frequencies corresponding to the gradual overall variation in brightness.

As with smoothing kernels, there are many different sets of integers and different-size kernels that can be used to apply a Laplacian to an image. The simplest just uses the four immediately touching pixels that share a side with the central pixel

$$
\begin{array}{ccc}
 & -1 & \\
-1 & +4 & -1 \\
 & -1 & \\
\end{array}
$$

Larger kernels may combine a certain amount of smoothing by having positive weights for pixels in a small region near the central pixel, surrounded by negative weights for pixels farther away. Several examples are shown below. Because of the shape of these kernels when they are plotted as isometric views (**Figure 23**), they are sometimes described as a Mexican hat or sombrero filter; this name is usually reserved for kernels with more than one positive-weighted pixel at the center.

Figure 23. *Isometric and contour plot views of the 17×17 Mexican hat kernel.*

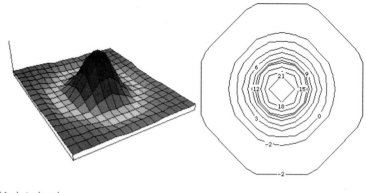

5×5 Laplacian kernel

```
 0   0  -1   0   0
 0  -1  -2  -1   0
-1  -2  16  -2  -1
 0  -1  -2  -1   0
 0   0  -1   0   0
```

7×7 Mexican hat kernel

```
 0   0  -1  -1  -1   0   0
 0  -1  -3  -3  -3  -1   0
-1  -3   0   7   0  -3  -1
-1  -3   7  24   7  -3  -1
-1  -3   0   7   0  -3  -1
 0  -1  -3  -3  -3  -1   0
 0   0  -1  -1  -1   0   0
```

13×13 Mexican hat kernel

```
 0   0   0   0   0  -1  -1  -1   0   0   0   0   0
 0   0   0  -1  -1  -2  -2  -2  -1  -1   0   0   0
 0   0  -2  -2  -3  -3  -4  -3  -3  -2  -2   0   0
 0  -1  -2  -3  -3  -3  -2  -3  -3  -3  -2  -1   0
 0  -1  -3  -3  -1   4   6   4  -1  -3  -3  -1   0
-1  -2  -3  -3   4  14  19  14   4  -3  -3  -2  -1
-1  -2  -4  -2   6  19  24  19   6  -2  -4  -2  -1
-1  -2  -3  -3   4  14  19  14   4  -3  -3  -2  -1
 0  -1  -3  -3  -1   4   6   4  -1  -3  -3  -1   0
 0  -1  -2  -3  -3  -3  -2  -3  -3  -3  -2  -1   0
 0   0  -2  -2  -3  -3  -4  -3  -3  -2  -2   0   0
 0   0   0  -1  -1  -2  -2  -2  -1  -1   0   0   0
 0   0   0   0   0  -1  -1  -1   0   0   0   0   0
```

17×17 Mexican hat kernel

```
 0   0   0   0   0   0  -1  -1  -1  -1  -1   0   0   0   0   0   0
 0   0   0   0  -1  -1  -1  -1  -1  -1  -1  -1  -1   0   0   0   0
 0   0  -1  -1  -1  -2  -3  -3  -3  -3  -3  -2  -1  -1  -1   0   0
 0   0  -1  -1  -2  -3  -3  -3  -3  -3  -3  -3  -2  -1  -1   0   0
 0  -1  -1  -2  -3  -3  -3  -2  -3  -3  -3  -3  -3  -2  -1  -1   0
 0  -1  -2  -3  -3  -3   0   2   4   2   0  -3  -3  -3  -2  -1   0
-1  -1  -3  -3  -3   0   4  10  12  10   4   0  -3  -3  -3  -1  -1
-1  -1  -3  -3  -2   2  10  18  21  18  10   2  -2  -3  -3  -1  -1
-1  -1  -3  -3  -3   4  12  21  24  21  12   4  -3  -3  -3  -1  -1
-1  -1  -3  -3  -2   2  10  18  21  18  10   2  -2  -3  -3  -1  -1
-1  -1  -3  -3  -3   0   4  10  12  10   4   0  -3  -3  -3  -1  -1
 0  -1  -2  -3  -3  -3   0   2   4   2   0  -3  -3  -3  -2  -1   0
 0  -1  -1  -2  -3  -3  -3  -2  -3  -2  -3  -3  -3  -2  -1  -1   0
 0   0  -1  -1  -2  -3  -3  -3  -3  -3  -3  -3  -2  -1  -1   0   0
 0   0  -1  -1  -1  -2  -3  -3  -3  -3  -3  -2  -1  -1  -1   0   0
 0   0   0   0  -1  -1  -1  -1  -1  -1  -1  -1  -1   0   0   0   0
 0   0   0   0   0   0  -1  -1  -1  -1  -1   0   0   0   0   0   0
```

Derivatives

The Laplacian is a good high-pass filter, but not a particularly good tool for demarcating edges (Berzins, 1984). In most cases, boundaries or edges of features or regions appear at least locally as a step in brightness, sometimes spread over several pixels. The Laplacian gives a larger response to a line than to a step, and to a point than to a line. In an image that contains noise, which is typically present as points varying in brightness due to counting statistics, detector characteristics, etc., the Laplacian will

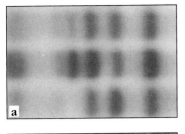

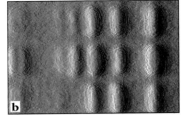

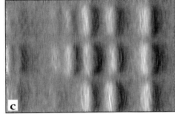

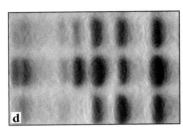

Figure 24. Image of a protein separation gel:
a) original;
b) difference between each pixel and its neighbor to the left;
c) vertical averaging of image **b** to reduce noise;
d) horizontal derivative using a 3×3 kernel as discussed in the text.

show such points more strongly than the edges or boundaries that are of interest.

Another approach to locating edges uses first derivatives in two or more directions. It will be helpful to first examine simple, one-dimensional first derivatives. Some images are essentially one-dimensional, such as chromatography preparations in which proteins are spread along lanes in an electrical field (**Figure 24**) or tree ring patterns from drill cores (**Figure 25**). Applying a first

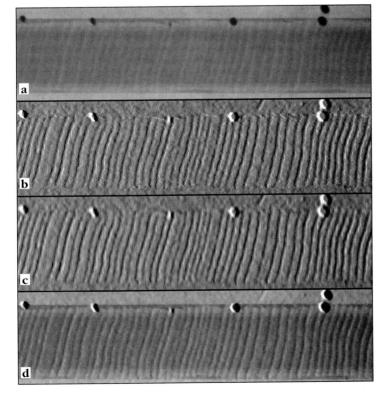

Figure 25. Image of tree rings in a drill core:
a) original;
b) difference between each pixel and its neighbor to the left;
c) vertical averaging of image **b** to reduce noise;
d) horizontal derivative using a 3×3 kernel as discussed in the text.

derivative to such an image, in the direction of important variation, demarcates the boundaries and enhances the visibility of small steps and other details, as shown in **Figures 24** and **25**.

Of course, for an image with digitized finite pixels, a continuous derivative cannot be performed. Instead, the difference value between adjacent pixels can be calculated as a finite derivative. This difference is also somewhat noisy, but averaging in the direction perpendicular to the derivative can smooth the result, as shown in **Figures 24** and **25**.

A derivative image with smoother appearance can be produced with fewer steps by applying an asymmetric kernel. Consider a set of kernels of the form shown below. There are 8 possible rotational orientations of this kernel about the center.

$$
\begin{array}{ccc}
1 & 0 & -1 \\
2 & 0 & -2 \\
1 & 0 & -1
\end{array}
\qquad
\begin{array}{ccc}
2 & 1 & 0 \\
1 & 0 & -1 \\
0 & -1 & -2
\end{array}
\qquad
\begin{array}{ccc}
1 & 2 & 1 \\
0 & 0 & 0 \\
-1 & -2 & -1
\end{array}
\quad \cdots
$$

Applying the first pattern of values shown to the tree ring and protein separation images is shown in **Figures 24** and **25**.

One improvement comes from averaging together the adjacent pixels in each vertical column before taking the difference; this reduces noise in the image. A second, more subtle effect is that these kernels are 3 pixels wide and thus replace the central pixel with the difference value. The simple subtraction described above causes a half-pixel shift in the image, which is absent with this kernel. The method shown here is fast, since it requires only a single pass through the image.

Obviously, other kernel values can be devised that will also produce derivatives. As the kernel size increases, more different directions are possible. Since this is fundamentally a one-dimensional derivative, it is possible to directly use the coefficients of Savitsky and Golay (1964), which were originally published for use with such one-dimensional data as spectrograms or other strip-chart recorder output. These coefficients, like the smoothing weights shown in Chapter 3, are equivalent to least-squares fitting a high-order polynomial to the data. In this case, though, the first derivative of the polynomial is evaluated at the central point. Both second degree (quadratic) and fourth degree (quartic) polynomials are shown.

Figure 26 shows a fragment of the brightness profile along the center of the tree ring image in **Figure 25**. The first derivative plots shown were obtained by using the pixel difference approximation, and by using these weights to fit quadratic and quartic polynomials over widths of 5, 9, and 13 pixels around each point. The fits produce much smoother results and suppress noise. However, by increasing the fitting width, the small-scale real variations in the data are suppressed. It is generally necessary, as in any fitting or smoothing operation, to keep the kernel size smaller than the features of interest.

Table of Coefficients for First Derivative Quadratic Fit

#	5	7	9	11	13	15	17	19	21	23	25
−12											−.0092
−11										−.0109	−.0085
−10									−.0130	−.0099	−.0077
−9								−.0158	−.0117	−.0089	−.0069
−8							−.0196	−.0140	−.0104	−.0079	−.0062
−7						−.0250	−.0172	−.0123	−.0091	−.0069	−.0054
−6					−.0330	−.0214	−.0147	−.0105	−.0078	−.0059	−.0046
−5				−.0455	−.0275	−.0179	−.0123	−.0088	−.0065	−.0049	−.0038
−4			−.0667	−.0364	−.0220	−.0143	−.0098	−.0070	−.0052	−.0040	−.0031
−3		−.1071	−.0500	−.0273	−.0165	−.0107	−.0074	−.0053	−.0039	−.0030	−.0023
−2	−.2000	−.0714	−.0333	−.0182	−.0110	−.0071	−.0049	−.0035	−.0026	−.0020	−.0015
−1	−.1000	−.0357	−.0250	−.0091	−.0055	−.0036	−.0025	−.0018	−.0013	−.0010	−.0008
0	0	0	0	0	0	0	0	0	0	0	0
+1	+.1000	+.0357	+.0250	+.0091	+.0055	+.0036	+.0025	+.0018	+.0013	+.0010	+.0008
+2	+.2000	+.0714	+.0333	+.0182	+.0110	+.0071	+.0049	+.0035	+.0026	+.0020	+.0015
+3		+.1071	+.0500	+.0273	+.0165	+.0107	+.0074	+.0053	+.0039	+.0030	+.0023
+4			+.0667	+.0364	+.0220	+.0143	+.0098	+.0070	+.0052	+.0040	+.0031
+5				+.0455	+.0275	+.0179	+.0123	+.0088	+.0065	+.0049	+.0038
+6					+.0330	+.0214	+.0147	+.0105	+.0078	+.0059	+.0046
+7						+.0250	+.0172	+.0123	+.0091	+.0069	+.0054
+8							+.0196	+.0140	+.0104	+.0079	+.0062
+9								+.0158	+.0117	+.0089	+.0069
+10									+.0130	+.0099	+.0077
+11										+.0109	+.0085
+12											+.0092

Table of Coefficients for First Derivative Quartic Fit

#	5	7	9	11	13	15	17	19	21	23	25
−12											+.0174
−11										+.0200	+.0048
−10									+.0231	+.0041	−.0048
−9								+.0271	+.0028	−.0077	−.0118
−8							+.0322	−.0003	−.0119	−.0159	−.0165
−7						+.0387	−.0042	−.0182	−.0215	−.0209	−.0190
−6					+.0472	−.0123	−.0276	−.0292	−.0267	−.0231	−.0197
−5				+.0583	−.0275	−.0423	−.0400	−.0340	−.0280	−.0230	−.0189
−4			+.0724	−.0571	−.0657	−.0549	−.0431	−.0335	−.0262	−.0208	−.0166
−3		+.0873	−.1195	−.1033	−.0748	−.0534	−.0388	−.0320	−.0219	−.0170	−.0134
−2	+.0833	−.2659	−.1625	−.0977	−.0620	−.0414	−.0289	−.0210	−.0157	−.0120	−.0094
−1	−.6667	−.2302	−.1061	−.0575	−.0346	−.0225	−.0154	−.0110	−.0081	−.0062	−.0048
0	0	0	0	0	0	0	0	0	0	0	0
+1	+.6667	+.2302	+.1061	+.0575	+.0346	+.0225	+.0154	+.0110	+.0081	+.0062	+.0048
+2	−.0833	+.2659	+.1625	+.0977	+.0620	+.0414	+.0289	+.0210	+.0157	+.0120	+.0094
+3		−.0873	+.1195	+.1033	+.0748	+.0534	+.0388	+.0320	+.0219	+.0170	+.0134
+4			−.0724	+.0571	+.0657	+.0549	+.0431	+.0335	+.0262	+.0208	+.0166
+5				−.0583	+.0275	+.0423	+.0400	+.0340	+.0280	+.0230	+.0189
+6					−.0472	+.0123	+.0276	+.0292	+.0267	+.0231	+.0197
+7						−.0387	+.0042	+.0182	+.0215	+.0209	+.0190
+8							−.0322	+.0003	+.0119	+.0159	+.0165
+9								−.0271	−.0028	+.0077	+.0118
+10									−.0231	−.0041	+.0048
+11										−.0200	−.0048
+12											−.0174

Using one-dimensional derivatives to extract one-dimensional data from two-dimensional images is a relatively unusual and specialized operation. However, extending the same principles to locating boundaries with arbitrary orientations in two-dimensional images is one of the most common of all image enhancement operations. The problem, of course, is finding a method that is insensitive to the (local) orientation of the edge.

One of the earliest approaches to this task was the Roberts' Cross operator (Roberts, 1965). It uses the same difference technique

Figure 26. Horizontal brightness profile for a line in the center of the tree ring image (Figure 25), and its derivatives:

a) *original brightness plotted for each pixel along a fragment of the line;*

b) *finite difference plot showing the difference between adjacent pixels;*

c) *derivative calculated using the weights for a quadratic polynomial fit to 5 points;*

d) *a quadratic fit to 9 points;*

e) *a quadratic fit to 13 points;*

f) *derivative calculated using the weights for a quartic polynomial fit to 5 points;*

g) *a quartic fit to 9 points;*

h) *a quartic fit to 13 points.*

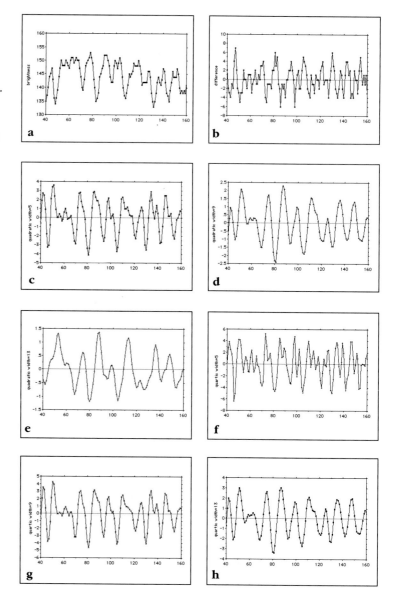

shown above for the one-dimensional case, but with two pixel differences at right angles to each other, as diagrammed in **Figure 27**. These two differences represent a finite approximation to the derivative of brightness. Two-directional derivatives can be combined to obtain a magnitude value that is insensitive to the orientation of the edge by squaring, adding, and taking the square root of the total.

This method has the same problems as the difference method used in one dimension. Noise in the image is magnified by the single-pixel differences, and the result is shifted by one-half of a pixel in both the x and y directions. In addition, the result is not invariant with respect to edge orientation. As a practical matter, the computers in common use when this model was first

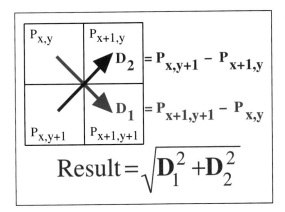

Figure 27. *Diagram of Roberts' Cross operator. Two differences in directions at right angles to each other are combined to determine the gradient.*

proposed were not very fast, nor were they equipped with separate floating-point math coprocessors. This made the square root of the sum of the squares impractical to calculate. Two alternatives were used: adding the absolute values of the two directional differences, or comparing the two absolute values of the differences and keeping the larger one. Both of these methods make the result quite sensitive to direction. In addition, even if the square root method is used, the magnitude of the result will vary because the pixel spacing is not the same in all directions, and edges in the vertical and horizontal directions spread the change in brightness over more pixels than edges in the diagonal directions.

In several of the comparison sequences that follow, the Roberts' Cross image will be shown (**Figures 30b** and **45c**). In all cases, the square root of the sum of squares of the differences was used. Even so, the images are characterized by varying sensitivity with respect to edge orientation, as well as a high noise level.

The Sobel and Kirsch operators

Just as for the example of the horizontal derivative above, the use of a larger kernel offers reduced sensitivity to noise by averaging several pixels and eliminating image shift. In fact, the derivative kernels shown above, or other similar patterns using different sets of integers, are widely used. Some common examples of these coefficients are shown in the table below.

+1	0	−1		+1	0	−1		+1	−1	−1		+5	−3	−3
+1	0	−1		+2	0	−2		+2	+1	−1		+5	0	−3
+1	0	−1		+1	0	−1		+1	−1	−1		+5	−3	−3

+1	+1	0		+2	+1	0		+2	+1	−1		+5	+5	−3
+1	0	−1		+1	0	−1		+1	+1	−1		+5	0	−3
0	−1	−1		0	−1	−2		−1	−1	−1		−3	−3	−3

+1	+1	+1		+1	+2	+1		+1	+2	+1		+5	+5	+5
0	0	0		0	0	0		−1	+1	−1		−3	0	−3
−1	−1	−1		−1	−2	−1		−1	−1	−1		−3	−3	−3

and so forth for eight rotations…

It actually makes little difference which of these patterns of values is used, as long as the magnitude of the result does not exceed the storage capacity of the computer being used. This is often a single byte per pixel, which, since the result of the above operation may be either negative or positive, can handle only values between −127 and +128. If large steps in brightness are present, this may result in the clipping of the calculated values, so that major boundaries are broadened or distorted in order to see smaller ones. The alternative is to employ automatic scaling, using the maximum and minimum values in the derivative image to set the white and dark values. To avoid loss of precision, though, requires two passes through the image: one to perform the calculations and find the extreme values and the second to actually compute the values and scale the results for storage.

As for the Roberts' Cross method, if the derivatives in two orthogonal directions are computed, they can be combined as the square root of the sums of their squares to obtain a result independent of orientation.

$$\text{Magnitude} = \sqrt{\left(\frac{\partial B}{\partial x}\right)^2 + \left(\frac{\partial B}{\partial y}\right)^2} \qquad (6$$

This is the Sobel (1970) method. It is one of the most commonly used techniques, even though it requires a fair amount of computation to perform correctly. (As for the Roberts' Cross, some computer programs attempt to compensate for hardware limitations by adding or comparing the two values, instead of squaring, adding, and taking the square root.)

With appropriate hardware, such as a shift register or array processor, the Sobel operation can be performed in essentially real time. This usually means 1/30th of a second per image, so that conventional video images can be processed and viewed. It often means viewing one frame while the following one is digitized, but in the case of the Sobel, it is even possible to view the image live, delayed only by two video scan lines. Two lines of data can be buffered and used to calculate the derivative values using the 3×3 kernels shown above. Specialized hardware to perform this real-time edge enhancement is used in some military applications, making it possible to locate edges in images for tracking, alignment of hardware in midair refueling, and other purposes.

At the other extreme, some general-purpose image analysis systems that do not have hardware for fast math operations perform the Sobel operation using a series of operations. First, two derivative images are formed, one using a horizontal and one a vertical orientation of the kernel. Then each of these is modified using a LUT to replace the value of each pixel with its square. The two resulting images are added together, and another LUT is used to convert each pixel value to its square root. No multiplication or square roots are needed. However, if this method is applied in a typical system with 8 bits per pixel, the

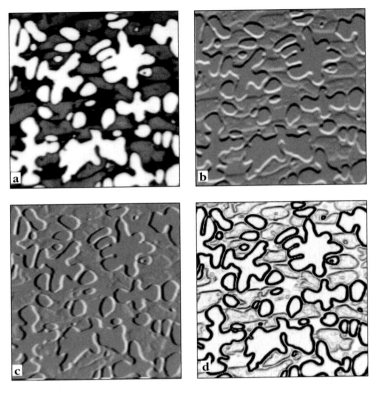

Figure 28. A metallographic image *(a)* with two directional derivatives *(b)* and *(c)*, and the Kirsch image *(d)* produced by keeping the maximum value from each direction.

loss of precision is severe, reducing the final image to no more than 4 bits of useful information.

A more useful method, when the mathematical operations needed to calculate the square root of the sum of squares for the Sobel must be avoided, is the Kirsch operator (1971). This method applies each of the eight orientations of the derivative kernel and keeps the maximum value. It requires only integer multiplication and comparisons. For many images, the results for the magnitude of edges are very similar to the Sobel. **Figure 28** shows an example. Vertical and horizontal derivatives of the image, and the maximum derivative values in each of eight directions, are shown.

Figures 29 and **30** illustrate the formation of the Sobel edge-finding image and compare it to the Laplacian, Roberts' Cross, and Kirsch operators. The example image contains many continuous edges running in all directions around the holes in the carbon film, as well as some straight edges at various orientations along the asbestos fibers. The Laplacian image is quite noisy, and the Roberts' Cross does not show all of the edges equally well. The individual vertical and horizontal derivatives are shown with the zero value shifted to an intermediate grey, so that both the negative and positive values can be seen. The absolute values are also shown.

Combining the two directional derivatives by a sum, or maximum operator, produces quite noisy and incomplete boundary enhancement. The square root of the sum of squares produces a

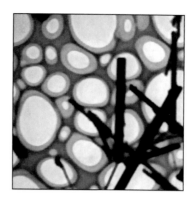

Figure 29. *Original image (asbestos fibers on a holey carbon film, imaged in a TEM. This image is the basis for the processing shown in Figure 30.*

good image, with little noise and continuous edge markings. The result from the Kirsch operator is very similar to the Sobel for this image.

In addition to the magnitude of the Sobel operator, it is also possible to calculate a direction value (Lineberry, 1982) for each pixel as

$$\text{Direction} = \text{Arc Tan} \left(\frac{\partial B / \partial y}{\partial B / \partial x} \right) \tag{7}$$

This assigns a value to each pixel for the gradient direction, which can be scaled to the grey scale of the image. **Figure 31** shows the vector results from applying the Sobel operator to the image of **Figure 29**. The magnitude and direction are encoded, but the vector field is too sparse to show any image details.

Figure 32 shows only the direction information for the image in **Figure 29**, using grey values to represent the angles. The progression of values around each more-or-less circular hole is evident. The use of a pseudo-color scale for this display is particularly suitable, since a rainbow of hues can show the progression without the arbitrary discontinuity required by the grey scale (in this example, at an angle of zero degrees). Unfortunately, the pixels within relatively homogeneous areas of the features also have colors assigned, because at every point there is some direction to the gradient, and these colors tend to overwhelm the visual impression of the image. A solution is to combine the magnitude of the gradient with the direction, as shown in **Figure 33**. This is the dendrite image from **Figure 28**, processed to show the magnitude and the direction of the Sobel edge gradient, the latter in color. These two images are then multiplied together so that the intensity of the color is proportional to the magnitude of the gradient. The result clearly shows the orientation of boundaries.

The magnitude and direction information can also be combined in an HSI representation of the image. In **Figure 34** the original grey scale image (the SEM image from **Figure 6**) has been

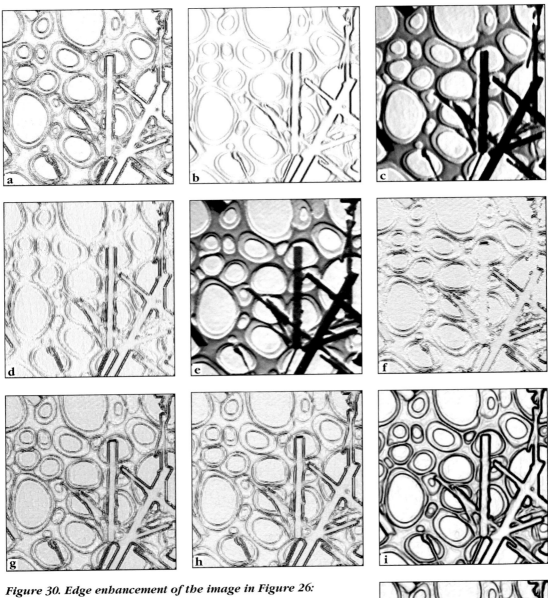

Figure 30. Edge enhancement of the image in Figure 26:

a) Laplacian operator;

b) Roberts' Cross operator;

c) horizontal derivative, scaled to full grey-scale range;

d) absolute value of image **c**;

e) vertical derivative, scaled to full grey-scale range;

f) absolute value of image **e**;

g) sum of absolute values from images **d** and **f**;

b) maximum of values in images **d** and **f**, pixel by pixel;

i) Sobel operator (square root of sum of squares of values);

j) Kirsch operator.

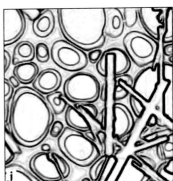

Figure 31. *Applying a Sobel operator to the image in Figure 28. Each vector has the direction and magnitude given by the operator, but even the fine vector field is too sparse to show any details of the image.*

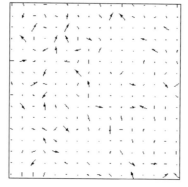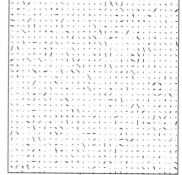

Figure 32. *Direction of the Sobel operator for the image in Figure 29.*

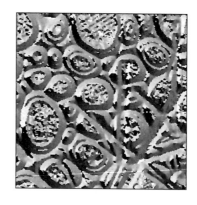

Figure 33. Combining the magnitude and direction information from the Sobel gradient operator:
a) *original grey scale image (from Figure 29);*
b) *Sobel gradient magnitude;*
c) *Sobel direction (color coded);*
d) *product of b times c.*

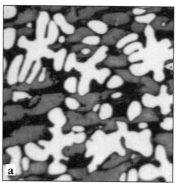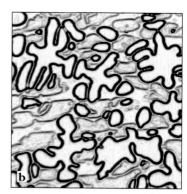

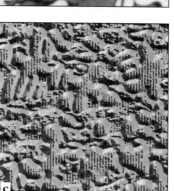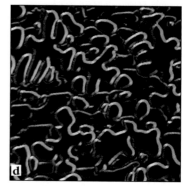

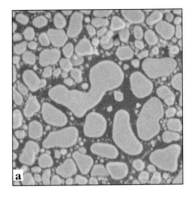
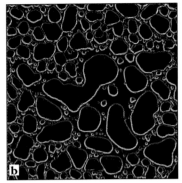

Figure 34. HSI representation of the gradient vector, with hue representing direction and the magnitude shown by saturation and intensity:
a) original image;
b) result.

processed to obtain the Sobel magnitude and direction. The direction information is then assigned to the hue plane and the magnitude to saturation and intensity.

Another way to improve the resulting image is to show the direction information only for those pixels which also have a strong magnitude for the brightness gradient. In **Figure 35** this is done by using the magnitude image as a mask, selecting (by thresholding as discussed in Chapter 6) the 40% of the pixels with the largest gradient magnitude, and showing the direction only for those pixels. This is more suitable for selecting pixels to be counted as a function of color (direction) for analysis purposes.

Figure 35 also shows a histogram plot of the preferred orientation in the image. This is constructed by sorting each pixel in **Figure 32** into one of 64 bins based on orientation, then summing up for all of the pixels in each bin the total of the gradient magnitude values. This kind of weighted plot is particularly common for interpreting the orientation of lines, such as dislocations in metals and the traces of faults in geographic maps. Further examples will be discussed below, as will the use of the direction image to reveal image texture, or to select regions of the image based on the texture or its orientation (Coppola et al., 1998).

Orientation determination using the angle calculated from the Sobel derivatives is not a perfectly isotropic or unbiased measure of boundary orientations because of the effects of the square

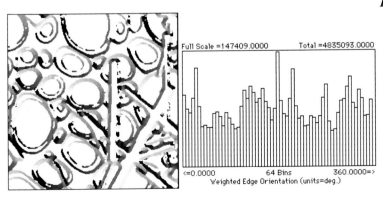

Figure 35. Uses of the edge orientation image in Figure 32: left) masking only those pixels whose edge magnitude is large (the 40% of the pixels with the largest magnitude); right) generating a histogram of weighted orientation, where each pixel is classified according to the local Sobel direction (horizontal axis) and the bins sum the Sobel magnitude (vertical axis).

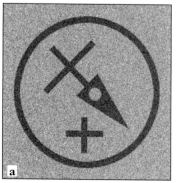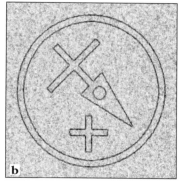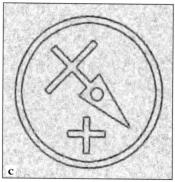

Figure 36. *Sobel magnitude images on a noisy test image* ***(a)*** *using 3×3* ***(b)*** *and 5×5* ***(c)*** *kernels.*

pixel grid and limited number of points sampled. With a larger kernel of values, weights can be assigned to better correspond to how far away the pixels are from the center. With a 5×5 array a more smoothly varying and isotropically uniform result can be obtained. **Figure 36** shows an example with a circle and some lines with superimposed image noise as a test object; the definition of the edge using the Sobel magnitude is improved by the larger neighborhood although the line breadth becomes greater. In **Figure 37** the direction values from a perfect circle are shown; the bias in favor of multiples of 90 degrees is evident. In real applications, measuring the orientation histogram from a perfect circle and using that to normalize the measurements from an irregular boundary of interest may be used to cancel the bias.

The use of an edge-enhancing operator to modify images is useful in many situations. We have already seen examples of sharpening using the Laplacian, to increase the contrast at edges and make images appear sharper to the viewer. Gradient or edge-finding methods also do this, but they also modify the image so that its interpretation becomes somewhat different. Since this contrast increase is selective, it responds to local information in the image in a way that manipulating the brightness histogram cannot.

For example, **Figure 38** shows several views of galaxy M51. In the original image, it is quite impossible to see the full range of

Figure 37. *Direction measurement with a 5×5 Sobel operator. Even with the larger kernel a histogram shows that orthogonal directions are overestimated.*

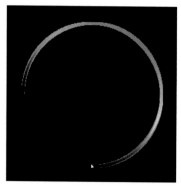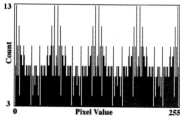

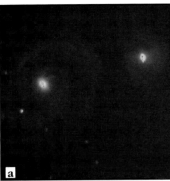 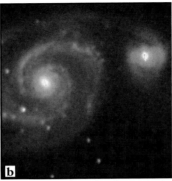 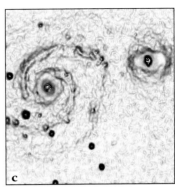

Figure 38. Enhancing an astronomical image (M51): a) original telescope image, with brightness range too great for printing; b) application of "unsharp masking" by subtracting a smoothed image to reduce contrast selectively and show detail; c) gradient of original image using a Sobel operator, which also shows the fine structure of the galaxy.

brightness, even on a high-quality photographic negative. It is even less possible to print it. The extremely light and dark areas simply cover too great a range. Compressing the range nonlinearly, using a logarithmic transfer function, can make it possible to see both ends of the scale at the same time. However, this is accomplished by reducing small variations, especially at the bright end of the scale, so that they are not visible.

A rather common approach to dealing with this type of image is called unsharp masking. Traditionally, it has been applied using photographic darkroom techniques. First, a contact print is made from the original negative onto film, leaving a small gap between the emulsion on the original and that on the film so that the image is blurred. After the film is developed, a new print is made with the two negatives clamped together. The light areas on the original negative are covered by dark areas on the printed negative, allowing little light to come through. Only regions where the slightly out-of-focus negative does not match the original are printed. This is functionally equivalent to the Laplacian, which subtracts a smoothed (out of focus) image from the original to suppress gradual changes and pass high frequencies or edges.

Applying the unsharp mask operator increases the visibility of fine detail, while suppressing overall variations in brightness. **Figure 39** shows an example using the same X-ray image from **Figure 2**. In the original image the bones in the fingers are thinner and hence not as dense as those in the wrist, and the written label is hardly visible. The filtered image makes these more readily visible.

Closely related to unsharp masking is the subtraction of one smoothed version of the image from another having a different degree of smoothing. This is called the Difference of Gaussians (D.O.G.) method and is believed to be similar to the way the human visual system locates boundaries (Marr, 1982) and other features (the effect of inhibition increasing contrast at boundaries was shown above). Smoothing an image using Gaussian kernels

Figure 39. Application of an unsharp mask to an X-ray image of a human hand:
a) *original;*
b) *processed.*

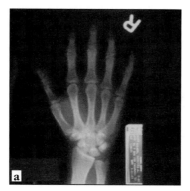
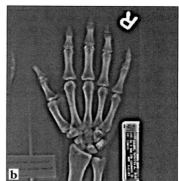

with different standard deviations suppresses high-frequency information, which corresponds to small details and spacing that are present. Large structures are not affected. The difference between the two images keeps only those structures (lines, points, etc.) that are in the intermediate size range between the two operators. Examples of this operation will be shown below in **Figure 44**. **Figure 40** shows a plot of two Gaussian curves with different standard deviations, and their difference, which is very similar to a cross section of the Laplacian. This edge extractor is also sometimes called a Marr-Hildreth operator.

The gradient enhancement shown in **Figure 38** uses a Sobel operator to mark edges. This shows the structure within the galaxy in a very different way, by emphasizing local spatial variations regardless of the absolute value of the brightness. This produces a distinctly different result than the Laplacian or unsharp masking.

Figure 41 shows another example requiring edge enhancement. The specimen is a polished aluminum metal. The individual grains exhibit different brightnesses because their crystallographic lattices are randomly oriented in space so that the etching procedure used darkens some grains more than others. It is the grain boundaries that are usually important in studying metal structures,

Figure 40. *The Difference-of-Gaussians ("D.O.G.") operator in one dimension. Two Gaussian curves with different standard deviations are shown, with their difference. The result is a sharpening operation much like the Laplacian.*

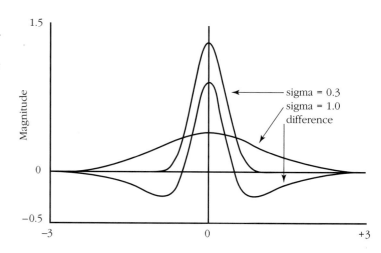

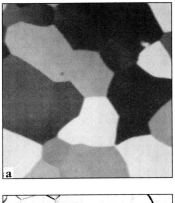

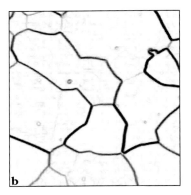

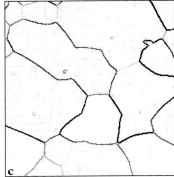

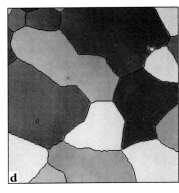

Figure 41. Delineating boundaries between grains:

a) aluminum metal, polished and etched to show different grains (contrast arises from different crystallographic orientation of each grain, so that some boundaries have less contrast than others);

b) variance edge-finding algorithm applied to image **a**;

c) grey scale skeletonization (ridge finding) applied to image **b** (points not on a ridge are suppressed);

d) thresholding and skeletonization of the boundaries to a single line of pixels produces the grain boundaries, shown superimposed on the original image.

since the configuration of grain boundaries results from prior heat treatment and processing and controls many mechanical properties. The human visual process detects the grain boundaries using its sensitivity to boundaries and edges. Most image analysis systems use a gradient operation, such as a Sobel, to perform a similar enhancement prior to measuring the grain boundaries.

In the example in **Figure 41**, another method has been employed. This is a variance operator, which calculates the sum of squares of the brightness differences for the 8 pixels surrounding each pixel in the original image. This value, like the other edge-enhancement operators, is very small in uniform regions of the image and becomes large whenever a step is present. In this example, the dark lines (large magnitudes of the variance) are further processed by thinning to obtain the single pixel lines that are superimposed on the original image. This thinning or ridge-finding method is discussed further below.

Performing derivative operations using kernels can be considered a template matching or cross-correlation process. The pattern of weights in the kernel is a template that gives the maximum response when it matches the pattern of brightness values in the pixels of the image. The number of different kernels used for derivative calculations indicates that there is no single best definition of what constitutes a boundary. Also, it might be helpful at the same time to look for other patterns that are not representative of an edge.

These ideas are combined in the Frei and Chen algorithm (1977), which applies a set of kernels to each point in the image. Each kernel extracts one kind of behavior in the image, only a few of which are indicative of the presence of an edge. For a 3×3 neighborhood region, the kernels, which are described as orthogonal or independent basis functions, are shown below.

number	kernel			number	kernel		
0	1	1	1	4	$\sqrt{2}$	-1	0
	1	1	1		-1	0	1
	1	1	1		0	1	$-\sqrt{2}$
1	-1	$-\sqrt{2}$	-1	5	0	1	0
	0	0	0		-1	0	1
	1	$\sqrt{2}$	1		0	-1	0
2	-1	0	1	6	-1	0	1
	$-\sqrt{2}$	0	$\sqrt{2}$		0	0	0
	-1	0	1		1	0	-1
3	0	-1	$\sqrt{2}$	7	1	-2	1
	1	0	-1		-2	4	-2
	$-\sqrt{2}$	1	0		1	-2	1
				8	-2	1	-2
					1	4	1
					-2	1	-2

Only kernels 1 and 2 are considered to indicate the presence of an edge. The results of applying each kernel to each pixel are therefore summed to produce a ratio. The cosine of the square root of this value is effectively the vector projection of the information from the neighborhood in the direction of "edgeness," and is assigned to the pixel location in the derived image.

The advantage compared to more conventional edge detectors such as the Sobel is sensitivity to a configuration of relative pixel values independent of the magnitude of the brightness, which may vary from place to place in the image. **Figure 42** shows an example of the Frei and Chen operator. This may be compared to other edge-finding processing, shown in **Figures 43** through **45**, which apply some of the other operations discussed in this chapter to the same image.

Figure 42. Application of the Frei and Chen edge detector:
a) original (light microscope image of head louse);
b) result of Frei and Chen operator.

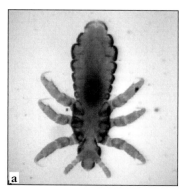 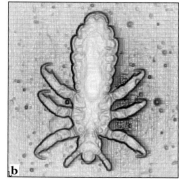

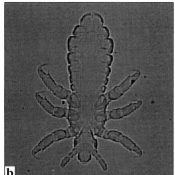

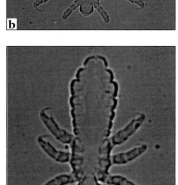

Figure 43. Application of Laplacian difference operations to the same image as in Figure 42:
a) *sharpening (addition of the 3×3 Laplacian to the original grey-scale image);*
b) *5×5 Laplacian;*
c) *7×7 Laplacian;*
d) *9×9 Laplacian.*

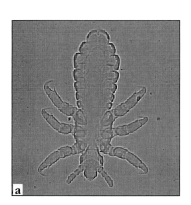

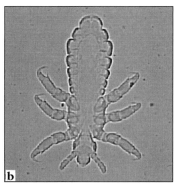

Figure 44. Difference of Gaussians applied to the same image as Figure 42:
a) *original image minus 3×3 Gaussian smooth;*
b) *difference between smoothing with* $\sigma = 0.625$ *and* $\sigma = 1.0$ *pixels;*
c) *difference between smoothing with* $\sigma = 1.6$ *and* $\sigma = 1.0$ *pixels;*
d) *difference between smoothing with* $\sigma = 4.1$ *and* $\sigma = 2.6$ *pixels.*

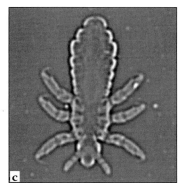

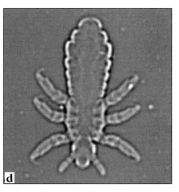

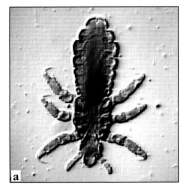

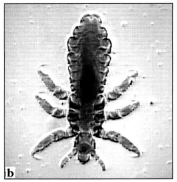

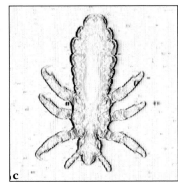

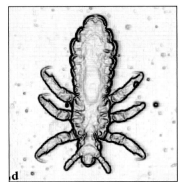

The noise or blurring introduced by the other operations is evident, as is the ability of the Frei and Chen procedure to reveal even the rather subtle edge information present in the original. **Figure 43** shows the application of a Laplacian operator, or high-pass filter, using different-sized kernels; **Figure 44** shows the difference of Gaussians, which is fundamentally similar. **Figure 45** shows the use of derivatives, including the Roberts' Cross and Sobel methods.

Most of the edge-finding processing operations involve square or circular neighborhoods, with a large number of multiplications and other operations. The Canny filter produces results similar to Kirsch or Sobel operators, but is separable (Canny, 1986; Olsson, 1993). This means that it can be performed in two passes, one of which requires only values from pixels in a horizontal line adjacent to the central pixel, and the other requires only values from pixels in a vertical line. From both a computational point of view, and in terms of the complexity of addressing a large number of neighbor pixels, this offers some advantages.

Rank operations

The neighborhood operations discussed in the preceding section use linear arithmetic operations to combine the values of various pixels. Another class of operators that also use neighborhoods instead performs comparisons. In Chapter 3, the median filter was introduced. This sorts the pixels in a region into brightness order, finds the median value, and replaces the central pixel with that value. Used to remove noise from images, this operation completely eliminates extreme values from the image.

Rank operations also include the maximum and minimum operators, which find the brightest or darkest pixels in each neighborhood and place that value into the central pixel. By loose analogy to the erosion and dilation operations on binary images, which are discussed in Chapter 7, these are sometimes called grey scale erosion and dilation (Heijmans, 1991). The erosion effect of this ranking operation was demonstrated in Chapter 3, in the context of removing features from an image to produce a background for leveling.

One of the important variables in the use of a rank operator is the size of the neighborhood. Generally, shapes that are squares (for convenience of computation) or approximations to a circle (to minimize directional effects) are used. As the size of the neighborhood is increased, however, the computational effort in performing the ranking increases rapidly. Also, these ranking operations cannot be easily programmed into specialized hardware, such as array processors. In consequence, it is not common to use regions larger than those shown in **Figure 46**.

Several uses of rank operators are appropriate for image enhancement and the selection of one portion of the information present in an image. For example, the top hat operator (Bright & Steel, 1987) has been implemented in various ways, but can be described using two different-size regions, as shown in **Figure 47**. If we assume that the goal of the operator is to find bright points, then the algorithm compares the maximum brightness value in a small central region to the maximum brightness value in a larger surrounding one. If the difference between these two values exceeds some arbitrary threshold, then the

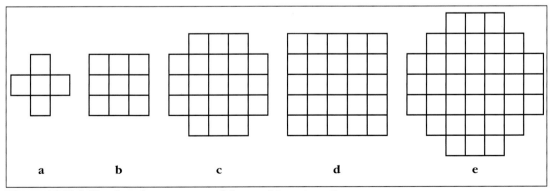

Figure 46. Neighborhood patterns used for ranking operations:
a) *4 nearest-neighbor cross;* *b)* *3×3 square containing nine pixels;*
c) *5×5 octagonal region with 21 pixels;* *d)* *5×5 square containing 25 pixels;*
e) *7×7 octagonal region containing 37 pixels.*

Figure 47. *Neighborhood patterns used for a top hat filter. The brightest value in the outer (white) region is subtracted from the brightest value in the inner (shaded) region. If the difference exceeds a threshold, then the central pixel is kept. Otherwise it is erased.*

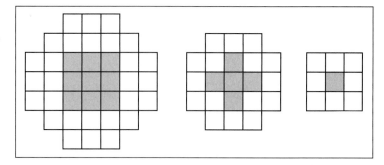

value of the central pixel is retained. Otherwise it is removed. This principle was also illustrated in Chapter 3.

Some systems contain specific programs to execute this algorithm, while others provide general-purpose ranking operations which can be combined to achieve this result. **Figure 48** shows the application of a top hat filter, in which the bright points in the diffraction pattern (calculated using a fast Fourier transform as discussed in Chapter 5) are retained and the overall variation in background brightness is suppressed. Performing the inverse transform on only the major points provides an averaged image, combining the repetitive information from many individually noisy atom images.

An equivalent result could be obtained by calculating two images from the original: one retaining the maximum brightness

Figure 48. Application of a top hat filter to select points in a diffraction pattern:

a) *high-resolution TEM image of silicon nitride, showing atomic positions;*

b) *FFT magnitude image calculated from image **a**;*

c) *application of a top hat filter to image **b**, selecting the locally bright points on a nonuniform background;*

d) *inverse transform using only the points selected in image **c**, enlarged to show detail.*

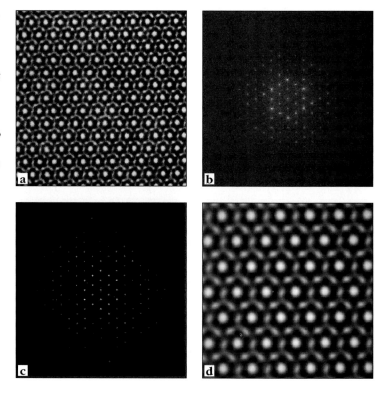

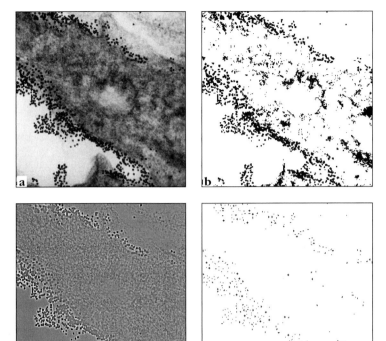

Figure 49. Application of a top hat filter:

a) *TEM image of Golgi-stained rat skeletal muscles, with gold particles (dark) on variable background;*

b) *thresholding of image **a** selects dark pixels, but cannot isolate the particles;*

c) *unsharp masking, produced by subtracting a smoothed version of the image from the original;*

d) *the top hat filter finds (most of) the particles in spite of the variation in the background.*

value in a 5-pixel-wide "brim" region, and the second doing the same for just the central pixel and its 4 edge-touching neighbors. Subtracting one from the other gives the difference between the maxima in the two regions. Next, thresholding to select only those points with a value greater than 12 would apply the same arbitrary threshold used in **Figure 49**. Not many systems allow creating a ranking neighborhood that omits the central pixels, to use as the brim of the hat.

The top hat filter is basically a point finder. The size of the point is defined by the smaller of the two neighborhood regions and may be as small as a single pixel in some cases. The larger region defines the local background, which the points of interest must exceed in brightness. Unlike the Laplacian, which subtracts the average value of the surrounding background from the central point, the top hat method finds the maximum brightness in the larger surrounding region (the "brim" of the hat) and subtracts that from the brightest point in the interior region. If the difference exceeds some arbitrary threshold (the "height" of the hat's crown), then the central pixel is kept.

In a description of the operation of the algorithm, the brim rests on the data and any point that pokes through the top of the hat is kept. If the central region is larger than a single pixel, though, this depiction is not quite accurate. When any of the points in the central region exceeds the brim value, the central pixel value (which may not be the bright one) is kept. This may produce

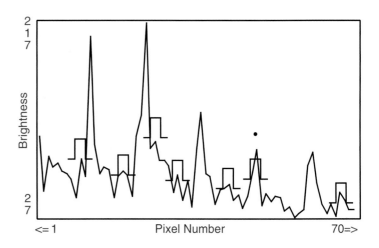

Figure 50. *Diagram of application of the top-hat filter to one-dimensional data (a brightness profile from the diffraction pattern in Figure 34). Several placements of the filter are shown. In only one (marked •) does the central value exceed the threshold.*

small haloes around single bright points that are smaller than the central neighborhood region. However, any bright point that is part of a feature larger than the central region will not be found by the top hat filter.

Of course, it should be noted that some images have features of interest that are darker rather than lighter than their surroundings. The logic of the top hat filter works just as well when it is inverted, and darkness rather than lightness is the test criterion. **Figure 50** shows such a case, in which the small (and quite uniformly sized) dark features are gold particles in Golgi stained muscle tissue. In this example, simply thresholding the dark particles does not work, because other parts of the image are just as dark. Similarly, a method such as unsharp masking, accomplished in the example by subtracting the average value (using a Gaussian smoothing filter with a standard deviation of 0.6 pixels) from the original, produces an image in which the particles are quite visible to a human viewer, but are still not distinguishable to a computer program.

It is possible to apply a top hat filter to one-dimensional data. The method is sometimes used, for instance, to select peaks in spectra. **Figure 51** shows an example. The brim of the hat rests

Figure 51. Grey-scale skeletonization (ridge finding):
a) *applied to the original image in Figure 42;*
b) *applied to the edge image produced by the Sobel operator shown in Figure 45.*

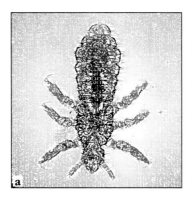
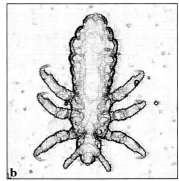

on the profile and in only a few places does the plot poke through the crown. Peaks that are too low, too broad, or adjacent to others are not detected.

It is also possible, in principle, to design a top hat filter that is not circularly symmetrical, but has regions shaped to select particular features of interest, even lines. Of course, the orientation of the feature must match that of the filter, so this is not a very general operation. When features with a well-defined shape and orientation are sought, cross-correlation in either the spatial or frequency domain is generally more appropriate.

A close relative of the top hat filter is the rolling ball filter. Instead of selecting points that exceed the local background, this filter eliminates them, replacing those pixel values with the neighborhood value. This is most easily described for an image in which the noise pixels are dark. The filter's name is meant to suggest an analogy to placing a ball on the image, again visualized as a surface in which elevation at each point is the brightness of the pixel.

As the ball rolls on the surface, it is in contact with several pixels (a minimum of three). An outer, large neighborhood and an inner, smaller one, both approximately circular, define the contact points by their minimum (darkest) values. The permitted difference value is a function of the radius of the ball. Any point that is darker and corresponds to points that the ball cannot touch is considered to be a noise point; its value is replaced with the darkest value in the outer region. Again, while the description here uses dark points as the targets to be removed, it is straightforward to reverse the logic and remove bright noise points.

The top hat filter is an example of a suppression operator. It removes pixels from the image if they do not meet some criteria of being "interesting" and leaves alone those pixels that do. Another operator of this type, which locates lines rather than points, is variously known as ridge-finding or grey scale skeletonization (by analogy to skeletonization of binary images, discussed in Chapter 7). We have already seen a number of edge-finding and gradient operators that produce bright or dark lines along boundaries. These lines are often wider than a single pixel and it may be desirable to reduce them to a minimum width (Bertrand et al., 1997).

The ridge-finding algorithm suppresses pixels (by reducing their value to zero) if they are not part of the center ridge of the line. This is defined as any pixel whose value is less than all of its 8 neighbors, or whose 8 touching neighbors have a single maximum that is greater than the pixel. **Figure 52** shows an example of the application of this operator to the image of the head louse in **Figure 52** and to the edges derived from that image in **Figure 45**. In both cases, the reduction of lines to single pixel

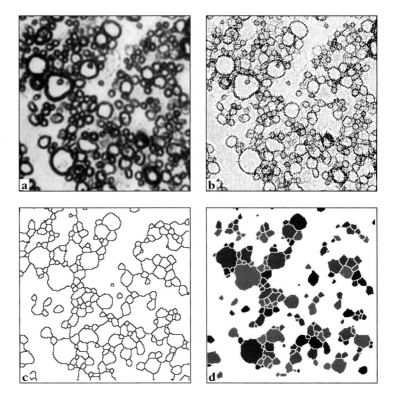

Figure 52. Converting boundaries to features:
a) *axons seen in cross section in a light microscope section;*
b) *grey-scale skeletonization of image a;*
c) *binary skeletonization and pruning of image b;*
d) *features within closed outlines of image c.*

width is accompanied by many smaller lines radiating from the principal ridge.

Figure 53 shows the direct application of ridge finding to an image of axons, which appear in the light microscope as dark outlines. Here, the grey scale skeleton of the outlines is converted to a binary image by thresholding (Chapter 6) and then reduced to a single line by binary image skeletonization (Chapter 7). The resulting image is then suitable for feature measurement, shown in **Figure 53d** by grey scale labeling of each feature.

Many structures are best characterized by a continuous network, or tesselation, of boundaries. **Figure 54** shows an example, a ceramic containing grains of two different compositions (the dark grains are alumina and the light ones zirconia). The grains are

Figure 53. *SEM image of thermally etched alumina-zirconia multiphase ceramic. The two phases are easily distinguished by brightness, but the boundaries between two light or two dark regions are not. (Image courtesy of Dr. K. B. Alexander, Oak Ridge National Labs, Oak Ridge, TN.)*

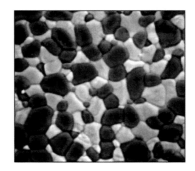

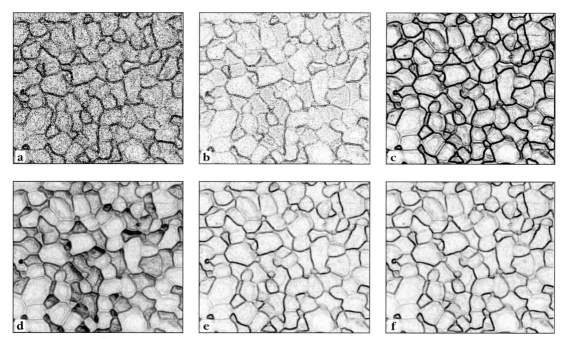

Figure 54. Processing of Figure 53 to enhance edges (all operations performed on 3 × 3 neighborhood regions):

a) *absolute value of the Laplacian;*
b) *absolute value of the difference between original and Gaussian smooth;*
c) *Sobel gradient operator;*
d) *Frei and Chen edge operator;*
e) *variance operator;*
f) *range operator.*

easily distinguishable by the viewer, but it is the grain boundaries that are important for measurement to characterize the structure, not just the boundaries between light and dark grains, but also those between light and light or dark and dark grains.

Figure 55 shows the application of various edge-finding operators to this image. In this case, the variance produces the best boundary demarcation without including too many extraneous lines due to the texture within the grains. Thresholding this image (as discussed in Chapter 6) and processing the binary image (as discussed in Chapter 7) to thin the lines to single pixel width produces an image of only the boundaries, as shown in **Figure 56**. It is then possible to use the brightness of the pixels in the original image to classify each grain as either *a* or *b*. Images of only those boundaries lying between *a* and *a*, *b* and *b*, or *a* and *b* can then be obtained (as shown in the figure and discussed in Chapter 7). It is also possible to count the number of neighbors around each grain and use a color or grey scale to code them, as shown in **Figure 56**. This goes beyond the usual scope of image processing, however, and into the realm of image measurement and analysis, which is taken up in Chapter 8.

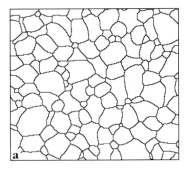
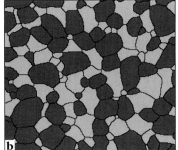
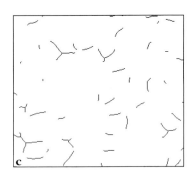

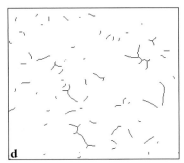
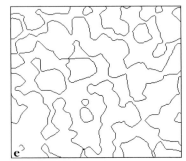

Figure 55. Grain boundary images derived from the variance image in Figure 54e by thresholding and skeletonization:

a) boundaries between the grains;

b) grains grey-scale coded to show phase identification;

c) only those boundaries between two dark (alumina) grains, making up 16.2% of the total;

d) only those boundaries between two light (zirconia) grains, making up 15.2% of the total;

e) only those boundaries between a light and dark grain, making up 68.6% of the total boundary.

A range image, such as those from the atomic force microscope (AFM) or interference microscope, or from radar imaging, assigns each pixel a brightness value representing elevations, so it is not necessary to arbitrarily imagine the grey scale brightness as such a structure. Rank operations are particularly well suited to such images, and can often be used to locate boundaries. **Figure 57** shows an example, an AFM image of the topography of a deposited coating. There is some variation in elevation from noise in the image, producing a local variation in grey levels that "roughens" the surface. This can be reduced with a rolling ball filter as shown.

Performing a grey-scale dilation (replacing each pixel with the brightest pixel in a 5-pixel wide neighborhood) and subtracting the original produces a set of bright lines along the boundaries. Thresholding and skeletonizing this image (using techniques discussed in Chapters 6 and 7) produce a network of lines as shown in the figure. Overlaying these lines on the original shows that the correspondence to the visual boundaries between regions is

Figure 56. *The grains from Figure 55 grey scale coded to show the number of neighbors touching each, and a plot of the frequency of each number of neighbors. Further analysis shows that both the size and the number of neighbor plots are different for the two different phases.*

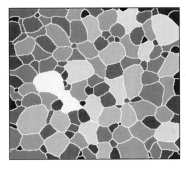
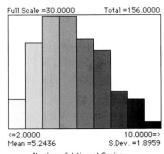

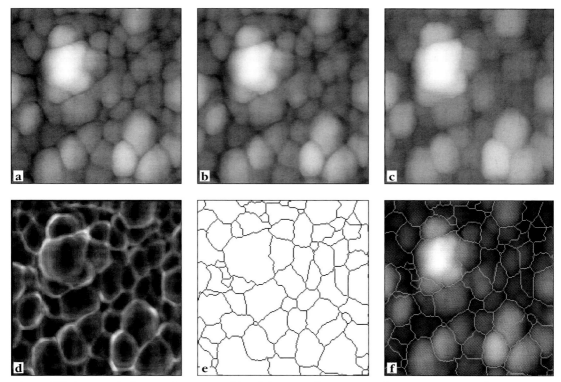

Figure 57. An atomic force microscope (AFM) image of a coating, showing a series of gently rounded bumps:

a) the original range image (grey scale proportional to elevation);
b) noise smoothed by the application of a rolling ball filter;
c) use of a rank filter to replace each pixel with its brightest neighbor;
d) difference between **b** and **c,** showing boundary delineation;
e) thresholding and skeletonizing image **d** to get lines;
f) boundary lines overlaid on the original image.

not perfect. This is due primarily to the fact that the surface slope on each side of the boundaries is different, and the subtraction process therefore produces an asymmetric border that has a midline that is offset from the boundary. Nevertheless, the tesselation of lines is useful for counting and measuring the individual structures in the coating.

For range images (particularly radar images used in surveillance), searching for a target pattern can be accomplished using a special class of adaptive operators. A top hat filter of the right size and shape would seem appropriate for the task, but better performance can be achieved by adjusting the parameters of size and especially height according to the local pixel values (Verly & Delanoy, 1993). In principle, the more knowledge available about the characteristics of the target and of the imaging equipment, the better an adaptive filter can be made to find the features and separate them from background. In practice, these approaches seem to be little used, and are perhaps too specific for general applications.

Figure 58. Enhancement of texture:

a) *transmission electron microscope image of liver thin section;*

b) *range image (difference between maximum and minimum brightness values in a 3×3 neighborhood);*

c) *root-mean-square (RMS) image (square root of the sum of squares of differences between the central pixel and its neighbors in a 3×3 neighborhood);*

d) *RMS image using a 5-pixel-wide octagonal neighborhood.*

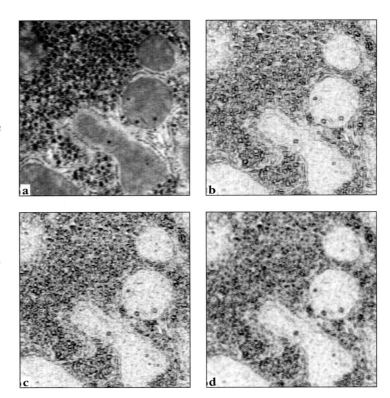

Texture

Many images contain regions characterized not so much by a unique value of brightness, but by a variation in brightness that is often called texture. This is a somewhat loosely defined term that refers to the local variation in brightness from one pixel to the next or within a small region. If the brightness is interpreted as elevation in a representation of the image as a surface, then the texture is a measure of the surface roughness, another term without an accepted or universal quantitative meaning.

Rank operations are also used to detect this texture in images. One of the simplest (but least versatile) of the texture operators is simply the range or difference between maximum and minimum brightness values in the neighborhood. For a flat or uniform region, the range is small. Larger values of the range correspond to surfaces with a larger roughness. The size of the neighborhood region must be large enough to include dark and light pixels, which generally means being larger than any small uniform details that may be present. **Figure 58** shows an example.

When visual examination of an image suggests that the basis for discriminating various structural regions is a texture rather than color or brightness, it may be possible to use a simple texture operator such as the range to extract it. This is often the case in biological specimens, and particularly in foods. **Figure 59** shows another example, a microscope image of the curds and protein in

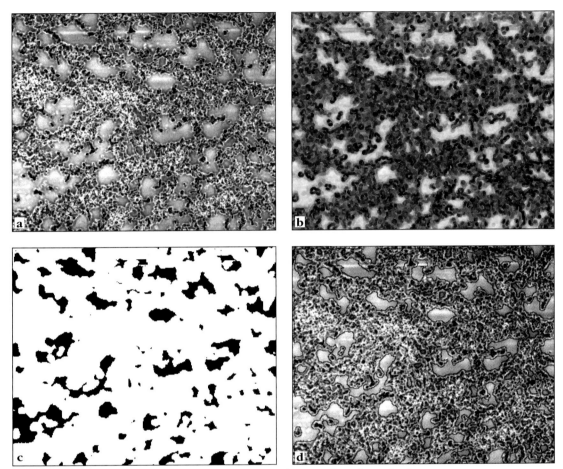

Figure 59. Application of a range operator to an image of curds and whey:
a) *original;*
b) *range operator applied (5-pixel-wide circular neighborhood);*
c) *thresholded;*
d) *region outlines superimposed on original.*

cheese. The smooth regions (curds) produce a low range value, while the highly textured protein produces a high value. The overall shading of the image has also been removed and it is not possible to use thresholding to delineate the regions.

The range operator converts the original image to one in which brightness represents the texture, the original feature brightness is gone, and different structural regions may be distinguished by the range brightness. As shown in **Figure 60**, the range operator also responds to the boundaries between regions that are of different average brightness and is sometimes used as an edge-defining algorithm. Comparison to other edge-finding methods discussed in this chapter shows that the Sobel and Frei and Chen are superior, but the range operation requires little arithmetic and is very fast.

Another estimator of texture is the variance in neighborhood regions. This is the sum of the squares of the differences between

Figure 60. Application of range and variance operators to the same image as in Figure 42:
a) range (3×3 neighborhood);
b) range (5-pixel-wide octagonal neighborhood);
c) variance (3×3 neighborhood);
d) variance (5-pixel-wide octagonal neighborhood).

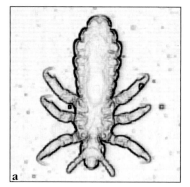
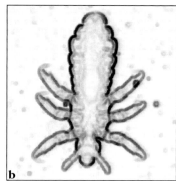
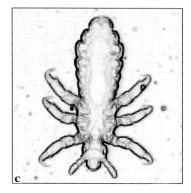
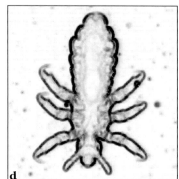

the brightness of the central pixel and its neighbors. Because the value can become quite large, the result is sometimes displayed as the square root of this difference. If the sum of squares is first normalized by dividing by the number of pixels in the neighborhood, this is just the root-mean-square (RMS) difference of values and corresponds to a similar RMS measure of roughness for surfaces.

Like the range, the variance also responds to the variation of pixels in the region. It is less sensitive to the individual extreme pixel values and produces an image with less noise than the range operator. **Figures 54** and **60** show the comparison between applying the RMS operator with a 3×3 pixel neighborhood or a 5-pixel-wide octagonal neighborhood, and the range operator. Like the range operator, the variance also responds to boundaries between regions of different brightnesses and is sometimes used as an edge detector.

Satellite images are especially appropriate for characterization by texture operators. Categorization of crops, construction, and other land uses produces distinctive textures that humans can recognize. Therefore, methods have been sought that duplicate this capability in software algorithms. In a classic paper on the subject, Haralick listed 14 such texture operators that utilize the pixels within a region and their brightness differences (Haralick et al., 1973; Haralick, 1979; Weszka et al., 1976). This region is not a neighborhood around each pixel, but comprises all of the pixels within a contiguous block delineated by some boundary or other identifying criterion such as brightness, etc. A table is constructed with the number of adjacent pixel pairs within the region as a function of their brightnesses. This pixel table is then used to calculate the texture parameters.

In the expressions below, the array $P(i,j)$ contains the number of nearest-neighbor pixel pairs (in 90-degree directions only) whose brightnesses are i and j, respectively. R is a renormalizing constant equal to the total number of pixel pairs in the image or any rectangular portion used for the calculation. In principle, this can be extended to pixel pairs that are separated by a distance d and to pairs aligned in the 45-degree direction (whose separation distance is greater than ones in the 90-degree directions). The summations are carried out for all pixel pairs in the region. Haralick applied this to rectangular regions, but it is equally applicable to pixels within irregular outlines.

The first parameter shown is a measure of homogeneity using a second moment. Since the terms are squared, a few large differences will contribute more than many small ones. The second one shown is a difference moment, which is a measure of the contrast in the image. The third is a measure of the linear dependency of brightness in the image, obtained by correlation.

$$f_1 = \sum_{i=1}^{N} \sum_{j=1}^{N} \left(\frac{P(i,j)}{R} \right)^2$$

$$f_2 = \sum_{n=0}^{N-1} n^2 \left\{ \sum_{|i-j|=n} \left(\frac{P(i,j)}{R} \right) \right\} \tag{8}$$

$$f_3 = \frac{\sum_{i=1}^{N} \sum_{j=1}^{N} \{ i \cdot j \cdot P(i,j) / R \} - \mu_x \cdot \mu_y}{\sigma_x \cdot \sigma_y}$$

In these expressions, N is the number of grey levels, and μ and σ are the mean and standard deviation, respectively, of the distributions of brightness values accumulated in the x and y directions. Additional parameters describe the variance, entropy, and information measure of the brightness value correlations. Haralick has shown that when applied to large rectangular areas in satellite photos, these parameters can distinguish water from grassland, different sandstones from each other, and woodland from marsh or urban regions.

Some of these operations are obviously easier than others to calculate for all of the pixels in an image. The resulting values can be scaled to create a useful derived image that can be discriminated with brightness thresholding. In any given instance, it sometimes requires experimentation with several texture operators to find

Figure 61. Application of
Haralick texture operators
to the image in Figure 58:
a) *3×3 neighborhood;*
b) *5×5 neighborhood.*

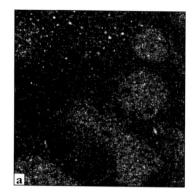 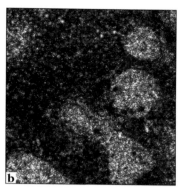

the one that gives the best separation between the features of interest and their surroundings.

Some of these same operations can be applied to individual pixels to produce a new image, in which the brightness is proportional to the local texture. **Figure 61** illustrates the use of the Haralick angular second moment operator (f_2 above) applied to 3×3 and 5×5 pixel neighborhoods centered on each pixel to calculate a texture value, which is then assigned to the pixel. This result can be compared to **Figure 58**.

Fractal analysis

The characterization of surface roughness by a fractal dimension has been applied to fracture surfaces, wear and erosion, corrosion, etc. (Mandelbrot et al., 1984; Underwood & Banerji, 1986; Mecholsky & Passoja, 1985; Mecholsky et al., 1986, 1989; Srinivasan et al., 1991; Fahmy et al., 1991). It has also been shown (Pentland, 1983; Peleg et al., 1984) that the brightness pattern in images of fractal surfaces is also mathematically a fractal and that this also holds for SEM images (Russ, 1990a). A particularly efficient method for computing the fractal dimension of surfaces from elevation images is the Hurst coefficient, or rescaled range analysis (Hurst et al., 1965; Feder, 1988; Russ, 1990c). This procedure plots the greatest difference in brightness (or elevation, etc.) between points along a linear traverse of the image or surface as a function of the search distance, on log-log axes. When the range is scaled by dividing by the standard deviation of the data, the slope of the resulting line is directly related to the fractal dimension of the profile.

Performing such an operation at the pixel level is interesting, because it may permit local classification that can be of use for image segmentation. Processing an image so that each pixel value is converted to a new brightness scale indicating local roughness (in the sense of a Hurst coefficient) permits segmentation by simple brightness thresholding. It uses two-dimensional information on the brightness variation, compared to the one-dimensional comparison used in measuring brightness profiles.

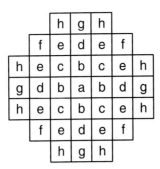

Figure 62. *Octagonal 7-pixel-wide neighborhood (37 pixels total) used for local rescaled-range (Hurst coefficient) calculation. Pixel labels identify groups with the same distance from the central pixel.*

Figure 62 shows a neighborhood region consisting of 37 pixels in a 7-pixel-wide octagonal shape. The size is a compromise between the desire to include many pixel values (for accurate results) and the need for fast calculation. Qualitatively similar results are obtained with 5-, 9-, and 11-pixel-wide regions. Unlike some neighborhood operators, such as smoothing kernels, the use of progressively larger neighborhood regions for the Hurst operator does not select information with different dimensions or scales in the image. Instead, it increases the precision of the fit and reduces the noise introduced by individual light or dark pixels, at least up to a region size as large as the defined structures in the image.

Each of the pixels in the diagram of **Figure 62** is labeled to indicate its distance from the center of the octagon. The distances (in pixel units) and the number of pixels at each distance are listed in **Table 1**. The distances range from 1 pixel (the 4 touching neighbors sharing a side with the central pixel) to 3.162 pixels ($\sqrt{10} = \sqrt{3 \times 3 + 1 \times 1}$).

Table 1. Distance of pixels labeled in Figure 54 from the center of the neighborhood.

Pixel class	Number	Distance from center
a	1	0
b	4	1
c	4	1.414 ($\sqrt{2}$)
d	4	2
e	8	2.236 ($\sqrt{5}$)
f	4	2.828 ($\sqrt{8}$)
g	4	3
h	8	3.162 ($\sqrt{10}$)

Application of the operator proceeds by examining the pixels in the neighborhood around each pixel in the original image. The brightest and darkest pixel values in each of the distance classes are found and their difference used to construct a Hurst plot. Performing a least-squares fit of the slope of the log (brightness difference) vs. log (distance) relationship is simplified because the distance values (and their logarithms) are unvarying and can be stored beforehand in a short table. It is also unnecessary to divide by the standard deviation of pixel brightnesses in the image, since this is a constant for each pixel in the image and the slope

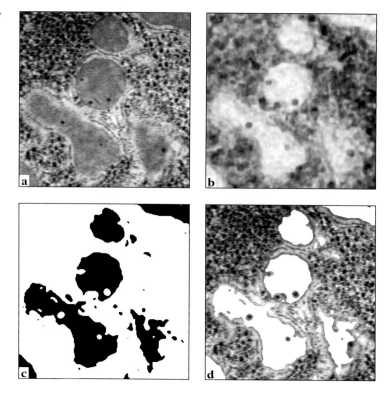

Figure 63. Segmentation based on texture using a Hurst operator:

a) liver (transmission electron micrograph of thin section);

b) Hurst transform image;

c) thresholded binary from image b;

d) high-texture regions in original using image c as a mask.

of the Hurst plot will be arbitrarily scaled to fit the brightness range of the display anyway.

Building the sums for the least-squares fit and performing the necessary calculations is moderately complex. Hence, it is time consuming compared to simple neighborhood operations such as smoothing, etc., but still well within the capability of typical desktop computer systems. Unfortunately, the comparison operations involved in this operator do not lend themselves to array processors or other specific hardware solutions.

Figure 63a shows a portion of a TEM of a thin section of liver tissue, used in **Figures 58** and **60**. The image contains many different structures at the organelle level, but for classification purposes the large, relatively uniform grey regions and the much more highly textured regions containing many small dark particles can be distinguished visually. Unfortunately, the average brightness level of the two areas is not sufficiently different to permit direct thresholding (discussed in Chapter 6). There are many pixels in the highly textured region that are brighter, the same, or darker than the average grey level of the smooth region. The conversion of the original image to one whose texture information permits thresholding of the regions is shown in the figure.

Figure 64 shows highly magnified images of two representative locations in each of these regions, with outlines showing specific locations of the octagonal neighborhood of **Figure 63** and

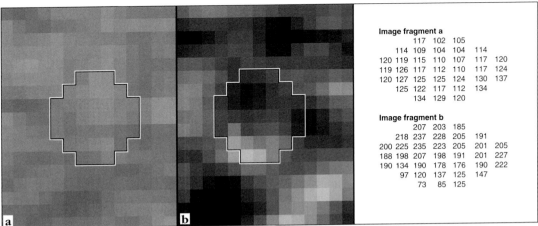

Image fragment a
```
        117 102 105
    114 109 104 104 114
120 119 115 110 107 117 120
119 126 117 112 110 117 124
120 127 125 125 124 130 137
    125 122 117 112 134
        134 129 120
```

Image fragment b
```
        207 203 185
    218 237 228 205 191
200 225 235 223 205 201 205
188 198 207 198 191 201 227
190 134 190 178 176 190 222
     97 120 137 125 147
         73  85 125
```

Figure 64. *Enlarged portions of smooth (**a**) and rough (**b**) areas of Figure 63a, showing individual pixels in representative 7-pixel-wide octagonal neighborhoods with the numerical values of the pixels (0 = white, 255 = black).*

the brightness values of those pixels. The convention for pixel values in these 8-bit monochrome images is white=0, black=255. Sorting through the pixels in each distance class, finding the brightest and darkest and their difference, and constructing a plot of log (brightness range) vs. log (distance) is shown for these two specific pixel locations in **Table 2** and **Figure 65**. Notice that the slopes of the Hurst plots are quite different and that the lines fit the points rather well as shown by the r-squared values.

Scaling the Hurst values to the brightness range of an image (in this example by multiplying arbitrarily by 64) and applying the

Table 2. Distance and brightness data for the neighborhoods in Figure 64.

Distance (pixels)	1	√2	2	√5	√8	3	√10
Image fragment a							
brightest	110	107	104	104	104	102	102
darkest	125	125	126	130	134	134	137
range	15	18	21	26	30	32	35
Image fragment b							
brightest	178	176	137	120	97	85	73
darkest	223	235	235	237	237	237	237
range	45	59	98	117	140	152	159

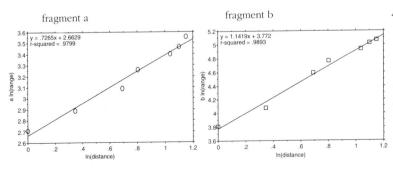

fragment a

$y = .7265x + 2.6629$
r-squared = .9799

fragment b

$y = 1.1419x + 3.772$
r-squared = .9893

Figure 65. *Hurst plots of the logarithm of the maximum brightness range vs. log of distance for the two neighborhoods shown in Figure 64.*

Figure 66. *Fracture surface of a steel test specimen. The smooth portion of the fracture occurred by fatigue, and the rougher portion by tearing.*

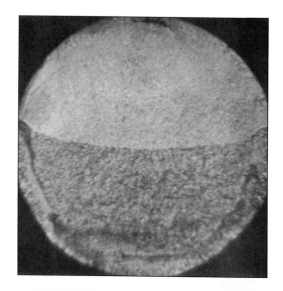

Figure 67. *Brightness histograms of two 100 × 100 pixel regions (marked) in Figure 66, showing greater variation in the rough area, but extensive overlap of brightness values with the smooth region.*

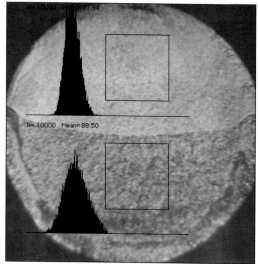

Figure 68. *Application of the local Hurst operator to the image in Figure 66, showing the larger values (darker pixels) for the rough portion of the fracture surface.*

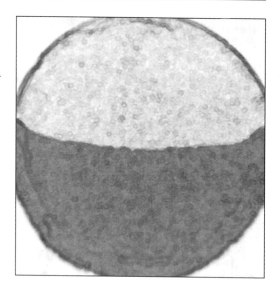

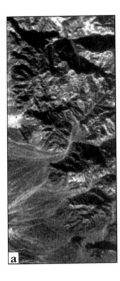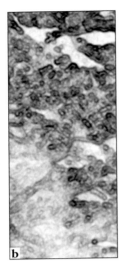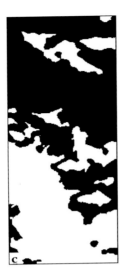

Figure 69. Aerial photograph (Death Valley, California):
a) original, showing differences in local texture;
b) application of the Hurst operator;
c) binary image formed by thresholding image *b* to select high values of roughness.

operation to each pixel in the image produces the result shown in **Figure 63b**. **Figures 63c** and **63d** show the use of the processed image for segmentation by thresholding (Chapter 6).

Figure 66 shows an image of the broken end of a steel test specimen. Part of the surface was produced by fatigue and part by the terminal tearing failure. Visual examination easily distinguishes the two regions based on texture. Measuring the area of the fatigue crack is important for determining the mechanical properties of the steel. However, the boundary is quite difficult to locate by computer processing.

Figure 67 shows the brightness histograms of two regions of the image, each 100 pixels square. The brightness values overlap extensively, although the variation of brightness values in the rough region is greater than in the smooth region. This means that simple thresholding is not useful. Applying the local Hurst operator to this image produces the result shown in **Figure 68**. The two regions are clearly delineated, in spite of some local variations within each.

On an even larger scale, **Figure 69a** shows an aerial photograph of part of Death Valley, California. The terrain consists of comparatively smooth regions of desert and alluvial fans from the mountains, as well as much rougher terrain produced by weathering. Applying the same local Hurst operator to this image produces the result shown in **Figure 69b**, which can be directly thresholded to distinguish the two regions shown in **Figure 69c**.

Figure 70 shows several other processing operations applied to the same image as **Figure 69** for comparison. Both the range and variance operators are sometimes used to characterize texture in images, but in this case, they do not perform as well as the Hurst operator. The Sobel operator highlights the edges and outlines the discontinuities in the image, but does not distinguish the smooth and rough regions.

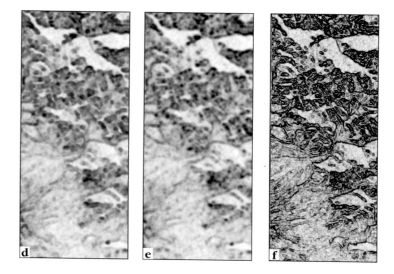

Figure 70. Other neighborhood operations applied to the image in Figure 69:

d) range;

e) variance;

f) Sobel.

Another comparison of different approaches to detecting texture is shown in **Figure 71**. This shows a light microscope image of curds and whey. The large smooth areas are the curds, while the more textured areas are the protein. Direct thresholding of the image does not produce good results, as shown in **Figure 71b**. In this example the image was first background leveled and then thresholded. Small features can be identified by their area and removed (in the example image they are just colored grey), to leave an approximation of the curds, but in this image there is considerable background clutter due to clumps of thresholded pixels that touch features or the edge of the frame.

Figures 71c, **e** and **g** show the original image processed with three different operators described above that respond to texture. All of the operations utilize the pixels within a 5-pixel-wide neighborhood. They range widely in complexity (and hence execution time). The range operator is just the difference in brightness between the lightest and darkest pixel in the neighborhood, while the Haralick operator calculates a difference moment, and the Hurst operator uses a table of the maximum differences as a function of pixel separation. In all cases, thresholding and removal of the small features (shaded grey in the images) gives the results shown in **Figures 71d**, **f** and **h**. These are cleaner images than direct thresholding, but still do not give nicely defined curd shapes and boundaries. Further examples using this very difficult image will be shown in Chapters 6 and 7.

Implementation notes

Many of the techniques discussed in this chapter and in Chapter 3 are neighborhood operators that access pixels in a small area around each central pixel, perform some calculation or comparison with those values, and then derive a new value for the central pixel. In all cases, this new value is used to produce a new

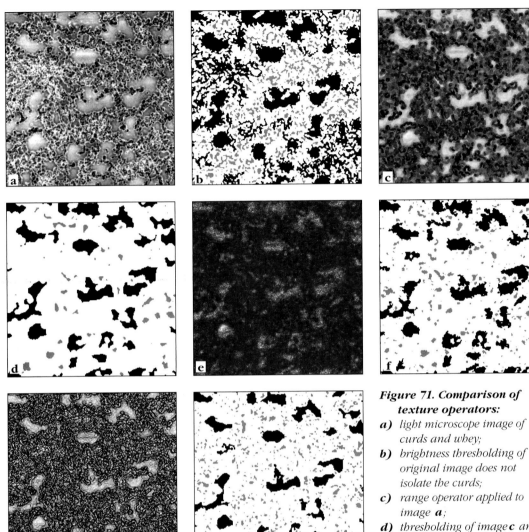

Figure 71. Comparison of texture operators:

a) light microscope image of curds and whey;

b) brightness thresholding of original image does not isolate the curds;

c) range operator applied to image **a**;

d) thresholding of image **c** and size selection to eliminate small groups of pixels (colored grey);

e) Haralick operator applied to image **a**;

f) thresholding of image **e** and size selection to eliminate small groups of pixels (colored grey);

g) Hurst operator applied to image **a**;

h) thresholding of image **g** and size selection to eliminate small groups of pixels (colored grey).

image, and it is the original values of pixels which are used in the neighborhood around the next pixel as the operation is repeated throughout the image.

Most image analysis systems, particularly those operating in desktop computers, have limited memory (particularly when the large size of images is considered). Creating a new image for every image processing operation is an inefficient use of this limited resource. Consequently, the strategy generally used is to perform the operation "in place," to process one image and replace it with the result.

This requires only enough temporary memory to hold a few lines of the image. The operations are generally performed left to right along each scan line and top to bottom through the image.

Duplicating the line that is being modified, and keeping copies of the preceding lines whose pixels are used, allows the new (modified) values to be written back to the original image memory. The number of lines is simply $(n+1)/2$ where n is the neighborhood dimension (e.g., 3×3, 5×5, etc.). Usually, the time required to duplicate a line from the image is small and by shuffling through a series of pointers, it is only necessary to copy each line once when the moving process reaches it, then reuse the array for subsequent vertical positions.

Some of the image processing methods described above create two or more intermediate results. For example, the Roberts' Cross or Sobel filters apply two directional derivatives whose magnitudes are subsequently combined. It is possible to do this pixel by pixel, so that no additional storage is required. However, in some implementations, particularly those that can be efficiently programmed into an array processor (which acts on an entire line through the image at one time), it is faster to obtain the intermediate results for each operator applied to each line and then combine them for the whole line. This requires a small amount of additional storage for the intermediate results.

Another consideration in implementing neighborhood operations is how to best treat pixels near the edges of the image. Many of the example images shown here are taken from the center of larger original images, so edge effects are avoided. In others, a band around the edge of the image is skipped, which is one of the most common ways to respond to the problem. With this approach, the programs skip pixels within a distance of $(n-1)/2$ pixels from any edge, where n is the total width of the neighborhood.

Other possibilities include having special neighborhood rules near edges to sort through a smaller set of pixels, duplicating rows of pixels at edges (i.e., assuming each edge is a mirror), or using wrap-around addressing (i.e., assuming that the left and right edges and the top and bottom edges of the image are contiguous). None of these methods is particularly attractive, in general. Since the largest and smallest brightness values are used to find the maximum range, the duplication of rows of pixels would not provide any extra information for range operations. In all cases, the use of fewer pixels for calculations would degrade the precision of the results. There is no reason whatsoever to assume that the image edges should be matched, and indeed, quite different structures and regions will normally occur there. The most conservative approach is to accept a small shrinkage in useful image size after processing, by ignoring near-edge pixels.

Image math

The image processing operations discussed so far in this chapter operate on one image and produce a modified result, which may be stored in the same image memory. Another class of operations uses two images to produce a new image (which may replace one of the originals). These operations are usually described as image arithmetic, since operators such as addition, subtraction, division, and multiplication are included. They are performed pixel by pixel, so that the sum of two images simply contains pixels whose brightness values are the sums of the corresponding pixels in the original images. There are some additional operators used, as well, such as comparing two images to keep the brighter (or darker) pixel. Other operations, such as Boolean OR or AND logic, are generally applied to binary images; they will be discussed in that context in Chapter 7.

Actually, image addition has already been used in a method described previously. In Chapter 3, the averaging of images to reduce noise was discussed. The addition operation is straightforward, but a decision is required about how to deal with the result. If two 8-bit images (with brightness values from 0 to 255 at each pixel) are added together, the resulting value can range from 0 to 510. This exceeds the capacity of the image memory. One possibility is simply to divide the result by two, obtaining a resulting image that is correctly scaled to the 0 to 255 range. This is what is usually applied in image averaging, in which the N images added together produce a total, which is then divided by N to rescale the data.

Another possibility is to find the largest and smallest actual values in the sum image, and then dynamically rescale the result to this maximum and minimum, so that each pixel is assigned a new value B = range × (sum − minimum) / (maximum − minimum), where range is the capacity of the image memory, typically 255. This is superior to performing the division by two and then subsequently performing a linear expansion of contrast, as discussed in Chapter 3, because the precision of the resulting values is higher. When the integer division by two is performed, fractional values are truncated and some information may be lost.

On the other hand, when dynamic ranging or automatic scaling is performed, it becomes more difficult to perform direct comparison of images after processing, since the brightness scales may not be the same. In addition, autoscaling takes longer, since two complete passes through the image are required: one to determine the maximum and minimum and one to apply the autoscaling calculation. Many of the images printed in this book have been autoscaled in order to maximize printed contrast. Whenever possible, this operation has been performed as part of the processing operation to maintain precision.

Adding together images superimposes information and can in some cases be useful to create composites, which help to communicate complex spatial relationships. We have already seen that adding the Laplacian or a derivative image to the original can help provide some spatial guidelines to interpret the information from the filter. Usually, this kind of addition is handled directly in the processing by changing the central value of the kernel. For the Laplacian, this modification is called a sharpening filter, as noted above.

Subtracting images

Subtraction is widely used and more interesting than the addition operation. In Chapter 3, subtraction was used to level images by removing background. This chapter has already mentioned uses of subtraction, such as that employed in unsharp masking, where the smoothed image is subtracted, pixel by pixel, from the original. In such an operation, the possible range of values for images whose initial range is 0 to 255 becomes −255 to +255. The data can be rescaled to fit into a single byte, replacing the original image, by adding 255 and dividing by two, or the same autoscaling method described above for addition may be employed. The same advantages and penalties for fixed and flexible scaling are encountered.

Subtraction is primarily a way to discover differences between images. **Figure 72** shows two images of coins and their difference. The parts of the picture that are essentially unchanged in the two images cancel out and appear as a uniform medium grey except for minor variations due to the precision of digitization, changes in illumination, etc. The coin that has been moved between the two image acquisitions is clearly shown. The dark image shows where the feature was; the bright one shows where it has gone.

Subtracting one image from another effectively removes from the difference image all features that do not change, while highlighting those that do. If the lighting and geometry of view is consistent, the only differences in pixel values where no changes occur are statistical variations in the brightness, due to camera or electronic noise. The bright and dark images show features that have been removed from or added to the field of view, respectively.

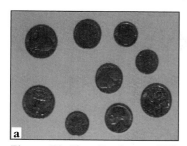 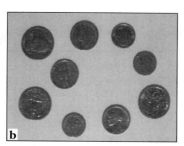 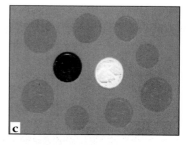

Figure 72. Showing image differences by subtraction:
a) original image; b) image after moving one coin; c) difference image after pixel-by-pixel subtraction.

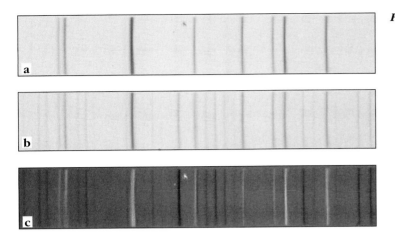

Figure 73. Image subtraction to enhance the visibility of details: a & b) scanned images of films from a Debye Scherer X-ray camera, taken with similar compounds; c) the difference between b and a showing the low intensity lines present in one film due to the presence of trace compounds in the sample.

Even in the presence of some noise, subtraction of two images can be an effective way to identify small differences that might otherwise escape notice. **Figure 73** shows an example. The image shows two films from a Debye-Scherer X-ray camera. The vertical lines show the exposure of the film by X-rays that were diffracted from a tiny sample, each line corresponding to reflection from one plane of atoms in the structure of the material. Comparing the films from these similar samples shows that most of the lines are similar in position and intensity, because the two samples are in fact quite similar in composition. The presence of trace quantities of impurities is revealed by additional faint lines in the image. Subtraction of one set of lines from the second increases the relative amount of noise, but reveals the presence of lines from the trace compounds. These can then be measured and used for identification.

A major use of image subtraction is quality control. A master image is acquired and stored that shows the correct placement of parts on circuit boards (**Figure 74**), the alignment of labels on packaging, etc. When the image is subtracted from a series of images acquired from subsequent objects, the differences are strongly highlighted, revealing errors in production. This subtraction is often carried out at video frame rates using dedicated

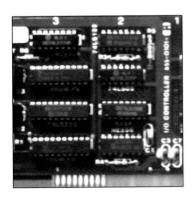
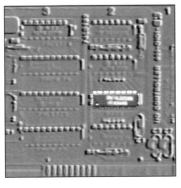

Figure 74. Difference images for quality control. A master image is subtracted from images of each subsequent part. In this example, the missing chip in a printed circuit board is evident in the difference image.

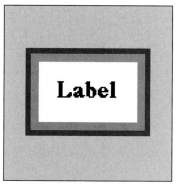 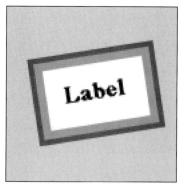 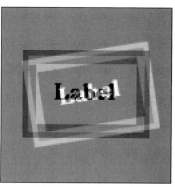

Figure 75. *Illustration of the use of image subtraction to detect misalignment in label positioning. The area of white and dark pixels measures the extent of positioning error.*

hardware. Since it is unrealistic to expect parts to be exactly aligned, a tolerance can be specified by the area of bright and dark (mismatched) pixels present after the subtraction. **Figure 75** shows this schematically.

The same technique is used in reconnaissance photos to watch for the appearance or disappearance of targets in a complex scene. Image warping, as discussed in Chapter 3, may be required to align images taken from different points of view before the subtraction can be performed. A similar method is used in astronomy. "Blinking" images taken of the same area of the sky at different times is the traditional way to search for moving planets or asteroids. This technique alternately presents each image to a human viewer, who notices the apparent motion of the point of light that is different in the two images. Some use of computer searching using subtraction has been used, but for dim objects in the presence of background noise has not proved as sensitive as a human observer.

Object motion can be measured using subtraction, if the features are large enough and the sequential images are acquired fast enough that they overlap in successive frames. In this case, the subtraction shows a bright area of mismatch that can be measured. The length of the unmatched region divided by the elapsed time gives the velocity; direction can be determined by the orientation of the region. This technique is used at microscopic scales to track the motion of cells on slides (**Figure 76**) in response to chemical cues.

At the other extreme, subtraction is used to track ice floes in the north Atlantic from satellite photos. For motion between two successive images that is too large for this method, it may be possible to identify the same objects in successive images based on size, shape, etc. and thus track motion. Or, one can assume that where paths cross, the points causing the least deviation of the path give the correct match (**Figure 77**). However, the direct subtraction technique is much simpler and more direct.

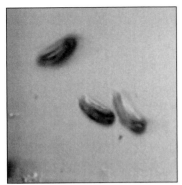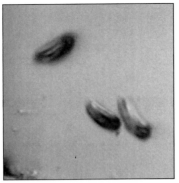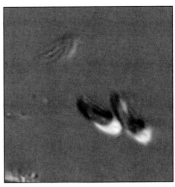

Figure 76. Two frames from a videotape sequence of free-swimming single-celled animals in a drop of pond water, and the difference image. The length of the white region divided by the time interval gives the velocity.

Multiplication and division

Image multiplication is perhaps the least used of the mathematics modes, but it is generally included for the sake of completeness in systems offering the other arithmetic operations. Multiplication was used above in **Figure 33** to combine the edge magnitude and direction data from the Sobel operator. Another possible use is superimposing one image on another in the particular case when the superimposed data are proportional to the absolute brightness of the original image. An example is texture; **Figure 78** shows an illustration. A Gaussian random brightness pattern is superimposed on the smooth polygonal approximation of a shaded sphere in order to provide an impression of roughness. Similar multiplicative superimposition may be used to add fluorescence or other emission images to a reflection or transmission image.

One of the difficulties with multiplication is the extreme range of values that may be generated. With 8-bit images whose pixels

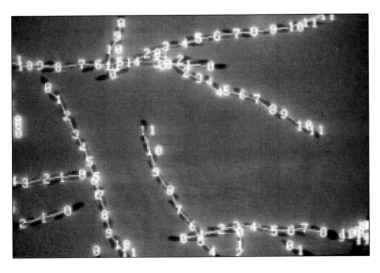

Figure 77. Analysis of motion in a more complex situation than shown in Figure 76. Where the paths of the swimming microorganisms cross, they are sorted out by assuming that the path continues in a nearly straight direction. (Gualtieri & Coltelli, 1992).

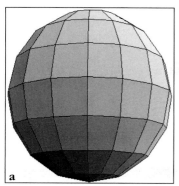 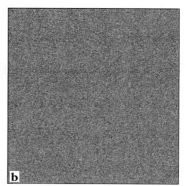 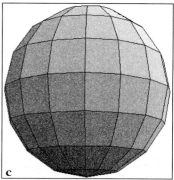

Figure 78. Multiplication of images can be used to superimpose texture on an image:
a) smooth faceted globe;
b) Gaussian random values;
c) product of a times b.

can have a range between 0 and 255, the possible products can range from 0 to more than 65,000. This is a 2-byte product, only the high byte of which can be stored back into the same image memory unless automatic scaling is used. A significant loss of precision may result for values in the resulting image.

The magnitude of the numbers also creates problems with division. First, division by 0 must be avoided. This is usually done by adding 1 to all brightness values, so that the values are interpreted as 1 to 256 instead of 0 to 255. Then it is necessary to first multiply each pixel in the numerator by some factor that will produce quotients covering the 0 to 255 range, while maintaining some useful precision for the ends of the range. Automatic scaling is particularly useful for these situations, but it cannot be used in applications requiring comparison of results to each other or to a calibration curve.

An example of division in which automatic scaling is useful is the removal of background (as discussed in Chapter 3) when linear detectors or cameras are used. An example of division when absolute values are required is calculating ratios of brightness from two or more Landsat bands (an example is shown in Chapter 1) or two or more filter images when examining fluorescent probes in the light microscope. In fluorescence microscopy, the time variation of emitted light intensity is normalized by alternately collecting images through two or more filters at different wavelengths above and below the line of interest, and calibrating the ratio against the activity of the element(s) of interest. In satellite imagery, ratios of intensities (particularly Band 4 = 0.5 to 0.6 μm, Band 5 = 0.6 to 0.7 μm, Band 6 = 0.7 to 0.8 μm, and Band 7 = 0.8 to 1.1 μm) are used for terrain classification and the identification of some rock types. The thermal inertia of different rock formations may also be determined by ratioing images obtained at different local times of day, as the formations heat or cool.

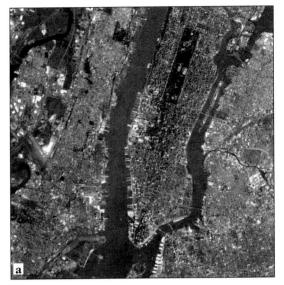

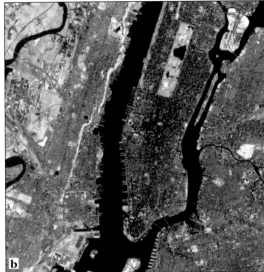

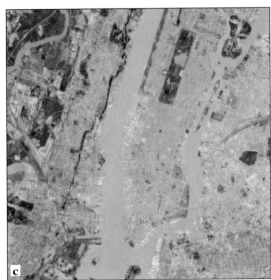

Figure 79. Landsat thematic mapper images of New York City:

a) Band 1 (visible blue);

b) Band 4 (near infrared);

c) ratio of Band 4 to Band 1 (showing vegetation areas).

As an example of mineral identification, silicates exhibit a wavelength shift in the absorption band with composition. Granites, diorites, gabbros, and olivene peridotes have progressively decreasing silicon content. The absorption band shifts to progressively longer wavelengths in the 8 to 12 µm thermal infrared band as the bond-stretching vibrations between Si and O atoms in the silicate lattice change. The Thermal Infrared Multispectral Mapper satellite records six bands of image data in this range, which are combined and normalized to locate the absorption band and identify rock formations. Carbonate rocks (dolomite and limestone) have a similar absorption response in the 6 to 8 µm range, but this is difficult to measure in satellite imagery because of atmospheric absorption. At radar wavelengths, different surface roughnesses produce variations in reflected intensity in

Figure 80. Combining views of NGC-2024 to show star-forming regions and dust.
a) *1.2-μm infrared image;*
b) *1.6-μm infrared image;*
c) *2.2-μm infrared image;*
d) *2.2-μm image minus 1.6-μm image;*
e) *1.6-μm image divided by 1.2-μm image.*

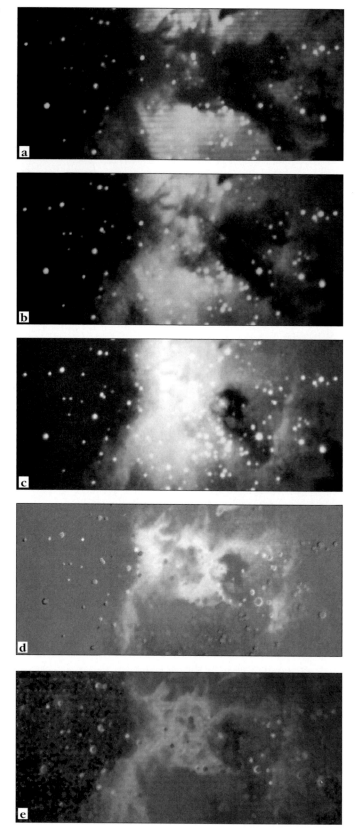

the Ka, X, and L bands and can be combined in the same ways to perform measurements and distinguish the coarseness of sands, gravels, cobbles, and boulders (Sabins, 1987).

In the same way, Bands 1 (0.55 to 0.68 μm, or visible red) and 2 (0.72 to 1.10 μm, or reflected infrared) from multispectral satellite imagery are used to recognize vegetation. Band 1 records the chlorophyll absorption and Band 2 gives the reflection from the cell structure of the leaves. The ratio $(B_2 - B_1) / (B_2 + B_1)$ eliminates variations due to differences in solar elevation (illumination angle) and is used to measure the distribution of vegetation in images. Typically, this approach also combines data from successive scans to obtain the spectral vegetation index as a function of time. Other ratios have been used to image and to measure chlorophyll concentrations due to phytoplankton in the ocean (Sabins, 1987). **Figure 79** shows a simplified approximation to this method using the ratio of near infrared to blue to isolate vegetation from satellite imagery.

Ratios are also used in astronomical images. **Figure 80** shows infrared images of the star-forming region in NGC-2024. Infrared light penetrates the dust that blocks much of the visible light. Ratios or differences of the different wavelength images show details in the dust and enhance the visibility of the young stars.

Figure 81 shows two fluorescence microscope images from tissue stained with Fura-2, excited using 340 and 385 nm light. This specific stain is used to localize the concentration of Ca+ in the material. The ionic concentration is calculated from the ratio of the two images, while the sum of the two (80% of the first and 20% of the second) gives an isobestic image that normalizes the data for the total amount of stain. A particularly useful way of visualizing the result is achieved by placing the results from the image math operations into a color display. **Figure 81c** shows the ratio displayed as hue and the isobestic image as intensity with saturation set to maximum (images and technique courtesy of P. J. Sammak, Univ. of Minnesota).

Image math also includes the logical comparison of pixel values. For instance, two images may be combined by keeping the brighter (or darker) of the corresponding pixels at each location. This is used, for instance, to build up a confocal scanning light microscope (CSLM) image with great depth of field. Normal light microscope images have limited depth of field because of the high numerical aperture of the lenses. In the CSLM, the scanning light beam and aperture on the detector reduce this depth of field even more by eliminating light scattered from any point except the single point illuminated in the plane of focus, as indicated in **Figure 82**.

A single, two-dimensional image is formed by scanning the light over the sample (or, equivalently, by moving the sample itself with the light beam stationary). For a specimen with an irregular

**Figure 81. Fura-2 fluorescence
microscope images:**

a) *340 nm excitation;*

b) *385 nm excitation;*

c) *colored result with hue = ratio
of 340/385 nm images,
intensity = 0.8 × 340 + 0.2 ×
385 images, saturation =
100%.*

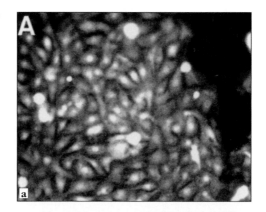

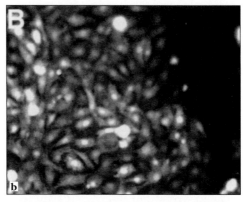

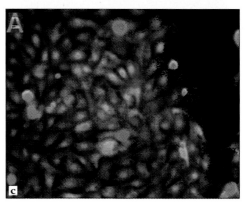

Figure 82. *Principle of the
confocal scanning light
microscope. Light reflected
from out-of-focus planes or
points does not reach the
detector.*

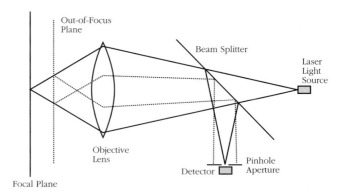

Figure 83. *Combining CSLM images by keeping the brightest value at each pixel location. Images **a** and **b** are two individual focal plane images from a series of 25 on an integrated circuit. Only the portion of the surface which is in focus is bright. Since the in-focus point is brightest, combining all of the individual planes produces image **c,** which shows the entire surface in focus.*

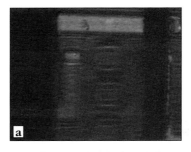

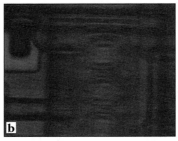

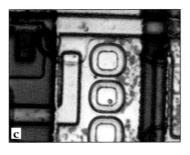

surface, this image is very dark, except at locations where the surface lies in the plane of focus. By moving the specimen vertically, many such planar images can be acquired. The display of a complete three-dimensional set of such images is discussed in Chapter 10. However, at each pixel location, the brightest value of light reflectance occurs at the in-focus point. Consequently, the images from many focal depths can be combined by keeping only the brightest value at each pixel location to form an image with an unlimited depth of field. **Figure 83** shows an example.

An additional effect can be produced by shifting each image slightly before performing the comparison and superposition. **Figures 84** and **85** show an example. The 26 individual images, four of which are shown in **Figure 84**, are combined in this way to produce a perspective view of the surface (this image was also shown in Chapter 1 as an example of one mode of collecting and displaying three-dimensional imaging information).

Another use of combining several images arises in polarized light microscopy. As shown in **Figure 86**, the use of polarizer and analyzer with specimens such as mineral thin sections produces images in which some grains are colored and others dark, as a function of analyzer rotation. Combining images from many rotations

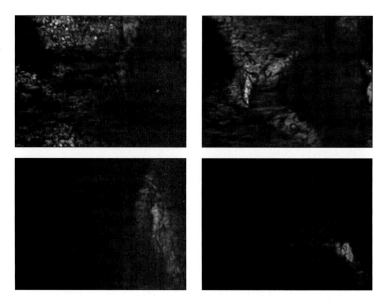

Figure 84. *Four individual focal sections from a confocal light microscope series on a ceramic fracture surface. The images are 40 μm wide, and the images in the stack of 26 images are spaced 1 μm apart in depth.*

and keeping just the brightest pixel value produces an image that shows all of the grains. The same technique can be used with transmission electron microscope images of thin metal foils, to combine images in which some grains are darkened due to electron diffraction effects, or to remove dark contours that result from bending of the foil.

Figure 85. *Surface reconstruction from the images shown in Figure 76. Each image is shifted two pixels to the right and up, and combined by keeping the brightest value at each pixel location. The result is a perspective view of the entire surface.*

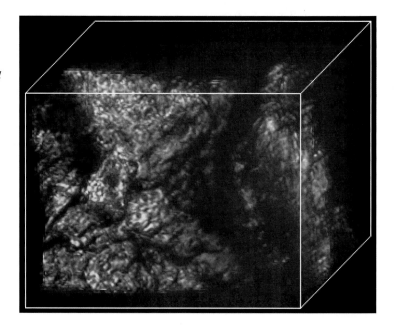

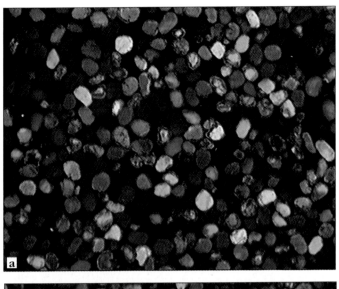

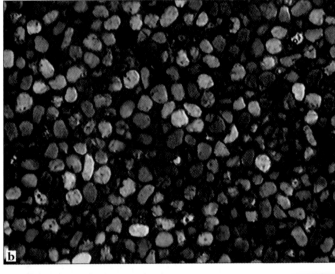

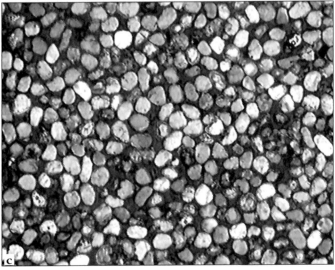

Figure 86. Thin section of sandstone viewed by polarized light. a , b) *different orientations of the analyzer;* **c)** *maximum brightness image from 6 rotations.*

5

Processing Images in Frequency Space

Some necessary mathematical preliminaries

What frequency space is all about

It is unusual to pick up a book on image analysis without finding at least a portion of it devoted to a discussion of Fourier transforms (see especially Pratt, 1991; Gonzalez & Wintz, 1987; Jain, 1989). In part, this is due to the utility of working in frequency space to perform certain image measurement and processing operations. Many of these same operations can be performed in the original (spatial domain) image only with significantly greater computational effort. Another reason for the lengthy sections on these methods is that the authors frequently come from a background in electrical engineering and signal processing and so are familiar with the mathematics and the use of these methods for other types of signals, particularly the one-dimensional (time varying) electrical signals that make up much of our modern electronics.

However, the typical image analyst interested in applying computer methods to images for purposes of enhancement or measurement is often not comfortable with the pages of mathematics (and intimidating notation) used in these discussions. Furthermore, he or she may not have the fortitude to relate these concepts to the operation of a dedicated image analysis computer. Unable to see the connection between the topics discussed and the typical image problems encountered in real life, the potential user might therefore find it easier to skip the subject. This is a loss, because the use of frequency space methods can offer benefits in many real-life applications, and it is not essential to deal deeply with the mathematics to arrive at a practical working knowledge of these techniques.

The Fourier transform and other frequency space transforms are applied to two-dimensional images for many different reasons. Some of these have little to do with the purposes of enhancing visibility and selection of features or structures of interest for measurement. For instance, some of these transform methods are used as a means of image compression, in which less data than the original image must be transmitted or stored. In this type of application, it is necessary to reconstruct the image (bring it back from the frequency to the spatial domain) for viewing. It is desirable to be able to accomplish both the forward and reverse transform rapidly and with a minimum loss of image quality. Image quality is a somewhat elusive concept that certainly includes the alteration of grey levels, definition of feature boundaries, and introduction or removal of fine-scale texture in the image. Usually, the greater the degree of compression, the greater the loss of image fidelity.

Speed is usually a less important concern to image measurement applications, since the acquisition and subsequent analysis of the images are likely to require some time anyway, but the computational advances (both in hardware and software or algorithms) made to accommodate the requirements of the data compression application help to shorten the time for some other processing operations, as well. On the other hand, the amount of image degradation that can be tolerated by most visual uses of the compressed and restored images is far greater than is usually acceptable for image analysis purposes. Consequently, the amount of image compression that can be achieved with minimal loss of fidelity is rather small, as discussed in Chapter 2.

Since in most cases the transmission of an image from the point of acquisition to the computer used for analysis is not a major concern, we will ignore this entire subject here and assume that the transform retains all of the data, even if this means that there is no compression at all. Indeed, most of these methods are free from any data loss. The transform encodes the image information completely and it can be exactly reconstructed, at least to within the arithmetic precision of the computer being used (which is generally better than the precision of the original image sensor or analog-to-digital converter).

Although there are many different types of image transforms that can be used, the best known (at least, the one with the most recognizable name) is the Fourier transform. This is due in part to the availability of a powerful and very efficient algorithm for computing it, known as the Fast Fourier Transform or FFT (Cooley & Tukey, 1965; Bracewell, 1989), which we will encounter in due course. Although many of the examples in this text were actually computed using a newer approach (the Fast Hartley Transform or FHT [see Hartley, 1942; Bracewell, 1984, 1986; Reeves, 1990]), the frequency space images are presented in the same form that the Fourier method would yield. For the sake of explanation, it is probably easiest to describe the better-known method.

The usual approach to developing the mathematical background of the Fourier transform begins with a one-dimensional waveform and then expands to two dimensions (an image). In principle, this can also be extended to three dimensions, although it becomes much more difficult to visualize or display. Three-dimensional transforms between the spatial domain (now a volume image constructed of voxels instead of pixels) and the three-dimensional frequency space are used, for example, in some tomographic reconstructions.

The mathematical development that follows has been kept as brief as possible, but if you suffer from "integral-o-phobia" then it is permitted to skip this section and go on to the examples and discussion, returning here only when (and if) a deeper understanding is desired.

The Fourier transform

Using a fairly standard nomenclature and symbology, let us begin with a function $f(x)$, where x is a real variable representing either time or distance in one direction across an image. It is very common to refer to this function as the spatial or time domain function and the transform F introduced below as the frequency space function. The function f is a continuous and well-behaved function. Do not be disturbed by the fact that in a digitized image, the values of x are not continuous but discrete (based on pixel spacing), and the possible brightness values are quantized as well. These values are considered to sample the real or analog image that exists outside the computer.

Fourier's theorem states that it is possible to form any one-dimensional function $f(x)$ as a summation of a series of sine and cosine terms of increasing frequency. The Fourier transform of the function $f(x)$ is written $F(u)$ and describes the amount of each frequency term that must be added together to make $f(x)$. It can be written as

$$F(u) = \int_{-\infty}^{+\infty} f(x)e^{-2\pi iux}\,dx \qquad (1$$

where i is (as usual) $\sqrt{-1}$. The use of the exponential notation relies on the mathematical identity (Euler's formula)

$$e^{-2\pi iux} = \cos(2\pi ux) - i\sin(2\pi ux) \qquad (2$$

One of the very important characteristics of this transform is that given $F(u)$, it is possible to recover the spatial domain function $f(x)$ in the same way.

$$f(x) = \int_{-\infty}^{+\infty} F(u)e^{2\pi i u x} du \qquad (3$$

These two equations together comprise the forward and reverse Fourier transform. The function $f(x)$ is generally a real function, such as a time-varying voltage or a spatially-varying image brightness. However, the transform function $F(u)$ is generally complex, the sum of a real part R and an imaginary part I.

$$F(u) = R(u) + i\,I(u) \qquad (4$$

It is usually more convenient to express this in polar rather than Cartesian form

$$F(u) = |F(u)|\ e^{i\phi(u)} \qquad (5$$

where $|F|$ is called the magnitude and ϕ is called the phase. The square of the magnitude $P(u) = |F(u)|^2$ is commonly referred to as the power spectrum, or spectral density of $f(x)$.

The integrals from minus to plus infinity will in practice be reduced to a summation of terms of increasing frequency, limited by the finite spacing of the sampled points in the image. The discrete Fourier transform is written as

$$F(u) = \frac{1}{N} \sum_{x=0}^{N-1} f(x)e^{-i2\pi u x/N} \qquad (6$$

where N is the number of sampled points along the function $f(x)$, which are assumed to be uniformly spaced. Again, the reverse transform is similar (but not identical; note the absence of the $1/N$ term and the change in sign for the exponent).

$$f(x) = \sum_{u=0}^{N-1} F(u)e^{i2\pi u x/N} \qquad (7$$

The values of u from 0 to N–1 represent the discrete frequency components added together to construct the function $f(x)$. As in the continuous case, $F(u)$ is complex and may be written as real and imaginary or as magnitude and phase components.

The summation is normally performed over terms up to one-half the dimension of the image (in pixels), since it requires a minimum of two pixel brightness values to define the highest frequency present. This limitation is described as the Nyquist frequency. Because the summation has half as many terms as the width of the original image, but each term has a real and imaginary part, the total number of values produced by the Fourier transform is the same as the number of pixels in the original image width, or the number of samples of a time-varying function.

In both the continuous and the discrete cases, a direct extension from one-dimensional functions to two- (or three-) dimensional ones can be made by substituting $f(x,y)$ for $f(x)$ and $F(u,v)$ for $F(u)$, and performing the summation or integration over two (or three) variables instead of one. Since the dimensions x,y,z are orthogonal, so are the u,v,w dimensions. This means that the transformation can be performed separately in each direction. For a two-dimensional image, for example, it would be possible to perform a one-dimensional transform on each horizontal line of the image, producing an intermediate result with complex values for each point. Then a second series of one-dimensional transforms can be performed on each vertical column, finally producing the desired two-dimensional transform.

The program fragment listed below shows how to compute the FFT of a function. It is written in Fortran, but can be translated into any other language (you may have to define a type to hold the complex numbers). On input to the subroutine, F is the array of values to be transformed (usually the imaginary part of these complex numbers will be 0) and LN is the power of 2 (up to 10 for the maximum 1024 in this implementation). The transform is returned in the same array F. The first loop reorders the input data, the second performs the successive doubling that is the heart of the FFT method, and the final loop normalizes the results.

```
        SUBROUTINE FFT(F,LN)
        COMPLEX F(1024),U,W,T,CMPLX
        PI=3.14159265
        N=2**LN
        NV2=N/2
        NM1=N-1
        J=1
        DO 3 I=1,NM1
                IF (I.GE.J) GOTO 1
                T=F(J)
                F(J)=F(I)
                F(I)=T
1               K=NV2
2               IF (K.GE.J) GOTO 3
                J=J-K
                K=K/2
                GOTO 2
3               J=J+K
        DO 5 L=1,LN
                LE=2**L
                LE1=LE/2
                U=(1.0,0.0)
                W=CMPLX(COS(PI/LE1),-SIN(PI/LE1))
                DO 5 J=1,LE1
                        DO 4 I=J,N,LE
                                IP=I+LE1
                                T=F(IP)*U
                                F(IP)=F(I)-T
4
5                               F(I)=F(I)+T
                        U=U*W
        DO 6 I=1MN
6               F(I)=F(I)/FLOAT(N)
        RETURN
        END
```

Applying this one-dimensional transform to each row and then each column of a two-dimensional image is not the fastest way to perform the calculation, but it is by far the simplest and is actually used in many programs. A somewhat faster approach, known as a butterfly because it uses various sets of pairs of pixel

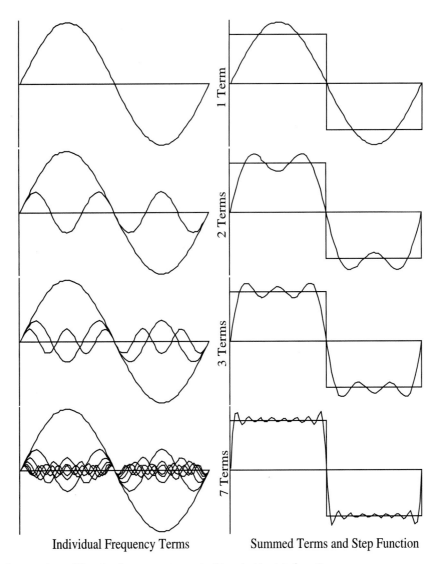

Individual Frequency Terms   Summed Terms and Step Function

Figure 1. *Summation of Fourier frequency terms to fit a simple step function.*

values throughout the two-dimensional image, produces identical results. Storing the array of W values can also provide a slight increase in speed.

The resulting transform of the original image into frequency space has complex values at each pixel. This is difficult to display in any meaningful way. In most cases, the display is based on only the magnitude of the value, ignoring the phase. If the square of the magnitude is used, this may be referred to as the image power spectrum, since different frequencies are represented at different distances from the origin, different directions represent different orientations in the original image, and the power at each location shows how much of that frequency and orientation is present in the image. This display is particularly useful for isolating periodic structures or noise, which is dis-

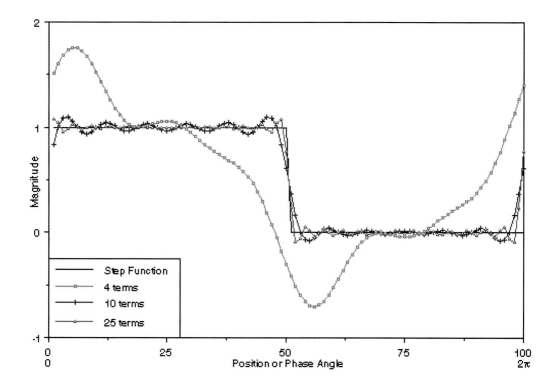

Figure 2. *Match between a step function and the first 4, 10, and 25 Fourier terms.*

cussed below. However, the power spectrum by itself cannot be used to restore the original image. The phase information is also needed, although it is rarely displayed and is usually difficult or impossible to interpret visually.

Fourier transforms of real functions

A common illustration in introductory-level math textbooks on the Fourier transform (which usually deal only with the one-dimensional case) is the quality of the fit to an arbitrary, but simple, function by the sum of a finite series of terms in the Fourier expansion. **Figure 1** shows the familiar case of a step function, illustrating the ability to add up a series of sine waves to produce the desired step. The coefficients in the Fourier series are the magnitudes of each increasing frequency needed to produce the fit. **Figure 2** shows the result of adding together the first 4, 10, and 25 terms. Obviously, the greater the number of terms included, the better the fit (especially at the sharp edge). **Figure 3** shows the same comparison for a ramp function.

Notice in both of these cases that the function is actually assumed to be repetitive or cyclical. The fit goes on at the right and left ends of the interval as though the function were endlessly repeated in both directions. This is also the case in two dimensions; the image in the spatial domain is effectively one tile in an endlessly repeating pattern. If the right and left edges or the top

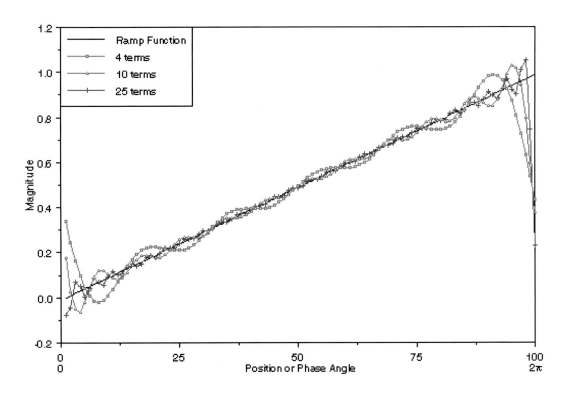

Figure 3. *Match between a ramp function and the first 4, 10, and 25 Fourier terms.*

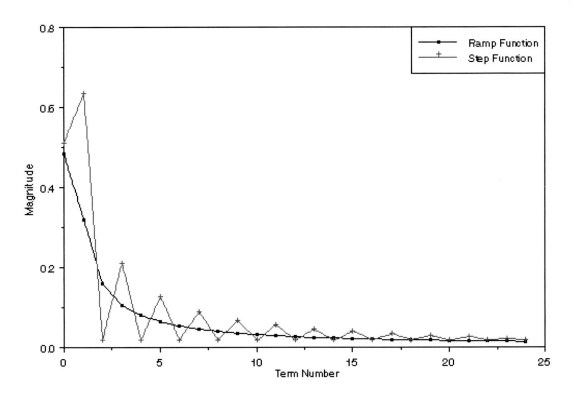

Figure 4. *Magnitude of the first 25 Fourier terms fit to the step and ramp in Figures 2 and 3.*

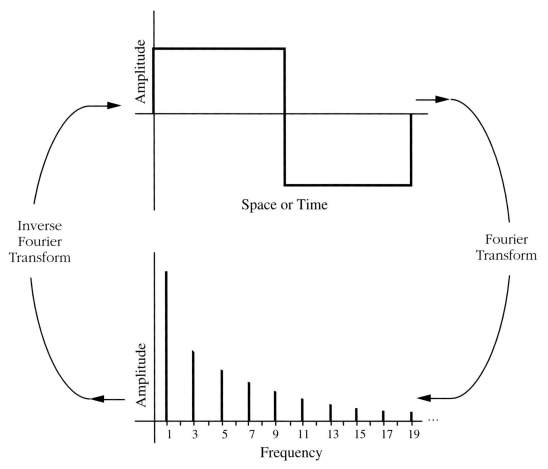

Figure 5. *Role of the forward and inverse transform and the spatial and frequency domain representations of a step function.*

and bottom edges of the image are different, this can produce very noticeable effects in the resulting transform. One solution is to embed the image in a larger one consisting of either zeroes or the average brightness value of the pixels. This kind of padding makes the image twice as large in each direction, requiring four times as much storage and calculation. It is needed particularly when correlation is performed, as discussed below.

The magnitude of the Fourier coefficients from the fit shown in **Figures 2** and **3** is plotted as amplitude vs. frequency (**Figure 4**). Notice that the step function consists only of odd terms, while the magnitudes for the ramp function transform decrease smoothly. Rather than the magnitudes, it is somewhat more common to plot the power spectrum of the transform, and to plot it as a symmetric function extending to both sides of the origin (zero frequency, or the DC level). As noted above, the power is simply the square of the magnitude. Because the range of values can be very large, the power spectrum is sometimes plotted with

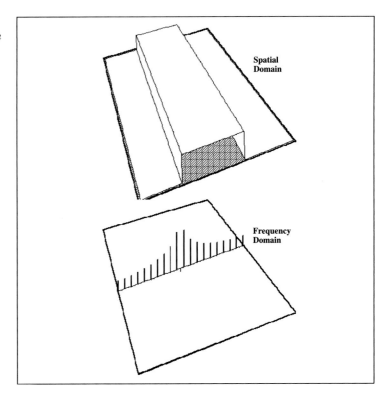

Figure 6. Two-dimensional presentation of a step function and its frequency transform.

Spatial Domain

Frequency Domain

a logarithmic or other compressed vertical scale to show the smaller terms usually present at high frequencies, along with the lower frequency terms.

Figure 5 reiterates the duality of the Fourier transform process. The spatial and frequency domains show the information in very different ways, but the information is the same. Of course, the plot of amplitude in the frequency transform does not show the important phase information, but we understand that the values are actually complex.

It is important to recall, in examining these transforms, that the axes represent frequency. The low-frequency terms near the origin of the plot provide the overall shape of the function, while the high-frequency terms are needed to sharpen edges and provide fine detail. The second point to be kept in mind is that these terms are independent of each other (this is equivalent to the statement that the basis functions are orthogonal). Performing the transform to determine coefficients to higher and higher frequencies does not change the previous ones, and selecting any particular range of terms to reconstruct the function will do so to the greatest accuracy possible with those frequencies.

Proceeding to two dimensions, **Figure 6** shows the square wave simply extended uniformly in one direction. This produces a Fourier transform consisting of exactly the same frequency terms in the direction perpendicular to the step and nothing in any

other direction. **Figure 7** shows the transform of an image in which the brightness values vary in one direction as a linear ramp. Since the ramp varies in only one direction, the power spectrum consists of a single line of values whose brightness profile is the same as that for the one-dimensional function shown in **Figure 3**. The same power spectrum is obtained from the shifted ramp image shown in the figure (although the phase image is different). This image is 256 pixels wide, so a total of 128 terms are calculated. If only the first 25 of these terms are used in the reconstruction, the resulting ramp image, shown with grey scale coding in **Figure 8** and plotted isometrically in **Figure 9**, exhibits the same variation from the ideal ramp as shown in the one-dimensional case.

Figure 10 shows four images of perfectly sinusoidal variations in brightness. The first three vary in spacing (frequency) and orientation; the fourth is the superposition of all three. For each, the two-dimensional frequency transform is particularly simple. Each of the pure tones has a transform consisting of a single point (identifying the frequency and orientation). Because of the redundancy of the plotting coordinates, the point is shown in two symmetrical locations around the origin. The superposition of the three sinusoids produces an image whose frequency transform is simply the sum of the three individual transforms. This principle of additivity will be important for much of the discus-

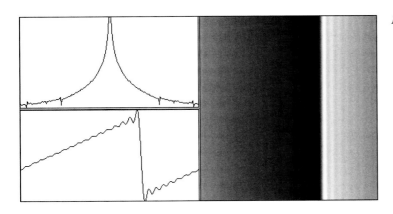

Figure 8. *The horizontal profile of the transform power spectrum from Figure 7 (top left), the retransformed image using the first 25 terms (right), and its horizontal brightness profile (bottom left).*

Figure 9. *Isometric plot of a reconstructed two-dimensional image of the results shown in Figure 8, based on the first 25 terms in the Fourier transform of the shifted linear ramp.*

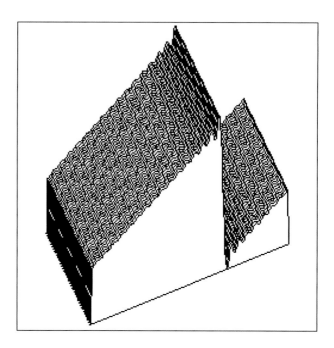

sion below. Subtracting the information from a location in the frequency transform is equivalent to removing the corresponding information from every part of the spatial-domain image.

Figure 11 shows two images with the same shape in different orientations. The frequency transforms rotate with the feature. Two-dimensional power spectra are easiest to describe using polar coordinates, as indicated in **Figure 12** for the frequency transform of the step function. The frequency increases with

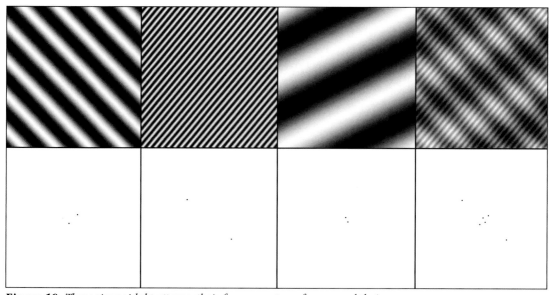

Figure 10. *Three sinusoidal patterns, their frequency transforms, and their sum.*

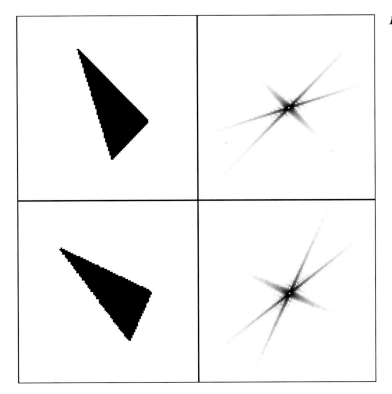

Figure 11. *Figure 11. Rotation of a spatial-domain image (left), and the corresponding rotation of the frequency transform (right).*

radius ρ, and the orientation depends on the angle θ. It is common to display the two-dimensional transform with the frequencies plotted from the center of the image, which is consequently redundant (the top and bottom or left and right halves are simply duplicates, with symmetry about the origin). In some cases, this image is shifted so that the origin is at the corners of the image and the highest frequencies are in the center. One format can be converted to the other by swapping quadrants of the display. For most of the purposes of interest here (removing or selecting specific frequencies, etc.) the display with the origin centered will be simplest to use and has been adopted here.

Figure 13 shows a two-dimensional step consisting of a rectangle. The two-dimensional frequency transform of this image produces

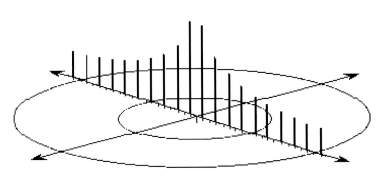

Figure 12. Frequency transform of a step function rotates with orientation of the spatial image.

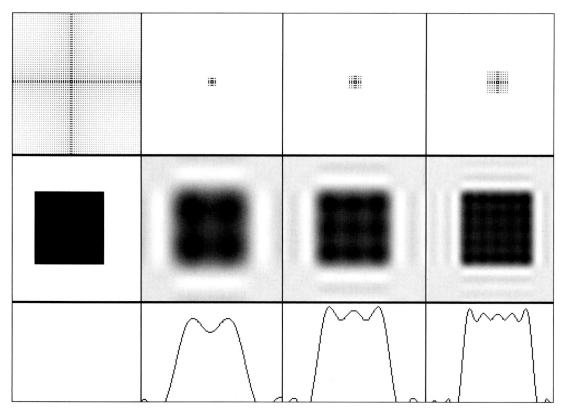

Figure 13. *A two-dimensional step function and its frequency transform (left), and reconstructions with different numbers of terms (shown as a portion of the frequency transform). Bottom row shows horizontal line profiles through the center of the reconstructed spatial image.*

the same series of diminishing peaks in the x and y axis directions as the one-dimensional step function. Limiting the reconstruction to only the central (low frequency) terms produces the reconstructions shown. Just as for the one-dimensional case, this limits the sharpness of the edge of the step and produces some ringing in the overall shape. The line profiles through the image show the same shape as previously discussed for the one-dimensional case. This can also be seen in **Figures 14** and **15**, where the magnitude, as well as the power spectrum with a logarithmic vertical scale, is shown. With a linear scale, the power spectrum would show only the central peak of this sine function, and the outer lobes would be virtually invisible. Notice also the different spacing of the lobes in the vertical and horizontal directions, resulting from the different dimensions of the original rectangle.

Frequencies and orientations

It is helpful to develop a little familiarity with the power spectrum display of the frequency-space transform of the image using simple images. **Figure 16** shows several shapes, more complex than the simple rectangular step function, with their two-dimensional frequency transforms. For each, the displayed power spectrum shows the orientation of the various edges, and the various

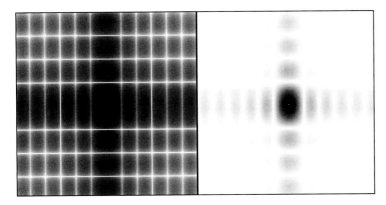

Figure 14. The two-dimensional frequency transform of a rectangular step function shown as a logarithmic display of the power spectrum (left) and the magnitude (right).

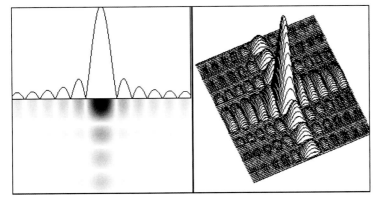

Figure 15. The magnitude image from Figure 14 shown with its cross section (left) and isometric display (right).

frequencies show the terms needed to represent them. In only a few simple cases can a visual examination of the power spectrum identify the original generating shape.

In **Figure 17**, the lines can be represented by a single peak because their brightness profile is perfectly sinusoidal (as in **Figure 10** above); thus only a single frequency is present. If the line profile is different, more terms are needed to represent the shape and consequently more peaks appear in the power spectrum. **Figure 18** shows an example in which the frequency transform consists of a series of peaks in the same orientation (perpendicular to the line angle).

In **Figure 19**, the lines have the aliasing common in computer displays (and in halftone printing technology), in which the lines at a shallow angle on the display are constructed from a series of steps corresponding to the rows of display pixels. This further complicates the frequency transform, which now has additional peaks representing the horizontal and vertical steps in the image that correspond to the aliasing, in addition to the main line of peaks seen in **Figure 18**.

It is possible to select only the peaks along the main row and eliminate the others with a mask or filter, as will be discussed below. After all, the frequency-domain image can be modified just like any other image. If this is done and only the peaks in the

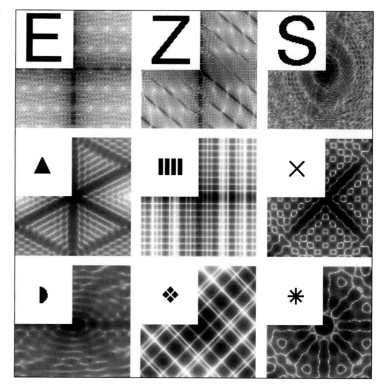

Figure 16. *Nine two-dimensional black and white shapes (insets) with their frequency transforms. (Image courtesy Arlo Reeves, Dartmouth Univ.)*

main row used for the inverse transformation (back to the spatial domain), the aliasing of the lines is removed. In fact, that is how the images in **Figures 17** and **18** were produced. This will lead naturally to the subject of filtering (discussed in a later section): removing unwanted information from spatial-domain images by operating on the frequency transform.

Measuring images in the frequency domain
Orientation and spacing

The idealized examples shown in the preceding tutorial show that any periodic structure in the original spatial-domain image will be represented by a peak in the power spectrum image at a radius corresponding to the spacing and a direction corresponding to the orientation. In a real image, which also includes non-periodic information, these peaks will be superimposed on a broad and sometimes noisy background. However, finding the peaks is generally much easier than finding the original periodic structure. Also, measuring the peak locations accurately is much easier and more accurate than trying to extract the same information from the original image, because all of the occurrences are effectively averaged together in the frequency domain.

Figure 20 shows an example of this kind of peak location measurement. The spatial-domain image is a high-resolution TEM image of the lattice structure in pure silicon. The regular spacing

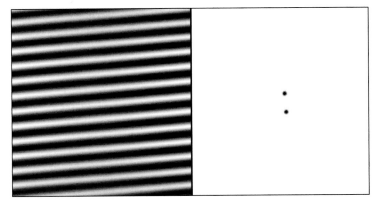

Figure 17. A set of sinusoidal lines (left) and the frequency transform (right).

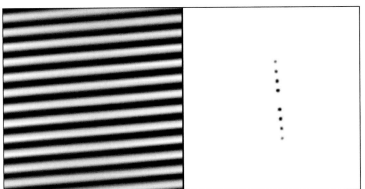

Figure 18. The same lines as Figure 17 with a non-sinusoidal brightness profile.

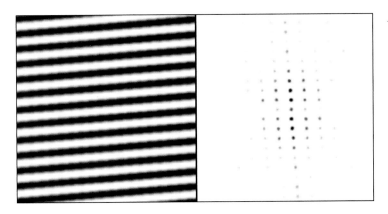

Figure 19. The same lines as Figure 18 with aliasing.

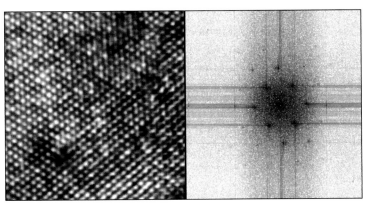

Figure 20. High-resolution TEM image of atomic lattice in silicon (left), with the frequency transform (right). (Image courtesy Sopa Chevacharoenkul, Microelectronics Center of North Carolina.)

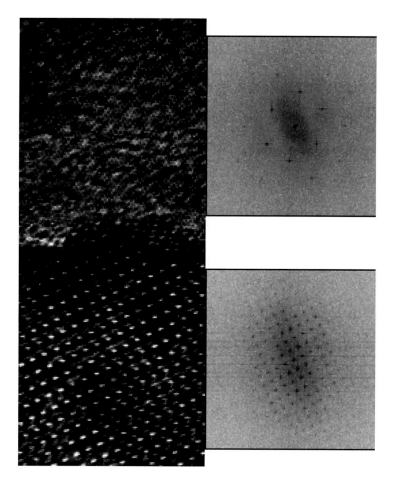

Figure 21. High-resolution TEM image of two adjacent grains in mullite (left), with their frequency transforms (right). (Image courtesy Sopa Chevacharoenkul, Microelectronics Center of North Carolina.)

of the bright spots represents the atomic structure of the lattice. Measuring all of the individual spacings of the spots would be very time-consuming and not particularly accurate. The frequency-domain representation of this image shows the periodicity clearly. The series of peaks indicates that the variation of brightness is not a simple sine wave, but contains many higher harmonics. The first-order peak gives the basic atomic spacing (and orientation), which can be measured by interpolating the peak position to a fraction of a pixel width, corresponding to an accuracy for the atom spacing of a few parts in ten thousand.

To the electron microscopist, the power spectrum image of the frequency-domain transform looks just like an electron diffraction pattern, which in fact it is. The use of microscope optics to form the diffraction pattern is an analog method of computing the frequency-domain representation. This can be done with any image by setting up suitable optics. While it is a fast way to obtain the frequency-domain representation, this method has two serious drawbacks for use in image processing.

First, the phase information is lost when the diffraction pattern is recorded, so it is not possible to reconstruct the spatial-domain image from a photograph of the diffraction pattern. It is possible to perform the reconstruction from the actual pattern by using suitable lenses (indeed, that is what happens in the microscope), so in principle it is possible to insert the various masks and filters discussed below. However, making these masks and filters is difficult and exacting work that must usually be performed individually for each image to be enhanced. Consequently, it is much easier (and more controllable) to use a computer to perform the transform and to apply any desired masks.

It is also easier to perform measurements on the frequency-domain representation using the computer. Locating the centers of peaks by curve fitting would require recording the diffraction pattern (typically with film, which may introduce nonlinearities or saturation over the extremely wide dynamic range of many patterns), followed by digitization to obtain numerical values. Considering the speed with which a spatial-domain image can be recorded, the frequency transform calculated, and interactive or automatic measurement performed, the computer is generally the tool of choice.

Figure 21 shows an electron microscope image of two adjacent grains in a ceramic (mullite) structure. The calculated diffraction patterns from each region can be analyzed to determine the orientation difference between the grains. This analysis is made easier by the ability to adjust the display contrast so that both brighter and dimmer spots can be seen. Contrast adjustments can be made with much more flexibility than photographic film recording of the patterns can afford.

When spots from a periodic structure are superimposed on a general background, the total power in the spots expressed as a fraction of the total power in the entire frequency transform gives a useful quantitative measure of the degree of periodicity in the structure. This may also be used to compare different periodicities (different spacings or orientations) by comparing summations of values in the power spectrum. For electron diffraction patterns, this is a function of the atomic density of various planes and the atomic scattering cross sections.

While the display of the power spectrum corresponds to a diffraction pattern and is the most familiar presentation of frequency-space information, it must not be forgotten that the phase information is also needed to reconstruct the original image. **Figure 22** shows a test image, consisting of a regular pattern of spots, and its corresponding power spectrum. If the phase information is erased (all phases set to zero), the reconstruction (**Figure 23**) shows some of the same periodicity, but the objects are no longer recognizable. The various sine waves have been shifted in phase, so that the feature boundaries are not reconstructed.

The assumption that the image is one repetition of an endless sequence is also important. Most real images do not have perfectly

Figure 22. *Test image consisting of a regular pattern and its frequency transform power spectrum.*

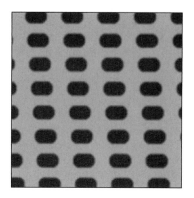 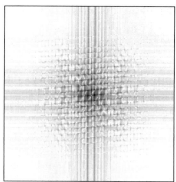

matching left and right or top and bottom edges. This produces a large step function at the edge, which would be more apparent if the image were shifted by an arbitrary offset (**Figure 24**). As in the ramp example shown earlier, this does not alter the power spectrum image, although the phase image is shifted. The discontinuity requires high-frequency terms to fit, and since the edges are precisely horizontal and vertical, the power spectrum display shows a central cross superimposed on the rest of the data. For the test pattern of **Figure 22**, the result of eliminating these lines from the original frequency transform and then retransforming is shown in **Figure 25**. The central portion of the image is unaffected, but at the edges the discontinuity is no longer fit. The pattern from each side has been reproduced on the other side of the boundary, superimposed on the correct data.

Preferred orientation

Figure 26 shows another example of a periodic structure, only much less perfect and larger in scale than the lattice images above. The specimen is a thin film of magnetic material viewed in polarized light. The stripes are oppositely oriented magnetic domains in the material that are used to store information in the film. The frequency transform of this image clearly shows the width and spacing of the domains. Instead of a single peak, there are arcs that show the variation in orientation of the stripes, which is evident in the original image but difficult to quantify.

The length of the arcs and the variation of brightness (power) with angle along them can be easily measured to characterize the preferred orientation in the structure. Even for structures that are not perfectly periodic, the integrated power as a function of angle can be used to measure the preferred orientation. This is identical to the results of autocorrelation operations carried out in the spatial domain, in which an image is shifted and combined with itself in all possible displacements to obtain a matrix of fractional values, but it is much faster to perform with the frequency-domain representation. Also, this makes it easier to deal with grey scale values.

Reconstructing periodic structures that are not perfectly aligned can be performed by selecting the entire arc in the frequency

Figure 23. *Retransformation of Figure 22 with all phase information set to zero.*

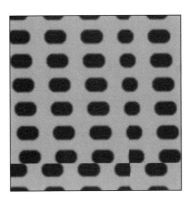

Figure 24. *The test image of Figure 22 with an arbitrary spatial shift, showing the discontinuities at the image boundaries*

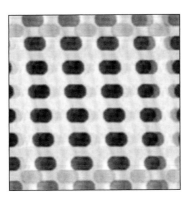

Figure 25. *Retransformation of Figure 22 with the central cross (horizontal and vertical lines) reduced to zero magnitude, so that the left and right edges of the image, and the top and bottom edges, are forced to match.*

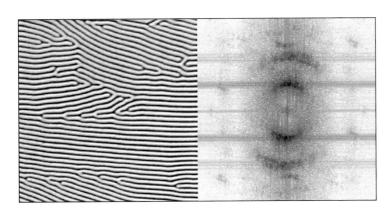

Figure 26. *Polarized light image of magnetic domains in thin film material (left), with the frequency transform (right).*

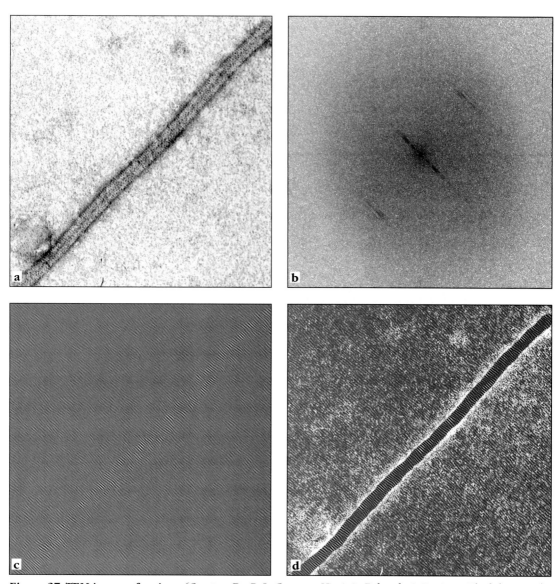

Figure 27. TEM image of a virus *(Courtesy Dr. R. L. Grayson, Virginia Polytechnic Institute, Blacksburg, VA):*
a) original image, in which the internal helical structure is difficult to discern;
b) frequency transform of image a, in which the regular repeating structure of the virus and its angular variation in orientation is evident;
c) retransformation of just the peaks in the frequency transform, in which the periodic lines are not limited to the virus;
d) using the virus particle as a mask, the helical pattern becomes evident.

transform. **Figure 27** illustrates this with a virus particle. The TEM image hints at the internal helical structure, but does not show it clearly. In the frequency transform, the periodic spacing and the variation in direction is evident. The spacing can be measured (2.41 nm) and the helix angle determined from the length of the arc. Retransforming only these arcs shows the periodicity but this is not limited spatially to the virus particle. Using the spatial-domain image as a mask (as discussed in Chapter 7) makes the helical pattern evident.

One particular type of preferred orientation in images, which arises not from the specimen but rather from the imaging system

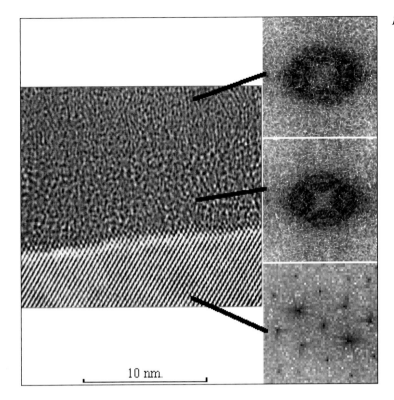

itself, is astigmatism. This is a particular problem with electron microscopes because of the operating principles of electromagnetic lenses. Even skilled operators devote considerable time to making adjustments to minimize astigmatism, and it is often very difficult to recognize it in images in order to correct it. Astigmatism results in the defocusing of the image and a consequent loss of sharpness in one direction, sometimes with an improvement in the perpendicular direction. This becomes immediately evident in the frequency transform, since the decrease in brightness or power falls off radially (at higher frequencies) and the asymmetry can be noted.

Figure 28 shows an example. The specimen is a cross section with three layers. The bottom is crystalline silicon, above which is a layer of amorphous (noncrystalline) silicon, followed by a layer of glue used to mount the sample for thinning and microscopy. The glue is difficult to distinguish by eye from the amorphous silicon. Frequency transforms for the three regions are shown. The bright spots in the pattern from the crystalline silicon give the expected diffraction pattern. While the two regions above do not show individual peaks from periodic structures, they are not the same. The amorphous silicon has short-range order in the atomic spacings based on strong covalent bonding that is not visible to the human observer because of its chaotic overall pattern. This shows up in the frequency transform as a white cross in the dark ring, indicating that in the 45-degree

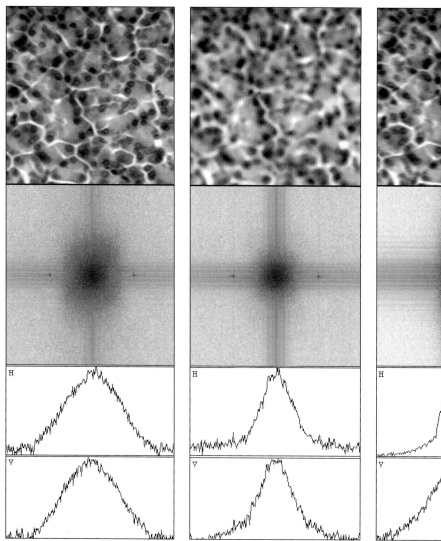

Figure 29. *Out-of-focus image with its power spectrum and horizontal and vertical line profiles, showing presence of high-frequency information as compared to Figure 30.*

Figure 30. *Out-of-focus image with its power spectrum and horizontal and vertical line profiles, showing loss of high-frequency information as compared to Figure 29.*

Figure 31. *Astigmatic image produced by misaligning lens, with its power spectrum and horizontal and vertical line profiles showing different high-frequency components.*

directions there is a characteristic distance and direction to the next atom. This pattern is absent in the glue region, where there is no such structure.

In both regions, the dark circular pattern from the amorphous structure is not a perfect circle, but an ellipse. This indicates astigmatism. Adjusting the microscope optics to produce a uniform circle will correct the astigmatism and provide uniform resolution in all directions in the original image. It is much easier to observe the effects of small changes in the frequency-space display than in the spatial-domain image.

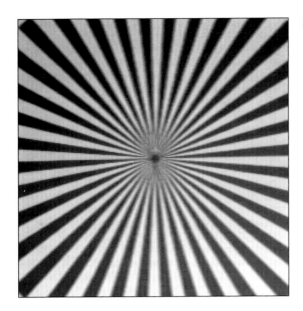

Figure 32. *Test pattern image.*

The frequency transform of an image can be used to optimize focus and astigmatism. When an image is in focus, the high-frequency information is maximized in order to sharply define the edges. This provides a convenient test for sharpest focus. **Figure 29** shows a light microscope image that is in focus. The line profiles of the power spectrum in both the vertical and horizontal directions show a more gradual dropoff at high frequencies than **Figure 30**, which is the same image out of focus. When astigmatism is present (**Figure 31**), the power spectrum is asymmetric, as shown by the profiles.

Figure 32 shows a test pattern of radial lines. Due to the finite spacing of detectors in the video camera used, as well as limitations in electronics bandwidth that eliminate the very high frequencies required to resolve small details, these lines are incompletely resolved where they are close together. **Figure 33** shows the two-dimensional Fourier transform power spectrum of this image, plotted isometrically to emphasize the magnitude values. The low-frequency information is at the center and the frequencies increase radially. This is the usual presentation of the magnitude information, plotted as log (magnitude^2) and ignoring the phase. **Figure 34** shows the complete set of data, using color. One image shows the real and imaginary components of the transform and the other the magnitude and phase, encoded in different color planes. While technically complete, these displays are rarely used because the randomness of much of the phase information is simply confusing to the viewer.

In the grey scale power spectrum, it is evident that there is a well-defined boundary, different in the x and y directions, beyond which the magnitude drops abruptly. This corresponds to the spacing of the individual detectors in the camera, which is

Figure 33. *Frequency transform of image in Figure 32, presented as an isometric view.*

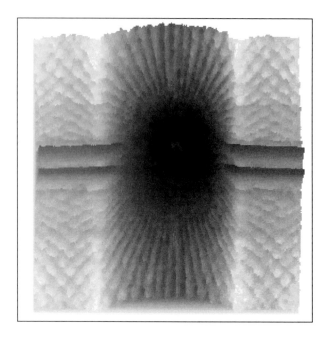

different in the horizontal and vertical directions. In many cases, it is not so obvious where the physical source of resolution limitation lies. However, the Fourier transform power spectrum will still show the limit, permitting the resolution of any imaging system to be ascertained.

Texture and fractals

Besides the peaks in the power spectrum resulting from periodic structures that may be present and the ultimate limitation at high

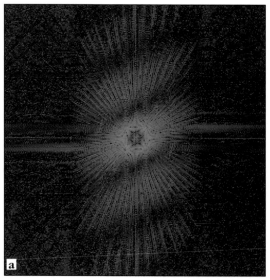

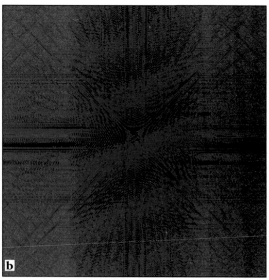

Figure 34. Color representations of the FT power spectrum from Figure 32:
a) *YUV image in which U=Real,V=Imaginary;*
b) *RGB image in which Red=Magnitude, Blue=Phase.*

frequencies due to finite image resolution, it may seem as though there is only a noisy background containing little useful information. This is far from true. Many images represent the brightness of light scattered from surfaces, or other data such as surface elevation. In these images, the roughness or texture of the surface is revealed and may be measured from the power spectrum.

The concept of a fractal surface dimension will not be explained here in detail, but is discussed in Chapter 11. Surfaces that are fractal have an area that is mathematically undefined. It is greater than the projected area covered by the irregular surface and increases as the measurement scale becomes finer. The fractal dimension is the slope of a line on a log-log plot of measured area vs. the size of the measuring tool. Many naturally occurring surfaces resulting from wear, erosion, agglomeration of particles, or fracture are observed to have this character. It has also been shown that images of these surfaces, whether produced by the scattering of diffuse light or the production of secondary electrons in an SEM, are also fractal. That is, the variation of brightness with position obeys the same mathematical relationship. The fractal dimension is an extremely powerful and compact representation of the surface roughness, which can often be related to the history of the surface and the properties that result.

Measuring surface fractals directly is rarely practical. The most common approach is to reduce the dimensionality and measure the fractal dimension of a boundary line produced by intersecting the surface with a sampling plane. This may either be produced by cross sectioning or by polishing down into the surface to produce islands. In either case, the rougher the surface, the more irregular the line. This line also has a fractal dimension (the slope of a log-log plot relating the measured line length and the length of the measurement tool), which is just 1.0 less than that of the surface.

A closely related approach to measuring the fractal dimension of a line is the Hurst coefficient (also known as the rescaled range). First applied to time-series data, it plots the maximum difference between any two points in the sequence as a function of the temporal difference. The slope on a log-log scale is the coefficient K. If the values are elevation values along a traverse across a physical surface, then the fractal dimension is just $F = 2 - K$.

For many images, it is easy to perform this determination along a single line profile across the image. However, it is difficult to obtain a meaningful average value for the entire surface or to study systematically the variation in roughness with orientation that is often present, depending on the history of the surface.

Earlier figures showed the linear addition of frequency terms to construct a square or sawtooth wave. For a fractal profile, we expect that terms of increasingly higher frequency will continue to contribute to the summation, since by definition a fractal curve

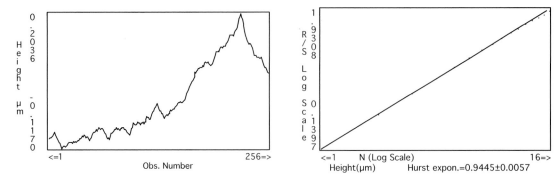

Figure 35. *A one-dimensional computer-generated line (left) with the rescaled range plot showing its Hurst coefficient (right).*

is self-similar and has detail extending to ever-finer scales (or higher frequencies). This also implies that the proportion of amplitudes of higher frequency terms must be self-similar. An exponential curve satisfies this criterion. The magnitudes of the coefficients in a Fourier transform of a fractal curve decrease exponentially with the log of frequency, while the phases of the terms are randomized.

Figure 35 shows a computer-generated fractal line and its rescaled range plot, whose slope gives the Hurst coefficient. The plot of Fourier magnitudes shown in **Figure 36** shows the expected exponential decrease. **Figure 37** shows a plot correlating the slope observed in the Fourier magnitude plot with the Hurst coefficient of ten such lines. This implies that there is a simple relationship between the fractal dimension of a profile and the exponential decrease in magnitude of the terms in a Fourier expansion, as indeed had been predicted by Feder (1989). This correlation makes it practical to use the radial decrease of magnitude in a two-dimensional Fourier-transform

Figure 36. *Log-log plot of FFT magnitude vs. frequency for the line in Figure 34.*

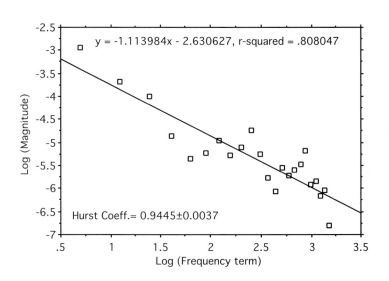

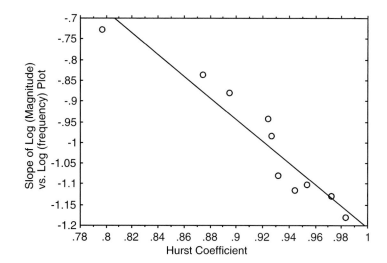

Figure 37. *Correlation between slope of the plot of log magnitude vs. log frequency curves for the frequency transform, and Hurst coefficient, for ten generated test lines.*

image as a measure of roughness and the directional variation of that decrease as a measure of orientation (Mitchell & Bonnell, 1990; Russ, 1990; Russ, 1994).

Measuring the two-dimensional Fourier transform is more efficient than measuring and averaging Hurst coefficients along many individual brightness profiles in the original image. It also allows any periodic structures that may be present to be ignored, since these show up as discrete points in the frequency-transform image and can be skipped in determining the overall exponential decrease in the magnitude values. In other words, it is possible to look beyond the periodic structures or noise (e.g., arising from electronic components) in the images and still characterize the underlying chaotic nature of the surface.

Figure 38 shows an image of surface elevation as measured with a scanning tunneling microscope (STM). The sample is a machined metal surface with a more-or-less periodic grooved structure that reflects the motion of the tool across the material. Individual line profiles of the brightness (elevation) values in the image can be fit to determine a Hurst coefficient, as long as the bright points (atoms) are avoided. However, these are only samples of the surface; we would like to characterize the average roughness and its directional variation.

Figure 39 shows the two-dimensional Fourier transform of this image. The power spectrum image is shown with a logarithmic intensity scale, so we expect to find a linear decrease in brightness with the log of radius (frequency). **Figure 40** shows a rose plot of the slope of the log magnitude vs. log frequency relationship as a function of direction. The anisotropy of the surface is evident. These values are being studied as an indicator of the fractal characteristics of the machined surface, and correlated with variables such as material properties, cutting conditions, and so forth.

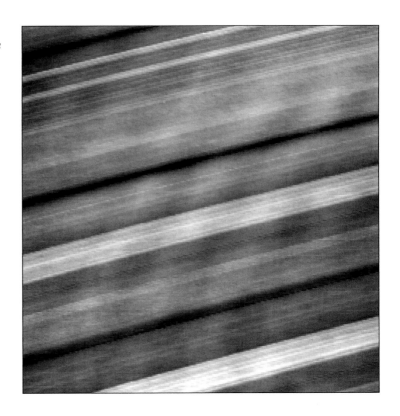

Figure 38. Atomic force microscope (AFM) image of a machined surface of nickel.

Filtering images

Isolating periodic noise

Figure 41 shows two spatial-domain features having grey scales that together would add up to the same rectangular step function shown in **Figure 13**. The power spectrum displays of these two images are shown along with their sum (**Figure 42**). The sum is identical to that shown in **Figure 13** for the original rectangle. In other words, the frequency transform has a property of separability and additivity. Adding together the transforms of two original images or functions produces the same result as the transform of the sum of the originals.

This idea opens the way to using subtraction to remove unwanted parts of images. It is most commonly used to remove periodic noise, which can be introduced by the devices used to record or transmit images. We will see some examples below. If the image of the noise or its Fourier transform can be determined, then subtracting the transform from that of the noisy image will leave only the desired part of the information. This can then be transformed back to the spatial domain (usually described as the inverse transform) to produce a noise-free image.

Figures 32 and **33** showed a resolution test pattern (as digitized by a video camera) and its two-dimensional Fourier transform power spectrum. If a circle is used to limit the portion of the power spectrum to the center (low frequencies less than

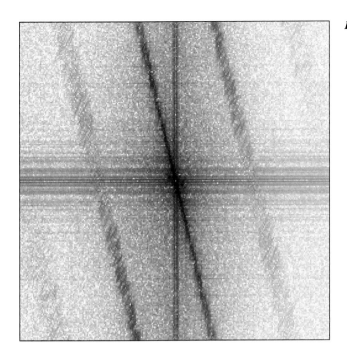

Figure 39. The Fourier transform power spectrum of Figure 38.

9 pixels^{-1}), then the reconstruction shows the coarse spacings in the original, as shown in **Figure 43**, but it does not show the central portion of the original pattern, where the spacings are smaller and higher-frequency information is present. Conversely, reconstructing the portion of the power spectrum outside the same circle shows only the high-frequency portion of the origi-

FFT plot
Mean D = 1.196
Ratio = 0.688

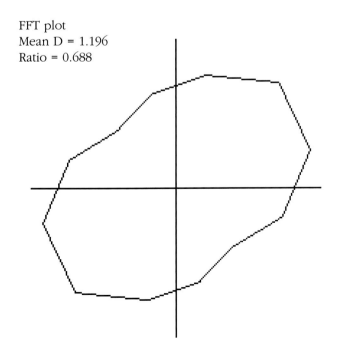

Figure 40. A rose plot of the slope of the log magnitude vs. log frequency relationship as a function of direction. The mean fractal dimension is 1.196, with considerable anisotropy.

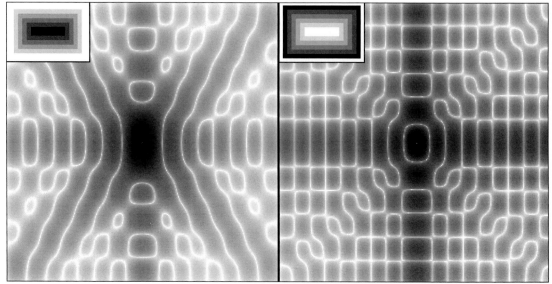

Figure 41. Stepped (grey scale) rectangles (insets) and their frequency transforms.

Figure 42. The sum of the two rectangles in Figure 41 (a black and white rectangle, inset) and the sum of the individual frequency transforms.

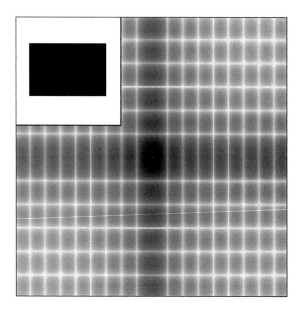

nal image (**Figure 43**). This consists of the central portion of the original pattern and the edges of the wider portions of the lines.

In this illustration of filtering, portions of the Fourier-transform image were selected based on frequency, which is why these filters are generally called low-pass and high-pass filters. Usually, selecting arbitrary regions of the frequency domain for reconstruction produces artefacts, unless some care is taken to shape the edges of the filter region to attenuate the data smoothly. This can be seen in the one-dimensional example of the step function in **Figure 1**. If only the first few terms are used then, in addition to not modeling the steepness of the step, the reconstruc-

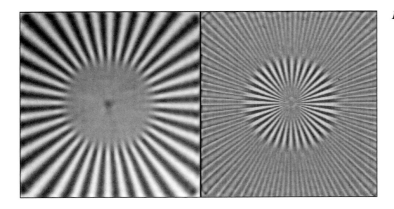

Figure 43. Reconstructions of the image in Figure 32 through low-pass (left) and high-pass (right) filters.

tion has oscillations near the edge, which are generally described as ringing.

It is necessary to shape the edge of the filter to prevent ringing at sharp discontinuities. This behavior is well-known in one-dimensional filtering (used in digital signal processing, for example). Several different shapes are commonly used. Over a specified width (usually given in pixels, but of course ultimately specified in terms of frequency or direction), the filter magnitude can be reduced from maximum to minimum using a weighting function. The simplest function is linear interpolation (also called a Parzen window function). Better results can be obtained using a parabolic or cosine function (also called Welch and Hanning window functions, respectively, in this context). The most elaborate filter shapes do not drop to the zero or minimum value, but extend a very long tail beyond the cutoff point. One such shape is a Gaussian. **Figure 44** shows several of these shapes. In **Figure 43**, a cosine cutoff 6 pixels wide was used.

Another filter shape often used in these applications is a Butterworth filter, whose magnitude can be written as

$$H = 1 \ / \ [1 + C \cdot (R/R_0)^{2n}] \tag{8}$$

where R is the distance from the center of the filter (usually the center of the frequency transform image, or zero-frequency point), and R_0 is the nominal filter cutoff value. The constant C is often set equal to 1.0 or to 0.414; the value defines the magnitude of the filter at the point where $R=R_0$ as either 50% or $1/\sqrt{2}$. The integer n is the order of the filter; its most common value is 1. **Figure 45** shows comparison profiles of several Butterworth low-pass filters (ones that attenuate high frequencies). The converse shape having negative values of n passes high frequencies and attenuates low ones.

To illustrate the effects of these filters on ringing at edges, **Figure 46** shows a simple test shape and its two-dimensional FFT power spectrum image. The orientation of principal terms perpendicular to the major edges in the spatial-domain image is

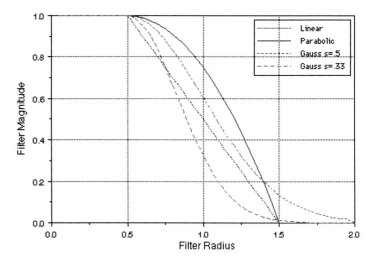

Figure 44. Some common filter edge profiles.

evident. Performing a reconstruction using a simple aperture with a radius equal to 25 pixels (called an ideal filter) produces the result shown in **Figure 47a**. The oscillations in brightness near the edges are quite visible.

Ringing can be reduced by shaping the edge of the filter, as discussed above. The magnitudes of frequency terms near the cutoff value are multiplied by factors less than one, whose values are based on a simple function. If a cosine function is used, which varies from 1 to 0 over a total width of 6 pixels, the result is improved (**Figure 47b**). In this example, the original 25-pixel radius used for the ideal filter (the sharp cutoff) is the point at which the magnitude of the weighting factor drops to 50%. The weights drop smoothly from 1.0 at a radius of 22 pixels to 0.0 at a radius of 28 pixels.

Increasing the distance over which the transition takes place further reduces the ringing, as shown in **Figure 47c**. Here, the 50% point is still at 25 pixels but the range is from 15 to 35 pixels.

Figure 45. Shapes for Butterworth filter profiles of order 1, 2, and 3.

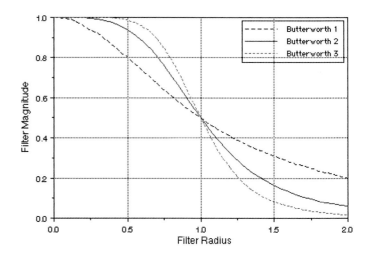

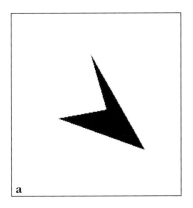

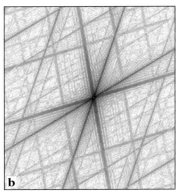

Note that the improvement is not achieved simply by increasing the high-frequency limit, which would improve the sharpness of the feature edges but would not by itself reduce the ringing. **Figure 47d** shows the same reconstruction using a second-degree Butterworth filter shape whose 50% point is set at 25 pixels.

Figure 48 shows an image with both fine detail and some noise along with its frequency transform. Applying Butterworth low-pass filters with radii of 10 and 25 pixels in the frequency-domain image smooths the noise with some blurring of the high-frequency detail (**Figure 49**), while the application of Butterworth high-pass filters with the same radii emphasizes the edges and reduces the contrast in the large (low-frequency) regions (**Figure 50**). All of these filters were applied as multiplicative masks.

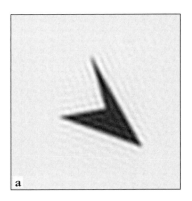

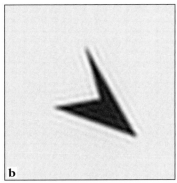

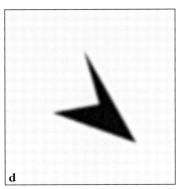

Figure 47. Reconstruction of shape from its frequency transform in Figure 46, using an aperture (mask or filter) diameter:
a) ideal filter in which the cutoff at 25 pixels is exact and abrupt;
b) cosine-weighted edge shape in which the 50% radius is 25 pixels with a half-width of 3 pixels;
c) cosine-weighted edge shape in which the 50% radius is 25 pixels with a half-width of 10 pixels;
d) Butterworth second-degree shape with a 50% radius of 25 pixels.

Figure 48. *Image and its transform used for filtering in Figures 49 and 50.*

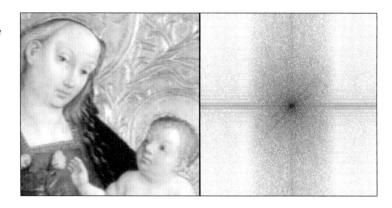

Figure 49. *Filtering of Figure 48 with low-pass Butterworth filters having 50% cutoff diameters of 10 (left) and 25 pixels (right).*

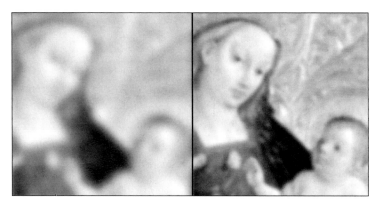

Figure 50. *Filtering of Figure 48 with high-pass Butterworth filters having 50% cutoff diameters of 10 (left) and 25 pixels (right).*

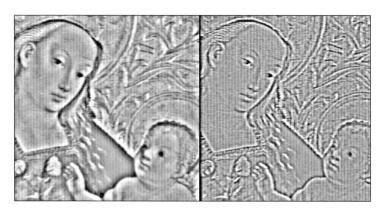

Of course, it is not necessary for the variation in magnitude to be from 1 to 0. Sometimes the lower limit is set to a fraction, so that the high (or low) frequencies are not completely attenuated. It is also possible to use values greater than 1. A high-frequency emphasis filter with the low-frequency value set to a reduced value, such as 0.5, and a high-frequency value greater than 1, such as 2, is called a homomorphic filter. It is usually applied to an image whose brightness values have previously been converted to their logarithms (using a LUT). This filtering operation will simultaneously increase the high-frequency information (sharpening edges) while reducing the overall brightness range

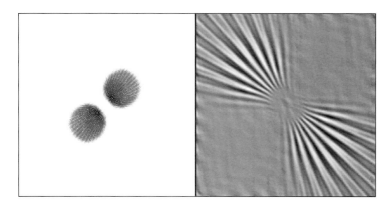

Figure 51. *Retransformation of Figure 32 (right) through a filter centered at a nonzero frequency and direction (left).*

to allow edge brightness values to show. The physical reasoning behind the homomorphic filter is a separation of illumination and reflectance components in the image. As with most of these filters, though, the real justification is that it improves the appearance of many images of practical interest.

It is also possible to select a region of the Fourier transform image that is not symmetrical. **Figure 51** shows a selection of intermediate frequency values lying in a particular direction on the transform in **Figure 33**, along with the resulting reconstruction. This kind of filtering may be useful to select directional information from images. It also demonstrates the basic characteristic of Fourier transform images: locations in the Fourier transform image identify periodicity and orientation information from any or all parts of the spatial-domain image.

Masks and filters

Once the location of periodic noise in an original image is isolated into a single point in the Fourier-transform image, it becomes possible to remove it. A filter removes selected frequencies and orientations by reducing the magnitude values for those terms, either partially or to zero, while leaving the phase information alone (which is important in determining where in the image that information appears).

There are many different ways to specify and to apply this reduction. Sometimes it is practical to specify a range of frequencies and orientations numerically, but most often it will be convenient to do so directly, using the magnitude or power spectrum display of the Fourier transform image. Drawing circular or pie-shaped regions on this display allows specific peaks in the power spectrum, corresponding to the periodic information, to be selected.

Properly, the regions should be shaped either as circles symmetrically centered on the origin (zero frequency point) or as pie-shaped regions of annuli bounded on the inside and outside by concentric circles whose radii specify frequencies and bounded on the other two sides by radial lines specifying direc-

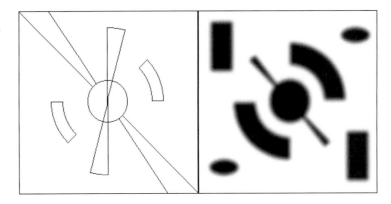

Figure 52. *Illustration of circular, annular, and wedge filter shapes (left) and edge shaping of similar regions (right).*

tions. **Figure 52** illustrates several such wedges; note their symmetry about the origin. In practice, it is often more convenient to draw arbitrary shapes such as circles or rectangles to select the regions of the Fourier transform to be filtered. Such arbitrary choices usually require eliminating a bit more of the original image information than the purely periodic noise. Except in those few cases in which the important information is very close in frequency and orientation to the noise, however, nothing of importance in the original image is lost.

More important is the use of a smoothing function to ease the transition in magnitudes from outside the filtered region to inside. Instead of an abrupt cutoff, a variety of transition functions ranging from simple linear interpolation to cosine curves, Gaussian curves, etc. may be used, as mentioned before. When the transition takes place over a distance of only a few pixels, the differences between these transition curves are of little importance.

It can be difficult to calculate the reduction of magnitude in the transition edge zone of a filter region if the region is complex in shape, making it simpler to apply circular or rectangular filter regions. However, if the filter is considered as another image containing a mask of values to be multiplied by the original magnitude component of the Fourier transform (leaving the phase information untouched), then it becomes possible to modify the edges of the region using standard image processing tools, such as smoothing (Chapter 3), constructing a Euclidean distance map (Chapter 7), or manipulating the values with a nonlinear LUT (Chapter 4). **Figure 52** shows several regions of different shapes which have had their edge values reduced in this way. Multiplying this image (scaled to the range 0 to 1) by the original Fourier transform magnitude, followed with retransformation, will remove any periodic information with the selected frequency and direction.

Usually, it is only by first examining the transform-image power spectrum that the presence and exact location of these points can be determined. **Figure 53** shows an image of a halftone print from a magazine. The pattern results from the halftone

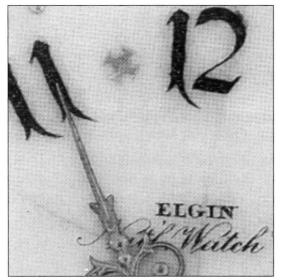
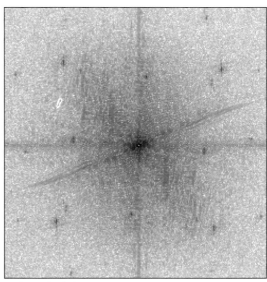

Figure 53. *A halftone image (left) and its frequency transform (right).*

screen used in the printing process. In the frequency transform of the image, this regular pattern shows up as well-defined narrow peaks or spikes. Filtering removes the peaks by setting the magnitude at those locations to zero (but not altering any of the phase information). This allows the image to be retransformed without the noise. The filtered Fourier transform image power spectrum shown in **Figure 54** shows the circular white spots where filtering was performed.

It is interesting to note that image compression does not necessarily remove these noise spikes in the Fourier transform. Com-

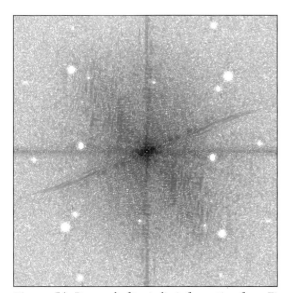
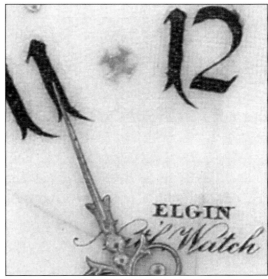

Figure 54. *Removal of periodic information from Figure 53 by reducing the magnitude (left) and retransforming (right).*

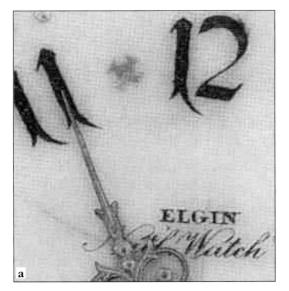

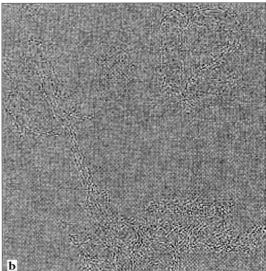

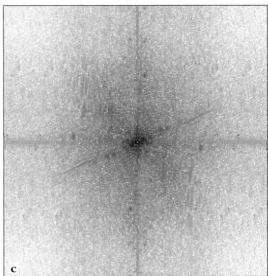

Figure 55. Clock image (from Figure 53)
a) after JPEG compression (from 67K to 5K);
b) differences from the original image;
*c) FT power spectrum of image **a**, showing the spikes due to periodic noise.*

pression is generally based on discarding the terms in the transform (Fourier, Cosine, etc.) whose magnitudes are small. The halftone pattern is interpreted as an important feature of the image by these compression methods. **Figure 55** shows the same image after it has been compressed and restored using the JPEG method discussed in Chapter 2, its transform, and the difference between the original image and the compressed version. The need to preserve the periodic noise spikes actually reduces the amount of other useful detail that can be retained.

The effects of compression are best examined in the frequency transform. **Figure 56** shows a portion of the image of Saturn used in Chapter 4, before and after compression by the JPEG algorithm. Some differences, particularly in the rings, can be seen. The frequency transforms of the two images show that this is due

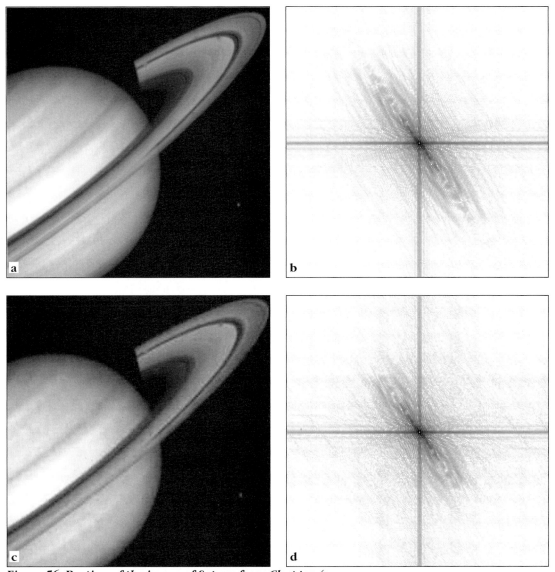

Figure 56. Portion of the image of Saturn from Chapter 4:
a) original;
b) FT power spectrum showing high frequencies needed for detail in rings;
c) image after maximum JPEG compression (from 60K to 5K);
d) FT power spectrum of *c* showing loss of high frequency information.

to the loss of lines of high frequency information that are needed to define the profiles of the rings and the detail within them.

Figure 57 shows another example, this time a light microscope image that was also digitized from a printed brochure with halftone noise. The filtering and retransformation shown in **Figure 58** shows the use of notch filters, which remove large rectangular (or ideally, pie-shaped) regions of the power spectrum to clean up the noise. The same notch filter is also applied in some cases to *keep* only a narrow range of frequencies or

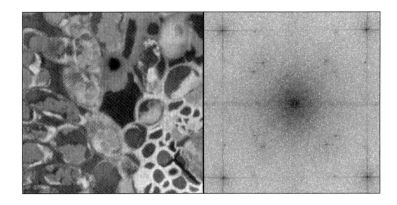

Figure 57. A digitized microscope image (left) and its frequency transform (right).

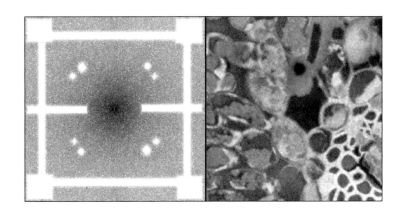

Figure 58. Application of filters to Figure 57 (left) and retransformation (right).

Figure 59. Removal of periodic transmission noise from a reconnaissance photo (left: original; right: filtered).

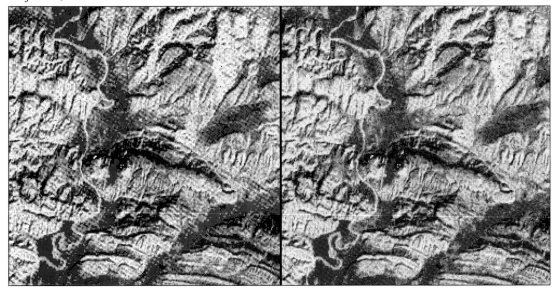

directions, rather than eliminate them. Discussed below, this simply requires the filter mask values to be inverted before multiplying. **Figure 59** illustrates the same removal of periodic noise from a reconnaissance photograph, in which the interference is due to electronic noise from transmission or recording. The principles are identical for macroscopic or microscopic images.

The preceding examples relied on human observation of the peaks in the Fourier transform image, recognition that the peaks were responsible for the periodic noise, and outlining them to produce the filter. In some cases, it is possible to construct an appropriate image filter automatically from the Fourier transform power spectrum. The guiding principle is that peaks in the power spectrum that are narrow and rise significantly above the local background should be removed. If the Fourier transform magnitude image is treated like an ordinary spatial-domain grey scale image, this peak removal is easily accomplished using a rank filter.

The rank filter replaces each pixel value with the minimum (or maximum) value found anywhere within some small defined region, such as a 5×5 or 7×7 square or an octagon (approximating a circle). It will not change values in uniform or gradually varying regions, but will effectively erase any large variations that are smaller than the radius of the neighborhood. Since many Fourier transform magnitude images are rather grainy, particularly at high frequencies, the direct application of a rank filter to the magnitude image may cause other artefacts to appear in the image. Consequently, it is more common to construct a mask by copying the magnitude image, performing some smoothing to reduce the graininess, and then using a rank filter. The difference between the original smoothed image and the rank-filtered one should contain just the peaks. The inverse of this difference image can be used as a multiplicative mask to completely remove the peaks due to periodic noise.

This sequence is demonstrated in **Figure 60** for the same image as in **Figures 53** and **54**. A region of halftone periodic noise is selected and tiled (repeated in horizontal and vertical directions) to fill the entire image area. The transform of this image is then processed using a maximum rank filter of size 9×9 (octagonal) to produce the mask shown in **Figure 60**, in which the peaks due to periodicity are clearly delineated. By tiling the image fragment, the phase information from the position of the periodic structure is correctly preserved. The inverse of this mask is then multiplied by the frequency transform of the original image to produce the filtered result.

The example in **Figure 61** shows an example of an image scanned in from a newspaper; the halftone dots are very evident. The dark spots ("spikes") in the power spectrum (**Figure 61b**) correspond to the periodic structure in the image. They align with the repetitive pattern of dots, and their darkness indicates how much of various frequencies are present. Removing them is

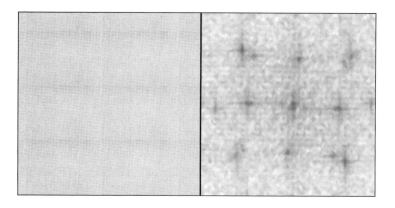

Figure 60. *Construction of a mask from the frequency transform of a tiled noise region. Left: repeated tiling of one section of noise in the original image; right: transform after rank filtering.*

equivalent to removing the periodic component. In this case a top hat filter was used to locate the spikes and create a mask (**Figure 61c**). The result of applying this mask as a filter to remove the spikes shows that the periodic noise has been removed without affecting any of the other information present (**Figure 61d**). There is still some pixel-to-pixel noise because the image has been scanned at a higher magnification than it was printed.

An additional filter can be employed to remove the remaining pixel noise. A Butterworth second-order high-frequency cut-off filter keeps low frequencies (gradual variations in grey scale) while progressively cutting off higher ones (the more rapid variations associated with pixel noise). In this case the mid-point of the cutoff was set to the spacing of the half-tone dots in the original image (**Figure 61e**). The final version of the power spectrum (**Figure 61f**) shows the periodic spots removed and the high frequencies attenuated. An inverse transform produces the final image (**Figure 61g**). Note that even the cat's whiskers which are barely discernible in the original image can be clearly seen. The use of a smoothing or blur function would have erased these fine lines long before the halftone dots were smoothed out.

Selection of periodic information

In some types of images, it is the periodic information that is useful and the nonperiodic noise that must be suppressed. The methods for locating the periodic peaks, constructing filters, smoothing the filter edges, and so forth are unchanged. The only difference is that the filter sense is changed and in the case of a multiplicative mask, the values are inverted.

Figure 62 shows a one-dimensional example. The image is a light micrograph of stained skeletal muscle, in which there is a just-visible band spacing that is difficult to measure because of the spotty staining contrast (even with contrast expansion). The FT image shows the spots that identify the band structure. Reconstruction with only the first harmonic shows the basic band structure, and adding the second and third harmonics defines the band shape fairly well.

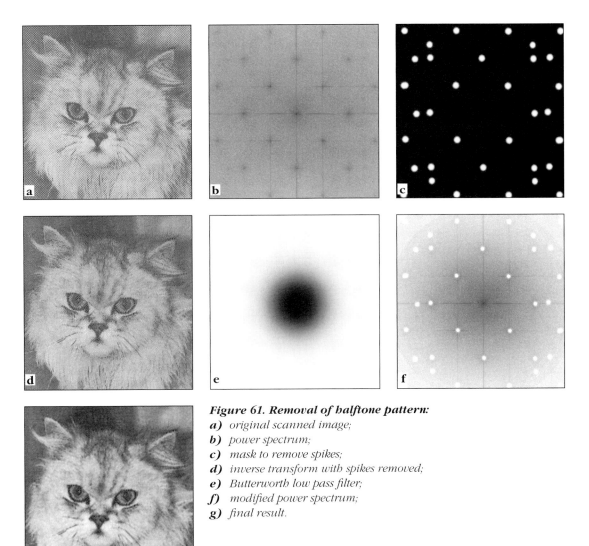

Figure 61. Removal of halftone pattern:
a) original scanned image;
b) power spectrum;
c) mask to remove spikes;
d) inverse transform with spikes removed;
e) Butterworth low pass filter;
f) modified power spectrum;
g) final result.

Figure 63 shows a high-resolution TEM lattice image from a crystalline ceramic (mullite). The periodicity of the lattice can be seen, but it is superimposed on a variable and noisy background that results from local variations in the thickness of the sample. This background alters the local contrast, making it more difficult to observe the details in the rather complex unit cell of this material. The figure shows the Fourier transform image, in which the peaks corresponding to the periodic structure can be seen. As noted before, this image is essentially the same as would be recorded photographically using the TEM to project the diffraction pattern of the specimen to the camera plane. Of course, retransforming the spatial-domain image from the photographed diffraction pattern is not possible because the phase information has been lost. In addition, more control over the Fourier trans-

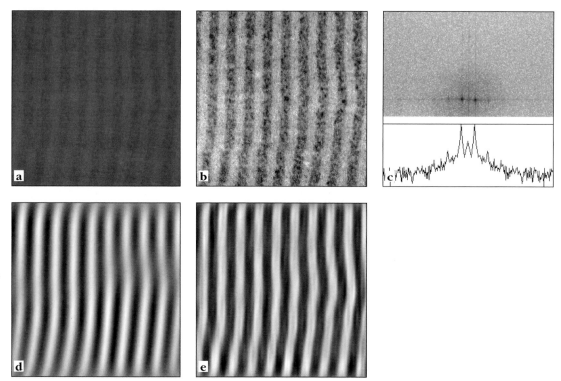

Figure 62. Light micrograph of stained (toluidine blue)1μm section of skeletal muscle. a) *original image;* *b)* *expanded contrast (the band spacing is still difficult to measure due to spotty stain contrast);* *c)* *the FT power spectrum shows spots that identify the band spacing;* *d)* *reconstruction with just the first harmonic shows the basic band structure;* *e)* *adding the 2nd and 3rd harmonics defines the band shape well.*

form display is possible because a log scale or other rule for converting magnitude to screen brightness can be selected.

A filter mask is constructed in **Figure 64** to select a circular region around each of the periodic spots. Multiplying this region by the magnitude values reduces them to zero everywhere else. Retransforming this image produces the spatial-domain image shown. Filtering has removed all of the nonperiodic noise, both the short-range (high-frequency) graininess and the gradual (low-frequency) variation in overall brightness. The resulting image shows the lattice structure clearly.

Figure 65 shows an even more dramatic example. In the original image (a cross section of muscle myofibrils) it is practically impossible to discern the periodic structure due to the presence of noise. There are isolated locations where a few of the fibrils can be seen to have a regular spacing and arrangement, but human observers do not easily see through the noise and variability to find this regularity. The Fourier transform image shows the peaks from the underlying regularity, however. Selecting only these peak points in the magnitude image (with their original phase information) and reducing all other magnitude values to zero produces the result shown in **Figure 66**. The retransformed

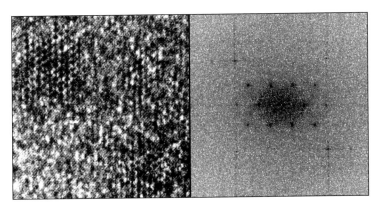

Figure 63. High resolution TEM lattice image (left) and its frequency transform (right).

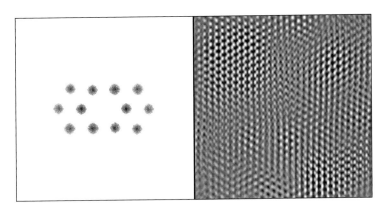

Figure 64. Filtering of Figure 63 to keep the periodic signal (left) and retransformation (right).

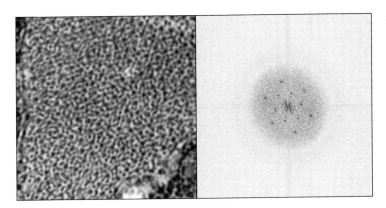

Figure 65. Transmission electron microscope image of cross section of muscle myofibrils (left) and the frequency transform (right). (Image courtesy Arlo Reeves, Dartmouth Univ.)

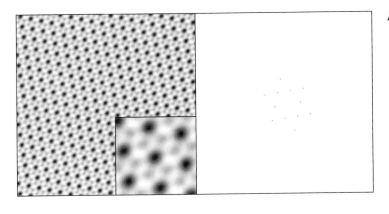

Figure 66. Retransformation of Figure 65 (left) with only the six principal periodic peaks in the frequency transform (right).

image clearly shows the six-fold symmetry expected for the myofibril structure. The inset shows an enlargement of this structure in even finer detail, with both the thick and thin filaments shown. The thin filaments, especially, cannot be seen clearly in the original image.

A caution is needed in using this type of filtering to extract periodic structures. It is possible to construct a mask that will eliminate real information from the image while keeping artefacts and noise. Selecting points in the power spectrum with six-fold symmetry insured that the filtered and retransformed spatial image would show that type of structure. This means that the critical step is the recognition and selection of the peaks in the Fourier transform image. Fortunately, there are many suitable tools for finding and isolating such points, since they are narrow peaks that rise above a gradually varying local background. The top hat filter discussed in Chapter 4 is an example of this approach.

It is also possible to construct a filter to select a narrow range of spacings, such as the interatomic spacing in a high-resolution image. This annular filter makes it possible to enhance a desired periodic structure selectively. **Figure 67** shows a high-resolution TEM image of an atomic lattice. Applying an annular filter that blocks both the low and high frequencies produces the result shown, in which the atom positions are more clearly defined. However, if the filter also selects a particular orientation (a slit or pie-wedge filter), then the dislocation that is difficult to discern in the original image becomes clearly evident.

As for removing periodic noise, a filter that selects periodic information and reveals periodic structure can often be designed by examining the Fourier transform power spectrum image itself to locate peaks. The mask or filter can be constructed either manually or automatically. In some cases, there is *a priori* information available (such as lattice spacings of crystalline specimens).

Figures 68 and **69** compare two methods for masking the frequency transform. The original is a TEM image of a silicon lattice. Setting a threshold to choose only points in the transform above a certain level tends to reject high-frequency points, producing some image smoothing, as shown in **Figure 68**. However, selection of the discrete periodic points with a mask produces a superior result, as shown in **Figure 69**.

In **Figure 70**, the structure (of graphitized carbon in particles used for tire manufacture) shows many atomic lattices in different orientations. In this case, the diffraction pattern shows the predominant atom plane spacing of 3.5 Ångstroms, in the form of a ring of spots. Applying an annular filter to select just that spacing, retransforming and adding the atom positions to the original image, enhances the visibility of the lattice structure.

The use of filtering in FT space is also useful for isolating structural information when the original image is not perfectly regular.

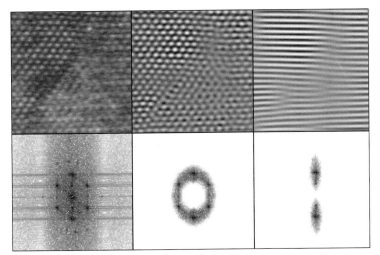

Figure 67. Noisy high-resolution TEM image (left), and the results of applying an annular filter to select atomic spacings (center), and a slit filter to select vertical spacings only (right). Top images show the spatial domain, and bottom row shows frequency domain.

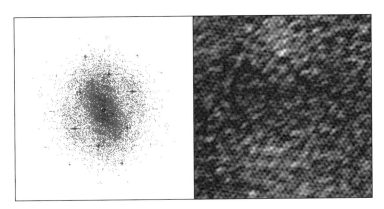

Figure 68. Thresholding of a frequency transform to select only points with a high magnitude (left) and retransformation (right).

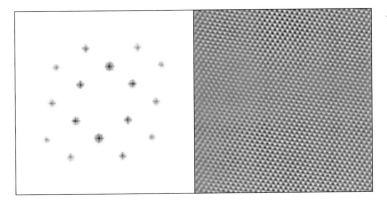

Figure 69. Masking of discrete periodic points (left) and retransformation (right); compare to Figure 68.

Figure 71 shows the same skeletal muscle tissue shown in **Figure 62**, but cross-sectioned and stained with uranyl acetate/lead citrate. The black dots are immunogold labeling for fast myosin, involved in muscle contraction. The spots are more or less regularly spaced because of the uniform diameters of the muscle fibers, but have no regular order to their arrangement. Sharpening the image using a top hat filter, as discussed above

Figure 70.

a) *Transmission electron microscope (TEM) image of graphitized carbon;*

b) *the FT power spectrum from image **a** showing the broken ring of spots corresponding to the plane spacing in the graphite;*

c) *the power spectrum plotted as a perspective drawing to emphasize the ring of peaks;*

d) *inverse transform of just the ring of spots;*

e) *image **d** added to the original image **a** to enhance the visibility of the lattice.*

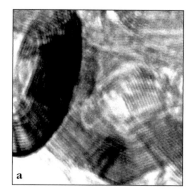

a

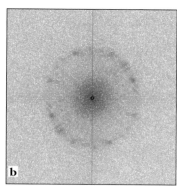

b

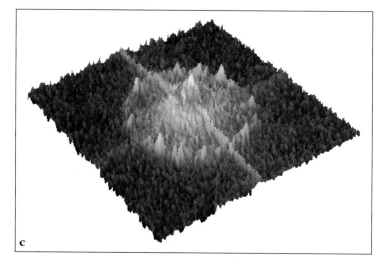

c

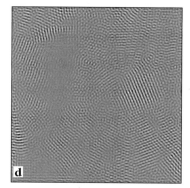

d

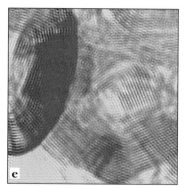

e

and in Chapter 4, improves the visibility of the spots as compared to the original image. So does the use of an annular Fourier filter that selects just the ring of spots corresponding to the fiber diameter.

Convolution and correlation
Fundamentals of convolution

One of the most common operations on images that is performed in the spatial domain is convolution, in which a kernel of

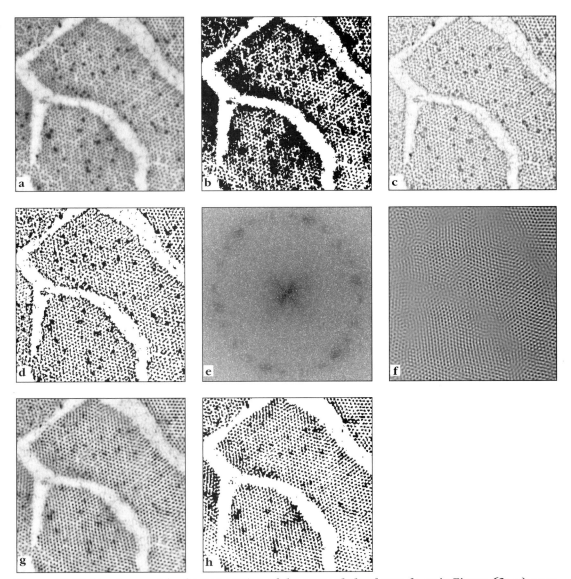

Figure 71. Light micrograph of cross section of the same skeletal muscle as in Figure 62: a) *cross sectioned and uranyl acetate/lead citrate stained. Black dots are immunogold labeling for fast myosin.* **b)** *Thresholding the dark spots in* **a** *does not cleanly delineate the fibers;* **c)** *applying a top hat filter by subtracting the brightest pixel value within a 5-pixel-wide circle;* **d)** *the procedure in* **c** *improves the ability to threshold the gold particles;* **e)** *the power spectrum from the Fourier transform, showing a broken ring of spots corresponding to the average diameter of the fibers;* **f)** *retransforming the ring of spots with an annular filter selects just the spacings of the gold particles;* **g)** *adding this back to the original image increases the contrast;* **h)** *thresholding the image in* **g** *delineates the fibers.*

numbers is multiplied by each pixel and its neighbors in a small region, the results summed, and the result placed in the original pixel location. This is applied to all of the pixels in the image. In all cases, the original pixel values are used in the multiplication and addition, and the new derived values are used to produce a new image. Sometimes this operation is performed a few lines at a time, so that the new image ultimately replaces the old one.

This type of convolution is particularly common for smoothing and derivative operations. For instance, a simple smoothing kernel might contain the following values:

1/16	2/16	1/16
2/16	4/16	2/16
1/16	2/16	1/16

In practice, the fastest implementation would be to multiply the pixel and its 8 immediate neighbors by the integers 1, 2, or 4, sum the products, then divide the total by 16. In this case, using integers that are powers of 2 allows the math to be extremely fast (involving only bit shifting), and the small size of the kernel (3×3) makes the application of the smoothing algorithm on the spatial-domain image very fast, as well.

There are many spatial-domain kernels, including ones that take first derivatives (for instance, to locate edges) and second derivatives (for instance, the Laplacian, which is a nondirectional operator that acts as a high-pass filter to sharpen points and lines). They are usually presented as a set of integers, with it understood that there is a divisor (usually equal to the sum of all the positive values) that normalizes the result. Some of these operators may be significantly larger than the 3×3 example shown above, involving the adding together of the weighted sum of neighbors in a much larger region that is usually, but not necessarily, square.

Applying a large kernel takes time. **Figure 72** illustrates the process graphically for a single placement of the kernel. Even with very fast computers and with careful coding of the process to carry out additions and multiplications in the most efficient order, performing the operation with a 25×25 kernel on a 512×512 image would require a significant amount of time (and

Figure 72. *Illustration of applying a convolution kernel to an image in the spatial domain.*

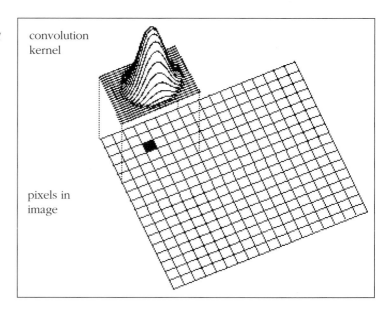

convolution kernel

pixels in image

even larger kernels and images are often encountered). Though it can be speeded up somewhat by the use of special hardware, such as a pipelined array processor, a special-purpose investment is required. A similar hardware investment can be used to speed up the Fourier transform. Our interest here is in the algorithms, rather than in their implementation.

For any computer-based system, increasing the kernel size eventually reaches a point at which it is more efficient to perform the operation in the Fourier domain. The time needed to perform the FFT or FHT transformation from the spatial domain to the frequency domain and back is more than balanced by the speed with which the convolution can be carried out. If there are any other reasons to perform the transformation to the frequency-domain representation of the image, then even small kernels can be most efficiently applied there.

This is because the equivalent operation to spatial-domain convolution is a simple multiplication of each pixel in the magnitude image by the corresponding pixel in a transform of the kernel. The transform of the kernel can be obtained and stored beforehand just as the kernel is stored. If the kernel is smaller than the image, it is padded with zeroes to the full image size. Without deriving a proof, it can be simply stated that convolution in the spatial domain is exactly equivalent to multiplication in the frequency domain. Using the notation presented before, in which the image is a function $f(x,y)$ and the kernel is $g(x,y)$, we would describe the convolution operation in which the kernel is positioned everywhere on the image and multiplied by it as

$$g(x,y) * f(x,y) = \iint (f(\alpha,\beta) \cdot g(x - \alpha, y - \beta) \, d\alpha \, d\beta \qquad (9$$

where α and β are dummy variables for the integration, the range of which is across the entire image, and the symbol $*$ indicates convolution. If the Fourier transforms of $f(x,y)$ and $g(x,y)$ are $F(u,v)$ and $G(u,v)$ respectively, then the convolution operation in the Fourier domain is simple point-by-point multiplication, or

$$g(x,y) * f(x,y) <=> G(u,v) \, F(u,v) \qquad (10$$

There are a few practical differences between the two operations. The usual application of a kernel in the spatial domain avoids the edge pixels (those nearer to the edge than the halfwidth of the kernel), since their neighbors do not exist. As a practical alternative, a different kernel that is one-sided and has different weights can be applied near edges. In transforming the image to the frequency domain, the tacit assumption is made that the image wraps around at edges, so that the left edge is contiguous with the right and the top edge is contiguous with the bottom. Applying a convolution by multiplying in the frequency domain is equivalent to addressing pixels in this same wraparound manner when applying the kernel to the spatial image. It will usually produce some artefacts at the edges.

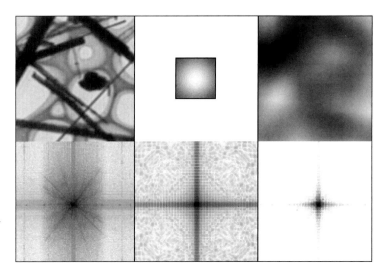

Figure 73. Smoothing by applying a large kernel in the spatial domain, and convolution in the frequency domain. *Top left: original image; bottom left: its frequency transform; top center: smoothing kernel; bottom center: its frequency transform; bottom right: convolution (product of the transforms); top right: smoothed image produced by spatial convolution with kernel, or retransformation of product.*

Figure 73 shows the equivalence of convolution in the spatial domain and multiplication in the frequency domain, for the case of a large smoothing kernel. The kernel is shown along with its transform. Applying the kernel to the image in the spatial domain produces the result shown in the example. Multiplying the kernel transform by the image transform produces the frequency-domain image whose power spectrum is shown. Retransforming this image produces the identical result to the spatial-domain operation. Large kernels such as this one are often used to smooth images in order to eliminate small features and obtain a varying background that can then be subtracted to isolate the features.

Notice that the equivalence of frequency-domain multiplication to spatial-domain convolution is restricted to multiplicative or linear filters. Other neighborhood operations, such as rank filtering (saving the brightest, darkest, or median brightness value in a neighborhood), are nonlinear and have no frequency-domain equivalent.

Imaging system characteristics
Convolution can also be used as a tool to understand how imaging systems alter or degrade images. For example, the blurring introduced by imperfect lenses can be described by a function $H(u,v)$ which is multiplied by the frequency transform of the image (**Figure 74**). The operation of physical optics is readily modeled in the frequency domain. Sometimes it is possible to determine the separate characteristics of each component of the system; sometimes it is not. In a few cases, determining the point-spread function of the system (the degree to which a perfect point in the object plane is blurred in the image plane) may make it possible to sharpen the image by removing some of the blur. This is done by dividing by $H(u,v)$, the transform of the point-spread image.

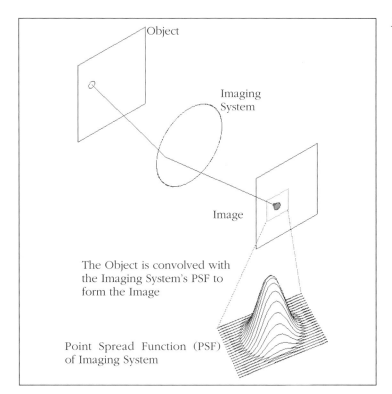

Object

Imaging
System

Image

The Object is convolved with
the Imaging System's PSF to
form the Image

Point Spread Function (PSF)
of Imaging System

Figure 74. *System characteristics
introduce a point spread
function into the acquired
image.*

To illustrate this sharpening we can use the simple resolution
test pattern shown before. The radial lines become unresolved at
the center of the pattern, even in the best-focus image shown in
Figure 32. This is largely due to the limited resolution of the
video camera used (a solid-state CCD array). The image was digitized as a 256×256 square. **Figure 33** showed the power spectrum (using a log scale) for the original in-focus image. The
falloff in power at high frequencies is in agreement with the
visual loss of resolution at the center of the pattern.

An intentionally out-of-focus image was obtained (**Figure 75**) by
misadjusting the camera lens. In addition to blurring the lines,
this defocus also reduces the image contrast slightly. The point-
spread function of the camera system was determined by placing
a single black point in the center of the field of view, without
disturbing the lens focus, and acquiring the image shown in
Figure 75.

Power spectra (using a logarithmic display scale) for the out-of-
focus and point-spread images are shown in **Figures 75** and **76**,
respectively. The magnitude of the point-spread function is sometimes called the imaging system's Modulation Transfer Function
(MTF). The reduction in medium and high frequencies for the
out-of-focus pattern is evident. For the symmetric point-spread
function, the white ring at about one-third of the image width is
a ring of zero values that will become important in performing
the deconvolution.

Figure 75. *Blurred (out-of-focus) image of test pattern in Figure 32 (left), and its frequency transform (right).*

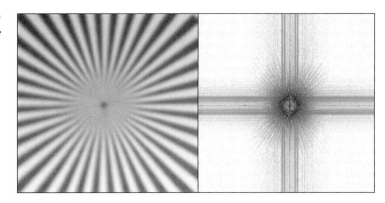

Figure 76. *Blurred (out-of-focus) image of a single point (left) and its frequency transform (right).*

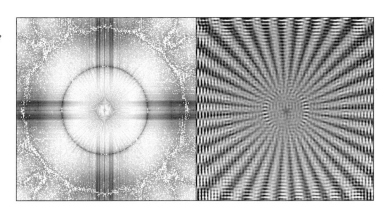

Figure 77. *Result of dividing the frequency transform in Figure 76 by that in Figure 75 (left), and retransforming (right).*

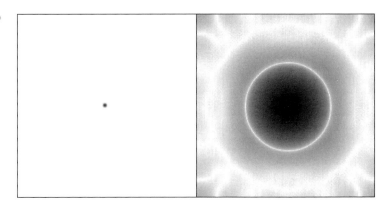

Figure 78. *Same procedure as in Figure 77 but restricting the range to avoid zeroes.*

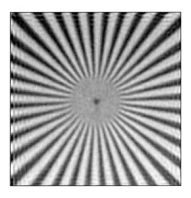

For deconvolution, we divide the complex frequency-domain image from the out-of-focus test pattern by that for the point-spread. Actually, this is done by dividing the magnitude values and subtracting the phase values. The result of retransformation after performing the complex division is shown in **Figure 77**. While some hint of the test pattern is evident, the retransformed image is dominated by a noise pattern. This results from the zeroes in the divisor, which cause numeric overflow problems for the program.

There are two approaches to dealing with this effect, both of which seek to restrict the division operation to those pixels in the complex transform images that will not cause overflow. One is to place a physical restriction, such as a filter or mask, on the image (this is often described as apodization). The other is to define a zero result for any division that causes numerical overflow. By defining a circular band along the line of zeroes, with cosine edge-weighting over a six-pixel-wide region, the zeroes were avoided. Retransformation produced the result shown in **Figure 78**. Most of the artefacts have been removed and the radial lines appear well-defined, although they are not as sharp as the original in-focus image of the test pattern.

There are potential pitfalls in this method. One problem is the finite representation of the complex numbers in the frequency-domain image. Division by small values can produce numerical overflow that can introduce serious artefacts into the image. Also, it is often very difficult to obtain a good point-spread function by recording a real image. If the noise content of that image and the one to be sharpened are different, it can exacerbate the numerical precision and overflow problems. Removal of more than a small fraction of the blurring in a real image is almost never possible, but of course there are some situations in which even a small improvement may be of considerable practical importance.

Division by the frequency transform of the blur is referred to as an inverse filter. Using the notation introduced previously, it can be written as

$$F(u,v) \approx \left[\frac{1}{H(u,v)}\right] \cdot G(u,v) \qquad (11$$

An approach to limiting the damage caused by very small values of H is to add a weighting factor, so that zeroes are avoided.

$$F(u,v) \approx \left[\frac{1}{H(u,v)}\right] \cdot \left[\frac{|H(u,v)|^2}{|H(u,v)|^2 + K}\right] \cdot G(u,v) \qquad (12$$

Ideally, K should be calculated from the statistical properties of the transforms (in which case this is known as a Wiener filter). However, when this is impractical, it is common to approximate K by trial and error to find a satisfactorily restored image in which the sharpness of edges from high-frequency terms is balanced against the noise from dividing by small numbers.

This approach to blur removal is applied to light microscope imaging of optical sections in thick samples. The blurring is produced by the passage of light through the portions of the sample above and below the plane of focus. It is not possible to know the exact details of the blur function, which changes from point to point in the image and from section to section. But by making some assumptions about the image, usually that edges should be sharp and that approximately uniform regions have the same shade of grey, unfolding the blur function with a Wiener-type filter in which the K value is adjusted for visual effect does produce improved images.

There are other ways to remove blur from images. One is the maximum entropy method discussed in Chapter 4. This assumes some foreknowledge about the image, such as its noise properties. This information is expressed in a different way than the filter shape, but both methods represent practical compromises.

Removing motion blur and other defects

Additional defects besides out-of-focus optics can be corrected in the frequency domain as well. One of the most common defects is blur caused by motion. This is rarely a problem in microscopy applications, but can be very important in remote sensing, in which light levels are low and the exposure time must be long enough for significant camera motion to occur with respect to the scene. Fortunately, in most of these circumstances the amount and direction of motion is known. That makes it possible to draw a line in the spatial domain that defines the blur. The frequency transform of this line is then divided into the transform of the blurred image. Retransforming the resulting image restores the sharp result. **Figures 79** to **81** illustrate this method. **Figure 79** is the blurred image, **Figure 80** is the blur vector and its transform, and **Figure 81** is the reconstructed (deblurred) result.

It is important to note the similarity and the difference between this example and the removal of out-of-focus blur. Both involve dividing the transform of the blurred image by that of the defect. This follows directly from the equation presented for convolution, in which the transform of the convolved image is the product of those from the original image and the defect. The major difference is that in the motion blur case we can calculate the exact blurring vector to be removed, while in the out-of-focus blur case we must estimate the blur from an actual image. This estimation introduces unavoidable noise in the image, which is greatly magnified by the division. Using a filter mask to limit the range of application of the division restricts the correction to lower frequencies, and the amount of restoration is consequently limited. The greater the uncertainty in the defects introduced by the imaging system, the less the degree of restoration possible.

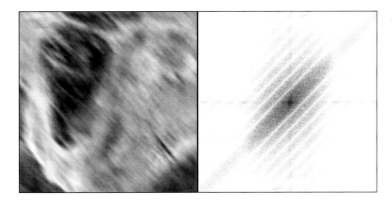

Figure 79. Aerial photo blurred by motion (left), and its frequency transform (right).

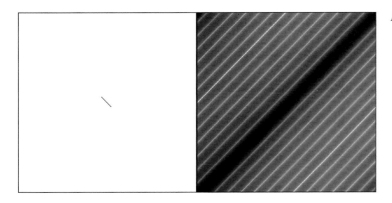

Figure 80. The blur vector for Figure 79 (left) and its frequency transform (right).

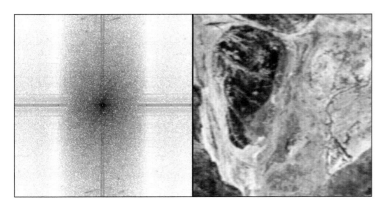

Figure 81. The result of dividing the transform in Figure 79 by the one in Figure 80 (left), and retransforming (right).

Additional limitations arise from the finite internal precision in computer implementation of the FFT or FHT and the storage of the complex frequency-transform image. Programs may use either floating-point or fixed-point notation, the latter requiring less storage space and offering somewhat greater speed. However, the minimum magnitude values that can be accurately recorded generally occur at higher frequencies, controlling how sharp edges appear in the spatial-domain image. Too small a precision also limits the ability to sharpen images by removing degrading blur due to the imaging system.

If the blur is not known *a priori*, it can often be estimated from the direction and spacing of the lines of zeroes in the frequency-domain power spectrum. To avoid the limitations shown above in attempting to remove out-of-focus blur using a measured point-spread function, it may be necessary to iteratively divide by several assumed blur directions and magnitudes to find an optimum result.

One of the most important areas for these image restoration techniques is deblurring the images formed by optical sectioning. This is the technique in which a series of images are recorded from different depths of focus in a semitransparent specimen using a light microscope. The passage of light through the overlying layers of the specimen cause a blurring that adversely affects the sharpness and contrast of the images, preventing their being assembled into a three-dimensional stack for visualization and measurement of the three-dimensional structures present.

The confocal light microscope overcomes some of these problems by rejecting light from points away from the point of focus, which improves the contrast of the images (it also reduces the depth of field of the optics, producing higher resolution in the depth axis, but this is important only at the highest magnifications). But the scattering and diffraction of light by the upper layers of the specimen still degrades the image resolution.

In principle, the images of the upper layers contain information that can be used to deconvolute those from below. This would allow sharpening of those images. The entire process is iterative and highly computer intensive, the more so because the blurring of each point on each image may be different from other points. In practice, it is usual to make some assumptions about the blurring and noise content of the images which are used as global averages for a given specimen or for a given optical setup.

Even with these assumptions, the computations are still intensive and iterative. There is a considerable theoretical and limited practical literature in this field (Carrington, 1990; Holmes et al., 1991; Monck et al., 1992; Joshi & Miller, 1993; Richardson, 1972; Snyder et al., 1992) A review of several of the leading methods can be found in Van Kempen et al., 1997. The examples shown deal only with idealized structures and averaging assumptions about the noise characteristics of the images and the point spread function of the microscope, which suggests that restoration of real images will not be as good as the examples shown. Similar concerns and methods can in principle be applied to other in situ three-dimensional imaging techniques such as tomography and seismic imagery.

The deconvolution of tip shape artefacts in scanned probe microscopy is a different field, usually not performed in frequency space. It is discussed in Chapter 11.

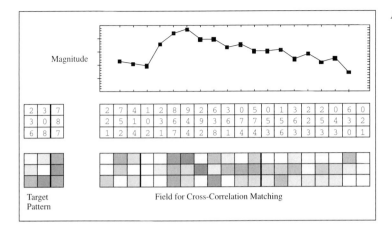

Figure 82. *Diagram of template matching. The target pattern is shifted across the image fragment and the cross-correlation value at each location is recorded as brightness.*

Template matching and correlation

Closely related to the spatial-domain application of a kernel for smoothing, etc. is the idea of template matching. In this case, a target pattern is shifted to every location in the image, the values are multiplied by the pixels that are overlaid, and the total is stored at that position to form an image showing where regions identical or similar to the target are located. **Figure 82** illustrates this process.

This method is used in many contexts to locate features within images. One is searching reconnaissance images for particular objects such as vehicles. Tracking the motion of hurricanes in a series of weather satellite images or cells moving on a microscope slide can also use this approach. Modified to deal optimally with binary images, it can be used to find letters in text. When the target is a pattern of pixel brightness values from one image in a stereo pair and the searched image is the second image from the pair, the method has been used to perform fusion (locating matching points in the two images) to measure parallax and calculate range.

For continuous two-dimensional functions, the cross-correlation image is calculated as

$$c(i,j) = \int_{-\infty}^{+\infty} \int_{-\infty}^{+\infty} f(x,y)\, g(x-i,\, y-j)\, dx\, dy \qquad (13$$

Replacing the integrals by finite sums over the dimensions of the image gives the expression below. In order to normalize the result of this template matching or correlation without the absolute brightness value of the region of the image biasing the results, the operation in the spatial domain is usually calculated as the sum of the products of the pixel brightnesses divided by their geometric mean.

$$\frac{\displaystyle\sum_i \sum_j f_{x+i,\,y+j} \cdot g_{i,j}}{\sqrt{\displaystyle\sum_i \sum_j f^2_{x+i,\,y+j} \cdot \sum_i \sum_k g^2_{i,j}}} \qquad (14$$

When the dimensions of the summation are large, this is a slow and inefficient process compared to the equivalent operation in frequency space. The frequency-space operation is simply

$$C(u,v) = F(u,v)\ G^*(u,v) \qquad (15$$

where * indicates the complex conjugate of the function values. The complex conjugate of the pixel values affects only the imaginary part (or, when magnitude and phase are used, the phase). The operation is thus seen to be very similar to convolution, and indeed it is often performed using many of the same program subroutines. Operations that involve two images (division for deconvolution, multiplication for convolution, and multiplication by the conjugate for correlation) are sometimes called dyadic operations, to distinguish them from filtering and masking operations (monadic operations) in which a single frequency transform image is operated on (the mask image is not a frequency-domain image).

Usually, when correlation is performed, the wraparound assumption joining the left and right edges and the top and bottom of the image is not acceptable. In these cases, the image should be padded by surrounding it with zeroes to bring it to the next larger size for transformation (the next exact power of two, required for FFT and FHT calculations). Since the correlation operation also requires that the actual magnitude values of the transforms be used, slightly better mathematical precision can be achieved by padding with the average values of the original image brightnesses rather than with zeroes. It may also be useful to subtract the average brightness value from each pixel, which removes the zeroth (DC) term from the transformation. Since this value is usually the largest in the transform (it is the value at the central pixel), its elimination allows the transform data more dynamic range.

Correlation is primarily used for locating features in one image that appear in another. **Figures 83** to **85** show an example. The first image contains text, while the second contains the letter "e" by itself. The frequency transforms of the two images are shown in each figure. Since neither image has text crossing the image boundaries, no padding to a larger size was needed in this case. **Figure 85** shows the result of the cross-correlation after retransforming the image to the spatial domain and also shows the same image presented as an isometric display.

Note that the brightest points in the correlation image correspond to the occurrences of the letter "e." These have been found by

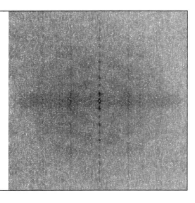

Figure 83. *Sample of text (left), and its frequency transform (right).*

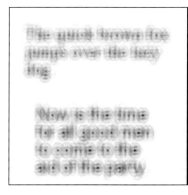

Figure 84. *The target letter "e" (left) and its frequency transform (right).*

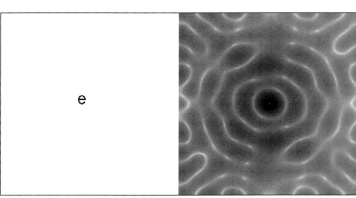

Figure 85. *The cross-correlation of Figures 83 and 84, shown as brightness (left) and as a perspective display (right).*

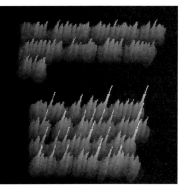

the autocorrelation process. Note also that there are lower but still significant peaks corresponding to other letters with some similarity to the "e," particularly the "a" and the "o." Finally, note that the letter "e" in the upper sentence is not found by this method. This is because that text is set in a different font (sans serif Helvetica instead of serif Times Roman). Cross-correlation is sensitive to feature shape (and also size and orientation).

Autocorrelation

In the special case when the image functions f and g (and their transforms F and G) are the same, the correlation operation is called autocorrelation. This is used to combine together all parts

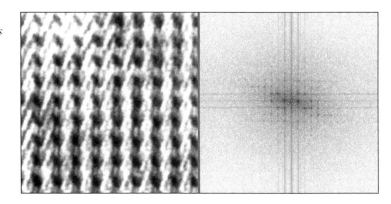

Figure 86. *High resolution TEM image of mullite (left), and its frequency transform (right). (Image courtesy Sopa Chevacharoenkul, Microelectronics Center of North Carolina.)*

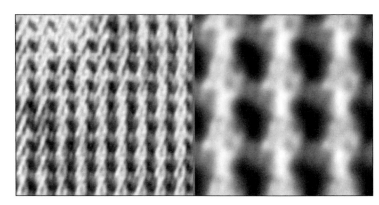

Figure 87. *Autocorrelation image from Figure 86 (left) and an enlarged view (right).*

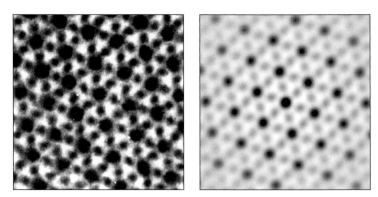

Figure 88. *TEM image of cross section of insect flight muscle (left), and the autocorrelation image (right). (Image courtesy of Mike Lamvik, Duke Univ.)*

of the image, in order to find and average repetitive structures. **Figures 86** and **87** show one of the classic uses of this method applied to a TEM image of a lattice structure (mullite). Each individual repeating unit in the image contains some noise, but by averaging all repeats together, a better image of the fine structural details can be obtained.

The process is carried out as described above. The frequency transform of the image is multiplied by its own conjugate and the result retransformed, so that fine details down to atomic positions in this complex lattice can be seen. **Figure 88** shows another example, in which the repeating structure of muscle

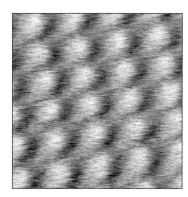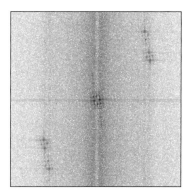

Figure 89. *STM image of pyrolytic graphite. (Image courtesy Richard Chapman, Microelectronics Center of North Carolina) and its Fourier transform.*

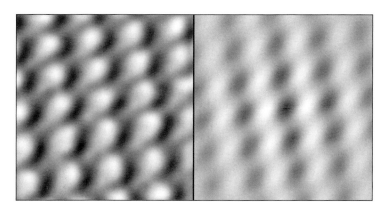

Figure 90. *Processing of Figure 89: comparison of smoothing with a low-pass filter (left), and autocorrelation (right).*

fibers in an insect flight muscle is averaged in the same way by autocorrelation. In both these cases, padding was needed because the images do not wrap around at the edges.

To compare this method of removing noise with filtering, we can use the (quite noisy) STM image shown in **Figure 89** with its frequency transform. **Figure 90** compares the results of filtering by setting a mask to accept only the central (low-frequency) portion of the transform (12 pixels in diameter plus a 6-pixel-wide cosine edge shaping), with the result of autocorrelation. The filtered image is certainly smoother, since all high-frequency information (some of which has produced significant peaks in the transform image) is removed. The autocorrelation image shows more details of the shape of the response at the regularly spaced atoms by averaging all of the repetitions and keeping high-frequency information.

Figure 91 shows another use of the autocorrelation function, to measure preferred orientation. The image is a felted textile material. Due to the fabrication process the fibers have neither a randomized nor uniform orientation; neither are they regularly arranged. The frequency transform shown indicates a slightly asymmetric shape. Performing the cross-correlation and retransforming to the spatial domain gives the image shown in **Figure 92**. The brightness profiles of the central spot show the preferred orientation quantitatively. This is the same result

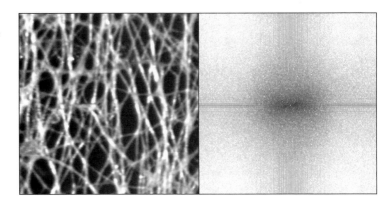

Figure 91. *Image of felted textile fibers (left) and the frequency transform (right).*

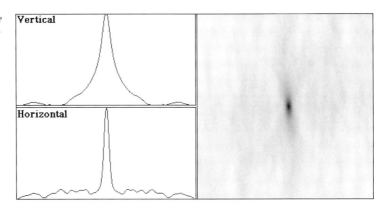

Figure 92. *Autocorrelation image from Figure 91 (right), and its horizontal and vertical brightness profiles (left).*

achieved by cross-correlation in the spatial domain (sliding the image across itself and recording the area of feature overlap as a function of relative offset) to determine preferred orientation.

Conclusion

Processing images in the frequency domain is useful for removing certain types of noise, applying large convolution kernels, enhancing periodic structures, and locating defined structures in images. It can also be used to measure images to determine periodicity or preferred orientation. All of these operations can be carried out in the spatial domain, but are often much more efficient in the frequency domain. The FFT (or FHT) operation is limited to images that are powers of two in size, but they can be efficiently computed in small (desktop) systems. This makes frequency-domain operations useful and important tools for image analysis.

6

Segmentation and Thresholding

One of the most widely used steps in the process of reducing images to information is segmentation: dividing the image into regions that hopefully correspond to structural units in the scene or distinguish objects of interest. Segmentation is often described by analogy to visual processes as a foreground/background separation, implying that the selection procedure concentrates on a single kind of feature and discards the rest.

This is not quite true for computer systems, which can generally deal much better than humans with scenes containing more than one type of feature of interest. **Figure 1** shows a common optical illusion that can be seen as a vase or as two facing profiles, depending on whether we concentrate on the white or black areas as the foreground. It seems that humans are unable to see both interpretations at once, although we can flip rapidly back and forth between them once the two have been recognized.

This is true in many other illusions as well. **Figure 2** shows two others. The cube can be seen in either of two orientations, with the dark corner close to or far from the viewer; the sketch can be seen as either an old woman or a young girl. In both cases, we can switch between versions very quickly but we cannot perceive them both at the same time.

Thresholding

Selecting features within a scene or image is an important prerequisite for most kinds of measurement or understanding of the

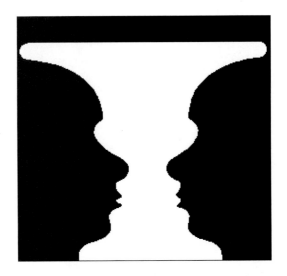

Figure 1. *The "vase" illusion. Viewers may see either a vase or two human profiles in this image, and can alternate between them, but cannot see both interpretations at the same time.*

scene. Traditionally, one simple way thresholding has been accomplished is to define a range of brightness values in the original image, select the pixels within this range as belonging to the foreground, and reject all of the other pixels to the background. Such an image is then usually displayed as a binary or two-level image, using black and white or other colors to distinguish the regions. (There is no standard convention on whether the features of interest are white or black; the choice depends on the particular display hardware in use and the designer's preference; in the examples shown here the features are black and the background is white.)

This operation is called thresholding. Thresholds may be set interactively by a user watching the image and using a colored overlay to show the result of turning a knob or otherwise adjusting the settings. As a consequence of the ubiquitous use of a mouse as the human interface to a graphical computer display, the user may adjust virtual sliders or mark a region on a histogram to select the range of brightness values. The brightness histogram of the image (or a region of it) is very useful for making adjustments. As discussed in earlier chapters, this is a plot of the number of pixels in the image having each brightness level. For a typical 8-bit monochrome image, this equals 2^8 or 256 grey scale values. The plot may be presented in a variety of formats, either vertical or horizontal, and some displays use color or grey scale coding to assist the viewer in distinguishing the white and black sides of the plot.

Examples of histograms have been shown in earlier chapters. In the figures that follow, most are shown with a grey scale to identify the pixel brightness and with lines whose length is proportional to the number of pixels with that brightness. Note that the histogram counts pixels in the entire image (or in a defined region of interest), losing all information about the original location of the pixels or the brightness values of their neighbors. Peaks in the histogram often identify the various homogeneous

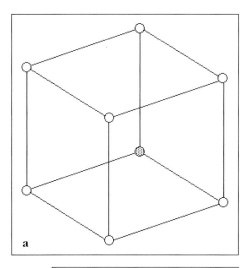

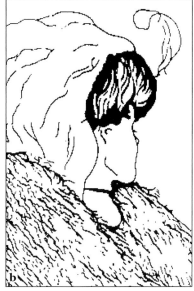

Figure 2. Examples of either/or interpretation:
a) *the Necker cube, in which the dark corner may appear close to or far from the viewer;*
b) *the "Old woman/ Young girl" sketch.*

regions (often referred to as phases, although they correspond to a phase in the metallurgical sense only in a few applications) and thresholds can then be set between the peaks. There are also automatic methods to adjust threshold settings (Prewitt & Mendelsohn, 1966; Weszka, 1978; Otsu, 1979; Kittler et al., 1985; Russ & Russ, 1988a; Rigaut, 1988; Lee et al., 1990; Sahoo et al., 1988; Russ, 1995c), using either the histogram or the image itself as a guide, as we will see below. Methods that compare to *a priori* knowledge the measurement parameters obtained from features in the image at many threshold levels (Wolf, 1991) are too complex and specialized for this discussion.

There are many images in which no clear-cut set of histogram peaks corresponds to distinct phases or structures in the image. In some of these cases, direct thresholding of the image is still possible. In most, however, the brightness levels of individual

Figure 3. Example of terrain classification from satellite imagery using multiple spectral bands.

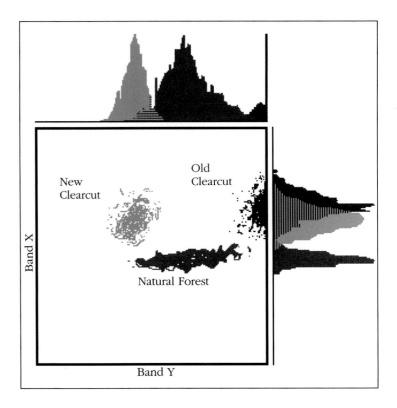

pixels are not uniquely related to structure. In some of these instances, prior image processing can be used to transform the original brightness values in the image to a new image, in which pixel brightness represents some derived parameter such as the local brightness gradient or direction.

Multiband images

In some cases, segmentation can be performed using multiple original images of the same scene. The most familiar example is that of color imaging, which uses different wavelengths of light. For satellite imaging in particular, this may include several infrared bands containing important information for selecting regions according to vegetation, types of minerals, and so forth (Haralick & Dinstein, 1975). **Figure 3** shows an example. It is more difficult to visualize, but a series of images obtained by performing different processing operations on the same original image can also be used in this way. Examples include combining one image containing brightness data, a second containing local texture information, etc.

In general, the more independent color bands or other images that are available, the easier and better the job of segmentation that can be performed. Points that are indistinguishable in one image may be fully distinct in another. However, with multi-spectral or multilayer images, it can be difficult to specify the selection criteria. The logical extension of thresholding is simply

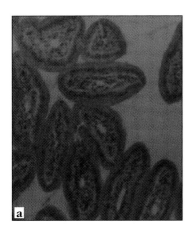 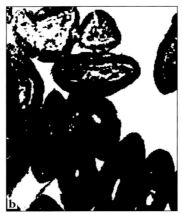 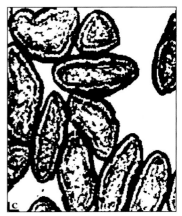

Figure 4. Thresholding a color image:

a) *original stained biological thin section;*

b) *thresholding performed on the intensity image is not very satisfactory;*

c) *thresholding on the hue image delineates the stained structures.*

to place brightness thresholds on each image, for instance to specify the range of red, green, and blue intensities. These multiple criteria are then usually combined with an AND operation (i.e., the pixel is defined as part of the foreground if its three RGB components all lie within the selected ranges). This is logically equivalent to segmenting each image plane individually, creating separate binary images, and then combining them with a Boolean AND operation afterward. Such operations to combine multiple binary images are discussed in Chapter 7.

The reason for wanting to combine the various selection criteria in a single process is to assist the user in defining the ranges for each. The optimum settings and their interaction are not particularly obvious when the individual color bands or other multiple image brightness values are set individually. Indeed, simply designing a user interface which makes it possible to select a specific range of colors for thresholding a typical visible light image (usually specified by the RGB components) is not easy. A variety of partial solutions are available for use.

This problem has several aspects. First, while red, green, and blue intensities represent the way the detector works and the way the data are stored internally, they do not correspond to the way that people recognize or react to color. As discussed in Chapter 1, a system based on hue, saturation, and intensity or lightness (HSI) is more familiar. It is sometimes possible to perform satisfactory thresholding using only one of the hue, saturation or intensity planes as shown in **Figure 4**, but in the general case it is necessary to use all of the information. A series of histograms for each of the RGB color planes may show peaks, but the user is not often able to judge which of the peaks correspond to individual features of interest.

Even if the RGB pixel values are converted to the equivalent HSI values and histograms are constructed in that space, the use of three separate histograms and sets of threshold levels still does nothing to help the user see which pixels have various combinations of values. For a single monochrome image, various inter-

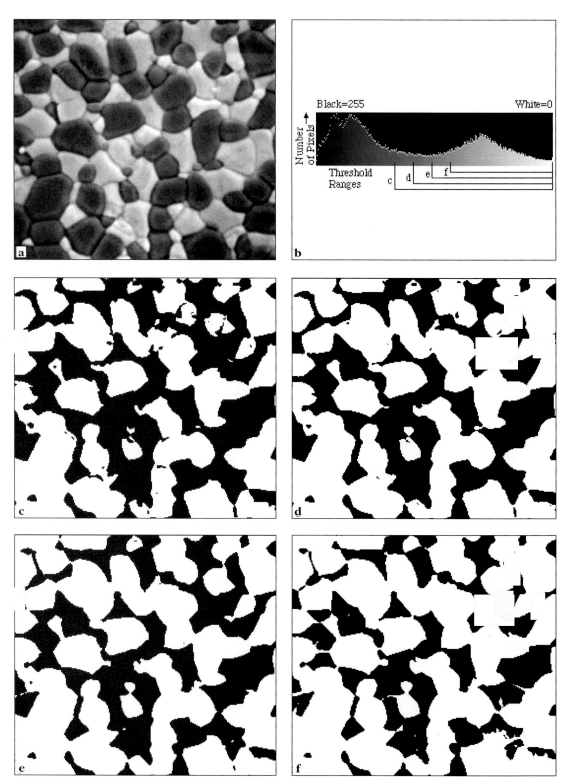

Figure 5. A grey scale image (a) *with its brightness histogram* **(b)** *and several binary images* **(c, d, e, f)** *produced by changing the settings of the threshold values used to select pixels, as shown on the histogram. The area fraction of the light phase varies with these settings from about 33 to 48%.*

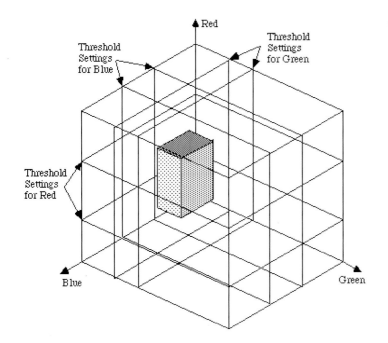

Figure 6. *Illustration of the combination of separate thresholds on individual color planes. The shaded area is the AND of the three threshold settings for red, green, and blue. The only shape that can be formed in the three-dimensional space is a rectangular prism.*

active color-coded displays allow the user either to see which pixels are selected as the threshold levels are adjusted or to select a pixel or cluster of pixels and see where they lie in the histogram. **Figure 5** shows an example, though because it consists of still images, it cannot show the live, real-time feedback possible in this situation.

For a three-dimensional color space, either RGB or HSI, this is not possible. There is no way with present display or control facilities to interactively enclose an arbitrary region in three-dimensional space and see which pixels are selected, or to adjust that region and see the effect on the image. It is also difficult to mark a pixel or region in the image and see the color values (RGB or HSI) labeled directly in the color space. For more than three colors (e.g., the multiple bands sensed by satellite imagery), the situation is even worse.

Using three one-dimensional histograms and sets of threshold levels, for instance in the RGB case, and combining the three criteria with a logical AND selects pixels that lie within a portion of the color space that is a simple prism, as shown in **Figure 6**. If the actual distribution of color values has some other shape in the color space, for instance if it is elongated in a direction not parallel to one axis, then this simple rectangular prism is quite inadequate to enclose some values and exclude others.

Two-dimensional thresholds

A somewhat better bound can be set by using a two-dimensional threshold. This can be done in any color coordinates

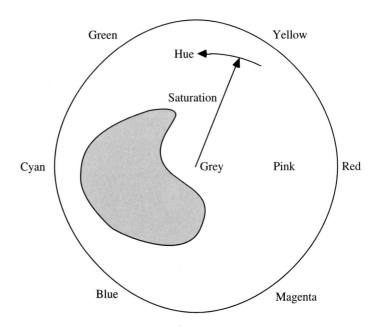

Figure 7. Illustration of selecting an arbitrary region in a two-dimensional parameter space (here the hue/saturation plane) to define a combination of color in two image planes to be selected for thresholding.

(RGB, HSI, etc.), but in RGB space it is difficult to interpret the meaning of the settings. This is one of the (many) arguments against the use of RGB for color images. However, the method is well-suited for color images encoded by hue and saturation. The HS plane is usually represented as a circle, in which direction (angle) is proportional to hue and radius is proportional to saturation (**Figure 7**). The intensity or lightness of the image is perpendicular to this plane and requires another dimension to show or to control.

Similar histogram displays and threshold settings can be accomplished using other planes and coordinates. For color images, the HS plane is sometimes shown as a hexagon (with red, yellow, green, cyan, blue, and magenta corners). The CIE color diagram shown in Chapter 1 is also a candidate for this purpose. For some satellite images, the near and far infrared intensities form a plane in which combinations of thermal and reflected IR can be displayed and selected.

As a practical matter, the HS plane is sometimes plotted as a square face on a cube that represents the HSI space. This is simpler for the computer graphics display and is used in several of the examples that follow. However, the HSI cube with square faces is topologically different from the cone or bi-cone used to represent HSI space in Chapter 1, and the square HS plane is topologically different from the circle in **Figure 7**. In the square, the minimum and maximum hue edges (400 nm = red and 700 nm = violet) are far apart, whereas in the circle, hue is a continuous function that wraps around. This makes using the square for thresholding somewhat less intuitive, but it is still superior in most cases to the use of RGB color space.

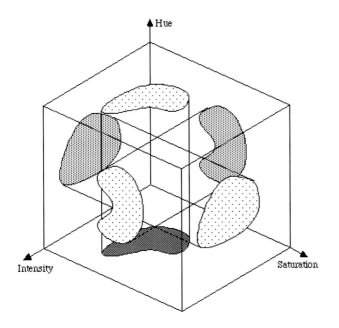

Figure 8. *Illustration of the combination of two-parameter threshold settings. Outlining of regions in each plane defines a shape in the three-dimensional space which is more adjustable than the Boolean combination of simple one-dimensional thresholds in Figure 5, but still cannot conform to arbitrary three-dimensional cluster shapes.*

An analog to a one-dimensional histogram of brightness in a monochrome image is a two-dimensional display in the HS plane. The number of pixels with each pair of values of hue and saturation can be plotted on this plane using brightness or color. Thresholds can be set by drawing an outline that is not necessarily simple or even convex, and so can be adapted to the distribution of the actual data. **Figure 8** illustrates this schematically. Automatic methods are available for drawing or adjusting the boundary based on the data. Indeed, they are very similar to methods for locating clusters for feature recognition, which is discussed below.

It is also possible to mark locations in this plane of individual pixels or regions of pixels in the image, as a guide to the user in the process of defining the boundary. This is often done by having the user point to or encircle pixels in the image so that the program can highlight the location of the color values on the various display planes.

For the two-dimensional square plot, the axes may have unusual meanings, but the ability to display a histogram of points based on the combination of values and to select threshold boundaries based on the histogram is a significant advantage over multiple one-dimensional histograms and thresholds, even if it does not generalize easily to the n-dimensional case.

The dimensions of the histogram array are usually somewhat reduced from the actual resolution (typically one part in 256) of the various RGB or HSI values for the stored image. This is not only because the array size would become very large ($256^2 = 65,536$ for the square, $256^3 = 16,777,216$ for the cube). Another reason is that for a typical real image, there are simply not that many distinct pairs or triples of values present, and a useful display

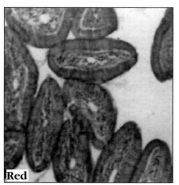 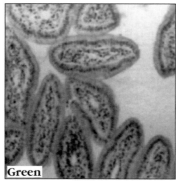 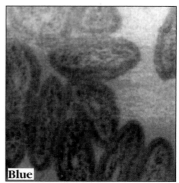

Figure 9. *Red, green, and blue color planes from the image in Figure 4 (discussed in Chapter 1).*

Figure 10. *Brightness histograms for the color plane images in Figure 9.*

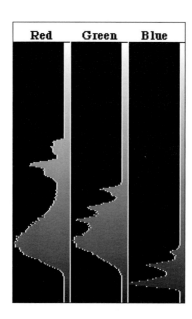

Figure 11. *Pairs of values for the pixels in the images of Figure 9, projected onto RG, BG, and RB planes.*

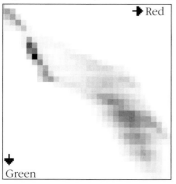 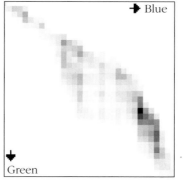 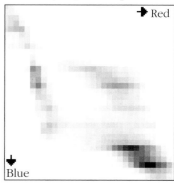

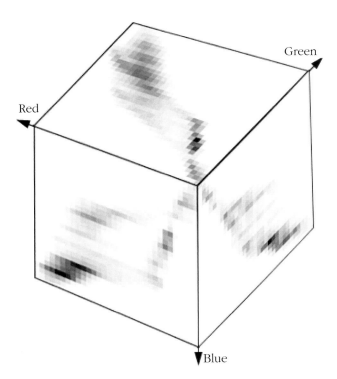

Figure 12. *The data from Figure 11 projected onto the faces of a cube.*

showing the locations of peaks and clusters can be presented using fewer bins. The examples shown below use 32×32 bins for each of the square faces of the RGB or HSI cubes, each of which thus requires $32^2 = 1024$ storage locations.

It is possible to imagine a system in which each of the two-dimensional planes defined by pairs of signals is used to draw a contour threshold, then project all of these contours back through the multidimensional space to define the thresholding, as shown in **Figure 8**. However, as the dimensionality increases, so does the complexity for the user, and the AND region defined by the multiple projections still cannot fit irregular or skewed regions very satisfactorily.

Multiband thresholding

Figure 4 shows a color image from a light microscope. The microtomed thin specimen of intestine has been stained with two different colors, so that there are variations in shade, tint, and tone. **Figure 9** shows the individual red, green, and blue values. The next series of figures illustrates how this image can be segmented by thresholding to isolate a particular structure using this information.

Figure 10 shows the individual brightness histograms of the red, green, and blue color planes in **Figure 9**. **Figure 11** shows the histograms of pixel values in the image, projected onto the red/green, green/blue, and blue/red faces of the RGB color cube. **Figure 12** presents these data as a perspective view on the cube.

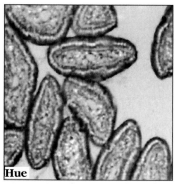 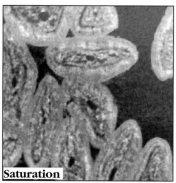 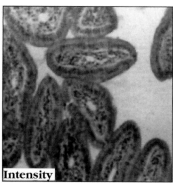

Figure 13. *The same color information as in Figure 9, converted to hue, saturation, and intensity components.*

Figure 14. *Brightness histograms for the color plane images in Figure 13.*

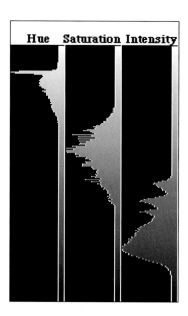

Figure 15. *Hue, saturation, and intensity values for the pixels in Figure 13, projected onto HI, HS, and SI planes. Note that the hue-saturation plane is topologically different from the usual HS circle.*

  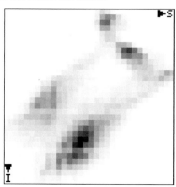

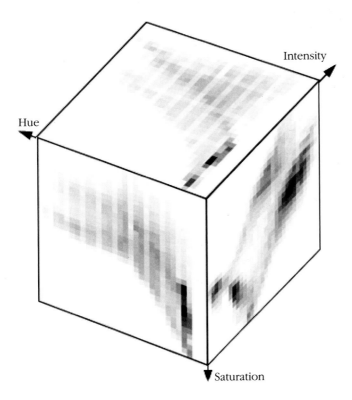

Figure 16. The data from Figure 15 projected onto the faces of a cube. Note that this cube is topologically different from the usual HSI biconical space (see text).

Notice that there is a trend on all faces for the majority of pixels in the image to cluster along the central diagonal in the cube. In other words, for most pixels, the trend toward more of any one color is part of a general increase in brightness by increasing the values of all colors. This means that RGB space poorly disperses the various color values and does not facilitate setting thresholds to discriminate the different regions present.

Figure 13 shows the conversion of the color information from Figure 9 into hue, saturation, and intensity images, and **Figure 14** shows the individual brightness histograms for these planes. **Figure 15** shows the values projected onto individual two-dimensional hue/saturation, saturation/intensity, and intensity/hue square plots. **Figure 16** combines these values into the total cube. Notice how the much greater dispersion of peaks in the various histograms uses more of the color space and separates several different clusters of values.

Figure 17 compares two different thresholded binary images. The pixels selected from their hue values alone include both the general background of the slide and the structures in the villi. However, a two-dimensional threshold set using the saturation and intensity values allows only the villi to be selected, eliminating the general background. This is a more specific image and hence is more useful for further measurement.

In general, for stains used in biological samples, the hue image identifies where a particular stain is located while the saturation

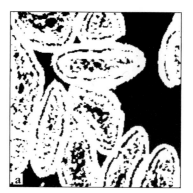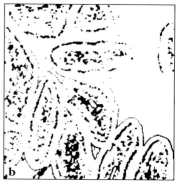

Figure 17. Thresholded binary images from the color figure represented in Figures 9 and 13:
a) *thresholded on hue, which includes both the structures within the villi and the background in the slide;*
b) *thresholded by a region in the two-dimensional saturation/intensity histogram, which selects just the villi.*

image corresponds to the amount of the stain, and the intensity image indicates the overall density of the stained specimen. Combining all three planes as shown in **Figure 18** can often select particular regions that are not well delineated otherwise.

Multiband images are not always simply different colors. A very common example is the use of multiple elemental X-ray maps from the SEM, which can be combined to select phases of interest based on composition. In many cases, this combination can be accomplished simply by separately thresholding each individual image and then applying Boolean logic to combine the images. Of course, the rather noisy original X-ray maps may first require image processing (such as smoothing) to reduce the statistical variations from pixel to pixel (as discussed in Chapters 3 and 4), and binary image processing (as illustrated in Chapter 7).

Using X-rays or other element-specific signals, such as secondary ions or Auger electrons, essentially the entire periodic table can be detected. It becomes possible to specify very complicated combinations of elements that must be present or absent, or the approximate intensity levels needed (since intensities are generally roughly proportional to elemental concentration) to specify the region of interest. Thresholding these combinations of elemental images produces results that are sometimes described as chemical maps. Of course, the fact that several elements may be present in the same area of a specimen, such as a metal, mineral, or block of biological tissue, does not directly imply that they are chemically combined.

In principle, it is possible to store an entire analytical spectrum for each pixel in an image and then use appropriate computation to derive actual compositional information at each point, which is eventually used in a thresholding operation to select regions of interest. At present, this approach is limited in application by the large amount of storage and lengthy calculations required. However, as faster and larger computers and storage devices become common, such methods will become more widely used.

Visualization programs used to analyze complex data may also employ Boolean logic to combine multiple parameters. A simple

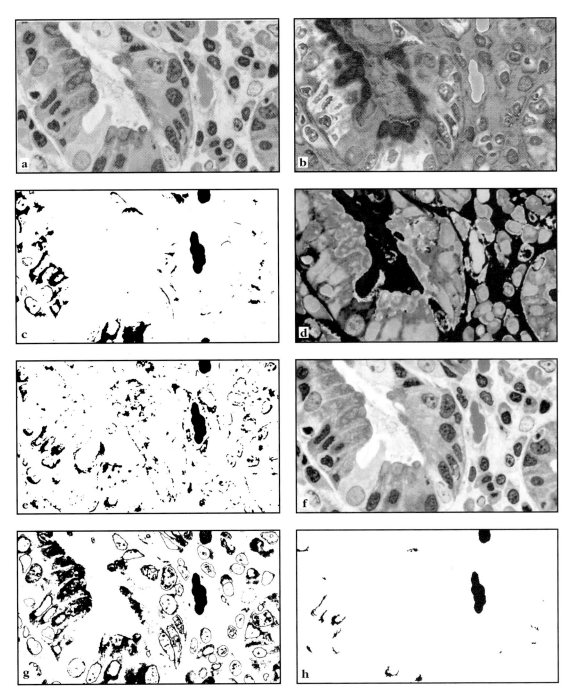

Figure 18. Light micrograph of stomach epithelium with a polychromatic stain, showing thresholding and color separations in HSI space:

a) original;

b) hue image;

c) thresholded hue image;

d) saturation image;

e) thresholded saturation image;

f) intensity image;

g) thresholded intensity image;

h) Boolean AND applied to combine three binary images produced by thresholding H, S and I planes.

example would be a geographical information system, in which such diverse data as population density, mean income level, and other census data were recorded for each city block (which would be treated as a single pixel). Combining these different values to select regions for test marketing commercial products is a standard technique. Another example is the rendering of calculated tensor properties in metal beams subject to loading, as modeled in a computer program. Supercomputer simulations of complex dynamical systems, such as evolving thunderstorms, produce rich data sets that may benefit from such analysis.

There are other uses of image processing that derive additional information from a single original grey scale image to aid in performing selective thresholding of a region of interest. The processing produces additional images that can be treated as multiband images useful for segmentation.

Thresholding from texture

Few real images of practical interest can be satisfactorily thresholded using simply the original brightness values in a monochrome image. The texture information present in images is one of the most powerful additional tools available. Several kinds of texture may be encountered, including different ranges of brightness, different spatial frequencies, and different orientations (Haralick et al., 1973). The next few figures show images that illustrate these variables and the tools available to utilize them.

Figure 19 shows a test image containing five irregular regions that can be visually distinguished by texture. The average brightness of each of the regions is identical, as shown by the brightness histograms in **Figure 20**. Region (e) contains pixels with uniformly random brightness values covering the entire 0 to 255

Figure 19. Test image containing five different regions to be distinguished by differences in the textures. The average brightness of each region is the same.

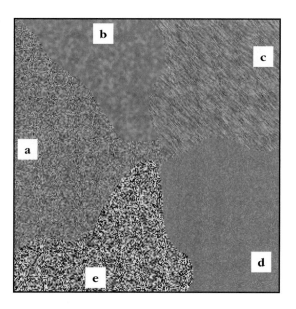

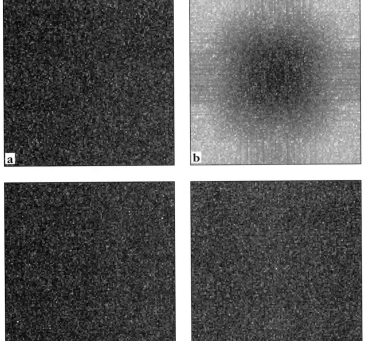

Figure 20. Brightness histograms of each area in Figure 19.

range. Regions (a) through (d) have Gaussian brightness variations, which for regions (a) and (d) are also randomly assigned to pixel locations. For region (b) the values have been spatially averaged with a Gaussian smooth, which also reduces the amount of variation. For region (c) the pixels have been averaged together in one direction to create a directional texture.

One tool that is often recommended (and sometimes useful) for textural characterization is the two-dimensional frequency transform. **Figure 21** shows these power spectra for each of

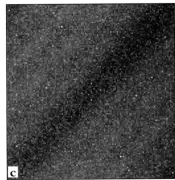

Figure 21. 2D FFT power spectra of the pattern in each area of Figure 19. While some minor differences are seen (e.g., the loss of high frequencies in region **b** and the directionality in region **c**, these cannot be used with a filter for segmentation.

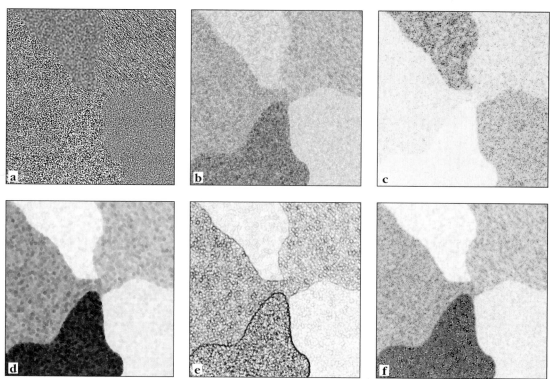

Figure 22. Application of various texture-sensitive operators to the image in Figure 19:
a) Laplacian; b) Frei & Chen; c) Haralick; d) range; e) Hurst; f) variance.

the patterns in **Figure 19**. The smoothing in region (b) acts as a low-pass filter, so the high frequencies are attenuated. In region (c) the directionality is visible in the frequency transform image. For the other regions, the random pixel assignments do not create any distinctive patterns in the frequency transforms. They cannot be used to select the different regions in this case.

Several spatial-domain texture-sensitive operators are applied to the image in **Figure 22**. The Laplacian shown in (a) is a 3×3 neighborhood operator; it responds to very local texture values and does not enhance the distinctions between the textures present here. All of the other operators act on a 5×5 pixel octagonal neighborhood and transform the textures to grey scale values with somewhat different levels of success. Range (d) and variance (f) give the best distinction between the different regions.

There is still some variation in the grey values assigned to the different regions by the texture operators, because they work in relatively small neighborhoods where only a small number of pixel values control the result. Smoothing the variance image (**Figure 23a**) produces an improved image that has unique grey scale values for each region. **Figure 24** shows the brightness histogram of the original variance image and the result after smoothing. The spatial smoothing narrows the peak for each region by reducing the variation within it. The five peaks are

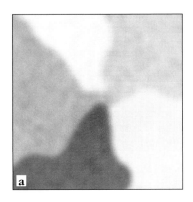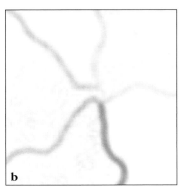

Figure 23. *Result of smoothing the variance image (Figure 22f) with a Gaussian kernel with standard deviation equal to 1.6 pixels (a), and the Sobel edge detector applied to the smoothed image (b).*

separated and allow direct thresholding. **Figure 25** shows a composite image with each region selected by thresholding the smoothed variance image.

Figure 23b shows the application of a Sobel edge (gradient) operator to the smoothed gradient image. Thresholding and skeletonizing (as discussed in Chapter 7) produces a set of boundary lines, which are shown superimposed on the original image in **Figure 26**. Notice that because the spatial scale of the texture is several pixels wide, the location of the boundaries of regions is necessarily uncertain by several pixels. It is also difficult to estimate the proper location visually, for the same reason.

Figure 27 shows an image typical of many obtained in microscopy. The preparation technique has used a chemical etch to reveal the microstructure of a metal sample. The lamellae indicate islands of eutectic structure, which are to be separated from the uniform light regions to determine the volume fraction of each. The brightness values in regions of the original image are not distinct, but a texture operator is able to convert the image to one that can be thresholded.

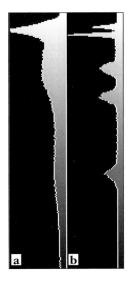

Figure 24. *Histograms of the variance image (Figure 22f) before (a) and after (b) smoothing the image with a Gaussian kernel with 1.6 pixel standard deviation. The five regions are now different in brightness and can be thresholded.*

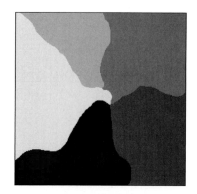

Figure 25. *Thresholding the smoothed variance image for each of the peaks in the histogram delineates the different texture regions.*

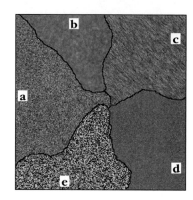

Figure 26. *Results of segmentation by skeletonizing the edge from the Sobel operator in Figure 23b.*

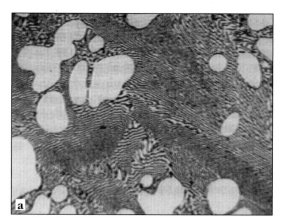

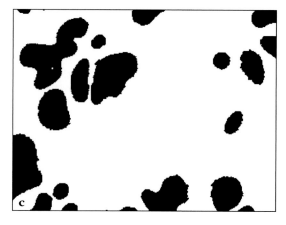

Figure 27. Application of the Hurst texture operator to a microscope image of a metal containing a eutectic:

a) *original image, with light single-phase regions and lamellae corresponding to the eutectic;*

b) *application of a Hurst operator (discussed in Chapter 4) to show the local texture in image **a**;*

c) *binary image formed by thresholding image **b** to select the low-texture (single phase) regions.*

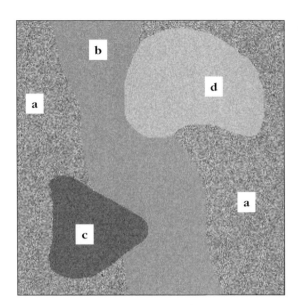

Figure 28. Another segmentation test image, in which some regions have different textures and some different mean brightness.

Multiple thresholding criteria

Figure 28 shows a somewhat more complex test image, in which some of the regions are distinguished by a different spatial texture and some by a different mean brightness. No single parameter can be used to discriminate all four regions. The texture values are produced by assigning Gaussian random values to the pixels. As before, a variance operator applied to a 5×5 octagonal neighborhood produces a useful grey scale distinction. **Figure 29** shows the result of smoothing the brightness values and the variance image.

It is necessary to use both images to select individual regions. This can be done by thresholding each region separately and then using Boolean logic (discussed in Chapter 7) to combine the two binary images in various ways. Another approach is to use the same kind of two-dimensional histogram as described above for color images (Panda & Rosenfeld, 1978). **Figure 30** shows the individual image-brightness histograms and the two-dimensional histogram. In each of the individual histograms, only three peaks are present because the regions are not all distinct in either brightness or variance. In the two-dimensional histogram, individual peaks are visible for each of the four regions.

Figure 31a shows the result of thresholding the intermediate peak in the histogram of the brightness image, which selects two of the regions of medium brightness. **Figure 31b** shows the result of selecting a peak in the two-dimensional histogram to select only a single region. The outlines around each of the regions selected in this way are shown superimposed on the original image in **Figure 32**.

The different derived images used to successfully segment an image such as this one are sometimes displayed using different

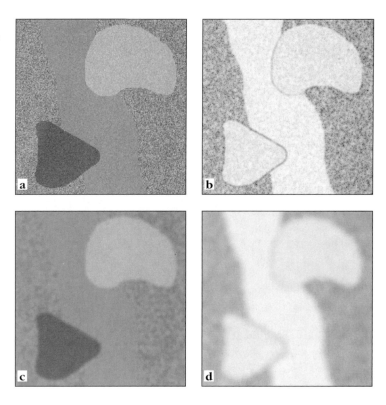

Figure 29. The brightness *(a)* and variance *(b)* images from Figure 28, and the results of smoothing each with a Gaussian filter, standard deviation = 1.6 pixels *(c* and *d)*.

color planes. This is purely a visual effect, of course, since the data represented have nothing to do with color. However, it does take advantage of the fact that human vision uses color information for segmentation. **Figure 33** shows the information from the image in **Figures 28** and **29**, with the original image in the intensity plane, the smoothed brightness values in the hue plane, and the texture information from the variance operator in the saturation plane of a color image.

Figure 30. Histograms of the individual images in Figure 29c (average or smoothed brightness) and 29d (variance as a measure of texture) and the two way histogram of the pixels showing the separation of the four regions.

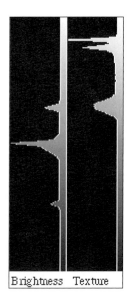

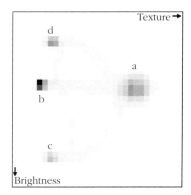

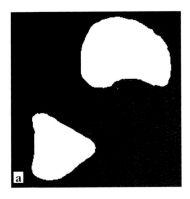
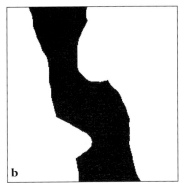

*Figure 31. Thresholding of
images in Figure 29:*
a) selecting intermediate
brightness values (regions *a*
and *b*);
b) selecting only region *b* by its
brightness AND texture.

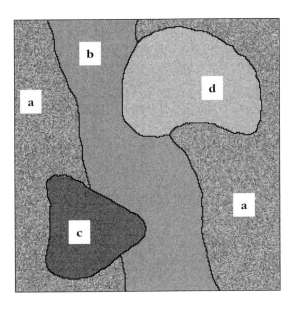

Figure 32. Result of segmenting
Figure 28 by thresholding on
the two-dimensional
histogram, or by ANDing
binary images thresholded
individually.

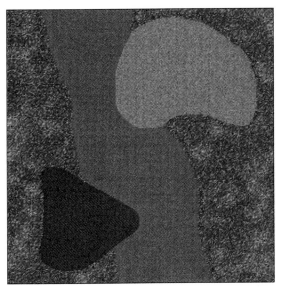

Figure 33. Multiband coding of
data from the image in
Figure 28. The intensity plane
shows the original image, the
hue plane contains smoothed
brightness values, and the
saturation plane contains the
texture information from a
variance operator.

Figure 34. Texture thresholding of curds and whey:

a) original image;

b) application of the Haralick texture operator;

c) thresholding image **b** and applying an opening (erosion and dilation);

d) measuring feature area to select just the large regions (outlines superimposed on original).

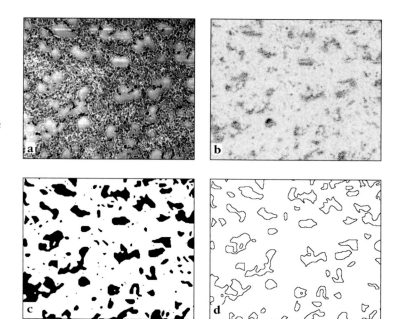

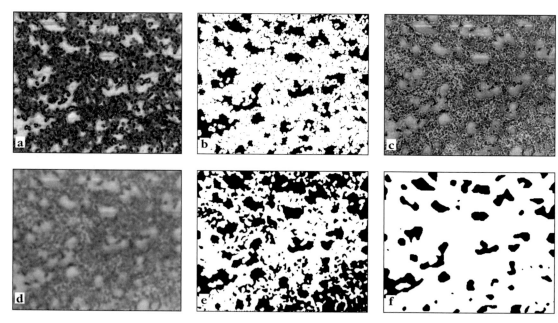

Figure 35. Texture and brightness thresholding of the curds and whey image from Figure 34:

a) range image;

b) thresholding image **a**;

c) leveled original image;

d) smoothing of image **c**;

e) thresholding image **d**;

f) Boolean AND of images **b** and **e**;

g) comparison of outlines from image **f** with those produced in Figure 34.

Figures **34** and **35** show an application of thresholding with two criteria, one of them texture, to a real image. The curds and whey image was used in Chapter 4 to show processing methods that respond to texture. Additional steps were needed to isolate just the curds (the large, light-colored, smooth areas), such as measurement of size and elimination of small features. **Figure 34** shows a typical procedure, using the Haralick texture operator, followed by thresholding, application of erosion and dilation, followed by area measurement and selection of the curds. In **Figure 35**, we instead apply two different thresholding criteria. The curds are smooth and bright, so these will be the criteria used for selection. The range image responds to the texture in the image, while smoothing the original image eliminates the texture and shows just the average brightness. Thresholding each of these images and then combining them with a Boolean AND (discussed in Chapter 7) to select pixels that are both bright and have a low texture, selects the curds.

Textural orientation

Figure 36 shows another test image containing regions having different textural orientations but identical mean brightness, brightness distribution, and spatial scale of the local variation. This rather subtle texture is evident in a two-dimensional frequency transform, as shown in **Figure 37a**. The three ranges of spatial-domain orientation are revealed in the three spokes in the transform.

Using a selective wedge-shaped mask with smoothed edges to select each of the spokes and retransform the image produces the three spatial-domain images shown in **Figure 37**. Each texture orientation in the original image is isolated, having a uniform grey

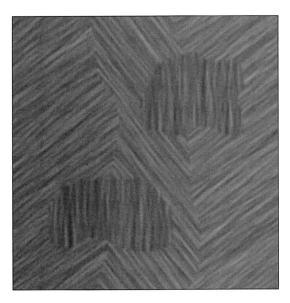

Figure 36. An image containing regions that have different textural orientations, but the same average brightness, standard deviation and spatial scale.

Figure 37. Isolating the directional texture in frequency space:

a) two-dimensional frequency transform of the image in Figure 32, showing the radial spokes corresponding to each textural alignment;

b, c, & d) retransformation using masks to select each of the orientations.

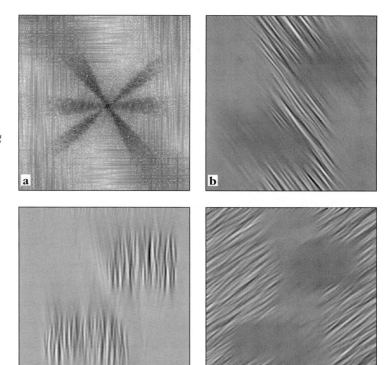

background in other locations. These images cannot be directly thresholded because the brightness values in the textured regions cover a range that includes the surroundings. Applying a range operator to a 5×5-pixel octagonal neighborhood, as shown in **Figure 38**, suppresses the uniform background regions and highlights the individual texture regions.

Thresholding these images and applying a closing operation (a dilation followed by an erosion, as discussed in Chapter 7) to fill in internal gaps and smooth boundaries, produces images of each region. **Figure 39** shows the composite result. Notice that the edges of the image are poorly delineated, a consequence of the inability of the frequency transform to preserve edge details, as discussed in Chapter 5. Also, the boundaries of the regions

Figure 38. *Application of a range operator to the images in Figure 37 b, c, and d.*

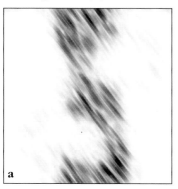
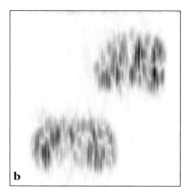
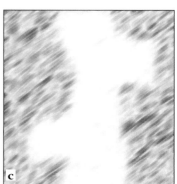

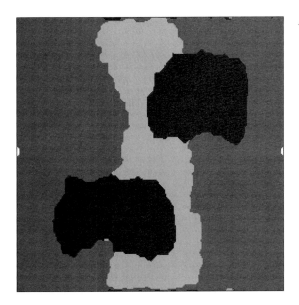

Figure 39. Regions from Figure 36 selected by thresholding the images in Figure 38.

are rather irregular and only approximately rendered in this result.

In many cases, spatial-domain processing is preferred for texture orientation. **Figure 40** shows the result from applying a Sobel operator to the image, as discussed in Chapter 4. Two directional first derivatives in the x and y directions are obtained using a 3×3 neighborhood operator. These are then combined using the arc tangent function to obtain an angle that is the direction of maximum brightness gradient. The resulting angle is scaled to fit the 0 to 255 brightness range of the image.

The brightness histogram shown in **Figure 40** shows six peaks. These occur in pairs 180 degrees apart, since in each texture

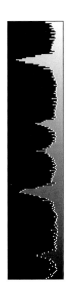
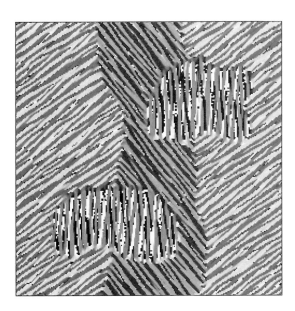

Figure 40. Application of the Sobel operator to the image in Figure 36, calculating the orientation of the gradient at each pixel by assigning a grey level to the arc tangent of $(\partial B/\partial y)/(\partial B/\partial x)$. The brightness histogram shows six peaks, in pairs for each principal textural orientation, since the directions are complementary.

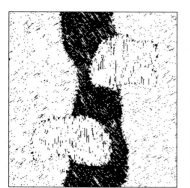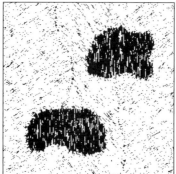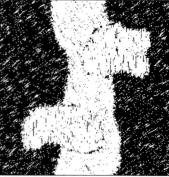

Figure 41. *Thresholding binary images from Figure 40, selecting the grey values corresponding to each pair of complementary directions (or performing two separate thresholds and ORing the results).*

region the direction of maximum gradient may lie in either of two opposite directions. This image can be reduced to three directions in several ways. One is to use a grey scale LUT, as discussed in Chapter 4, which assigns the same grey scale values to the highest and lowest halves of the original brightness (or angle) range, followed by thresholding the single peak for each direction. A second method is to set two different threshold ranges on the paired peaks and then combine the two resulting binary images using a Boolean OR operation (see Chapter 7). A third approach is to set a multiple-threshold range on the two complementary peaks. All of these are functionally equivalent.

Figure 41 shows the results of three thresholding operations to select each of the three textural orientations. There is some noise in these images, consisting of white pixels within the dark regions and vice versa, but these are much fewer and smaller than in the case of thresholding the results from the frequency-transform method shown above. After applying a closing operation (a dila-

Figure 42. *Outlines showing the regions defined by applying a closing (dilation and erosion) operation to each of the images in Figure 41.*

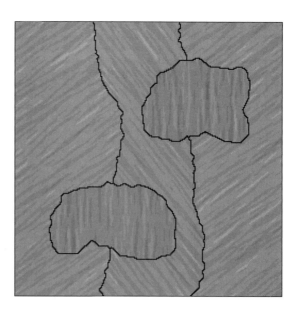

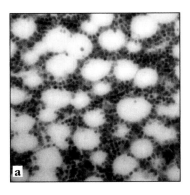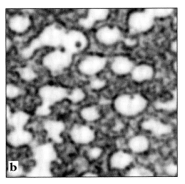

Figure 43. Light microscope image of bone marrow (*a*) and the result of applying a variance operator to characterize the texture in the image (*b*).

tion followed by an erosion, as discussed in Chapter 7), the regions are well delineated, as shown by the superposition of the outlines on the original image (**Figure 42**). This result is superior to the frequency transform and has smoother boundaries, better agreement with the visual judgment of location, and no problems at the image edges.

A more concrete example of the use of texture is shown in **Figure 43**. This is a light microscope image of bone marrow with a second image of the same area produced by applying a variance operator, as discussed in Chapter 4. The variance operator responds to the local texture in the image, rather than absolute brightness. **Figure 44** shows the individual histograms of the two images and the two-dimensional histogram of pixel values in both images.

Simple thresholding on the bright pixels in the original image does not select the large white areas, because the small spaces between the dark cells are equally bright (**Figure 45**). However,

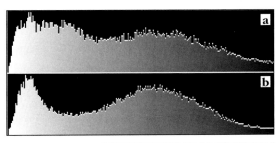
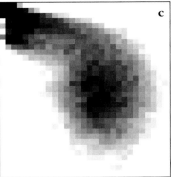

Figure 44. Brightness histograms (*a* and *b*) for the images in Figure 43, and the two-dimensional histogram showing the frequency of pairs of values of brightness (vertical) and texture (horizontal) for pixels at the same location in both images (*c*).

Figure 45. *Binary image produced by thresholding Figure 43a to select white areas.*

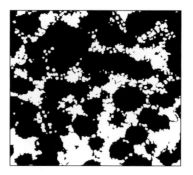

these regions are also low in texture (relatively smooth in appearance, with little local change in brightness).

Thresholding on the texture image and combining that result with the binary image from **Figure 45** produces a better representation, as shown in **Figure 46a**. This is equivalent to selecting pixels whose brightness and texture values fall within a rectangle in the texture/brightness histogram. Selecting a nonrectangular region in that plane produces an improved result, as shown in **Figure 46b**. Additional examples of thresholding a derived texture image to produce a binary image are shown in Chapter 4.

Figure 47 shows another example, a metallographic sample with a lamellar structure. This requires several steps to segment into the various regions. Brightness thresholding can delineate one region directly. Applying the Sobel orientation operator produces an image that can be thresholded to delineate the other two regions, but as before each region has pairs of grey scale values that are 180 degrees or 128 grey values apart. This requires setting two threshold ranges and combining the selected pixels with a Boolean OR operation.

Accuracy and reproducibility

In one or more dimensions, the selection of threshold values discussed so far has been manual. An operator interactively sets the cutoff values so that the resulting image is visually satisfying and the correspondence between what the user sees in the image and the pixels the thresholds select is as close as possible. This

Figure 46. Two-dimensional thresholding to select regions in Figure 43:

a) *ANDing together binary images selected by thresholding the two images individually;*

b) *using a nonrectangular threshold region directly on the two-dimensional histogram.*

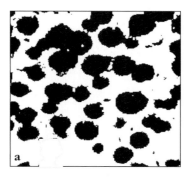
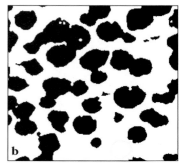

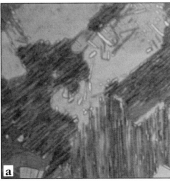

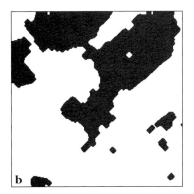

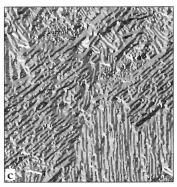

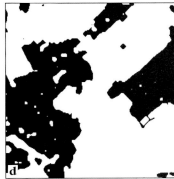

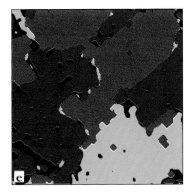

Figure 47. Thresholding on multiple criteria:

a) *original metallographic image;*

b) *one region selected by brightness thresholding (closing applied as discussed in Chapter 7);*

c) *Sobel orientation operator applied;*

d) *region selected by combining two thresholding angle values (closing applied);*

e) *final segmentation result with regions arbitrarily color coded.*

is not always consistent from one operator to another, or even for the same person over a period of time. The difficulty and variability of thresholding represents a serious source of error for further image analysis.

There are two slightly different requirements for setting threshold values. Both have to do with the typical use of binary images for feature measurement. One is to achieve reproducibility, so that variations due to the operator, lighting, etc. do not affect the results. The second goal of setting threshold values is to achieve accurate boundary delineation. For quality-control work, as one example, this latter requirement of accuracy is somewhat less important than precision.

Since pixel-based images represent at best an approximation to the continuous real scene being represented, and since thresholding classifies each pixel as either part of the foreground or the background, only a certain level of accuracy can be achieved. An alternate representation of features based on the boundary line can be more accurate. This is a polygon with many sides and corner points defined as x,y coordinates of arbitrary accuracy, as compared to the comparatively coarse pixel spacing.

The boundary-line representation is superior for accurate measurement because the line itself has no width. However, determining the line is far from easy. The location of individual points can be determined by interpolation between pixels, perhaps fitting mathematical functions to pixels on either side of the boundary to improve the results. This type of approach is commonly used in metrology applications, such as measuring dimensions of microelectronic circuit elements on silicon wafers. This type of application goes beyond the typical image processing operations dealt with in this text.

Thresholding produces a pixel-based representation of the image that assigns each pixel to either the feature(s) or the surroundings. The finite size of the pixels allows the representation only a finite accuracy, but we would prefer to have no bias in the result. This means that performing the same operation on many repeated images of the same scene should produce an average result that approaches the true value for size or other feature measurements. This is not necessary for quality-control applications in which reproducibility is of greater concern than accuracy, and some bias (as long as it is consistent) can be tolerated.

Many things can contribute to bias in setting thresholds. Human operators are not very good at setting threshold levels without bias. In most cases, they are more tolerant of settings that include additional pixels from the background region along with the features than they are of settings that exclude some pixels from the features. They are also not particularly consistent at choosing a brightness value for the threshold that is midway between two levels characteristic of feature and background. This is particularly true if the brightness scale is not logarithmic, either because of the detector or camera response, or prior image processing.

As indicated at the beginning of this chapter, the brightness histogram from the image is an important tool for setting threshold levels. In many cases, it will show distinct and separated peaks from the various phases or structures present in the field of view, or it can be made to do so by prior image processing steps. In this case, it seems that setting the threshold level midway between the peaks should produce consistent, and perhaps even accurate, results.

Unfortunately, this idea is easier to state than to accomplish. In many real images, the peaks corresponding to particular structures are not perfectly symmetrical or ideally sharp, particularly when there may be shading either of the entire image or within the features (e.g., a brightness gradient from center to edge). Changing the field of view or even the illumination may cause the peak to shift and/or to change shape. Nonlinear camera response or automatic gain circuits can further distort the brightness histogram. If the area fraction of the image that is the bright (or dark) phase changes from one field of view to another, some method is needed to maintain a threshold setting that adapts to these changes and preserves precision and accuracy.

If the peaks are consistent and well-defined, then choosing an arbitrary location at some fixed fraction of the distance between them is a rapid method often satisfactory for quality-control

Figure 48. *Example of finite pixels straddling a boundary line, with brightness values that average those of the two sampled regions.*

work. In many cases, it is necessary to consider the pixels whose brightness values lie between the peaks in the brightness histogram. In most instances, these are pixels that straddle the boundary and have averaged together the two principal brightness levels in proportion to the area subtended within the pixel, as indicated in **Figure 48**.

Asymmetric boundaries (for example, a metallographic specimen in which etching has attacked the softer of two phases so that the boundary is skewed) can introduce bias in these brightness values. So can prior processing steps, such as those responding to texture in the image. Many of these operations work on a finite and perhaps rather large neighborhood, so the boundary position becomes somewhat uncertain. If the processing operation responds nonlinearly to differences, as the variance operator does, the apparent boundary location will shift toward the most different pixel in the neighborhood.

Including position information

The histogram display shows only the frequency of occurrence of different values and does not preserve any information about position, the brightness of neighboring pixels, and other factors. Yet it is this spatial information that is important for determining boundary location. It is possible, in principle, to build a co-occurrence matrix for the image in which all possible combinations of pixel brightness are counted in terms of the distance between them. This information is used to select the pixels that are part of the feature instead of simply the pixel brightness values, but this is equivalent to a processing operation that uses the same co-occurrence matrix to construct a texture image for which simple thresholding can be used.

Another possible algorithm for threshold settings is to pick the minimum point in the histogram (**Figure 49**). This should correspond to the value that affects the fewest pixels and thus gives the lowest expected error in pixel classification when the image is segmented into features and background. The difficulty is that because this region of the histogram is (hopefully) very low, with

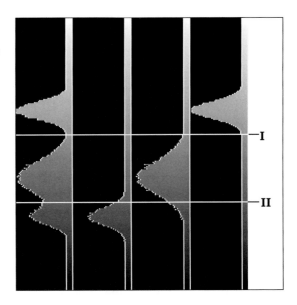

Figure 49. An example histogram from a specimen with three distinct regions. The minimum at level I cleanly separates the two peaks, while the one at level II does not because the brightness values in the two regions have variations that overlap.

few pixels having these values, the counting statistics are poor and the shape of the curve in the histogram is poorly defined. Consequently, the minimum value is hard to locate and may move about considerably with only tiny changes in overall illumination, a change in the field of view to include objects with a different shape, or more or fewer pixels along the boundary.

Figure 50 shows an image having two visibly obvious regions. Each contains a Gaussian noise pattern with the same standard deviation but a different mean, though the brightness values in the two regions overlap. This means that setting a threshold value at the minimum between the two peaks causes some pixels in each region to be misclassified, as shown in the figure.

This type of image often results from situations in which the total number of photons or other signals is low and counting statistics cause a variation in the brightness of pixels in uniform areas. Counting statistics produce a Poisson distribution, but when moderately large numbers are involved, this is very close to the more convenient Gaussian function used in these images. For

Figure 50. A test image containing two regions whose mean brightness levels are different, but which have variations in individual pixels that overlap:

a) original image (enlarged to show pixels);

b) result of setting a simple threshold at the minimum point.

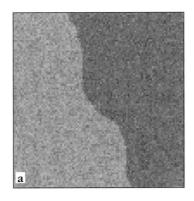
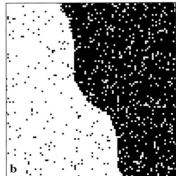

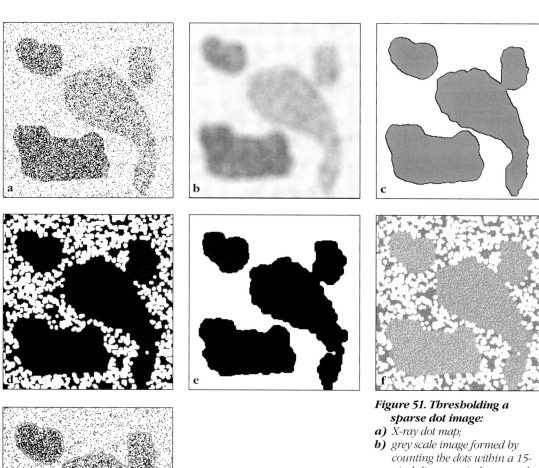

Figure 51. Thresholding a sparse dot image:

a) X-ray dot map;

b) grey scale image formed by counting the dots within a 15-pixel-diameter circle centered on each pixel;

c) boundary determined by thresholding image *b* at 4 standard deviations above the mean background level;

d) application of a closing operation (dilation followed by erosion) to fill the gaps between closely spaced pixels in image *a*;

e) application of an opening operation (erosion followed by dilation) to remove small dark regions in the background in image *d*;

f) overlay of the opening and closing operations with color coding to show the original dots (green), the pixels added by closing (red), and those subsequently removed by opening (blue);

g) comparison of the feature outlines determined by the smoothing and thresholding (red) vs. closing and opening (blue) methods.

extremely noisy images, such as X-ray dot maps from the SEM, some additional processing in the spatial domain may be required before attempting thresholding (O'Callaghan, 1974).

Figure 51 shows a typical sparse dot map. Most of the pixels contain 0 counts, and a few contain 1 count. The boundaries in the image are visually evident, but their exact location is at best approximate, requiring the human visual computer to group the dots together. Image processing can do this by counting the number of dots in a circular neighborhood around each pixel. Convolution with a kernel consisting of 1's in a 15-pixel-diameter circle accomplishes this, producing the result shown. This grey scale image can be thresholded to locate the boundaries shown, but there are inadequate data to decide whether the small regions, voids, and irregularities in the boundaries are real or simply due to the limited counting statistics. Typically, the threshold level will be set by determining the mean brightness level in the background region, and then setting the threshold several standard deviations above this to select just the significant regions.

The figure compares this approach to one based on the binary editing operations discussed in Chapter 7. Both require making some assumptions about the image. In the smoothing and thresholding case, some knowledge about the statistical meaning of the data is required. For X-rays, the standard deviation in the count rate is known to vary in proportion to the square root of the number of counts, which is the brightness in the smoothed image. Erosion and dilation are based on assumptions about the distances between dots in the image. Closing (dilation followed by erosion) fills in the gaps between dots to create solid areas corresponding to the features, as shown in **Figure 51d**. In the background regions, this does not produce a continuous dark region and so an opening (erosion followed by dilation) can remove it (**Figure 51e**). Adding and then removing pixels produces the final result shown. The boundaries are slightly different from those produced by smoothing and thresholding, but the original image does not contain enough data to distinguish between them.

Several possible approaches may be used to improve the segmentation of noisy regions, using **Figure 50** as a test case. Chapter 7 discusses binary image editing operations, including morphological processing. The sequence of a dilation followed by an erosion, known as a closing, fills holes, erases isolated pixels, and smooths the boundary line to produce the result shown in **Figure 52a**. By contrast, a much more complicated operation reassigns pixels from one region to the other to achieve minimum entropy in both regions. Entropy methods are generally a very computer-intensive approach to image restoration when a blur function is known. They function to improve degraded grey scale images, as discussed in Chapter 3.

In this case, the collection of pixels into two regions can be described as an entropy problem as follows (Kanpur et al., 1985):

Figure 52. The boundary in the image of Figure 50:

a) Thresholding at the minimum point in the histogram followed by closing (dilation and erosion);

b) Iteratively setting the minimum entropy point.

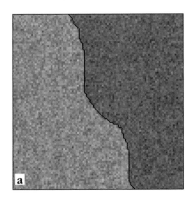
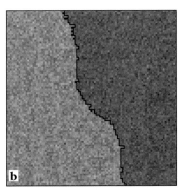

The total entropy in each region is calculated as $-\Sigma p_i \log_e p_i$, where p_i is the number of pixels having brightness i. Solving for the boundary that classifies each pixel into one of two groups to minimize this function for the two regions (subject to the constraint that the pixels in each region must touch each other) produces the boundary line shown in **Figure 52b**. Additional constraints, such as minimizing the number of touching pixels in different classes, would smooth the boundary. The problem is that such constraints are ad hoc, make the solution of the problem very difficult, and can usually be applied more efficiently in other ways (for instance by smoothing the binary image).

Setting a threshold value at the minimum in the histogram is sometimes described as selecting for minimum area sensitivity in the value (Weszka, 1978; Wall et al., 1974). This means that changing the threshold value causes the least change in the feature (or background) area, although as noted above this says nothing about the spatial arrangement of the pixels that are thereby added to or removed from the features. Indeed, the definition of the histogram makes any minimum in the plot a point of minimum area sensitivity.

For the image shown in **Figure 50**, the histogram can be changed to produce a minimum that is deeper, broader, and has a more stable minimum value by processing the image. **Figure 53** shows the results of smoothing the image (using a Gaussian kernel with a standard deviation of 1 pixel) or applying a median filter (both methods are discussed in Chapters 3 and 4). The peaks are narrower and the valley is broader and deeper. The consequences for the image, and the boundary that is selected by setting the threshold level between the peaks, are shown in **Figure 54**.

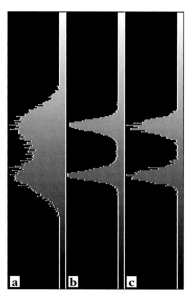

Figure 53. Histogram of the image in Figure 50:
a) *original, with overlapped peaks;*
b) *after smoothing;*
c) *after median filtering.*

Figure 54. Processing the image in Figure 50 to modify the histogram:

a) *Smoothing with a Gaussian kernel, standard deviation = 1 pixel;*

b) *The boundary produced by thresholding image **a**, superimposed on the original;*

c) *Median processing (iteratively applied until no further changes occurred);*

d) *The boundary produced by thresholding image **c**, superimposed on the original.*

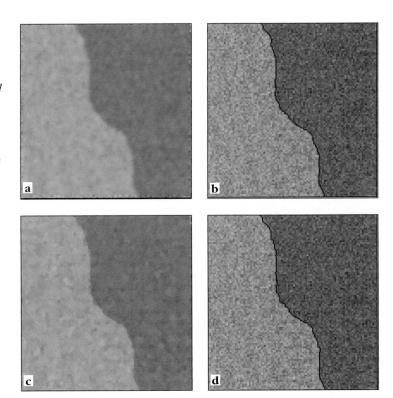

This seems not to be the criterion used by human operators, who can watch an image and interactively adjust a threshold value. Instead of the total area of features changing least with adjustment, which is difficult for humans to judge, we can instead use the total change in perimeter length around the features (Russ & Russ, 1988a). This may in fact be the criterion actually used by skilled operators. The variation in total perimeter length with respect to threshold value provides an objective criterion that can be efficiently calculated. The minimum in this response curve provides a way to set the thresholds that is reproducible, adapts to varying illumination, etc., and mimics to some extent the way humans set the values. For the case in which both upper and lower threshold levels are to be adjusted, this produces a response surface in two dimensions (the upper and lower values), which can be solved to find the minimum point as indicated in **Figure 55**.

Figure 55 shows an image whose brightness threshold has been automatically refined to minimize the variation in total boundary length. The brightness histogram shown in the figure has a very long valley between the two phase peaks, neither of which has a symmetric or Gaussian shape. The lowest point in the histogram does not necessarily correspond to the best threshold setting.

Figure 57 shows several plots derived from the histogram and image of **Figure 56**. Graphs plotting the area of the dark phase

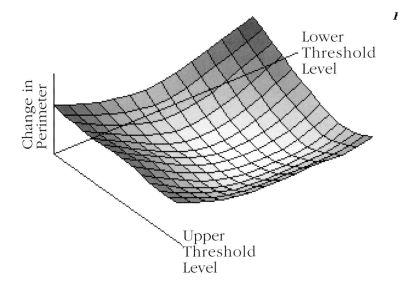

Change in Perimeter

Lower Threshold Level

Upper Threshold Level

Figure 55. *A two-way plot of the change in perimeter length vs. the settings of upper and lower level brightness thresholds. The minimum indicates the optimal settings.*

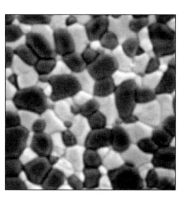

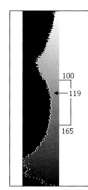

100

119

165

Figure 56. *A test image for automatic threshold adjustment, and its brightness histogram. The range from brightness values 100 through 165 is used in the plots of Figure 57.*

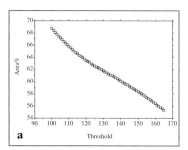

a

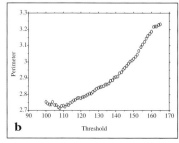

b

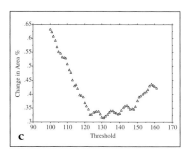

c

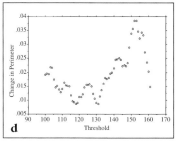

d

Figure 57. Plots of
a) *total area of the dark phase;*
b) *total boundary perimeter;*
c) *change in area; and*
d) *change in perimeter, for threshold settings from 100 to 165 on the image of Figure 56.*

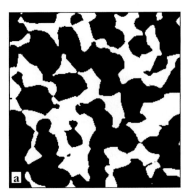
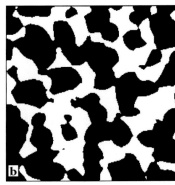

Figure 58. Binary images produced from Figure 56 by the application of thresholds at brightness levels of
a) *119 and*
b) *131, which are the minima in the plot of Figure 57d.*

vs. the threshold setting and the total boundary perimeter vs. the threshold setting are not helpful in finding an optimum or stable setting, but the derivatives of these curves are. The minimum point in the plot of change of area vs. setting occurs at a brightness value of 131. The two minima in the plot of change of perimeter vs. setting occur at 119 and 131. The two binary images produced by thresholding at these levels are shown in **Figure 58**. The 119 value appears to produce good representation of the phase boundaries, as shown in **Figure 59**.

Repeated measurements using this algorithm on many images of the same objects show that the reproducibility in the presence of finite image noise and changing illumination is rather good. Length variations for irregular objects varied less than 0.5%, or 1 pixel in 200 across the major diameter of the object.

Selective histograms

Most of the difficulties with selecting the optimum threshold brightness value between two peaks in a typical histogram arise from the intermediate brightness values of the histogram. These pixels lie along the boundaries of the two regions, so methods that eliminate them from the histogram will contain only peaks from the uniform regions and can be used to select the proper threshold value (Weszka & Rosenfeld, 1979; Milgram & Herman, 1979).

Figure 59. Superposition of the boundary selected with a threshold setting of 119 (minimum perimeter sensitivity) on the original image from Figure 56.

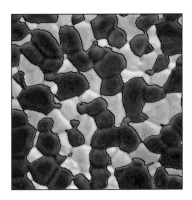

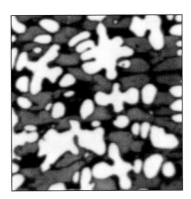

Figure 60. *A test image containing three visually distinct phase regions with different mean grey levels.*

One way to perform this selection is to use another derived image, such as the Sobel gradient or any of the other edge-finding operators discussed in Chapter 4. Pixels having a high gradient value can be eliminated from the histogram of the original image to reduce the background level in the range between the two phase peaks. **Figure 60** shows an example. The original image contains three phases with visually distinct grey levels.

Several methods can be used to eliminate edge pixels. A two-dimensional histogram of the original and gradient images is not a good choice here, because the coarser bins may distort the peak shape and reduce resolution in the histogram. Instead, it is more straightforward to threshold the gradient image, selecting pixels with a high value. This produces a binary image that can be used as a mask, as discussed in Chapter 7. This mask either restricts which pixels in the original image are to be used or replaces their brightness values with black or white so that they are effectively removed from the portion of the histogram to be analyzed.

As an example, using the image from **Figure 60**, the 20% of the pixels with the largest magnitude in the Sobel gradient image are selected by thresholding to produce a mask, which is used to remove those pixels from the original image (**Figure 61**). The result, shown in **Figure 62**, is the reduction of those portions of the histogram between peaks, with the peaks themselves little affected. This makes it easier to characterize the shapes of the peaks from the phases and select a consistent point between them.

Of course, this method requires setting a threshold on the gradient image to select the pixels to be bypassed. As shown in the example of **Figure 61**, this histogram rarely contains a peak, since the gradient magnitudes in the image vary widely. The most often used technique is simply to choose some fixed percentage of the pixels with the highest gradient value and eliminate them from the histogram of the original image.

In this case, however, the gradient operator responds more strongly to the larger difference between the white and grey

Figure 61.

a) *Application of a gradient operator (Sobel) to the image of Figure 60.*

b) *The histogram of the gradient does not show any useful structure.*

c) *Thresholding image **a** to select the 20% of the pixels with the largest gradient produces a mask which can be used*

d) *to eliminate many of the edge-straddling pixels in the original image.*

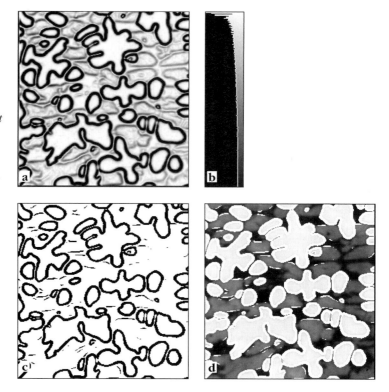

regions than to the smaller difference between the grey and dark regions. Hence the edge-straddling pixels (and their background in the histogram) are reduced much more between the white and grey peaks than between the grey and black peaks. **Figure 63** shows another method which alleviates the problem in this image. Beginning with a range image (the difference between the darkest and brightest pixels in a 5-pixel-wide octagonal neighborhood), nonmaximum suppression (also known as grey

Figure 62. *Brightness histograms from the original image in Figure 60 and the masked images in Figures 57d (mask 1) and 59d (mask 2), showing the reduction of number of pixels with brightness values in the ranges between the main peaks.*

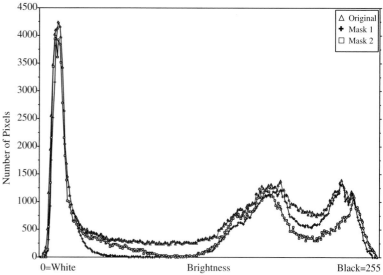

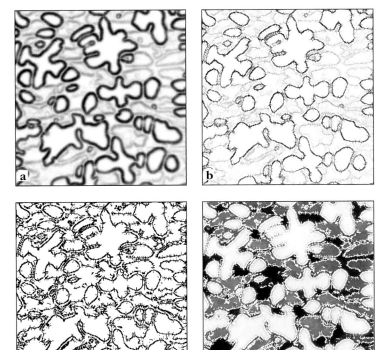

Figure 63. Another gradient mask for the image in Figure 60:

a) *Application of a 5-pixel wide octagonal range operator;*

b) *Nonmaximum suppression (grey scale skeletonization or ridge-finding) applied to image **a**;*

c) *Thresholding of image **b** to keep the darkest 20% of the pixels;*

d) *Masking of original image with image **c**.*

scale skeletonization, or ridge-finding) is used to narrow the boundaries and eliminate pixels that are not actually on the boundary. Then thresholding is used to select the darkest 20% of the remaining pixels to form a mask, which is applied to the original image.

The plot of the resulting histogram, also in **Figure 62**, shows a much greater suppression of the valley between the grey and black peaks. Since the same total fraction of pixels has been removed, this also affects the background near the white peak. All of these methods are somewhat ad hoc; the particular combination of different region brightnesses present in an image will dictate what edge-finding operation will work best and what fraction of the pixels should be removed.

Boundary lines

One of the shortcomings of thresholding is that the pixels are selected primarily by brightness, and only secondarily by location. This means that there is no requirement for regions to be continuous. Instead of defining a region as a collection of pixels whose brightness values are similar in one or more images, an alternate definition can be based on a boundary.

Manually outlining regions for measurement is one way to use this approach. Various interactive pointing devices, such as graphics tablets, touch screens, mice, or light pens, may be used and the drawing may take place while the viewer looks at the computer screen, at a photographic print on a tablet, or through the microscope, with the pointer device optically superimposed. None of these methods is without problems. Video displays have rather limited resolution. Drawing on the image in a microscope does not provide a record of where you have been. Mice are clumsy pointing devices, light pens lose precision in dark areas of the display, touch screens have poor resolution (and your finger gets in the way), and so on.

It is beyond our purpose here to describe the operation or compare the utility of these different approaches. Regardless of what physical device is used for manual outlining, the method relies on the human visual image processor to locate boundaries and produces a result that consists of a polygonal approximation to the region outline. Most people tend to draw just outside the actual boundary, making dimensions larger than they should be, and the amount of error is a function of the contrast at the edge. (There are exceptions to this, of course. Some people draw inside the boundary. But bias is commonly present in manually drawn outlines.)

Attempts to emulate the human outlining operation with a computer algorithm require a starting point, usually provided by the human. Then the program examines each adjoining pixel to find which has the characteristics of a boundary, usually defined as a step in brightness. Whichever pixel has the highest value of local gradient is selected and added to the growing polygon, and then the procedure is repeated. Sometimes a constraint is added to minimize sharp turns, such as weighting the pixel values according to direction.

Automatic edge following suffers from several problems. First, the edge definition is essentially local. People have a rather adaptable capability to look ahead various distances to find pieces of edge to be connected together. Gestalt psychologists describe this as grouping. Such a response is difficult for an algorithm that looks only within a small neighborhood. Even in rather simple images, there may be places along boundaries where the local gradient or other measure of edgeness drops.

In addition, edges may touch where regions abut. The algorithm is equally likely to follow either edge, which of course gives a nonsensical result. There may also be a problem of when to end the process. If the edge is a single, simple line, then it ends when it reaches the starting point. If the line reaches another feature that already has a defined boundary (from a previous application of the routine) or if it reaches the edge of the field of view, then there is no way to complete the outline.

The major problems with edge following are: a) it cannot by itself complete the segmentation of the image because it has to be given each new starting point and cannot determine whether there are more outlines to be followed and b) the same edge-defining

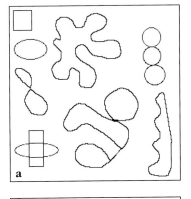
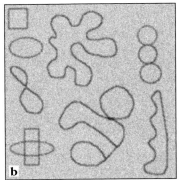

Figure 64. Test image for automatic line following:

a) *hand-drawn lines;*

b) *addition of random noise to a;*

c) *lines found by automatic tracing, showing the starting points for each (notice that some portions of crossing or branching line patterns are not followed);*

d) *lines found by thresholding and skeletonization.*

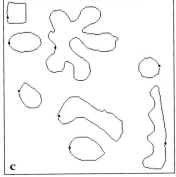
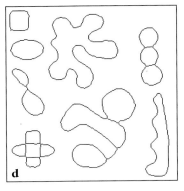

criteria used for following edges can be applied more easily by processing the entire image and then thresholding. This produces a line of pixels that may be broken and incomplete (if the edge following would have been unable to continue) or may branch (if several boundaries touch). However, there are methods discussed in Chapter 7 that apply erosion/dilation logic to deal with some of these deficiencies. The global application of the processing operation finds all of the boundaries.

Figure 64 illustrates a few of these effects. The image consists of several hand-drawn dark lines, to which a small amount of random noise is added and a ridge-following algorithm applied (Van Helden, 1994). Each of the user-selected starting points is shown with the path followed by the automatic routine. The settings used for this example instruct the algorithm to consider points out to a distance of 5 pixels in deciding which direction to move in at each point. Increasing this number produces artificially smooth boundaries, and also takes more time as more neighbors must be searched. Conversely, reducing it makes it more likely to follow false turnings. Many of the paths are successful, but a significant number are not. By comparison, thresholding the image to select dark pixels, and then skeletonizing the resulting broad outline as discussed in Chapter 7, produces good boundary lines for all of the regions at once.

The same comparison can be made with a real image. **Figure 65** shows a fluorescence image from a light microscope. In this

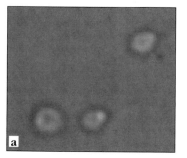

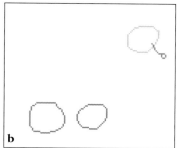

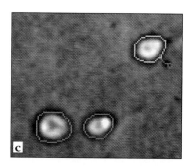

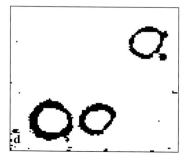

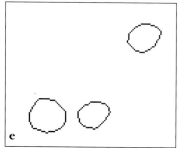

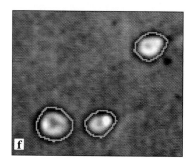

Figure 65. Light microscope fluorescence image with three features:

a) original;

b) edge-following algorithm (blue shows fully automatic results, purple shows a feature that required manual assistance to outline);

c) outlines from b superimposed on the original;

d) brightness thresholding the original image;

e) skeletonized outlines from figure d;

f) outlines from e superimposed on the original.

case, the inability of the fully automatic ridge-following method to track the boundaries has been supplemented by a manually assisted technique. The user draws a line near the boundary, and the algorithm moves the points onto the nearest (within some preset maximum distance) darkest point. This allows the user to overcome many of the difficulties in which the automatic method may wander away from the correct line, never to return. But it is still faster to use thresholding and skeletonizing to get the boundary lines, and while the details of the lines differ, it is not evident that either method is consistently superior for delineation.

Contours

One type of line that may provide boundary information and is guaranteed to be continuous is a contour line. This is analogous to the isoelevation contour lines drawn on topographic maps. The line marks a constant elevation, or in our case a constant brightness in the image. These lines cannot end, although they may branch or loop back upon themselves. In a continuous image or an actual topographic surface, there is always a point through which the line can pass. For a discrete image, the brightness value of the line may not happen to correspond to any specific pixel value. Nevertheless, if there is a pair of pixels with one value brighter than and one value darker than the contour level, then the line must pass somewhere between them.

The contour line can, in principle, be fit as a polygon through the points interpolated between pixel centers for all such pairs of pixels that bracket the contour value. This actually permits measuring the locations of these lines, and the boundaries that they may represent, to less than the dimensions of one pixel, called subpixel sampling or measurement. This is rarely done for an entire image because of the amount of work involved and the difficulty in representing the boundary by such a series of points, which must be assembled into a polygon.

Instead, the most common use of contour lines is to mark the pixels that lie closest to, or closest to and above, the line. These pixels approximate the contour line to the resolution of the pixels in the original image, form a continuous band of touching pixels (touching in an 8-neighbor sense, as discussed below), and can be used to delineate features in many instances. Creating the line from the image is simply a matter of scanning the pixels once, comparing each pixel and its neighbors above and to the left to the contour value, and marking the pixel if the values are above or below the test value.

Figure 66 shows a grey scale image with several contour lines, drawn at arbitrarily chosen brightness values, marked on the histogram. Notice that setting a threshold range at this same brightness level, even with a fairly large range, does not produce a continuous line, because the brightness gradient in some regions is quite steep and no pixels fall within the range. The brightness gradient is very gradual in other regions, so a gradient image (**Figure 67**) obtained from the same original by applying a Sobel operator does not show all of the same boundaries.

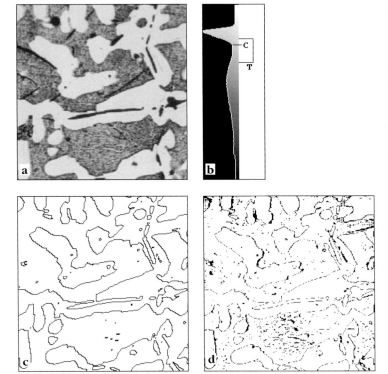

Figure 66. Cast iron (light micrograph) with ferrite (white) and graphite (black):

a) *original image;*

b) *brightness histogram showing levels used for contour (C) and threshold (T);*

c) *contour lines drawn using the value shown in **b**;*

d) *pixels selected by the threshold setting shown in **b**.*

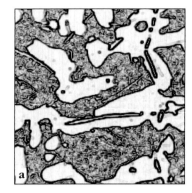

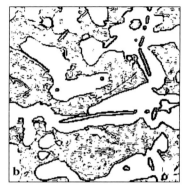

Figure 67. *Gradient image obtained by applying a Sobel operator to Figure 66 (**a**), and the pixels selected by thresholding the 20% darkest (highest gradient) values (**b**).*

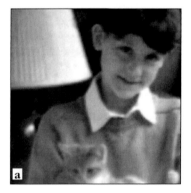

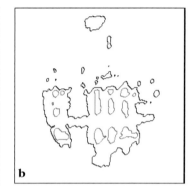

Figure 68. Ion microprobe image of boron implanted in a silicon wafer:

a) *original image, in which brightness is proportional to concentration;*

b) *two iso-brightness or iso-concentration contour values which make it easier to compare values in different parts of the image.*

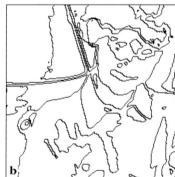

Figure 69. *Real-world image (**a**) and four contour lines drawn at selected brightness values (**b**). However irregular they become, the lines are always continuous and distinct.*

Drawing a series of contour lines on an image can be an effective way to show minor variations in brightness, as shown in **Figure 68**. Converting an image to a series of contour lines (**Figure 69**) is equivalent to creating a topographic map. Indeed, such a set of lines is a topographic map for a range image, in which the brightness values of pixels are their elevations. Such images may result from radar imaging, the CSLM, interferometry, the STM or AFM, and other devices.

They may also be produced by surface elevation measurements, as shown in **Figure 70**. This image has elevation contours cal-

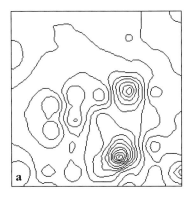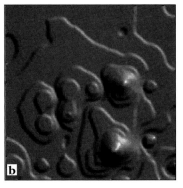

Figure 70. Elevation contour map from a range image *(a)* in which pixel brightness represents surface elevation, and a reconstructed and rendered view of the surface *(b)* as discussed in Chapters 10 and 11.

culated from stereo pair views of a specimen in the TEM, in which the "mountains" are deposited contamination spots. The information from the contour lines can be used to generate a rendered surface as shown in the figure and discussed in Chapters 10 and 11, to illustrate the surface topography.

Figure 71 shows an image containing features to be measured. The contours drawn by selecting a brightness value provide the same outline information as the edge pixels in regions determined by thresholding with the same value. The contour lines can be filled in to provide a pixel representation of the feature, using the logic discussed in Chapter 7. Conversely, the solid regions can be converted to an outline by a different set of binary image processes.

Figure 71. Selection of features in an image:

a) light micrograph of a cross section of a coating on a metal;

b) outlines of particles and voids obtained by setting a contour level;

c) features or regions obtained by thresholding with the same brightness value as in **b**;

d) regions obtained by automatically filling the boundaries from **b**;

e) outlines obtained by taking the custer of **c**.

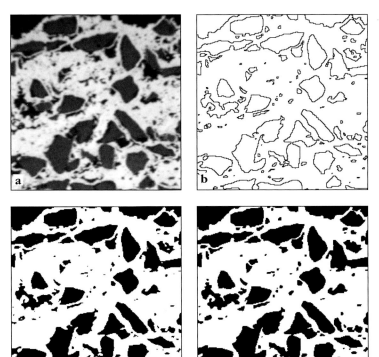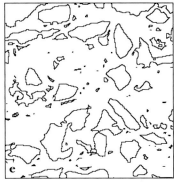

If the contour line is defined by pixel values, the information is identical to the thresholded regions. If subpixel interpolation has been used, then the resolution of the features may be better. The two formats for image representation are entirely complementary, although they have different advantages for storage, measurement, etc.

Image representation

Different representations of the binary image are possible; some are more useful than others for specific purposes. Most measurements, such as feature area and position, can be directly calculated from a pixel-based representation by simple counting procedures. This can be stored in less space than the original array of pixels by using run-length encoding (also called chord encoding). This treats the image as a series of scan lines. For each sequential line across each region or feature, it stores the line number, start position, and length of the line. **Figure 72** illustrates this schematically.

For typical images, the pixels are not randomly scattered, but collected together into regions or features so that the run-length encoded table is much smaller than the original image. This is the method used, for instance, to transmit fax messages over telephone lines. **Figure 73** shows how a black and white image is encoded for this purpose. In this example, the original image is 256×256 = 65,536 pixels, while the run-length table is only 1460 bytes long. The run-length table can be used directly for area

Figure 72. Encoding the same region in a binary image by run-length encoding, boundary polygonal representation, or chain code.

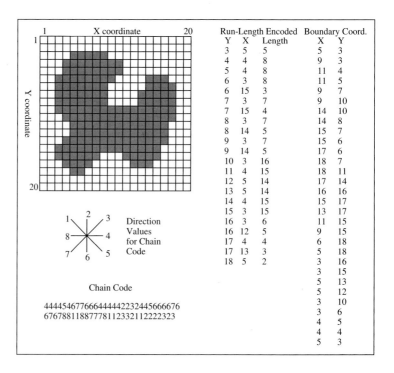

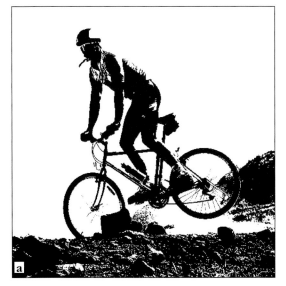

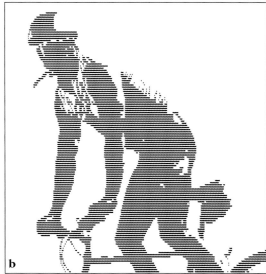

```
                gN̄
              N̄$H̄W
               NNN
              H$NN̄N̄
        /  #WNN$N̄qi
          $M#$NqN̄N$_
          NNWNN$NNNM̄_
          NW  ^N@NNNNN̄
          NN   N  NNNN$
          NW   N  NNNg$
          N'   N ,NNNN̄$gN
          $    g@NNNNN#$NN
       N$  NW̄  NNNNNL[W
       TW@@   NN  NNgJ̄
        ]^g__$NpwW̄$N(/ _wN#p̄_       =g
           W̄   NN  NNNJ$"  W̄p _gN̄N$N̄
          M̄Y9_#aN̄$  NL"$N,      ^ApN̄NNNNN
        _MNH$_ 9H$I # ]Ng6b . _HNNNNNNNN
     N̄"   $F$_   WNp$_NNNNMM̄$_N̄NNNNNNNNN
     N"     r #N̄  gNN̄N@NNW"]$8_]NNNNNNNNN
     N       0rN̄NNNN@ $,.L+W̄%4N$$NNNNNNN
     $    #F̄   _A_^ ^"  Nm_ 'gN̄A@NMENg#
     N    . gN̄N̄Ng$g'    ^W̄wwW̄" A$MONCĪ@
     NL       NNNNNNN̄MA_A              7
       Ng_ pNNN@hZNN$$̄       g=N̄N̄p=ggNN̄gN̄
N̄N̄NgN@NHNN̄N̄W̄H$$@@NNNNNNN̄NN̄N̄N̄N̄N̄NNNNNNNNNNN
NNNNNNMNNMNN$NMM$HMN$9$NN$NHNN$N$NN$N$I@
NNNNNN$NNNN#$NHNNg@MNNNNNNNNNN$NN@#KM@NNNN
ⁿNNNN$+g_MHMNN$$N̄N$W̄$N$$NNN#N$$$HN@$NN$N
ⁿₙNNN$$$HN̄$MNMMNNNNN$N$$NN$NMAM$HNN$NHN$N
```

Figure 73. Representing a black-and-white image for fax transmission:

a) *original;*

b) *run-length encoded (each horizontal line is marked with a red point at its start; just the position of the red point and the length of the line are sent);*

c) *representing the same image with formed characters, a trick commonly used two decades ago.*

and position measurements, with even less arithmetic than the pixel array. Since the chords are in the order in which the raster crosses the features, some logic is required to identify the chords with the features, but this is often done as the table is built.

The chord table is poorly suited for measuring feature perimeters or shape. Boundary representation, consisting of the coordinates of the polygon comprising the boundary, is superior for this task. However, it is awkward for dealing with regions containing internal holes, since there is nothing to relate the interior boundary to the exterior. Again, logic must be used to identify the internal boundaries, keep track of which ones are exterior and which are interior, and construct a hierarchy of features within features, if needed.

A simple polygonal approximation to the boundary can be produced when it is needed from the run-length table by using the end points of the series of chords, as shown in **Figure 72**. A special form of this polygon can be formed from all of the boundary points, consisting of a series of short vectors from one boundary point to the next. On a square pixel array, each of these lines is either 1 or $\sqrt{2}$ pixels long and can only have 1 of 8 directions. Assigning a digit from 0 to 7 (or 1 to 8) to each direction and writing all of the numbers for the closed boundary in order produces chain code, also shown in **Figure 72**.

This form is particularly well-suited for calculating perimeter or describing shape (Freeman, 1961, 1974; Cederberg, 1979). The perimeter is determined by counting the number of even and odd digits, multiplying the number of odd ones by $\sqrt{2}$ to correct for diagonal directions, and adding. The chain code also contains shape information, which can be used to locate corners, simplify the shape of the outline, match features independent of orientation, or calculate various shape descriptors. These measurement techniques are beyond the scope of this text.

Most current-generation imaging systems use an array of square pixels, because it is well suited both to raster-scan acquisition devices and to processing images and performing measurements. If rectangular pixels are acquired by using a different pixel spacing along scan lines than between the lines, processing in either the spatial domain with neighborhood operations or in the frequency domain becomes much more difficult, because the different pixel distances as a function of orientation must be taken into account. The use of rectangular pixels also impedes measurements.

With a square pixel array, there is a minor problem that we have already seen in the previous chapters on image processing: the four pixels diagonally adjacent to a central pixel are actually farther away than the four sharing an edge. An alternative arrangement that has been used in a few systems is to place the pixels in a hexagonal array. This has the advantage of equal spacing between all neighboring pixels, which simplifies processing and calculations. Its great disadvantage, however, is that standard cameras and other acquisition devices do not operate that way.

For a traditional square pixel array, it is necessary to decide whether pixels adjacent at a corner are actually touching. This will be important for the binary processing operations in Chapter 7. It is necessary in order to link pixels into features or follow the points around a boundary, as discussed above. While it is not evident whether one choice is superior to the other, whichever one is made, the background (the pixels which surround the features) must have the opposite relationship.

Figure 74 shows this dual situation. If pixels within a feature are assumed to touch any of their eight adjacent neighbors (called

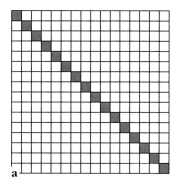 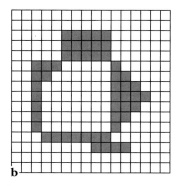

Figure 74. Ambiguous images:

a) *If the pixels are assumed to touch at their corners, then this shows a line which separates the background pixels on either side. But those pixels also touch at their corners. If 8-connectedness or 4-connectedness is selected for feature pixels, then the opposite convention applies to background pixels.*

b) *This shows either four separate features or one containing an internal hole, depending on the touching convention.*

eight-connectedness), then the line of pixels in **Figure 74a** separates the background on either side, and the background pixels that are diagonally adjacent do not touch. They are therefore four-connected. Conversely, if the background pixels touch diagonally, the pixels are isolated and only touch along their faces. For the second image fragment shown, choosing an eight-connected rule for features (dark pixels) produces a single feature with an internal hole. If a four-connected rule is used, there are four features and the background, now eight-connected, is continuous.

This means that simply inverting an image (interchanging white and black) does not reverse the meaning of the features and background. **Figure 75** shows a situation in which the holes within a feature (separated from the background) become part of a single region in the reversed image. This can cause confusion in measurements and binary image processing. When feature dimensions as small as one pixel are important, there is some basic uncertainty, and perhaps also some sensitivity to how the feature happens to lie along the raster orientation. This sensitivity is unavoidable and argues for using large arrays of small pixels to define small dimensions accurately.

Other segmentation methods

There are other methods used for image segmentation besides the ones based on thresholding discussed above. These are generally associated with fairly powerful computer systems and with

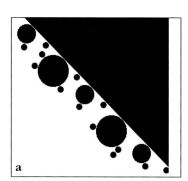 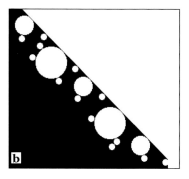

Figure 75. *Reversing an image (interchanging features and background) without changing the connectedness rules alters meaning. In image* *(a)* *the black pixels all touch at corners (8-connectedness) and so this is one feature with an irregular boundary. In image* *(b)* *the white pixels do not touch (4-connectedness) and so these are separate holes within the feature.*

attempts to understand images in the sense of machine vision and robotics (Ballard & Brown, 1982; Wilson & Spann, 1988). Two of the most widely described are split-and-merge and region growing, which seem to lie at opposite extremes in method.

Split-and-merge is a top-down method that begins with the entire image. Some image property is selected as a criterion to decide whether everything is uniform. This criterion is often based on the statistics from the brightness histogram. If the histogram is multimodal, or has a high standard deviation, etc., then the region is assumed to be nonuniform and is divided into four quadrants. Each quadrant is examined in the same way and subdivided again if necessary. The procedure continues until the individual pixel level is reached. The relationship between the parent region and the four quadrants, or children, is typically encoded in a quadtree structure, another name sometimes applied to this approach.

This is not the only way to subdivide the parent image and encode the resulting data structure. Thresholding can be used to divide each region into arbitrary subregions, which can be subdivided iteratively. This can produce final results having less blocky boundaries, but the data structure is much more complex, since all of the regions must be defined, and the time required for the process is much greater.

Subdividing regions alone does not create a useful image segmentation. After each iteration of subdividing, each region is compared to adjacent ones that lie in different squares at a higher level in the hierarchy. If they are similar, they are merged together. The definition of "similar" may use the same tests applied to the splitting operation, or comparisons may be made only for pixels along the common edge. The latter has the advantage of tolerating gradual changes across the image.

Figure 76 shows an example in which only four iterations have been performed. A few large areas have already merged, and their edges will be refined as the iterations proceed. Other parts of the image contain individual squares that require additional subdivision before regions become visible.

An advantage of this approach is that a complete segmentation is achieved after a finite number of iterations (for instance, a 512-pixel-square image takes 9 iterations to reach individual pixels, since $2^9 = 512$). Also, the quadtree list of regions and subregions can be used for some measurements, and the segmentation identifies all of the different types of regions at one time. By comparison, thresholding methods typically isolate one type of region or feature at a time. They must be applied several times to deal with images containing more than one class of objects.

On the other hand, the split-and-merge approach depends on the quality of the test used to detect inhomogeneity in each region. Small subregions within large uniform areas can easily

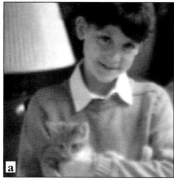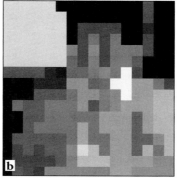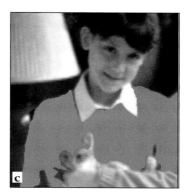

Figure 76. Other segmentation methods:
a) *original grey scale image;*
b) *split and merge after 4 iterations;*
c) *region growing from a point in the girl's sweater.*

be missed with this method. Standard statistical tests that assume, for example, a normal distribution of pixel brightness within regions are rarely appropriate for real images, so more complicated procedures must be used (Yakimovsky, 1976). Tests used for subdividing and merging regions can also be expressed as image processing operations. A processed image can reveal the same edges and texture used for the split-and-merge tests in a way that allows direct thresholding. This is potentially less efficient, since time-consuming calculations may be applied to parts of the image that are uniform, but the results are the same. Thresholding also has the advantage of identifying similar objects in different parts of the field of view as the same, which may not occur with split-and-merge.

Region growing starts from the bottom, or individual pixel level, and works upwards. Starting at some seed location (usually provided by the operator), neighboring pixels are examined one at a time and added to the growing region if they are sufficiently similar. Again, the comparison may be made to the entire region or just to the local pixels, with the latter method allowing gradual variations in brightness. The procedure continues until no more pixels can be added. **Figure 76c** shows an example in which one region has been identified; notice that it includes part of the cat as well as the girl's sweater. Then a new region is begun at another location. **Figure 77** shows an example of the application of this technique to a color image. The red boundary line shows the extent of the region grown from a starting point within the intestine.

If the same comparison tests are implemented to decide whether a pixel belongs to a region, the result of this procedure is the same as top-down split-and-merge. The difficulty with this approach is that the starting point for each region must be provided. Depending on the comparison tests employed, different starting points may not grow into identical regions. Also, there is

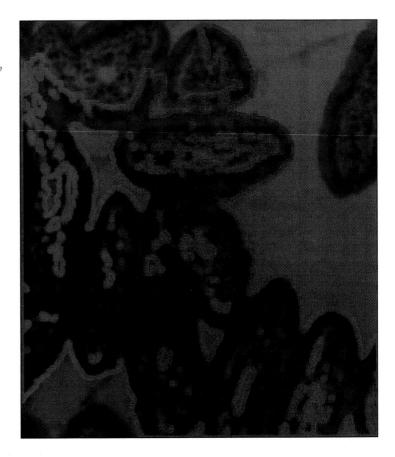

Figure 77. *Region growing applied to a color image (mouse intestine, Figure 48 in Chapter 1). The red lines show the boundaries of the region.*

no ideal structure to encode the data from this procedure, beyond keeping the entire pixel array until classification is complete; and the complete classification is slow, since each pixel must be examined individually.

Region growing also suffers from the conflicting needs to keep the test local, to see if an individual pixel should be added to the growing region, and to make it larger in scale, if not truly global, to ensure that the region has some unifying and distinct identity. If too small a test region is used, a common result is that regions leak out into adjoining areas or merge with different regions. This leaking or merging can occur if even a single pixel on the boundary can form a bridge.

Finally, there is no easy way to decide when the procedure is complete and all of the meaningful regions in the image have been found. Region growing may be a useful method for selecting a few regions in an image, as compared to manual tracing or edge following, for example, but it is rarely the method of choice for complex images containing many regions (Zucker, 1976).

Edge following was mentioned above in terms of an algorithm that tries to mimic a human drawing operation by tracing along a boundary, and at each point selecting the next pixel to step toward based on local neighborhood values. Human vision does not restrict itself to such local decisions, but can use remote information to bridge over troublesome points. A machine vision approach that does the same constructs outlines of objects as deformable polygons. The sides of the polygon may be splines rather than straight lines, to achieve a smoother shape. These deformable boundaries are referred to as "snakes" (Kass et al., 1987). The minimum length of any side, the maximum angular change at any vertex, and other arbitrary fitting constants must reflect some independent knowledge about the region that is to be fitted. They must generally be adjusted for each application until the results are acceptable as compared to visual judgment.

Since fitting is accomplished for all of the points on the boundary at once using a minimization technique, the snakes can accommodate some missing or confusing points. They are particularly useful for tracking moving boundaries in a sequence of images, since the deformation of the snake from one moment to the next must be small. This makes them useful for tracking moving objects in robotics vision. When applied to three-dimensional arrays of voxels, as in medical imaging, they become deformable polyhedra and are called balloons.

The general classification problem

The various methods described so far have relied on human judgment to recognize the presence of regions and to define them by delineating the boundary or selecting a range of brightness values. Methods have been discussed that can start with an incomplete definition and refine the segmentation to achieve greater accuracy or consistency. There are also fully automatic techniques that determine how many classes of objects are present and fully subdivide the image to isolate them. However, they are little used in small computer-based systems and are often much less efficient than using some human input. The task of general image segmentation can be treated as an example of a classification problem. Like most techniques involving elements or artificial intelligence, it may not use the same inputs or decision methods that a human employs, but it seeks to duplicate the results (and often succeeds).

One successful approach to general classification has been used with satellite imagery, in which many wavelength bands of data are available (Reeves, 1975). If each pixel in the image is plotted in a high-dimensionality space, where each axis is the measured brightness in one of the wavelength bands, it is expected that points corresponding to different classes of land use, crop type, soil or rock type, and so forth will cluster together and the clusters will be well separated from each other, as indicated in **Figure 78**. The problem then reduces to finding the clusters and fitting boundaries between them that can be used for classification.

Figure 78. *Schematic illustration of pixel classification in color space. Each pixel is plotted according to its color values, and clusters identify the various regions present.*

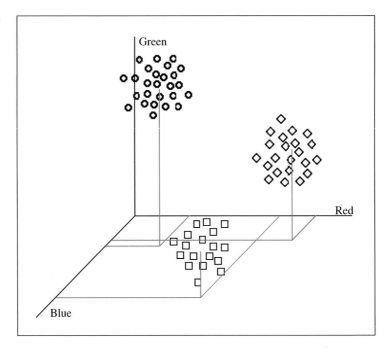

Reduced to a single dimension (a simple grey scale image), this classification begins with the brightness histogram. The cluster analysis looks for peaks and tries to draw thresholds between them. This is successful in a tiny handful of specialized tasks, such as counting cells of one type on a microscope slide. As the number of dimensions increases, for instance using the RGB or HSI data from color imagery or adding values from a derived texture or gradient image, the separation of the clusters usually becomes more distinct. Satellite imagery with several discrete visible and infrared wavelength bands is especially well suited to this approach.

Clusters are easier to recognize when they contain many similar points, but minor regions or uncommon objects may be overlooked. Also, the number of background points surrounding the clusters (or more often lying along lines between them) confuse the automatic algorithms. These points arise from the finite size of pixels that straddle the boundaries between regions. Finding a few major clusters may be straightforward. Being sure that all have been found is not.

Even after the clusters have been identified (and here some *a priori* knowledge or input from a human can be of great assistance), there are different strategies to using this information to classify new points. One is to surround each cluster with a boundary, typically either a polyhedron formed by planes lying perpendicular to the lines between the cluster centers, or n-dimensional ellipsoids. Points falling inside any of these regions are immediately classified.

Particularly for the ellipsoid case, it is also possible to have a series of concentric boundaries that enclose different percentages of the points in the cluster, which can be used to give a probability of classification to new points. This is sometimes described as a "fuzzy" classification method.

A third approach is to find the nearest classified point to each new point and assign that identity to the new one. This method has several drawbacks, particularly when there are some densely populated clusters and others with very few members, or when the clusters are close or overlapping. It requires considerable time to search through a large universe of existing points to locate the closest one, as well. An extension of this technique is also used, in which a small number of nearest neighbors are identified and "vote" for the identity of the new point.

Segmentation of grey scale images into regions for measurement or recognition is probably the most important single problem area for image analysis. Many novel techniques have been used that are rather ad hoc and narrow in their range of applicability. Review articles by Fu and Mui (1981) and Haralick and Shapiro (1988) present good guides to the literature. Most standard image analysis textbooks, such as Rosenfeld and Kak (1982), Castleman (1979), Gonzalez and Wintz (1987), Russ (1990b), and Pratt (1991) also contain sections on segmentation.

All of these various methods and modifications are used extensively in other artificial intelligence situations (see for example Fukunaga, 1990). They may be implemented in hardware, software, or some combination of the two. Only limited application of any of these techniques has been made to the segmentation problem. However, it is likely that the use of such methods will increase in the future as more color or multiband imaging is done and readily accessible computer power continues to increase.

7

Processing Binary Images

Binary images, as discussed in the preceding chapter, consist of groups of pixels selected on the basis of some property. The selection may be performed by thresholding brightness values, perhaps using several grey scale images containing different color bands, or processed to extract texture or other information. The goal of binarization is to separate features from background, so that counting, measurement, or matching operations can be performed.

However, as shown by the examples in Chapter 6, the result of the segmentation operation is rarely perfect. For images of realistic complexity, even the most elaborate segmentation routines misclassify some pixels as foreground or background. These may either be pixels along the boundaries of regions or patches of noise within regions. The major tools for working with binary images fit broadly into two groups: Boolean operations, for combining images, and morphological operations which modify individual pixels within images.

Boolean operations

In the section on thresholding color images, in Chapter 6, a Boolean operation was introduced to combine the data from individual color plane images. Setting thresholds on brightness values in each of the RGB planes allows pixels to be selected that fall into those ranges. This technique produces three binary images, which can then be combined with a logical AND opera-

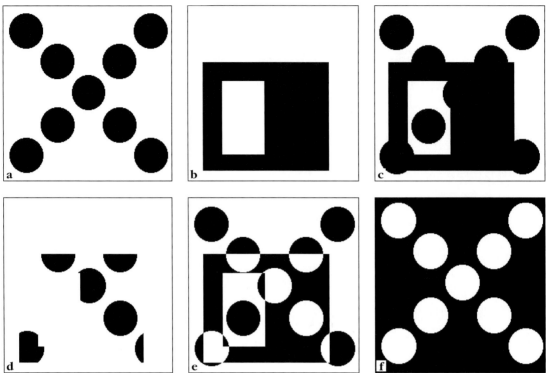

Figure 1. Simple Boolean operations: *a, b)* *two binary images;* *c)* *A OR B;* *d)* *A AND B;*
e) *A Ex-OR B;* *f)* *NOT A.*

tion. The procedure examines the three images pixel by pixel, keeping pixels for the selected regions if they are turned ON in all three images.

An aside: The terminology used here will be that of ON (pixels that are part of the selected foreground features) and OFF (the remaining pixels, which are part of the background). There is no universal standard for whether the selected pixels are displayed as white, black, or some other color. In many cases, systems that portray the selected regions as white on a black background on the display screen may reverse this and print hardcopy of the same image with black features on a white background. This reversal apparently arises from the fact that in each case, the selection of foreground pixels is associated with some positive action in the display (turning on the electron beam) or printout (depositing ink on the paper). It seems to cause most users little difficulty, provided that something is known about the image. Since many of the images used here are not common objects and some are made-up examples, we must try to be consistent in defining the foreground pixels (those of interest) in each case.

Returning to our desire to combine the information from several image planes, the AND operation requires that a pixel at location i,j be ON in each individual plane to show up in the result. Pixels having the correct amount of blue but not of red will be omit-

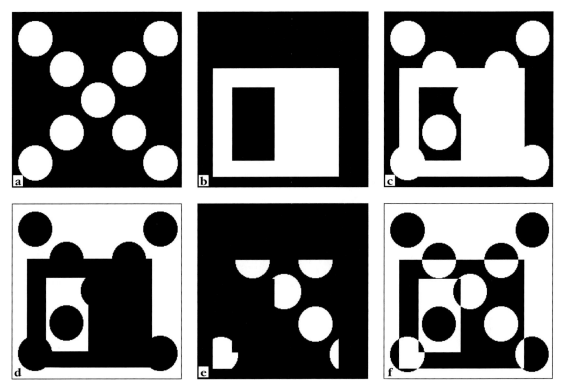

Figure 2. Combined Boolean operations: ***a)*** *NOT A;* ***b)*** *NOT B;* ***c)*** *(Image* ***a*** *) AND (Image* ***b*** *);* ***d)*** *NOT (Image* ***c*** *);* ***e)*** *NOT (A AND B);* ***f)*** *(Image* ***d*** *) AND (Image* ***e*** *), or (NOT (A AND B)) AND (NOT (NOT A) AND (NOT B))) . Compare this to A Ex-OR B in Figure 1e.*

ted, and vice versa. As was noted before, this marks out a rectangle in two dimensions, or a rectangular prism in higher dimensions, for the pixel values to be included. More complicated combinations of color values can be described by delineating an irregular region in n dimensions for pixel selection. The advantage of simply ANDing discrete ranges is that it can be performed very efficiently and quickly using binary images.

Other Boolean logical rules can be employed to combine binary images. The four possibilities are AND, OR, Ex-OR (Exclusive OR) and NOT. **Figure 1** illustrates each of these basic operations, and **Figure 2** shows a few of the possible combinations. All are performed pixel-by-pixel. The illustrations are based on combining two images at a time, since any logical rule involving more than two images can be broken down to a series of steps using just two at a time. The illustrations in the figures are identical to the Venn diagrams used in logic.

As described above, AND requires that pixels be ON in both of the original images in order to be ON in the result. Pixels that are ON in only one or the other original image are OFF in the result. The OR operator turns a pixel ON in the result if it is ON in either of the original images. Ex-OR turns a pixel ON in the result

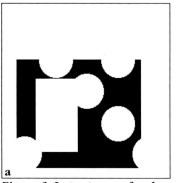 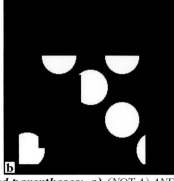 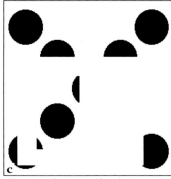

Figure 3. Importance of order and parentheses: **a)** *(NOT A) AND B;* **b)** *NOT (A AND B);* **c)** *A AND (NOT B).*

if it is ON in either of the original images, but not if it is ON in both. That means that combining (with an OR) the results of ANDing together two images with those from Ex-ORing them produces the same result as an OR in the first place. There are, in fact, many ways to arrange different combinations of the four Boolean operators to produce identical results (e.g., compare **Figure 2f** to **Figure 1e**).

AND, OR and Ex-OR require two original images and produce a single image as a result. NOT requires only a single image. It simply reverses each pixel, turning pixels that were ON to OFF and vice versa. Some systems implement NOT by swapping black and white values for each pixel. As long as we are dealing with pixel-level detail, this works correctly. Later, when feature-level combinations are described, the difference between an eight-connected feature and its four-connected background (discussed in Chapter 6) will have to be taken into account.

Given two binary images A and B, the combination (NOT A) AND B will produce an image containing pixels that lie within B but outside A. This is quite different from NOT (A AND B), which selects pixels that are not ON in both A and B. It is also different from A AND NOT B (**Figure 3**). The order of operators is important and the use of parentheses to clarify the order and scope of operations is crucial.

Combining Boolean operations

Actually, the four operations discussed above are redundant. Three would be enough to produce all of the same results. **Figure 2f** and **Figure 4** show ways that the results of an Ex-OR operation can also be produced by a sequence of AND, OR, and NOT operators. Consequently, some systems may omit one of them (usually Ex-OR). For simplicity, however, all four will be used in the examples that follow.

When multiple criteria are available for selecting the pixels to be kept as foreground, they may be combined using any of these

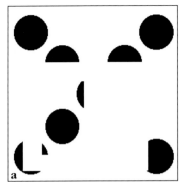 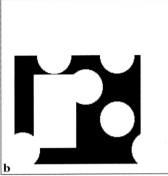 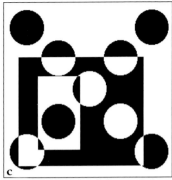

Figure 4. Equivalence of Boolean combinations: ***a)*** *A AND NOT B;* ***b)*** *B AND NOT A;* ***c)*** *Image* ***(a)*** *AND Image* ***(b)****, or ((A AND NOT B) OR (NOT A AND B)). Compare this to A Ex-OR B in Figure 1e.*

Boolean combinations. The most common situations are multi-band images, such as produced by a satellite or an SEM. In the case of the SEM, an X-ray detector is often used to create an image (called an X-ray dot map) showing the spatial distribution of a selected element. These images may be quite noisy (Chapter 3) and difficult to threshold (Chapter 6). However, by suitable long-term integration or spatial smoothing, they can lead to useful binary images that indicate locations where the concentration of the element is above some user-selected level.

This selection is usually performed by comparing the measured X-ray intensity to some arbitrary threshold, since there is a finite level of background signal resulting from the process of slowing down the electrons in the sample. The physical background of this phenomenon is not important here. The very poor statistical characteristics of the dot map (hence the name) make it difficult to directly specify a concentration level as a threshold. The X-ray intensity in one part of the image may vary from another region for several reasons: a) a change in that element's concentration, b) a change in another element that selectively absorbs or fluoresces the first element's radiation, or c) a change in specimen density or surface orientation. Comparison of one specimen to another is further hampered by the difficulty in exactly reproducing instrument conditions. These effects all complicate the relationship between elemental concentration and recorded intensity.

Furthermore, the very poor statistics of the images (due to the extremely low efficiency for producing X-rays with an electron beam and the low beam intensity required for good spatial resolution in SEM images) mean that these images often require processing, either as grey scale images (e.g., smoothing) or after binarization (using the morphological tools discussed below). For our present purpose, we will assume that binary images showing the spatial distribution of some meaningful concentration level of several elements can be obtained.

As shown in **Figure 5**, the SEM also produces more conventional images using secondary or backscattered electrons. These

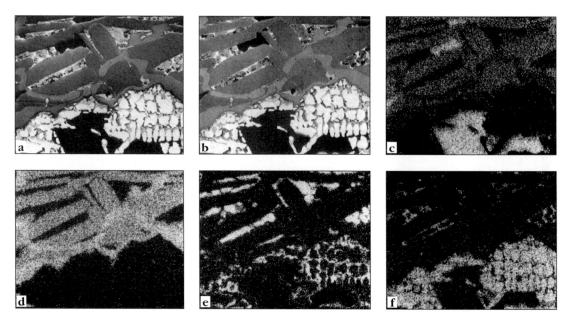

Figure 5. SEM results from a mineral: a) *backscattered electrons;* **b)** *secondary electrons;* **c)** *silicon (Si) X-ray map;* **d)** *iron (Fe) X-ray map;* **e)** *copper (Cu) X-ray map;* **f)** *silver (Ag) X-ray map.*

have superior spatial resolution and better feature shape definition, but with less elemental specificity. The binary images from these sources will also be combined with the X-ray or elemental information.

Figure 6 shows one example. The X-ray maps for iron (Fe) and silicon (Si) were obtained by smoothing and thresholding the grey scale image. Notice that in the grey scale images, there is a just-discernible difference in the intensity level of the Fe X-rays in two different areas. This is too small a difference for reliable thresholding. Even the larger differences in Si intensity are difficult to separate. However, Boolean logic easily combines the images to produce an image of the region containing Fe but not Si.

Figure 7 shows another example from the same data. The regions containing silver (Ag) are generally bright in the backscattered electron image, but some other areas are also bright. On the other hand, the Ag X-ray map does not have precise region boundaries because of the poor statistics. Combining the two

Figure 6:
a) iron;
b) iron AND NOT silicon.

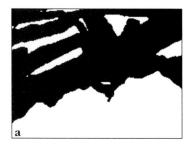

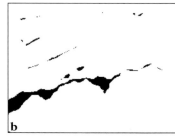

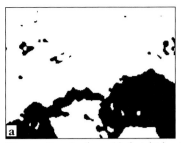 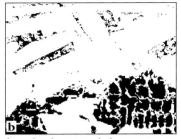 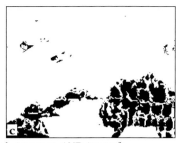

Figure 7: a) silver; b) bright levels from backscattered electron image; c) image a AND image b.

binary images with an AND produces the desired regions. More complicated sequences of Boolean logical operations can easily be imagined (**Figure 8**).

It is straightforward to imagine a complex specimen containing many elements. Paint pigment particles with a diverse range of compositions provide one example. In order to count or measure a particular class of particles (pigments, as opposed to brighteners or extenders), it might be necessary to specify those containing iron or chromium or aluminum, but not titanium or sulfur. This would be written as

$$(Fe \ OR \ Cr \ OR \ Al) \ AND \ (NOT \ (Ti \ OR \ S)) \tag{1}$$

The resulting image might then be ANDed with a higher-resolution binary produced by thresholding a secondary or backscattered electron image to delineate particle boundaries.

Most of the examples shown in earlier chapters that used multiple image planes (e.g., different colors or elements) or different processing operations (e.g., combining brightness and texture) use a Boolean AND to combine the separately thresholded binary images. The AND requires that the pixels meet all of the criteria in order to be kept. There are some cases in which the Boolean OR is more appropriate. One is illustrated in Chapter 4, **Figure 86**. This is an image of sand grains in a sandstone, viewed through polarizers. Each rotation of the analyzer causes different grains to become bright or colored. In the earlier figure, it was shown that keeping the brightest pixel value at each location as the analyzer is rotated gives an image that shows all of the grains.

Figure 9 shows an alternative approach to the same problem. Each individual image is thresholded to select those grains that

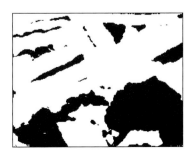

Figure 8. Further combination to delineate structure: (Cu OR Ag) AND NOT (Fe).

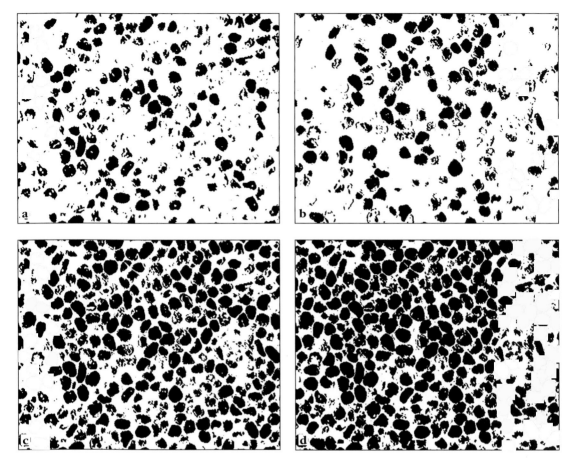

Figure 9. Combining multiple binary images.

a and *b)* binary images obtained by thresholding two of the polarized light images of a petrographic thin section of a sandstone (Figure 86 in Chapter 4);

c) the result of ORing together six such images from different rotations of the analyzer;

d) comparison binary image produced by thresholding the grey scale image obtained by combining the same six color images to keep the brightest pixel at each location.

are bright for that particular analyzer rotation angle. Then all of the binary images are combined using a Boolean OR. The resulting combination delineates most of the grains, although the result is not as good as the grey-level operation for the same number of analyzer rotations.

Masks

The above description of using Boolean logic to combine images makes the assumption that both images are binary (that is, black and white). It is also possible to use a binary image as a mask to modify a grey scale image. This is most often done to blank out (to either white or black, but generally to background) some portion of the grey scale image, either to create a display in which only the regions of interest are visible or to select regions whose brightness, density, and so forth are to be measured.

There are several physical ways that this operation can be performed. The binary mask can be used in an overlay, or alpha channel, in the display hardware to prevent pixels from being displayed, if the hardware supports that capability. It is also possible, and somewhat more common, to use the mask to modify

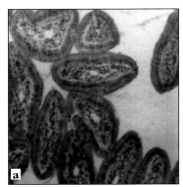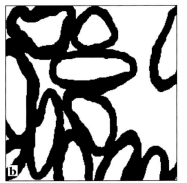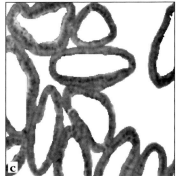

Figure 10. Masking to show a portion of a grey scale image. The displayed villi are selected with a mask obtained by thresholding a combination of the hue and saturation images.

the stored image. This can done using Boolean logic to set pixels in the grey scale image to the value of the binary image if it is nonzero. It is possible to produce the same result by multiplying the grey scale image by the binary image, with the convention that the binary image values are 0 (OFF) or 1 (ON) at each pixel. In some systems this result is implemented by combining the grey scale and binary images to keep whichever value is darker or brighter; if the mask is white for background and black for foreground pixels then the brighter pixel values at each location will erase all background pixels and keep the grey value for the foreground pixels.

This capability has been used extensively in earlier chapters to display the results of various processing and thresholding operations. It is easier to judge the performance of thresholding by viewing selected pixels with the original grey scale information, rather than just looking at the binary image. This format can be seen in the examples of texture operators in Chapter 4, for instance, as well as in Chapter 6 on Thresholding.

It is also possible to use a mask obtained by thresholding one version of an image to view another version. For instance, **Figure 10** shows the region along the villi of mouse intestine. The displayed pixels have the grey scale intensity values, but the thresholding to create the mask used to select these pixels is based on a combination of hue and saturation data.

Masking one derived image with another produces results such as those shown in **Figure 11**. Grey scale values represent the orientation angle (from the Sobel derivative) of grain boundaries in the aluminum alloy, masked by thresholding the magnitude of the gradient to isolate only the boundaries. A similar example was shown in **Figure 33** of Chapter 4.

Another use of masking and Boolean image combination is shown in **Figure 12**. An essentially cosmetic application, it is still useful and widely employed. A label superimposed on an image using either black or white may be difficult to read if the image

Figure 11. *Masking one image with another. The direction of a Sobel gradient applied to the light microscope image of an aluminum alloy is shown only in the regions where the magnitude of the gradient is large.*

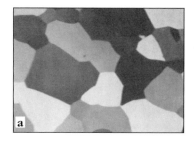

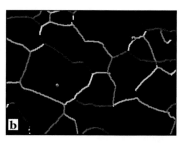

contains a full range of brightness values. In this example, the label is used to create a mask that is one pixel larger in all directions, using dilation (discussed below). This mask is then used to erase the pixels in the grey scale image to white before writing in the label in black (or vice versa). The result maintains legibility for the label while obscuring a minimum amount of the image.

Finally, a binary image mask can be used to combine portions of two (or more) grey scale images. This is shown in **Figure 13**. The composite image represents, in a very simple way, the kind of image overlays and combinations common in printing, advertising, and commercial graphic arts. While rarely suitable for scientific applications, this example will perhaps serve to remind us that modifying images to create things that are not real is very easy with modern computer technology. This justifies a certain skepticism in examining images, which were once considered iron-clad evidence of the truth.

From pixels to features

The Boolean operations described above deal with individual pixels in the image. For some purposes it is necessary to identify the pixels forming part of a connected whole. As discussed in Chapter 6, it is possible to adopt a convention for touching that is either eight-connected or four-connected for the pixels in a single feature (sometimes referred to as a blob to indicate that no

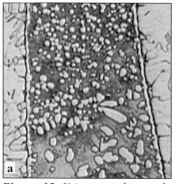

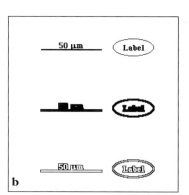

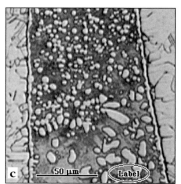

Figure 12. *Using a mask to apply a label to an image. The original image contains both white and black areas, so that simple superimposition of text will not be visible. A mask is created by dilating the label and Ex-ORing that with the original. The composite is then superimposed on the grey-scale image.*

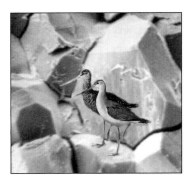

Figure 13. Hudsonian Godwits searching for a nesting site on an SEM image of an alumina fracture surface.

interpretation of the connected group of pixels has been inferred as representing anything specific in the image). Whichever convention is adopted, grouping pixels into features is an important step (Levialdi, 1992; Ritter, 1996).

It is possible to imagine starting with one pixel (any ON pixel, selected at random) and checking its 4- or 8-neighbor positions, labeling each pixel that is ON as part of the same feature, and then iteratively repeating the operation until no neighbors remain. Then a new unlabeled pixel would be chosen and the operation repeated, continuing until every ON pixel in the image was labeled as part of some feature. The usual way of proceeding with this deeply recursive operation is to create a stack to place pixel locations as they are found to be neighbors of already labeled pixels. Pixels are removed from the stack as their neighbors are examined. The process ends when the stack is empty.

It is more efficient to deal with pixels in groups. If the image has already been run-length or chord encoded, as discussed in Chapter 6, then all of the pixels within the chord are known to touch, touching any of them is equivalent to touching all, and the only candidates for touching are those on adjacent lines. This fact makes possible a very straightforward labeling algorithm that passes one time through the image. Each chord's end points are compared to those of chords in the preceding line; if they touch or overlap (based on a simple comparison of values), the label from the preceding line is attached to this chord. If not, then a new label is used.

If a chord touches two chords in the previous line that had different labels, then the two labels are identified with each other (this handles the bottom of a letter U for example). All of the occurrences of one label can be changed to the other, either immediately or later. When the pass through the image or the list of chords is complete, all of the chords, and therefore all of the pixels, are identified and the total number of labels (and therefore features) is known. **Figure 14** shows this logic in the form of a flow chart.

For boundary representation (including the special case of chain code), the analysis is partially complete, since the boundary

Figure 14. Flow chart for grouping touching pixels in a run-length or chord-encoded array into features and assigning ID numbers.

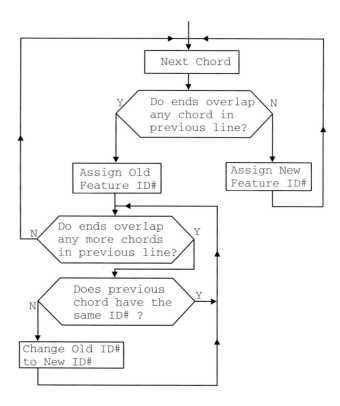

already represents a closed path around a feature. If features contained no holes and no feature could ever be surrounded by another, this would provide complete information. Unfortunately, this is not always the case. It is usually necessary to reconstruct the pixel array to identify pixels with feature labels (Kim et al., 1988).

In any case, once the individual features have been labeled, several additional Boolean operations are possible. One is to find and fill holes within features. Any pixel that is part of a hole is defined as OFF (i.e., part of the background) and is surrounded by ON pixels. For boundary representation, that means the pixel is within a boundary. For pixel representation, it means it is not connected to other pixels that eventually form a path to the edge of the field of view.

Recalling that the convention for touching (eight- or four-connectedness) must be different for the background than for the foreground, we can identify holes most easily by inverting the image (replacing white with black and vice versa) and labeling the resulting pixels as though they were features, as shown step-by-step in **Figure 15**. Features in this inverted image that do not touch any side of the field of view are the original holes. If the pixels are added back to the original image (using a Boolean OR), the result is to fill any internal holes in the original features.

One very simple example of the application of this technique is shown in **Figure 16**. In this image of spherical particles, the center of each feature has a brightness very close to that of the sub-

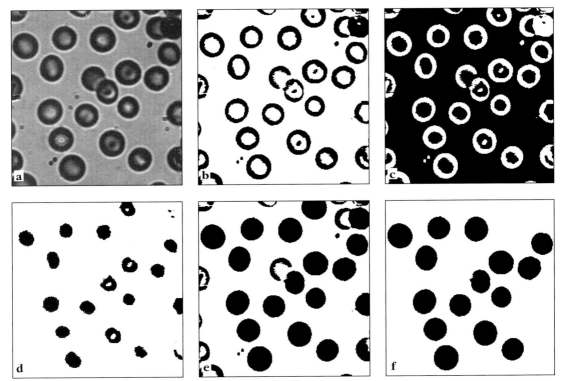

Figure 15. Light microscope image of red blood cells:
   a) original; b) thresholded, which shows the thicker outer edges of the blood cells but not the thinner central regions; c) image b inverted; d) features in image c that do not touch the edge of the field of view; e) adding the features in image d to those in image b using a Boolean OR; f) selecting just the features in image e that do not touch an edge, and are round and large enough to be a red blood cell.

strate due to the lighting. Thresholding the brightness values gives a good delineation of the outer boundary of the particles, but the centers have holes. Filling them as described produces a corrected representation of the particles, which can be measured. This type of processing is commonly required for SEM images, whose brightness varies as a function of local surface slope so that particles frequently appear with bright edges and dark centers (see for instance **Figure 77** in Chapter 1).

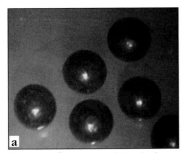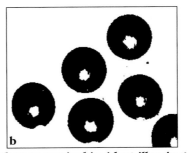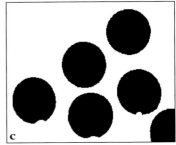

Figure 16. Image of buckshot with near-vertical incident illumination:
   a) original grey-scale image; b) brightness thresholded after leveling illumination; c) internal holes filled and small regions (noise) in background removed by erosion.

Figure 17. *Light microscope image of a polished section through an enamel coating on steel (Courtesy V. Benes, Research Inst. for Metals, Panenské Brezany, Czechoslovakia) shows bright spots of reflected light within many pores (depending on their depth).*

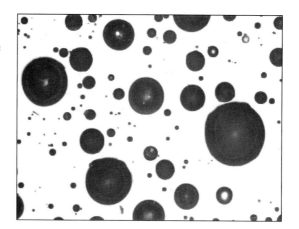

This problem is not restricted to convex surfaces. **Figure 17** shows a light microscope image of spherical pores in an enamel coating. The light spots in the center of many of the pores vary in brightness, depending on the depth of the pore. They must be corrected by filling the features in a thresholded binary image.

Figure 18 shows a more complicated situation requiring several operations. The SEM image shows the boundaries of the spores clearly to a human viewer, but they cannot be directly revealed by thresholding because the shades of grey are also present in the substrate. Applying an edge-finding algorithm (in this example, a Frei and Chen operator) delineates the boundaries, and it is then possible to threshold them to obtain feature outlines, as shown. These must be filled using the method described above. Further operations are then needed before measurement: erosion, to remove the other thresholded pixels in the image, and watershed segmentation, to separate the touching objects, are both described later in this chapter.

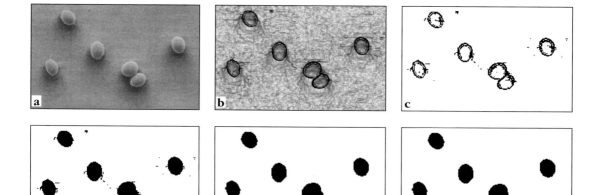

Figure 18. Segmentation of an image using multiple steps:
a) original SEM image of spores on a glass slide; b) application of a Frei and Chen edge operator to a; c) thresholding of image b; d) filling of holes in the binary image of the edges; e) erosion to remove the extraneous pixels in d; f) watershed segmentation to separate touching features in e.

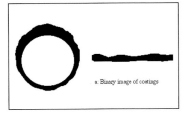

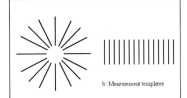

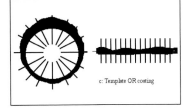

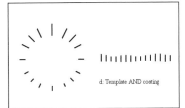

Figure 19. *Schematic diagram of ANDing a measurement template with a binary image of coating on a flat or round substrate to obtain a series of line segments which measure the coating thickness.*

The Boolean AND operation is also widely used to apply measurement templates to images. For instance, consider the measurement of coating thickness on a wire or plate viewed in cross section. We will presume for the moment that the coating can be readily thresholded, but it is not uniform in thickness. In order to obtain a series of discrete thickness values for statistical interpretation, it is easy to AND the binary image of the coating with a template or grid consisting of lines normal to the coating. **Figure 19** shows a schematic example, both for the case of a flat surface, in which the lines are vertical, and a wire, in which the lines are radial. The AND results in a series of line segments that sample the coating and are easily measured.

Figure 20 illustrates this for an actual case, consisting of coated particles embedded in a metallographic mount and sectioned. In this case, the distribution of the intercept lengths must be

Figure 20. Measuring coating thickness on particles:

a) *original grey-scale image of a random section through embedded, coated particles;*

b) *thresholded binary image of the coating of interest (note the additional lines of pixels which straddle the white and dark phase boundary);*

c) *removal of the straddle pixels by application of an opening (coefficient=4, depth=4) as discussed later in this chapter;*

d) *template consisting of random lines;*

e) *AND of image* *c* *and* *d* *showing line segments whose length distribution gives the actual coating thickness in a normal direction.*

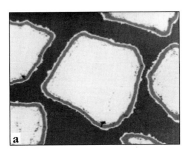

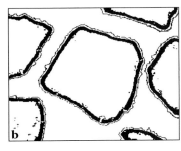

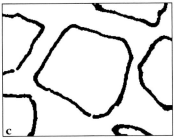

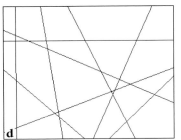

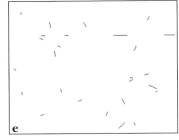

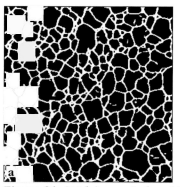
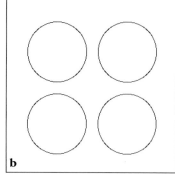
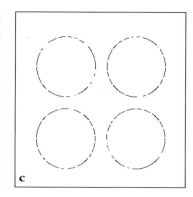

Figure 21. Applying a circle grid:

a) *thresholded image of grains in a metal;*

b) *original circle grid;*

c) *combination using a Boolean AND. From the number of arcs and total length of grid lines, the grain size can be calculated.*

interpreted stereologically to measure the actual boundary thickness, since the plane of polish does not go through the center of the particle. Therefore, the coating appears thicker than it actually is. This is handled by a set of random lines in the template. The distribution of line intercept lengths is directly related to that of the coating thickness in the normal direction, and the average coating thickness is just 3/2 divided by the average inverse intercept length.

Selection of an appropriate grid is crucial to the success of measurements. For a metallographic grain structure as shown in **Figure 21**, we do not know *a priori* that there is no preferred orientation and so a circle grid may be used to sample uniformly in all directions. Combining the grid of circles with the binary image using a Boolean AND leaves a series of arcs. The number of grains (and the number of boundaries) crossed by the lines is simply the number of separate line segments that are present, which can be determined by automatic counting. From this number and the total length of lines in the grid, the surface area per unit volume and the grain size can be determined.

Depending on the nature of the specimen and the problem to be solved, other grids may also be useful. **Figure 22** shows a macroscopic image of the root structure of a plant. Acquiring the image from at least three directions as the structure is rotated about the stem allows making a simple measurement of the total length of the roots, even though they are a complex three dimensional structure with lines that cross. The image is first converted to binary by thresholding and then skeletonization. In this case the required grid is a set of cycloid lines; ANDing them with the skeletonized image of the root gives a set of intersection points, most of them only a single pixel in size. These points are counted as in the previous example. Then the number of intersections are used with the length of the cycloid lines to determine the total root length. The principles behind these measurements methods

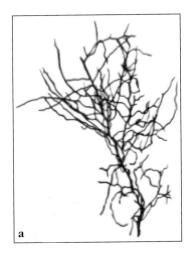
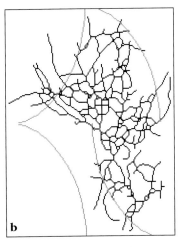

Figure 22. Measuring length:
a) *projected image of plant roots;*
b) *overlaying a cycloid grid on the thresholded and skeletonized root image to count the intersections, from which the total three-dimensional length can be determined.*

involve stereology (Dehoff & Rhines, 1968; Weibel, 1979; Kurzydlowski & Ralph, 1995; Reed & Howard, 1998) and lie beyond the scope of this text, but the use of image analysis is quite useful to apply the grids and perform the counting.

Even for very complex or subtle images for which automatic processing and thresholding cannot delineate the structures of interest, the superimposition of grids may be important. Many stereological procedures that require only counting of intersections of various types of grids with features of interest are extremely efficient and capable of providing unbiased estimates of valuable structural parameters. Combining image capture and processing to enhance the visibility of structures with overlays of the appropriate grids — arrays of points or lines, the latter including straight lines, circles and cycloids — allows the human user to recognize the important features and intersections (Russ, 1995a). The counting may be performed manually or the computer may also assist by tallying mouse-clicks or counting marks that the user places on the image. The combination of human recognition with computer assistance provides efficient solutions to many image analysis problems.

Boolean logic with features

Having identified or labeled the pixel groupings as features, it is possible to carry out Boolean logic at the feature level, rather than at the pixel level. **Figure 23** shows the principle of a feature-based AND. Instead of simply keeping the pixels that are common to the two images, entire features are kept if any part of them touches. This preserves the entire feature, so that it can be correctly counted or measured if it is selected by the second image.

Feature-AND requires a feature labeling operation to be performed on at least one of the images to be combined. Touching pixels in one image are identified as features as described in Chapter 6. Then each pixel that is "ON" in one of those features

Figure 23. Schematic diagram of feature-based AND.
a) and *b)* test images;
c) pixel-based Boolean AND of images *a* and *b*;
d) feature-based AND of image *a* with image *b*.

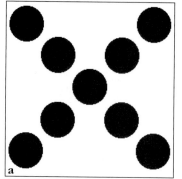
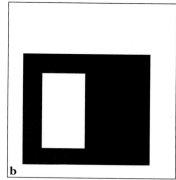
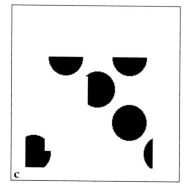
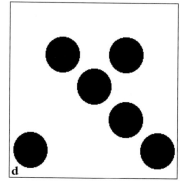

is checked against the second image. If any of the pixels in the feature match an "ON" pixel in the second image, the entire feature in the first image is copied to the result. This is not the only possible implementation. It would be equally possible to check each pixel in the second image against the first, but that would be less efficient. The method outlined limits the comparison to those pixels which are on, and halts the test for each feature whenever any pixel within it is matched.

Notice that unlike the more common pixel based AND, this statement does not commute; this means that (A Feature-AND B) does not produce the same result as (B Feature-AND A), as illustrated in **Figure 24**. The use of NOT with Feature-AND is straightforwardly implemented, for instance by carrying out the same procedure and erasing each feature in the first image that is matched by any pixel in the second. However, there is no Feature-OR statement, which would produce the identical result as the conventional pixel-based OR.

One use for the Feature-AND capability is to use markers within features to select them. For example, these might be cells containing a stained organelle or fibers in a composite containing a characteristic core. In any case, two binary images are produced by thresholding. In one image, the entire features are delineated, and in the second the markers are present. Applying the Feature-AND logic then selects all of the features which contain a marker.

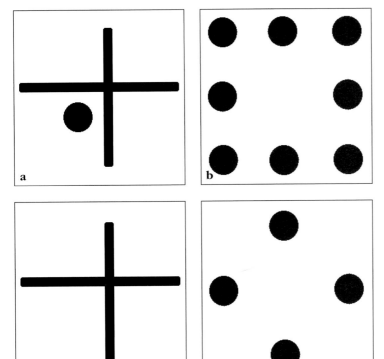

Figure 24. Feature-based
  Boolean logic used to combine
  two test images (*a* and *b*):
c) *a* Feature-AND *b* ;
d) *b* Feature-AND *a* .

This use of markers to select features is a particularly valuable capability in an image analysis system. **Figure 25** illustrates one way that it can be used. The original image has several red features, only some of which contain darker regions within. If one copy of the image is thresholded for dark spots and a second copy is thresholded for red features, then the first can be used as a set of markers to select the features of interest. A Feature-AND can be used to perform that operation. In real applications the marker image that selects the features of interest may be obtained by separate thresholding, by processing, or by using another plane in a multiplane image.

Figure 26 shows another example. Some of the bacteria (*E. coli*) contain one or more bright granules, which contain insulin produced by genetic engineering of the bacteria. For production control purposes, it is desired to count the number of bacteria that contain bright granules, which is not the same as counting the number of bright spots since more than one granule may lie within a single bacterium. As shown in the figure, thresholding can be used to isolate the bacteria. Applying a Laplacian operator and thresholding can select the bright spots. Feature-AND combination of these images selects those bacteria which contain the granules, so that they can be counted.

A similar procedure is applicable to the use of the nucleator (Gundersen et al., 1988), a stereological tool that counts cells in thin sections of tissue according to the presence of a unique

Figure 25. *Example of feature selection using markers. The red features and the dark spots in the original image* **(a)** *are thresholded to produce separate binary images (* **b** *and* **c** *). The dark spots are used as markers to select just those red features which contain dark markers* **(d)** *.*

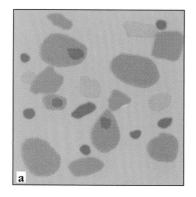
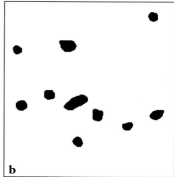
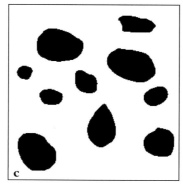
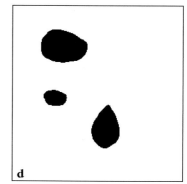

Figure 26. Selection of bacteria based on their containing one or more bright granules:
a) *original image;*
b) *thresholding the bacteria;*
c) *thresholding the granules;*
d) *Feature-AND combination.*

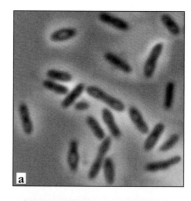
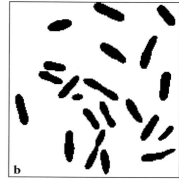
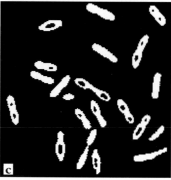
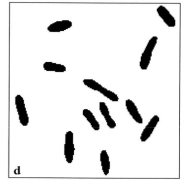

marker within the cell such as the nucleus. At a very different scale, the method might be used with aerial photographs to select and measure all building lots that contain any buildings, or fields that contain animals. The technique can also be used with X-ray images to select particles in SEM images, for instance, if the X-ray signal comes only from the portion of the particle which is visible to the X-ray detector. The entire particle image can be preserved if any part of it generates an identifying X-ray signal (which may require processing itself as discussed above in the context of combining images, and below in the context of merging isolated spots with dilation).

Selecting features by location

Feature-AND is also useful when used in conjunction with images that map regions according to distance. We will see below that dilating a line, such as a grain boundary or cell wall, can produce a broad line of selected thickness. Using this line to select features that touch it selects those features which, regardless of size or shape, come within that distance of the original boundary. Counting these for different thickness lines provides a way to classify or count features as a function of distance from irregular boundaries. **Figure 27** shows a diagram and **Figure 28** shows an actual image measuring grain-boundary depletion.

Figure 29 shows a similar situation, a metallurgical specimen of a plasma-sprayed coating applied to a turbine blade. There is

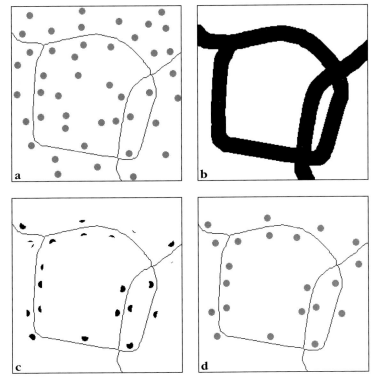

Figure 27. Comparison of pixel- and feature-AND:

a) *diagram of an image containing features and a boundary;*

b) *the boundary line, made thicker by dilation;*

c) *pixel-based AND of image **b** and **a** (incomplete features and one divided into two parts);*

d) *Feature-AND of image **b** and **a** (all features within a specified distance of the boundary).*

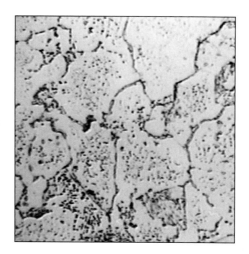

Figure 28. Light microscope image of polished section through a steel used at high temperature in boiler tubes. Notice the depletion of carbides (black dots) in the region near grain boundaries. This effect can be measured as discussed in the text.

always a certain amount of oxide present in such coatings, which in general causes no difficulties. But if the oxide, which is a readily identifiable shade of grey, is preferentially situated at the coating-substrate interface, it can produce a plane of weakness that may fracture and cause spalling of the coating. Thresholding the image to select the oxide, then ANDing this with the line representing the interface (itself obtained by thresholding the substrate phase, dilating, and Ex-ORing to get the custer, discussed more extensively later in this chapter) gives a direct measurement of the contaminated fraction of the interface.

An aperture or mask image can be used to restrict the analysis of a second image to only those areas within the aperture. Consider counting spots on a leaf: either spots due to an aerial spraying operation to assess uniformity of coverage, or perhaps spots of fungus or mold to assess the extent of disease. The acquired image is normally rectangular, but the leaf is not. There may well be regions outside the leaf that are similar in brightness to the spots. Creating a binary image of the leaf, then Feature-ANDing it with the total image selects those spots lying on the leaf itself. If the spots are small enough, this could be done as a pixel-based AND. However, if the spots can touch the edge of the leaf, the feature-based operation is safer. Counting can then provide the desired information, normally expressed as number-per-unit-area where the area of the leaf forms the denominator.

Figure 30 shows another situation, in which two different thresholding operations and a logical combination are used to select features of interest. The specimen is a polished cross section of an enamel coating on steel. The two distinct layers are different colored enamels containing different size distributions of spherical pores. Thresholding the darker layer includes several of the pores in the lighter layer, which have the same range of brightness values, but the layer can be selected by discarding features that are small or do not touch both edges of the field. This image then forms a mask that can be used to select only

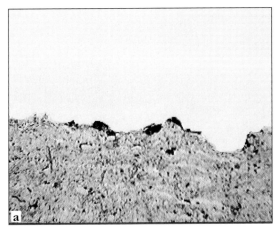

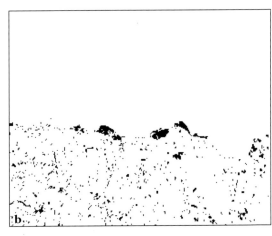

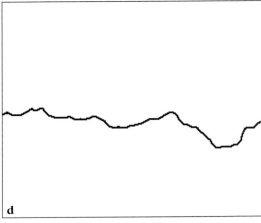

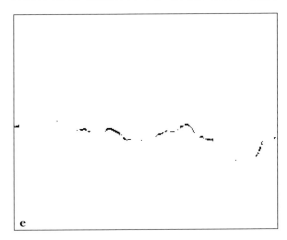

Figure 29. Isolating the oxide in a coating/substrate boundary:

a) *original grey-scale microscope image of a cross section of the plasma-sprayed coating (bottom) on steel;*

b) *thresholding of the dark oxide in the coating, including that lying in the interface;*

c) *thresholding of the substrate;*

d) *boundary line obtained by applying an opening (coefficient 3, depth 2) to remove noise pixels, then dilating the binary image (coefficient 0, depth 2) and Ex-ORing the result with the original;*

e) *AND of image* **d** *with image* **b**, *showing just the fraction of the interface occupied by oxide.*

the pores in the layer of interest. Similar logic can be employed to select the pores in the light layer. Pores along the interface will generally be included in both sets, unless additional feature-based logic is employed.

A similar application allows identifying grains in ores that are contained within other minerals, for instance, to determine the

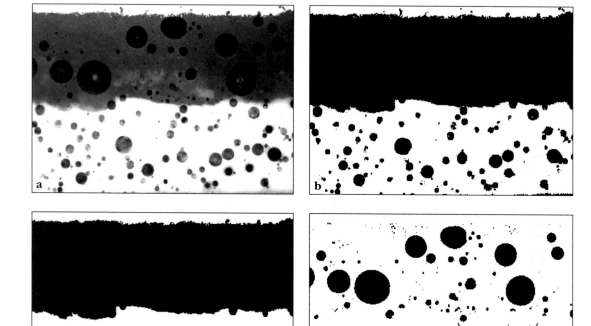

Figure 30. Selecting pores in one layer of enamel on steel:

a) original light microscope image (Courtesy V. Benes, Research Inst. for Metals, Panenské Brezany, Czechoslovakia);

b) image a thresholded to select dark pixels;

c) discarding all features from image b which do not extend from one side to the other leaves just the layer of interest;

d) thresholding the original image to select only dark pores produces a binary image containing more pores than those in the layer;

e) combining images b and d with a Boolean AND leaves only the pores within the dark layer.

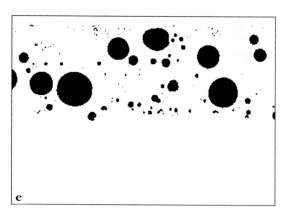

fraction which are "locked" within a harder matrix that cannot easily be recovered by mechanical or chemical treatment, as opposed to those that are not so enclosed and are easily liberated from the matrix.

A rather different use of feature-based Boolean logic implements the disector, a stereological tool that gives an unbiased and direct measure of the number of features per unit volume (Sterio, 1984). It requires matching features in two images that represent parallel planes separated by a distance T. The features represent the intersection of three-dimensional objects with those planes. Those objects which intersect both planes are ignored, but those which intersect only one plane or the other are counted. The total number of objects per unit volume is then

$$N_v = \frac{Count}{2 \cdot Area \cdot T} \tag{2}$$

where *Area* is the area of each of the images. This method has the advantage of being insensitive to the shape and size of the objects, but it requires that the planes be close enough together that no information is lost between the planes. In effect, this means that the distance T must be small compared to any important dimension of the objects.

When T is small, most objects intersect both planes. The features in those planes will not correspond exactly, but are expected to overlap at least partially. In the case of a branching three-dimensional object, both of the intersections in one plane are expected to overlap with the intersection in the second plane. Of course, since most of the objects do pass through both planes when T is small, and only the few that do not are counted, it is necessary to examine a large image area to obtain a statistically useful number of counts. That requirement makes the use of an automated method based on the Feature-AND logic attractive.

Since the features which overlap in the two images are those which are not counted, a candidate procedure for determining the value of N to be used in the calculation of number of objects per unit volume might be to first count the number of features in each of the two plane images (N_1 and N_2). Then the Feature-AND can be used to determine the features which are present in both images, and a count of those features (N_{common}) obtained, giving

$$N = N_1 + N_2 - 2 \cdot N_{common} \tag{3}$$

However, this is correct only for the case in which each object intersects each plane exactly once. For branching objects, it will result in an error.

A preferred procedure is to directly count the features in the two planes that are not selected by the Feature-AND. Since the logical operation does not commute, it is necessary to perform both operations: (#1 NOT F-AND #2) and (#2 NOT F-AND #1), and count the features remaining. This is illustrated schematically in **Figure 31**, along with a diagram showing how the features correspond to the three-dimensional objects.

Figure 32 shows a real application. The two images are separate slices reconstructed from X-ray tomography of a sintered ceramic sample. Each image is thresholded to generate a binary image of particle intersections. Each of the Feature-AND operations is performed, and the final image is the OR combination showing those features that appear in one (and only one) of the two slices. It would be appropriate to describe this image as a feature-based version of the exclusive-OR operation between the two images.

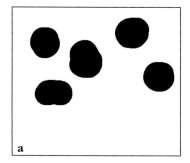

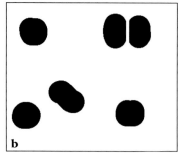

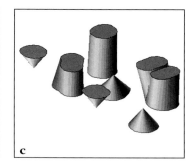

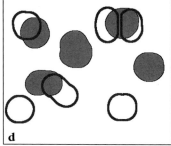

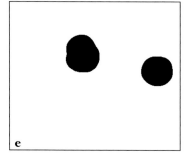

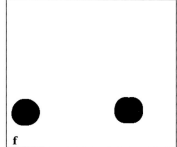

Figure 31. Implementation of the disector :

a) *bottom section;*

b) *top section;*

c) *perspective view of the objects represented by the two sections;*

d) *overlay of top section (outlines) on bottom section;*

e) *bottom NOT Feature-AND with top;*

f) *top NOT Feature-AND with bottom.*

Double thresholding

Another application for Feature-AND logic arises in the thresholding of difficult images such as grain boundaries in materials. As shown in **Figure 33**, it is unfortunately quite common to have nonuniform etching of the boundaries in specimen preparation, arising in part from the variation in the crystallographic mismatch at various boundaries. In addition, some etching often occurs within the grains due to the presence of precipitate or inclusion particles. The result is that direct thresholding of the image may not be able to produce a complete representation of the etched boundaries that does not also include "noise" within the grains.

A technique for dealing with such situations has been described as "double thresholding" by Olsson (1993), but can also be implemented by using Feature-AND. As illustrated in **Figure 33**, the procedure is first to threshold the image to select only the darkest pixels that are definitely within the etched boundaries, even if they do not form a complete representation of the boundaries. Then a second binary image is produced by thresholding the image again, to include more pixels. In this case the goal is to obtain a complete delineation of all the boundaries, accepting some noise within the grains. The increase in apparent width of the boundaries is not important, since skeletonization will subsequently be used to reduce the boundary lines to minimum width (the actual grain boundaries are only a few atoms thick).

The two binary images can then be combined with a Feature-AND to keep any feature in the second image that touches one in the first. This uses the few dark pixels that definitely lie within the boundaries as markers to select the broader boundaries,

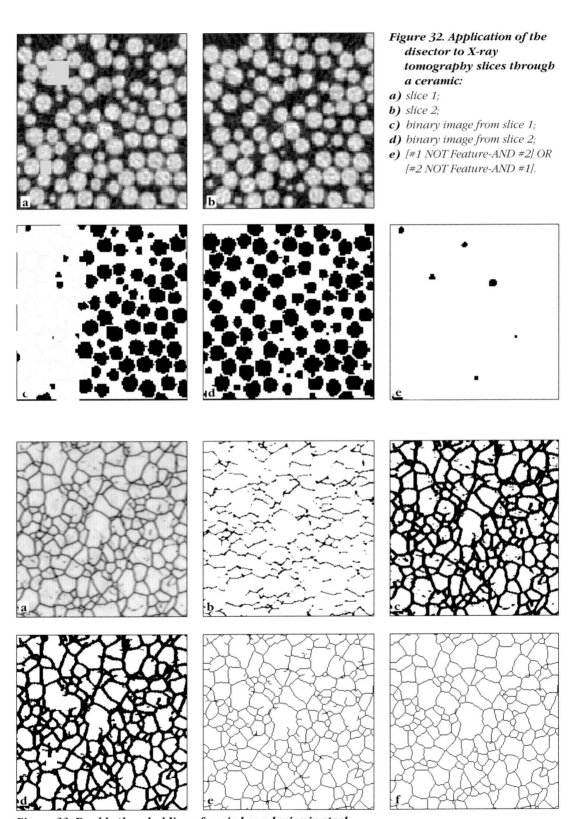

Figure 32. Application of the disector to X-ray tomography slices through a ceramic:
a) slice 1;
b) slice 2;
c) binary image from slice 1;
d) binary image from slice 2;
e) [#1 NOT Feature-AND #2] OR [#2 NOT Feature-AND #1].

Figure 33. Double thresholding of grain boundaries in steel:
a) original; b) first thresholding; c) second thresholding; d) Feature-AND; e) skeletonized; f) pruned.

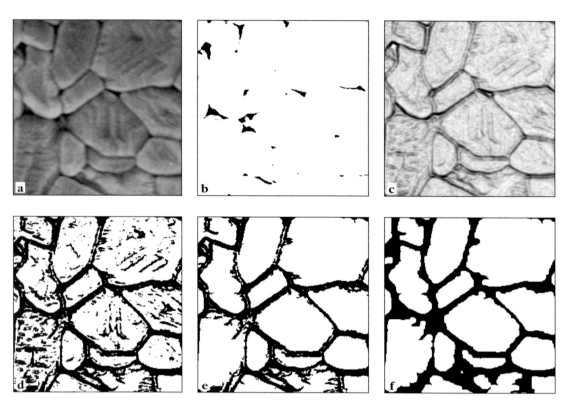

Figure 34. Double thresholding of grain boundaries in alumina:
a) *original image;*
b) *first thresholding;*
c) *variance operator;*
d) *second thresholding;*
e) *Feature-AND;*
f) *closing;*
g) *skeletonized and pruned.*

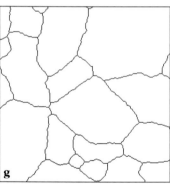

while rejecting the noise within the grains. Finally, as shown in the figure, the resulting image is skeletonized (reduced to a single pixel in width by a conditional erosion as discussed below) and branches are removed or "pruned" by repeatedly eliminating any pixels that touch only one neighbor. This produces an image useful for stereological measurements of grain boundary area, grain size, and so forth.

For more difficult images, additional processing steps may be required. **Figure 34** shows an image of a thermally etched ceramic material in which the grain boundaries are poorly delineated. There is also considerable structure evident within the grains, and the contrast in the scanning electron microscope image does not facilitate segmenting the image to show just the

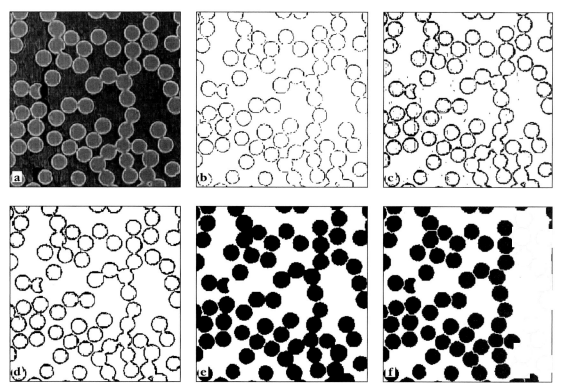

Figure 35. Double thresholding of fiber boundaries:
a) original; *b)* first thresholding; *c)* second thresholding; *d)* Feature-AND; *e)* filled boundaries;
f) segmented fibers.

grain boundaries. An initial thresholding selects just those darkest pixels that lie within the boundaries. Then an edge-finding algorithm (the variance operator, which calculates the sum of squares of differences of pixels in a moving local neighborhood) is applied to a copy of the original image to increase the contrast at edges. This process allows thresholding more of the boundaries, but also some of the intragrain structures.

Combining these images using Feature-AND followed by a morphological closing, skeletonization and pruning, gives a fair representation of the boundaries without the intragrain detail. In some applications, the additional use of a watershed segmentation (discussed below) to complete any missing boundary segments might be required to yield a final grain boundary image suitable for measurement.

In both of the preceding examples, the grain boundary network is a continuous tesselation of the image. Hence, it could be selected by using other criteria than the double-threshold method (for instance, touching multiple edges of the field). **Figure 35** shows an example requiring the double-threshold method. The acoustic microscope image shows a cross section through a fiber-reinforced material. These images are inherently noisy, but double-thresholding (in this example selecting the bright pixels) allows the boundaries around the fibers to be selected. Since the fibers touch each other, it is also necessary to separate them for measurement using a watershed segmentation as discussed below.

Erosion and dilation

The most extensive class of binary image processing operations is sometimes collectively described as morphological operations (Serra, 1982; Coster & Chermant, 1985; Dougherty & Astola, 1994). These include erosion and dilation, and modifications and combinations of these operations. All are fundamentally neighbor operations, as were discussed in Chapters 3 and 4 to process grey scale images in the spatial domain. Because the values of pixels in the binary images are restricted to 0 or 1, the operations are simpler and usually involve counting rather than weighted multiplication and addition. However, the basic ideas are the same, and it is possible to perform these procedures using the same specialized array-processor hardware sometimes employed for grey scale kernel operations.

There is a rich literature, much of it French, in the field of mathematical morphology. It has developed a specific notation for the operations and is generally discussed in terms of set theory. A much simpler and more empirical approach is taken here. Operations can be described simply in terms of adding or removing pixels from the binary image according to certain rules, which depend on the pattern of neighboring pixels. Each operation is performed on each pixel in the original image, using the original pattern of pixels. In practice, it may not be necessary to create an entirely new image; the existing image can be replaced in memory by copying a few lines at a time. None of the new pixel values are used in evaluating the neighbor pattern.

Erosion removes pixels from an image or, equivalently, turns pixels OFF that were originally ON. The purpose is to remove pixels that should not be there. The simplest example is pixels that have been selected by thresholding because they fell into the brightness range of interest, but do not lie within the regions of that brightness. Instead, they may have that brightness value either accidentally, because of finite noise in the image, or because they happen to straddle a boundary between a lighter and darker region and thus have an averaged brightness that happens to lie in the range selected by thresholding.

Such pixels cannot be distinguished by simple thresholding because their brightness value is the same as that of the desired regions. It may be possible to ignore them by using two-dimensional thresholding, for instance using the grey level as one axis and the gradient as a second one, and requiring that the pixels to be kept have the desired grey level and a low gradient. However, for our purposes here we will assume that the binary image has already been formed and that extraneous pixels are present.

The simplest kind of erosion, sometimes referred to as classical erosion, is to remove (set to OFF) any pixel touching another pixel that is part of the background (is already OFF). This removes a layer of pixels from around the periphery of all features and regions, which will cause some shrinking of dimensions and may create other problems if it causes a feature to break up into parts. We will deal with these difficulties below. Erosion will remove extraneous pixels altogether because these defects are normally only a single pixel wide.

Instead of removing pixels from features, a complementary operation known as dilation (or sometimes dilatation) can be used to add pixels. The classical dilation rule, analogous to that for erosion, is to add (set to ON) any background pixel which touches another pixel that is already part of a region. This will add a layer of pixels around the periphery of all features and regions, which will cause some increase in dimensions and may cause features to merge. It also fills in small holes within features.

Because erosion and dilation cause a reduction or increase in the size of regions, respectively, they are sometimes known as etching and plating or shrinking and growing. There are a variety of rules for deciding which pixels to add or remove and for forming combinations of erosion and dilation.

In the rather simple example described above and illustrated in **Figure 36**, erosion to remove the extraneous lines of pixels between light and dark phases also caused a shrinking of the features. Following the erosion with a dilation will more or less restore the pixels around the feature periphery, so that the dimensions are (approximately) restored. However, isolated pixels that have been completely removed do not cause any new pixels to be added. They have been permanently erased from the image.

Opening and closing

The combination of an erosion followed by a dilation is called an opening, referring to the ability of this combination to open up spaces between just-touching features, as shown in **Figure 37**. It is one of the most commonly used sequences for removing pixel noise from binary images. There are several parameters that can be used to adjust erosion and dilation operations, particularly the neighbor pattern and the number of iterations, as discussed below. In most opening operations, these are kept the same for both the erosion and the dilation.

In the example shown in **Figure 37**, the features are all similar in size. This fact makes it possible to continue the erosion until all features have separated but none have been completely erased. After the separation is complete, dilation grows the features back toward their original size. They would merge again unless logic is used to prevent it. A rule that prevents turning a pixel ON if its neighbors belong to different features maintains

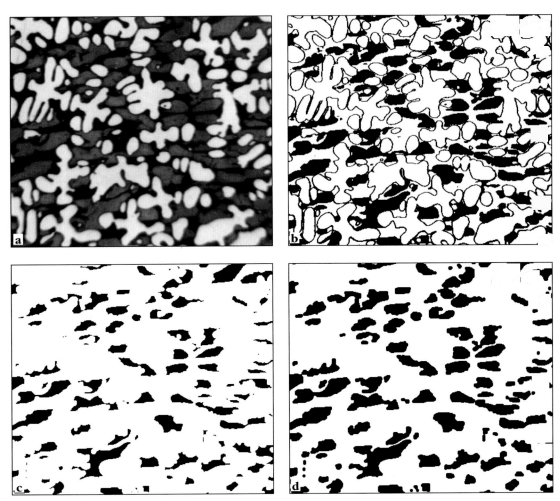

Figure 36: Removal of lines of pixels which straddle a boundary:

a) original grey-scale microscope image of a three-phase metal;

b) binary image obtained by thresholding on the intermediate grey phase;

c) erosion of image **b** using two steps (coefficient=0 and coefficient=1);

d) dilation of image **c** using the same coefficients.

the separation shown in the figure. This requires performing feature identification for the pixels, so the logic discussed above is required at each step of the dilation.

Notice also that the features do not revert to their original shape during dilation, but instead take on the shape imposed by the neighbor tests (in this case, an octagon). Continuing the dilation beyond the number of erosion cycles to make the features larger than their original size, followed by ANDing with the original to restore the feature outlines, produces an image with the original features separated. If the features had different original sizes, the separation lines would not lie correctly at the junctions. The watershed segmentation technique discussed later in this chapter performs better in such cases.

If the sequence is performed in the other order, that is, a dilation followed by an erosion, the result is not the same. Instead of removing isolated pixels that are ON, the result is to fill in places where isolated pixels are OFF, missing pixels within features or narrow gaps between portions of a feature. **Figure 38** shows an

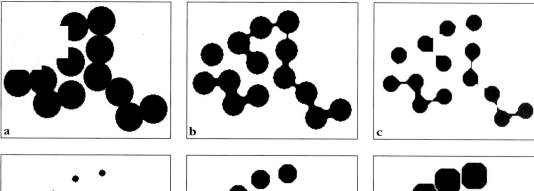

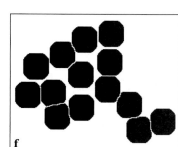

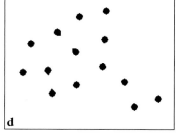

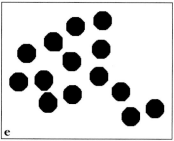

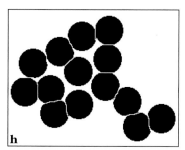

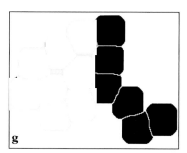

Figure 37. Separation of touching features by erosion/dilation:

a) *original test image;*

b) *after two cycles of erosion, alternating coefficient 0 and 1;*

c) *after four cycles;*

d) *after 7 cycles (features are now all fully separated);*

e) *four cycles of dilation applied to image **d** (features will merge on next cycle);*

f) *seven cycles of dilation using logic to prevent merging of features;*

g) *nine cycles of nonmerging dilation (features are larger than original);*

h) *dilated image ANDed with original to restore feature boundaries.*

example. Because of its ability to close up breaks in features, this combination is called a closing. The dilation and erosion operations are usually balanced in closings, as they are in openings.

Figure 39 shows an example of a closing used to connect together the parts of the cracked fibers shown in cross section. The cracks are all narrow, so dilation causes the pixels from either side to spread across the gap. The increase in fiber diameter is then corrected by an erosion, but the cracks do not reappear, since there are no OFF pixels there.

The classical erosion and dilation operations illustrated above turn a pixel ON or OFF if it touches any pixel in the opposite state. Usually, touching in this context includes any of the adjacent 8 pixels, although some systems deal only with the 4 edge-sharing neighbors. (These operations would also be much simpler and more isotropic on a hexagonal pixel array, but again, practical considerations lead to the general use of a grid of square pixels.)

A wide variety of other rules are possible. One approach is to count the number of neighbor pixels in the opposite state, compare this number to some threshold value, and only change the

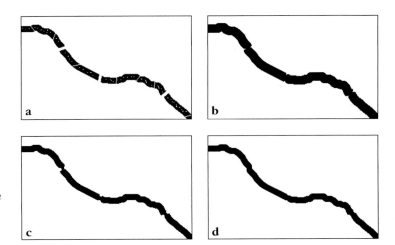

Figure 38. Using closing to connect parts of a broken feature:

a) *original test image;*

b) *application of two cycles of dilation, alternating coefficients 0 and 1;*

c) *application of two cycles of erosion (same coefficients) to image **b**;*

d) *the result of erosion and dilation with a depth of four cycles, showing more uniform width for the reconstructed line.*

state of the central pixel if that test coefficient is exceeded. In this method, classical erosion would use a coefficient of zero. One effect of different coefficient values is to alter the rate at which features grow or shrink and to some extent to control the isotropy of the result. This will be illustrated below.

It is also possible to choose a large coefficient, from 5 to 7, to select only the isolated noise pixels and leave most features alone. For example, choosing a coefficient of 7 will cause only single isolated pixels to be reversed (removed or set to OFF in an erosion, and vice versa for a dilation). Coefficient values of 5 or 6 may be able to remove lines of pixels (such as those straddling a boundary) without affecting anything else.

An example of this method is shown in **Figure 40**. Thresholding the original image of the pigment cell produces a binary image showing the features of interest and creates many smaller and irregular groups of pixels. Performing a conventional opening to remove them would also cause the shapes of the larger features to change and some of them to merge. Applying erosion with a coefficient of 5 removes the small and irregular pixel groups without affecting the larger and more rounded features, as shown. The erosion is repeated until no further changes take

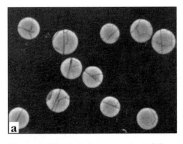
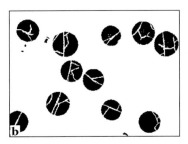
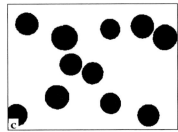

Figure 39. Joining parts of features with a closing:

a) *original image, cross section of cracked glass fibers;* **b)** *brightness thresholding, showing divisions within the fibers;* **c)** *after application of a closing.*

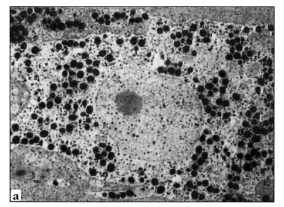

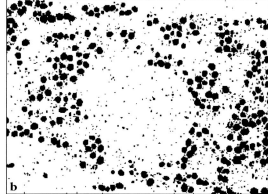

Figure 40. Removal of debris from an image:
a) *original image of a pigment cell;*
b) *brightness thresholding shows the pigment granules plus other small and irregular features;*
c) *erosion (coefficient=5) leaves the large and regular granules.*

place (the number of ON pixels in the binary image does not change). This procedure works because a corner pixel in a square has exactly 5 touching background neighbors and is not removed, while more irregular clusters have pixels with 6 or more background neighbors.

Isotropy

It is not possible for a small 3×3 neighborhood to define a really isotropic neighbor pattern. Classic erosion applied to a circle will not shrink the circle uniformly, but will proceed at a faster rate in the 45° diagonal directions because the pixel spacing is greater in those directions. As a result, a circle will erode toward a diamond shape, as shown in **Figure 41**. Once the feature reaches this shape, it will continue to erode uniformly, preserving the shape. However, in most cases, features are not really diamond shaped, which represents a potentially serious distortion.

Likewise, classic dilation applied to a circle also proceeds faster in the 45° diagonal directions, so that the shape dilates toward a square (also shown in **Figure 41**). Again, square shapes are stable in dilation, but the distortion of real images toward a block appearance in dilation can present a problem for further interpretation.

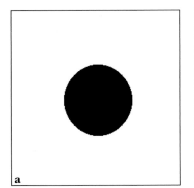
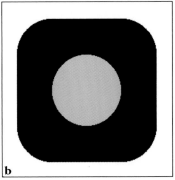
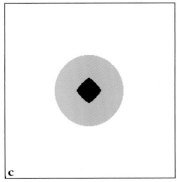

Figure 41. Testing the isotropy of classical (coefficient=0) dilation and erosion:
a) original circle; b) after 50 repetitions of dilation; c) after 25 repetitions of erosion.

Interestingly, a coefficient of 1 instead of 0 produces a very different result. For dilation, a background pixel that touches more than 1 foreground pixel (i.e., 2 or more out of the possible 8 neighbor positions) will be turned ON and vice versa for erosion. Eroding a circle with this procedure tends toward a square and dilation tends toward a circle, just the reverse of using a coefficient of 0. This is shown in **Figure 42**.

There is no possible intermediate value between 0 and 1, since the pixels are counted as either ON or OFF. If the corner pixels were counted as 2 and the edge-touching pixels as 3, it would be possible to design a coefficient that better approximated an isotropic circle. This would produce a ratio of 3/2 = 1.5, which is a reasonable approximation to $\sqrt{2}$, the distance ratio to the pixels. In practice, this is rarely done because of the convenience of dealing with pixels in binary images as a simple 0 or 1 value.

Another approach that is much more commonly used for achieving an intermediate result between the coefficients of 0 and 1 with their directional bias is to alternate the two tests. As shown in **Figure 43**, this alternating pattern produces a much better approximation to a circular shape in both erosion and dilation. This procedure raises the point that erosion or dilation need not be performed only once. The number of repetitions, also called the depth of the operation, corresponds roughly to the distance

Figure 42. Isotropy tests using a coefficient of 1:
a) the circle after 50 repetitions of dilation;
b) the circle after 25 iterations of erosion.

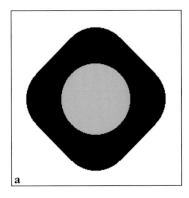
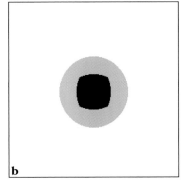

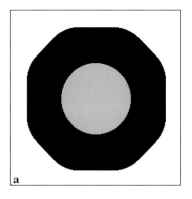

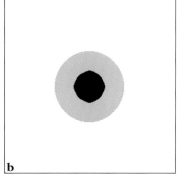

Figure 43. Improved isotropy by using alternating test coefficients of 0 and 1:
a) *the circle after 50 repetitions of dilation;*
b) *the circle after 25 repetitions of erosion.*

that boundaries will grow or shrink radially. It may be expressed in pixels or converted to the corresponding scale dimension.

Each neighbor pattern or coefficient has its own characteristic anisotropy. **Figure 44** shows the rather interesting results using a coefficient of 3. Like an alternating 0,1 pattern, this operation produces an 8-sided polygon. However, the rate of erosion is much lower, and in dilation the figure grows to the bounding octagon and then becomes stable, with no further pixels being added. This coefficient is sometimes used to construct bounding or convex polygons around features.

Measurements using erosion and dilation

Erosion performed n times (using either a coefficient of 0 or 1, or alternating them) will cause features to shrink radially by about n pixels (somewhat depending on the shape of the original feature). This will cause features whose smallest dimension is less than $2n$ pixels to disappear altogether. Counting the features that have disappeared (or subtracting the number that remain from the original) gives an estimate of the number of features smaller than that size. This means that erosion and counting can be used to get an estimate of size distributions without actually performing feature measurements (Ehrlich et al., 1984).

For irregularly shaped and concave features, the erosion process may cause a feature to subdivide into parts. Simply counting the

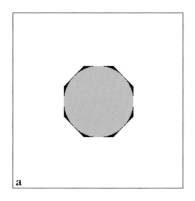

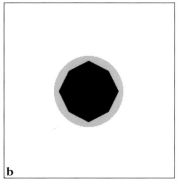

Figure 44. Octagonal shape and slow rate of addition or removal using a coefficient of 3:
a) *original circle after 50 repetitions of dilation (no further changes occur);*
b) *circle after 25 repetitions of erosion.*

number of features as a function of the number of iterations of erosion is therefore not a good way to determine the size distribution. One approach to this problem is to follow erosion by a dilation with the same coefficient(s) and number of steps. This will merge together many (but not necessarily all) of the separated parts and give a better estimate of their number. However, there is still considerable sensitivity to the shape of the original features. A dumbbell-shaped object will separate into two parts when the handle between the two main parts erodes; they will not merge. This separation may be desirable, if indeed the purpose is to count the two main parts.

A second method is to use Feature-AND, discussed above. After each iteration of erosion, the remaining features are used to select only those original features that touch them. The count of original features then gives the correct number. This is functionally equivalent to keeping feature labels on each pixel in the image and counting the number of different labels present in the image after each cycle of erosion. This method of estimating size distributions without actually measuring features, using either of these correction techniques, has been particularly applied to measurements in geology, such as mineral particle sizes or sediments.

The opposite operation, performing dilations and counting the number of separate features as a function of the number of steps, seems to be less common. It provides an estimate of the distribution of the nearest distances between features in the image. When this is done by conventional feature measurement, the x,y location of each feature is determined; then sorting in the resulting data file is used to determine the nearest neighbor and its distance. When the features are significantly large compared to their spacing or when their shapes are important, it can be more interesting to characterize the distances between their boundaries. This dilation method can provide that information directly and with less effort.

Instead of counting the number of features that disappear at each iteration of erosion, it is much easier simply to count the number of ON pixels remaining, which provides some information about the shape of the boundaries. Smooth Euclidean boundaries erode at a constant rate. Irregular and especially fractal boundaries do not, since many more pixels are exposed and touch opposite neighbors. This effect has been used to estimate fractal dimensions, although several more accurate methods are available with little or no extra computation (one comes from the Euclidean distance map, discussed below).

Fractal dimensions and the description of a boundary as fractal based on a self-similar roughness is a fairly new idea that is finding many applications in science and art (Mandelbrot, 1982; Feder, 1988). No description of the rather interesting background and uses of the concept is included here for want of space. The basic idea behind measuring a fractal dimension by erosion and dilation comes from the Minkowski definition of a fractal boundary dimension. By dilating a region and Ex-ORing the result with another image formed by eroding the region, the pixels along the boundary are obtained. For a minimal depth of erosion and dilation, this will be called the custer and is discussed below.

To measure the fractal dimension, the operation is repeated with different depths of erosion and dilation (Flook, 1978), and the effective width (total number of pixels divided by length and number of cycles) of the boundary is plotted vs. the depth on a log-log scale. For a Euclidean boundary, this plot shows no trend; the number of pixels along the boundary selected by the Ex-OR increases linearly with the number of erosion/dilation cycles. However, for a rough boundary with self-similar fine detail, the graph shows a linear variation on log-log axes whose slope gives the fractal dimension of the boundary directly. **Figure 45** shows an example.

It should perhaps be noted here, for lack of a better place, that another more efficient method for determining the boundary fractal dimension is known as box-counting or mosaic amalgamation (Kaye, 1986; Russ, 1990). This method is quite different from the classical structured walk method (Schwarz & Exner, 1980), which requires the boundary to be represented as a polygon instead of as pixels. The number of pixels through which the boundary passes (for boundary representation) are counted as the pixel size is increased by coarsening the image resolution (combining pixels in 2×2, 3×3, 4×4, ... blocks). For a fractal boundary, this also produces a straight line plot on a log-log scale which is interpreted as in the example above, although technically this is a slightly different fractal dimension.

Counting the number of pixels as a function of dilations also provides a rather indirect measure of feature clustering, since as nearby features merge, the amount of boundary is reduced and the region's rate of growth slows. Counting only the pixels and not the features makes it difficult to separate the effects of boundary shape and feature spacing. If all of the features are initially very small or if they are single points, this method can provide a fractal dimension (technically a Sierpinski fractal) for the clustering.

Extension to grey scale images

In Chapter 4, one of the image processing operations described was the use of a ranking operator, which finds the brightest or darkest pixel in a neighborhood and replaces the central pixel with that value. This operation is sometimes described as a grey scale erosion or dilation, depending on whether the use of the brightest or darkest pixel value results in a growth or shrinkage of the visible features.

Just as an estimate of the distribution of feature sizes can be obtained by eroding features in a binary image, the same technique

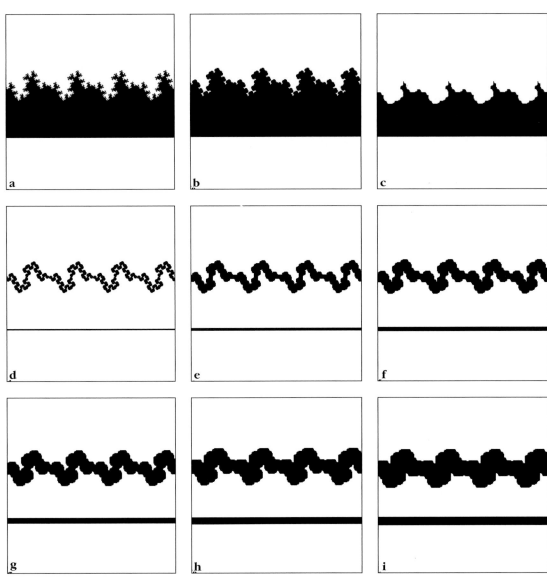

Figure 45. Measurement of Minkowski fractal dimension by erosion/dilation:

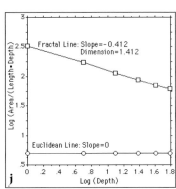

a) *test figure with upper boundary a classical Koch fractal and lower boundary a Euclidean straight line;*

b) *dilation of image **a** (1 cycle, coefficient=0);*

c) *erosion of image **a** (1 cycle, coefficient=0);*

d) *Ex-OR of **b** and **c**;*

e) *Ex-OR after 2 cycles;*

f) *Ex-OR after 3 cycles;*

g) *Ex-OR after 4 cycles;*

h) *Ex-OR after 5 cycles;*

i) *Ex-Or after 6 cycles;*

j) *plot of log of effective width (area of Ex-OR divided by length and number of cycles) vs. log of number of cycles.*

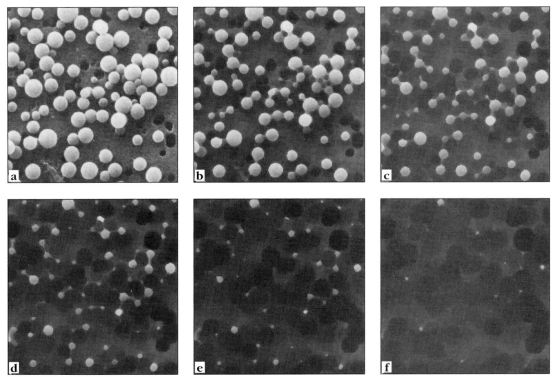

Figure 46. Use of grey scale erosion to estimate size distribution of overlapped spheres:
a) *original SEM image of lipid droplets;* ***b)–f)*** *result of applying 1, 2, 3, 4 and 5 repetitions of grey scale*
erosion (keeping darkest pixel value in a 5-pixel-wide octagonal neighborhood).

is also possible using grey scale erosion on a grey scale image.
Figure 46 shows an example. The lipid spheres in this SEM
image are partially piled up and obscure one another, which is
normally a critical problem for conventional image-measurement
techniques. Applying grey scale erosion reduces the feature sizes,
and counting the bright central points that disappear at each step
of repeated erosion provides a size distribution.

The assumption in this approach is that the features ultimately
separate before disappearing. This works for relatively simple
images with well-rounded convex features, none of which are
more than about half hidden by others. No direct image processing method can count the number of cannon balls in a pile
if the inner ones are hidden. It is possible to estimate the volume
of the pile and guess at the maximum number of balls contained,
but impossible to know whether they are actually there or
whether something else is underneath the topmost layer.

Coefficient and depth parameters

The important parameters for erosion and dilation are the neighborhood comparison test that is used and the number of times
the operation is repeated. The use of a simple test coefficient
based on the number of neighbors, irrespective of their location

Figure 47. *Effect of changing the neighborhood test in erosion, for coefficient values from 0 (classical erosion) to 7, and matching only to diagonal or orthogonal neighbors. Figure enlarged to show individual pixels.*

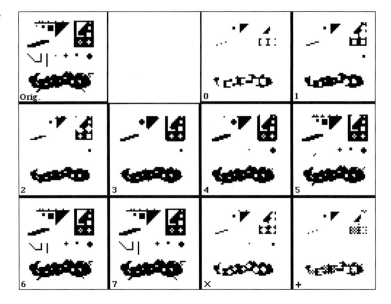

in the neighborhood, still provides considerable flexibility in the functioning of the operation. **Figures 47**, **48**, **49**, and **50** show several examples of erosion, dilation, opening, and closing operations using different coefficients and depths.

Notice that each coefficient produces results having a characteristic shape, which distorts the original features. Also, the greater the depth, or number of iterations in the operation, the greater this effect, in addition to the changes in the number of features present.

Specific neighbor patterns are also used for erosion and dilation operations. The most common are ones that compare the central pixel to its 4 edge-touching neighbors (usually called a "+" pattern

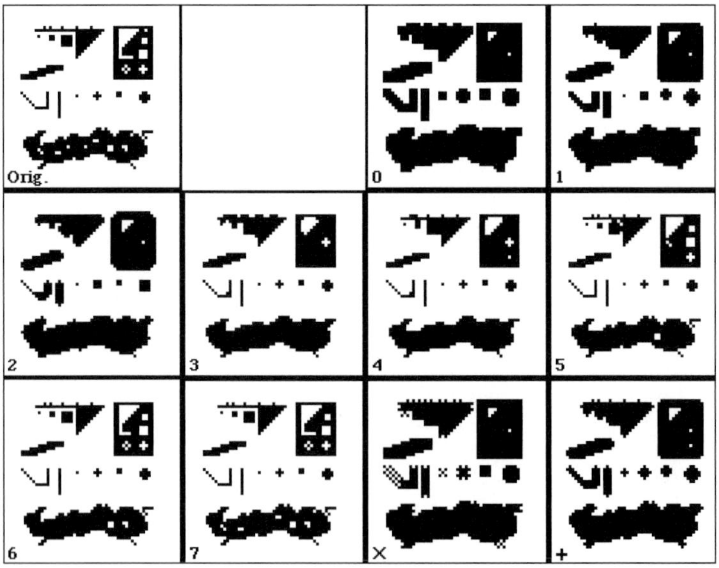

Figure 48. *Effect of changing the neighborhood test in dilation, for coefficient values from 0 (classical dilation) to 7, and matching only to diagonal or orthogonal neighbors. Figure enlarged to show individual pixels.*

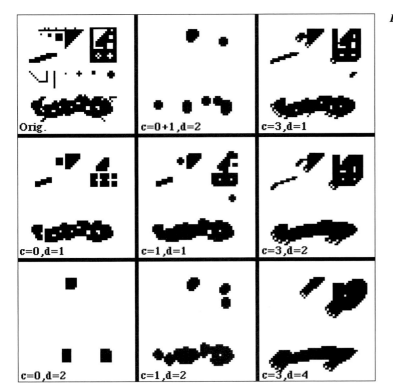

Figure 49. *Effect of changing the parameters in performing an opening: c=test coefficient, d=depth (c=0+1 indicates alternating test coefficients). Figure enlarged to show individual pixels.*

because of the neighborhood shape) or to the 4 corner-touching neighbors (likewise called an "x" pattern), changing the central pixel if any of the 4 neighbors is of the opposite type (ON or OFF). They are rarely used alone, but can be employed in an alternating pattern to obtain greater directional uniformity than classical erosion, as discussed above. **Figures 47** to **50** include some representative examples.

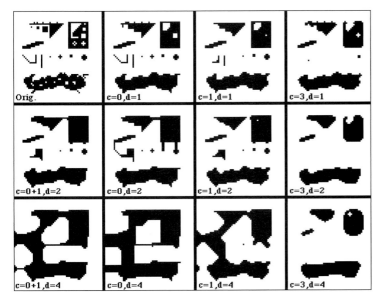

Figure 50. *Effect of changing the parameters in performing a closing: c=test coefficient, d=depth (c=0+1 indicates alternating test coefficients). Figure enlarged to show individual pixels.*

Any specific neighbor pattern can be used, of course. It is not even required to restrict the comparison to immediately touching neighbors. As for grey scale operations, larger neighborhoods make it possible to respond to more subtle textures and achieve greater control over directionality. The general case for this type of operation is called the hit-or-miss operator, which specifies any pattern of neighboring pixels divided into three classes: those that must be ON, those that must be OFF, and those that do not matter (are ignored). If the pattern is found, then the pixel is set to the specified state (Serra, 1982; Coster & Chermant, 1985).

This operation is also called template matching. The same type of operation carried out on grey scale images is called convolution and is a way to search for specific patterns in the image. This is also true for binary images; in fact, template matching with thresholded binary images was one of the earliest methods for optical character reading and is still used for situations in which the character shape, size, and location are tightly controlled (such as the characters at the bottom of bank checks). Much more flexible methods are needed to read more general text, however. In practice, most erosion and dilation is performed using only the 8 nearest-neighbor pixels for comparison.

One method for implementing neighborhood comparison that makes it easy to use any arbitrary pattern of pixels is the fate table. The 8 neighbors each have a value of 1 or 0, depending on whether the pixel is ON or OFF. Assembling these 8 values into a number produces a single byte, which can have any of 256 possible values. This value is used as an address into a table, which provides the result (i.e., turning the central pixel ON or OFF). **Figure 51** illustrates the relationship between the neighbor pattern and the generated address.

Efficient ways to construct the address by bitwise shifting of values, which takes advantage of the machine-language idiosyncrasies of specific computer processors, make this method very fast. The ability to create several tables of possible fates to deal with different erosion and dilation rules, perhaps saved on disk and loaded as needed, makes the method very flexible. However, it does not generalize well to larger neighborhoods or three-dimensional images (discussed in Chapter 10), because the tables become too large.

There are some applications for highly specific erosion/dilation operations that are not symmetrical or isotropic. These always

Figure 51. *Constructing an address into a fate table by assigning each neighbor position to a bit value.*

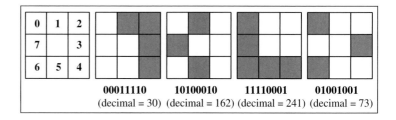

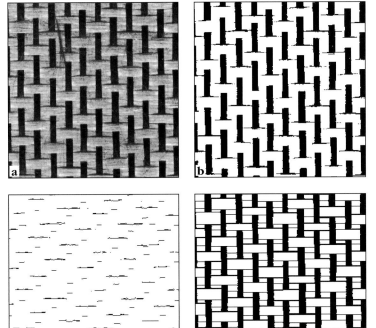

Figure 52. Using directional erosion and dilation to segment an image:

a) *original grey-scale image of a woven textile;*

b) *brightness thresholding of image a;*

c) *end pixels isolated by performing a vertical erosion and Ex-ORing with the original;*

d) *completed operation by repeated horizontal dilation of image c and then ORing with the original.*

require some independent knowledge of the image, the desired information, and the selection of operations that will selectively extract it. However, this is not as important a criticism as it may seem, since all image processing is to some extent knowledge-directed. The human observer tries to find operations to extract information he or she has some reason to know or expect to be present.

Figure 52 shows an example. The horizontal textile fibers vary in width as they weave above and below the vertical ones. Measuring this variation is important to modeling the mechanical properties of the weave, which will be embedded into a composite. The dark vertical fibers can be thresholded based on brightness, but delineating the horizontal fibers is very difficult. The procedure shown in the figure uses the known directionality of the structure.

After thresholding the dark fibers, an erosion is performed to remove only those pixels whose neighbor immediately below or above is part of the background. These pixels, shown in **Figure 52c**, can then be isolated by performing an Ex-OR with the original binary. They include the few points distinguishable between horizontal fibers and the ends of the vertical fibers where they are covered by horizontal ones.

Next, a directional dilation is performed in the horizontal direction. Any background pixel whose left or right touching neighbor is ON is itself set to ON, and this operation is repeated enough times to extend the lines across the distance between vertical fibers. Finally, the resulting horizontal lines are ORed with the original binary image to outline all of the individual fibers (**Figure 52d**). Inverting this image produces measurable features.

Examples of use

Some additional examples of erosion and dilation operations will illustrate typical applications and methods. One of the major areas of use is for X-ray maps from the SEM. These are usually so sparse that even though they are recorded as grey scale images, they are virtually binary images even before thresholding because most pixels have zero photons and a few pixels have one. Regions containing the element of interest are distinguished from those that do not by a difference in the spatial density of dots, which humans are able to interpret by a gestalt grouping operation. This very noisy and scattered image is difficult to use to locate feature boundaries. Dilation may be able to join points together to produce a more useful representation. An example was shown in **Figure 51** of Chapter 6, in comparison with grey scale image processing results.

Figure 53 shows a representative X-ray map from an SEM. Notice that the dark bands in the aluminum dot map represent the shadows where the gold grid blocks the incident electron beam or the emitted X-rays en route to the detector. **Figure 54** shows the result of thresholding the gold map and applying a closing to merge the individual dots. **Figure 55** illustrates the results for the aluminum map. Because it has more dots, it produces a somewhat better definition of the region edges.

Figure 53. X-ray "dot" maps from the SEM:
a) backscattered electron image of a gold grid above an aluminum stub;
b) secondary electron image;
c) gold X-ray dot image;
d) aluminum X-ray image (note shadows of grid).

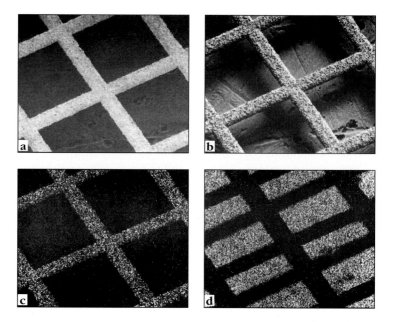

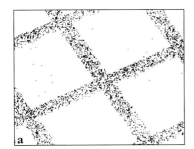 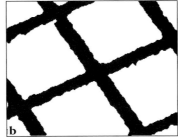 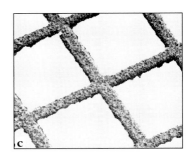

Figure 54. Delineating the gold grid:

a) *thresholded X-ray map;*

b) *image* ***a*** *after 2 repetitions of closing, alternating 0 and 1 coefficient;*

c) *the backscattered electron image masked to show the boundaries from image* ***b****; notice the approximate location of edges.*

Other images from the light and electron microscope sometimes have the same essentially binary image as well. Examples include ultrathin biological tissue sections stained with heavy metals and viewed in the TEM, and chemically etched metallographic specimens. The dark regions are frequently small, corresponding to barely resolved individual particles whose distribution and clustering reveal the desired microstructure (membranes in tissue, eutectic lamellae in metals, etc.) to the eye. As for the case of X-ray dot maps, it is sometimes possible to utilize dilation operations to join such dots to form a well-defined image.

In **Figure 56**, lamellae in a metal are etched to distinguish the regions with and without such structures. Dilation followed by erosion (a closing) merges together the individual lamellae, but there are also dark regions within the essentially white grains because of the presence of a few dark points in the original image. Following the closing with an opening (for a total sequence of dilation, erosion, erosion, dilation) produces a useful result.

In the example of **Figure 56**, the same coefficients and depths (alternating tests of 0 and 1 neighbors for approximate isotropy and two iterations for each dilation or erosion) were used. There is no fundamental reason for this symmetry. In **Figure 57**, a more difficult image is similarly processed, using different coefficients and depths for the initial closing and the final opening. Of course,

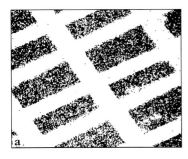 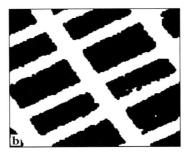

Figure 55. Delineating the aluminum map:

a) *simple thresholding. Notice the isolated continuum X-ray pixels within the grids;*

b) *after erosion with a coefficient of 7 to remove the isolated pixels and dilation (2 cycles) with an alternating 0 and 1 coefficient to fill the regions.*

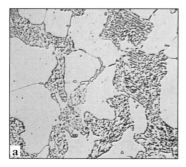

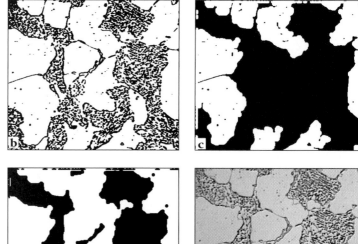

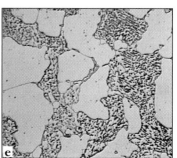

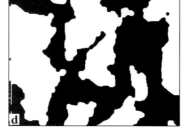

Figure 56. Combined closing and opening to delineate a region:

a) *original grey scale image of a chemically etched metallographic specimen;*

b) *brightness threshold applied to image **a**;*

c) *closing (alternating coefficient 0 and 1) applied to image **b**;*

d) *opening applied to image **c**;*

e) *region boundaries superimposed on original image.*

the choice of appropriate parameters is largely a matter of experience with a particular type of image and human judgment of the correctness of the final result. In other words, it takes trial and error to produce the image the human saw in the first place.

Notice the basic similarity between using these morphological operations on a thresholded binary image and various texture operators on the original grey scale image. In most cases, similar (but not identical) results can be obtained with either approach (provided the software offers both sets of tools). For instance, **Figure 58** shows the same image of curds and whey used earlier to compare several grey scale texture processing operations. Simply background leveling and thresholding the smooth, white areas (the curds) produces the result shown in **Figure 58b**. Clearly, there are many regions in the textured whey protein portion of the image that are just as bright as the curds. In grey scale

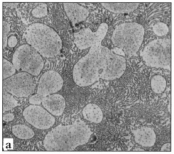

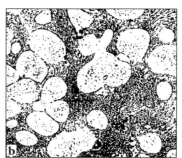

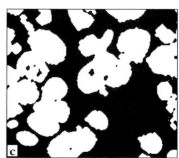

Figure 57. *Another example of combined closing and opening. In this case the closing used an alternating 0,1 coefficient with depth of 2, but the opening used a coefficient of 3 and depth of 4 to remove the small noise spots in the white phase regions.*

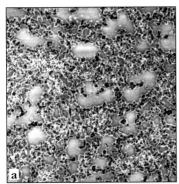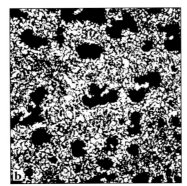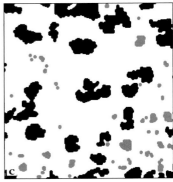

Figure 58. Segmenting the curds and whey image by erosion/dilation:
a) original image; b) thresholded; c) application of an opening followed by feature measurement (small features are shaded grey).

texture processing, these were eliminated based on some consideration of the local variation in pixel brightness. In this image, that variation produces narrow and irregular thresholded regions. An opening, consisting of an erosion to remove edge-touching pixels and a dilation to restore pixels smoothly to boundaries that still exist, effectively removes the background clutter as shown in **Figure 58c**. Small features are shaded grey and would normally be removed based on size to permit analysis of the larger curds. The erosion/dilation approach to defining the structure in this image amounts to making some assumptions about the characteristic dimensions of the features, their boundary irregularities, and their spacings.

Erosion/dilation procedures are often used along with Boolean combinations and feature identification and filling. **Figure 59** shows a representative sequence of operations, used in this case to produce a representation of particles in a plasma-sprayed coating. The original grey scale image (**Figure 59a**) shows a polished cross section through a complex, sprayed coating applied to a turbine blade. The dark grey particles with light interiors are hard, wear-resistant materials included to improve coating performance. Thresholding to select dark grey shows the periphery of the particles (**Figure 59b**), but does not include their central cores, which have the same average brightness as the matrix. Some of the particles do not show these cores, because the plane of sectioning has not passed through the core.

Inverting this image (**Figure 59c**) causes the interior cores to become features that do not touch the edges of the field of view. However, keeping only the features that do not touch the edge (**Figure 59d**) includes pores, as well as cores. The original image is thresholded again to select the light grey values characteristic of the matrix and the cores (**Figure 59e**). This result is ANDed with the inverted image to select only the cores (**Figure 59f**) identified as features in the inverted image (bright in the grey scale image) since the pores are dark.

Figure 59. Combined operations to isolate particles in a coating:

a) *original grey-scale image;*

b) *thresholded on dark grey showing periphery of particles;*

c) *inversion of image **b**;*

d) *elimination of edge-touching region to leave features corresponding to particle cores as well as pores;*

e) *thresholding of original image to select light grey characteristic of matrix and cores;*

f) *AND of image **e** with **d** to select cores;*

g) *OR of image **f** with **b**, to fill holes within particles;*

b) *application of opening (coefficient=3, depth=10) to remove boundary-straddling pixels.*

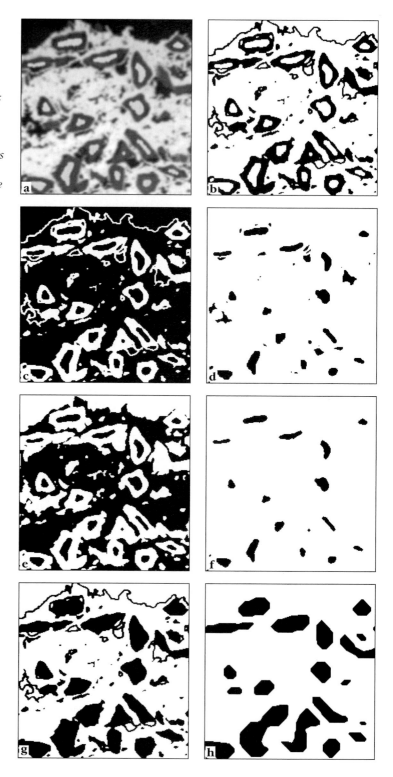

These cores are then ORed with the original binary image of the particle periphery (**Figure 59g**) to fill in the particles (but not the voids). Finally, an opening (coefficient = 3, depth = 10) removes

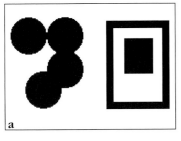
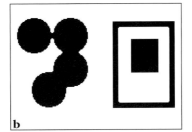
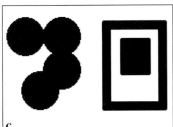
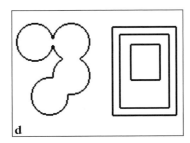

Figure 60. Schematic diagram of forming a custer:
a) *original image;*
b) *erosion of* **a** *;*
c) *dilation of* **a** *;*
d) *Ex-OR of* **b** *and* **c** *.*

the pixels straddling the boundaries between lighter and darker regions. The final result (**Figure 59h**) is a binary image of the particles suitable for counting or measurement. This may seem like a rather complicated procedure, and indeed it does require some human judgment to determine what characteristics of the desired features can be used to isolate them and how the necessary operations should be implemented, but the time required is minimal, since all of these operations are individually very simple.

The custer

In the discussion of fractal dimension measurement above, the Ex-OR combination of an erosion and a dilation was used to define the pixels along a boundary. The result is called the custer of a feature, apparently in reference to George Herbert Armstrong Custer, who was also surrounded. **Figure 60** shows the formation of a custer. In some cases, a custer is approximated by Ex-ORing the original binary image with the result of either a single erosion or dilation. This can be accomplished by performing an erosion with neighborhood rules, which keep only those pixels with at least one background neighbor (or similar rules for dilation).

The custer can be used to determine neighbor relationships between features or regions. As an example, **Figure 61** shows a three-phase metal alloy imaged in the light microscope. Each of the individual phases can be readily delineated by thresholding (and in the case of the medium grey image, an opening to remove lines of pixels straddling the white-black boundary). Then the custer of each phase can be formed as described.

Combining the custer of each phase with the other phases using an AND keeps only the portion of the custer that is common to

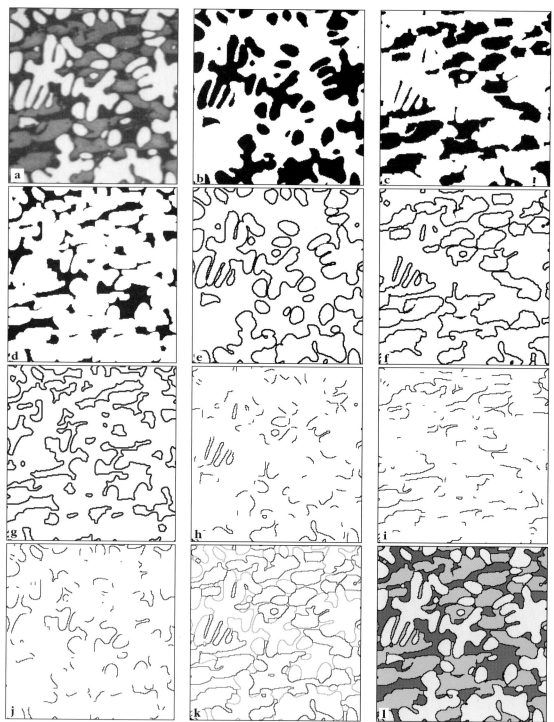

Figure 61. Use of Boolean logic to measure neighbor relationships:
   a) *an original light microscope image of a three-phase metal; **b)** thresholded white phase;*
   c) *thresholded grey phase; **d)** thresholded black phase; **e)** surrounding outline of white phase produced*
   *by dilation and Ex-OR with original; **f)** surrounding outline of grey phase produced by dilation and Ex-*
   *OR with original; **g)** surrounding outline of black phase produced by dilation and Ex-OR with original;*
   ***b)** AND of white outlines and grey features; **i)** AND of grey outlines with black features; **j)** AND of black*
   *outlines with white features; **k)** OR of all ANDed outlines using different colors to identify each*
   *phase/phase interface; **l)** outlines filled to show idealized phase regions.*

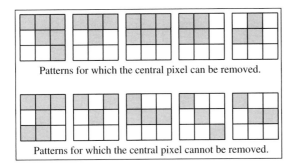

Figure 62. *Representative neighbor patterns which allow and do not allow the central pixel to be removed in skeletonization.*

Patterns for which the central pixel can be removed.

Patterns for which the central pixel cannot be removed.

the two phases. The result is to mark the boundaries as white-grey, grey-black, or black-white, so that the extent of each type can be determined by simple counting. In other cases, Feature-AND can be used to select the entire features that are adjacent to one region (and hence touch its custer).

Skeletonization

Erosion can be performed with special rules that remove pixels, except when doing so would cause a separation of one region into two. The rule for this is to examine the touching neighbors; if they do not form a continuous group, then the central pixel cannot be removed (Pavlidis, 1980; Nevatia & Babu, 1980; Davidson, 1991; Lan et al, 1992; Ritter & Wilson, 1996). The definition of this condition is dependent on whether four- or eight-connectedness is used, as shown in **Figure 62**. In either case, the selected patterns can be used in a fate table to conduct the erosion; for the four-connected case, only $2^4=16$ entries are needed (Russ, 1984).

Figure 63 shows several features with their (eight-connected) skeletons. The skeleton is a powerful shape factor for feature recognition, containing both topological and metric information. The topological values include the number of end points, the

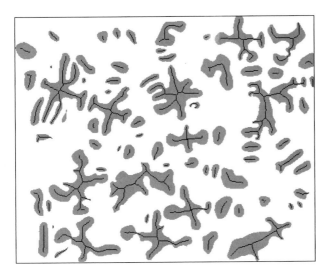

Figure 63. *A binary image containing multiple features, with their skeletons superimposed.*

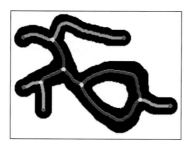

Figure 64. *The skeleton of a feature with 5 end points, 5 nodes, 5 branches, 5 links, and one loop (skeleton has been dilated for visibility).*

number of nodes where branches meet, and the number of internal holes in the feature. The metric values are the mean length of branches (both those internal to the feature and those having a free end) and the angles of the branches. These parameters seem to correspond closely to what human observers see as the significant characteristics of features. **Figure 64** shows the nomenclature used.

Locating the nodes and end points in a skeleton is simply a matter of counting neighbors. End points have a single neighbor, while nodes have more than two. Segment length can also be determined by counting, keeping track of the number of pixel pairs that are diagonally or orthogonally connected. Counting the number of nodes, ends, loops, and branches defines the topology of the feature. These topological events simplify the original image and assist in characterizing structure, as illustrated in **Figure 65**. Also, in many structures, measuring the distribution of link and branch lengths and their orientation provides metric information.

The problem with skeletonization is its sensitivity to minor changes in the shape of the feature. As shown in **Figure 66**, changing as little as a single pixel on the exterior boundary of a feature can alter the skeleton to add a branch and node. Changing a single pixel within the feature produces a loop and completely alters the topology. Considering the difficulty of obtaining a perfect binary representation of a feature or region and the need for the various operations discussed so far in this chapter to modify and attempt to correct them, it can be unwise to depend on a technique so sensitive to these variations.

Figure 65. *Simplification of a fingerprint image (a) by thresholding and skeletonization (b).*

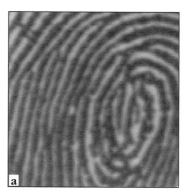
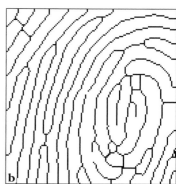

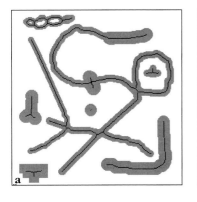

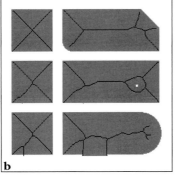

Figure 66. Examples of skeletons superimposed on features:
a) *for long and thin features the skeleton represents the shape well;*
b) *modifying the original feature by as little as a single pixel on the exterior or interior alters the skeleton by adding branches or loops.*

Just as the skeleton of features may be determined in an image, it is also possible to skeletonize the background. This is often called the "skiz" of the features. **Figure 67** shows an example. Consisting of points equidistant from feature boundaries, it effectively divides the image into regions of influence around each feature (Serra, 1982). It may be desirable to eliminate from the skiz those lines that are equidistant from two portions of the boundary of the same feature. This elimination is easily accomplished, since branches have an end; other lines in the skiz are continuous and have no ends except at the image boundaries. Pruning branches from a skeleton (or skiz) simply requires starting at each end point (points with a single neighbor) and eliminating touching pixels until a node (a point with more than two neighbors) is reached.

Boundary lines and thickening

Another use for skeletonization is to thin down boundaries that may appear broad or of variable thickness in images. This phenomenon is particularly common in light microscope images of

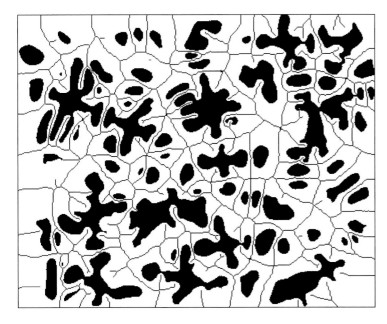

Figure 67. *The skiz of the features in the same image as Figure 63.*

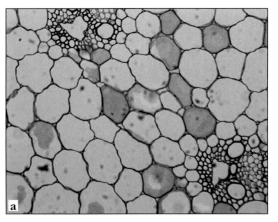

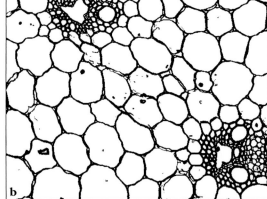

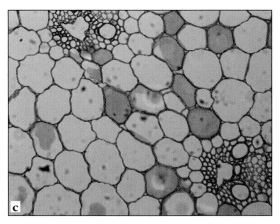

**Figure 68. Light microscope image of cells in
plant tissue:**

a) *original;*

b) *thresholded;*

c) *skeletonized (superimposed on original).*
(Image courtesy of Data Translations, Inc.)

metals whose grain boundaries are revealed by chemical etching. Such etching preferentially attacks the boundaries, but in order to produce continuous dark lines, it also broadens them. In order to measure the actual size of grains, the adjacency of different phases, or the length of boundary lines, it is preferable to thin the lines by skeletonization.

Figure 68 shows how this approach can be used to simplify an image and isolate the basic structure for measurement. The original image is a light micrograph of cells. It might be used to measure the variation in cell size with the distance from the two openings. This process will be greatly simplified by reducing the cell walls to single lines. Leveling the background brightness of the original image and then thresholding leaves boundary lines of variable width. Skeletonizing them produces a network of single-pixel-wide lines that delineate the basic cell arrangement.

Figure 69 shows another example. The original polished and etched metal sample has dark and wide grain boundaries, as well as dark patches corresponding to carbides and pearlite. Thresholding the image produces broad lines, which can be skeletonized to reduce them to single-pixel width. Since this is

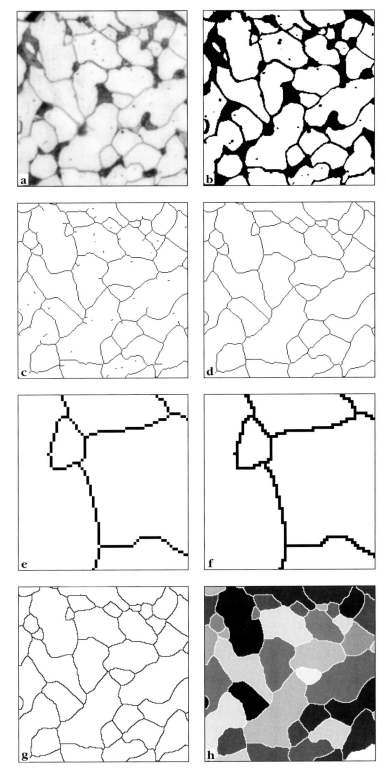

Figure 69. Skeletonization of grain boundaries:

a) metallographic image of etched 1040 steel;

b) thresholded image showing boundaries and dark patches of iron carbide (and pearlite);

c) skeletonized from image **b**;

d) pruned from image **c**;

e) enlarged to show eight-connected line;

f) converted to four-connected line;

g) grains separated by thickened lines;

h) identification of individual grains.

properly a continuous tesselation, it can be cleaned up by removing all branches that have end points, a process called pruning.

The resulting lines delineate the grain boundaries, but because they are eight-connected, they do not separate the grains for individual measurement. Converting the lines to four-connected, called thickening, can be accomplished with a dilation that adds pixels only for a few neighbor patterns corresponding to eight-connected corners (or the skeleton could have been produced using four-connected rules to begin with). The resulting lines do separate the grains, which can be identified and measured as shown.

Unfortunately, the grain boundary tesselation produced by simple thresholding and skeletonization is incomplete in many cases. Some of the boundaries may fail to etch because the crystallographic mismatch across the boundary is small or the concentration of defects or impurities is low. The result is a tesselation with some missing lines, which would bias subsequent analysis. **Figure 70** shows an example of this situation. The original image (obtained by thresholding and skeletonization) is complete, but a portion of the boundaries have been randomly erased. This primarily removes lines, rather than junctions (which tend to etch well).

Figure 71 shows one of the simplest approaches to dealing with this situation. Skeletonizing the incomplete network is used to identify the end points (points with a single neighbor). It is reasoned that these points should occur in pairs, so each is dilated by some arbitrarily selected distance which, it is hoped, will span half of the gap in the network. The resulting dilated circles are ORed with the original network and the result is again skeletonized. Wherever the dilation has caused the circles to touch, the result is a line segment that joins the corresponding end points.

This method is imperfect, however. Some of the points may be too far apart for the circles to touch, while in other places, the circles may obscure details by touching several existing lines, oversimplifying the resulting network. It is not easy to select an appropriate dilation radius, since the gaps are not all the same size (and not all of the grains are either). In addition, unmatched ends, or points due to dirt or particulates within the grains, can cause difficulties.

Other methods are also available. A computationally intensive approach locates all of the end points and uses a relaxation method to pair them up, so that line direction is maintained, lines are not allowed to cross, and closer points are matched first. This method suffers some of the same problems as dilation if unmatched end points or noise are present, but at least it deals well with gaps of different sizes. A third approach, though

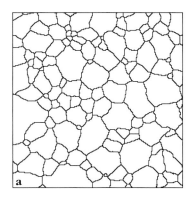

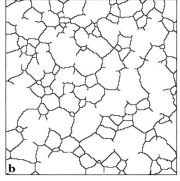

imperfect, is perhaps the most efficient and reasonably accurate method. It is shown below in conjunction with the Euclidean distance map (EDM).

Euclidean distance map

The image processing functions discussed in this and preceding chapters operate either on grey scale images (to produce other grey scale images) or on binary images (to produce other binary images). The Euclidean Distance Map (EDM) is a tool that works on a binary image to produce a grey scale image. The definition is simple enough: each pixel, in either the features or the background or both, is assigned a brightness value equal to its distance from the nearest boundary. This is normally interpreted to

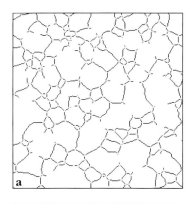

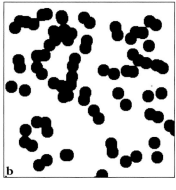

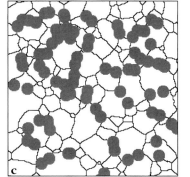

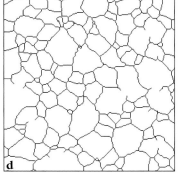

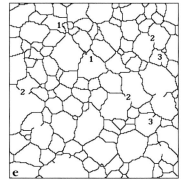

6	5	4	3	4	5	6
5	4	3	2	3	4	5
4	3	2	1	2	3	4
3	2	1	0	1	2	3
4	3	2	1	2	3	4
5	4	3	2	3	4	5
6	5	4	3	4	5	6

3	3	3	3	3	3	3
3	2	2	2	2	2	3
3	2	1	1	1	2	3
3	2	1	0	1	2	3
3	2	1	1	1	2	3
3	2	2	2	2	2	3
3	3	3	3	3	3	3

√18	√13	√10	3.0	3.2	3.6	4.2
√13	√8	√5	2.0	2.2	2.8	3.6
√10	√5	√2	1.0	1.4	2.2	3.2
√9	√4	√1	0	1.0	2.0	3.0
√10	√5	√2	1.0	1.4	2.2	3.2
√13	√8	√5	2.0	2.2	2.8	3.6
√18	√13	√10	3.0	3.2	3.6	4.2

Figure 72. *Arrays of pixels with their distance from the center pixel shown for the cases of 4- and 8-neighbor paths and in Pythagorean units.*

mean that the brightness of each point in the image encodes the straight line distance to the nearest point on any boundary. In a continuous image, as opposed to a digitized one containing finite pixels, this is unambiguous. In most pixel images, the distance is taken from each pixel in the feature to the nearest pixel in the background.

Searching through all of the background pixels to find the nearest one to each pixel in a feature and calculating the distance in a Pythagorean sense would be an extremely inefficient and time-consuming process for constructing the EDM. Furthermore, since the brightness values of the pixels are quantized, some round-off errors in distance must be accepted. Some researchers have implemented an EDM using distance measured in only a few directions. For a lattice of square pixels, this may either be restricted to the 90° directions, or it may also include the 45° directions (Rosenfeld and Kak, 1982). This measuring convention is equivalent to deciding to use a four-neighbor or eight-neighbor convention for considering whether pixels are touching. In either case, the distance from each pixel to one of its 4 or 8 neighbors is taken as 1, regardless of the direction. Consequently, as shown in **Figure 72**, the distance map from a point gives rise to either square or diamond-shaped artefacts and is quite distorted, as compared to the Pythagorean distance. These measuring conventions are sometimes described as city-block models (connections in 4 directions) or chessboard models (8 directions), because of the limited moves available in those situations.

A conceptually straightforward, iterative technique for constructing such a distance map can be programmed as follows.

1. Assign a brightness value of 0 to each pixel in the background.

2. Set a variable N equal to 0.

3. For each pixel that touches (in either the 4- or 8-neighbor sense, as described above) a pixel whose brightness value is N, assign a brightness value of $N + 1$.

4. Increment N and repeat step 3, until all pixels in the image have been assigned.

The time required for this iteration depends on the size of the features (the maximum distance from the background). A more efficient method is available that gives the same result with two passes through the image (Danielsson, 1980). This technique uses the same comparisons, but propagates the values through the image more rapidly.

1. Assign the brightness value of 0 to each pixel in the background and a large positive value (greater than the maximum feature width) to each pixel in a feature.

2. Proceeding from left to right and top to bottom, assign each pixel within a feature a brightness value one greater than the smallest value of any of its neighbors.

3. Repeat step 2, proceeding from right to left and bottom to top.

A further modification provides a better approximation to the Pythagorean distances between pixels (Russ & Russ, 1988b). The diagonally adjacent pixels are neither a distance 1 (8-neighbor rules) or 2 (4-neighbor rules) away, but actually $\sqrt{2} = 1.414\ldots$ pixels. This is an irrational number, but closer approximations than 1.00 or 2.00 are available. For instance, modifying the above rules so that a pixel brightness value must be larger than its 90° neighbors by 2 and greater than its 45° neighbors by 3 is equivalent to using an approximation of 1.5 for the square root of 2.

The disadvantage of this method is that all of the pixel distances are now multiplied by 2, increasing the maximum brightness of the EDM image by this factor. For images capable of storing a maximum grey level of 255, this represents a limitation on the largest features that can be processed in this way. However, if the EDM image is 16 bits deep (and can hold values up to 65,535), this is not a practical limitation. It also opens the way to selecting larger ratios of numbers to approximate $\sqrt{2}$, getting a correspondingly improved set of values for the distance map. For instance, $7/5 = 1.400$ and $58/41 = 1.415$.

It takes no longer to compare or add these values than it does any others, and they allow dimensions larger than 1024 pixels. Since this dimension is the half-width, features or background up to 2048 pixels wide can be processed ($1024 \cdot 41 = 41,984$, which is less than $2^{16} - 1 = 65,535$). Of course, the final image can be divided down by the scaling factor (41 in this example) to obtain a result in which pixel brightness values are the actual distance to the boundary (rounded or truncated to integers) and the total brightness range is within the 0 to 255 range that most displays are capable of showing.

The accuracy of an EDM constructed with these rules can be judged by counting the pixels whose brightness values place them within a distance s. This is just the same as constructing a

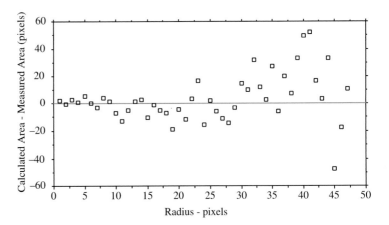

Figure 73. *Difference between theoretical area value (πr²) and the actual area covered by the EDM as a function of brightness (distance from boundary) shows increasing but still small errors for very large distances.*

cumulative histogram of pixel brightness in the image. **Figure 73** plots the error in the number of pixels vs. integer brightness for a distance map of a circle 99 pixels in diameter; the overall errors are not too large. Even better accuracy for the EDM can be obtained by performing additional comparisons to pixels beyond the first 8 nearest neighbors. Adding a comparison to the 8 neighbors in the 5×5 neighborhood whose Pythagorean distance is $\sqrt{5}$ produces values having even less directional sensitivity and more accuracy for large distances. If the integer values 58 and 41 mentioned above are used to approximate $\sqrt{2}$, then the path to these pixels consisting of a "knight's move" of one 90° and one 45° pixel step would produce a value of 58 + 41 = 99. Substituting a value of 92 gives a close approximation to the Pythagorean distance and produces more isotropic results.

It is interesting to compare each of the erosion methods discussed above to the ideal circular pattern provided by the EDM. Simple thresholding of the distance map can be used to select pixels that are farther from the edge than any desired extent of erosion. Similarly, the distance map of the background can be thresholded to perform a dilation. Both of these operations can be carried out without any iteration. The distance map is constructed noniteratively as well, so the execution time of the method does not increase with feature size (as do classical erosion methods) and is preferred for large features or depths. **Figure 74** shows the erosion and dilation of a circle using the distance map; compare this to **Figures 41** to **43** for classical erosion and dilation.

When more irregular shapes are eroded, the difference between the iterative methods and thresholding the EDM is less obvious visually. However, the directional bias of the iterative comparisons is still present and can be measured. **Figure 75** shows a binary image containing features with a variety of shapes. The dark pixels are those removed by thresholding the EDM to a depth of 6. Applying the various iterative erosion patterns described above removes some pixels that are at a greater distance than 6 pixels from the boundary or leaves ones which are closer to it.

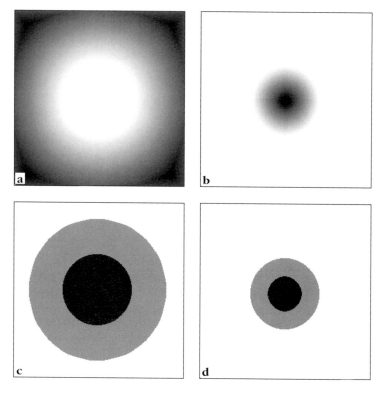

Figure 74. Isotropy achieved by using the Euclidean distance map for dilation and erosion (compare to Figures 41, 42, and 43):

a) the EDM of the background around the circle;

b) the EDM of the circle;

c) dilation achieved by thresholding the background EDM at a value of 50;

d) erosion achieved by thresholding the circle EDM at a value of 25.

Figure 76 shows the results in the form of a plot. The uppermost line in the plot shows the number of pixels present as a function of their distance from the boundary. This information comes directly from the brightness histogram of the EDM. Each of the other lines shows how many pixels were removed by various iterative erosion patterns, as a function of the pixel's distance from the boundary. The alternating cross-and-X or square-and-X

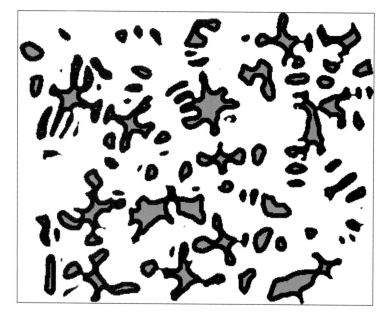

Figure 75. Binary test image showing the pixels removed by thresholding the EDM at a depth of 6.

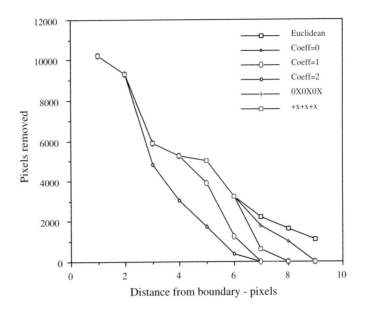

Figure 76. Plot of number of pixels removed in 6 cycles of erosion applied to Figure 73 using various iterative patterns, versus their actual distance from the boundary as given by the EDM. The OXOX and Coeff = 0 curves are superimposed exactly.

patterns and the unconditional erosion (coefficient = 0) remove all of the pixels at a distance up to 6 pixels from the boundary, but also remove additional pixels that are farther away. Coefficients of 1 or 2 remove no pixels farther than 6 pixels from the boundary, but do not remove all of the ones within 6 pixels of the boundary. None of the iterative methods accurately duplicates the results obtained by thresholding the EDM.

Similar results are obtained when dilations are performed or when combinations of erosions and dilations are carried out. Dilations are performed by first obtaining the EDM of the background. This can be accomplished either by inverting a copy of the image (reversing all of the black and white pixels in the binary image) or by constructing the EDM of the background at the same time as the features, by using complementary logic in the program. **Figures 77** and **78** compare the results of an opening applied to the same image as in **Figure 75**. In **Figure 77**, the opening of depth 6 is applied by thresholding a distance map of the features and then of the background. In **Figure 78**, the opening is performed using classical erosion and dilation. Notice the rather significant differences in pixels and even features that have been removed and also the resulting different feature shapes.

Watershed segmentation

A common difficulty in measuring images occurs when features touch, and therefore cannot be separately identified, counted, or measured. This situation may arise when examining an image of a thick section in transmission, where actual feature overlap may occur, or when particles resting on a surface tend to agglomerate and touch each other. One method for separating touching, but mostly convex, features in an image is known as watershed segmentation (Beucher & Lantejoul, 1979; Lantejoul & Beucher, 1981).

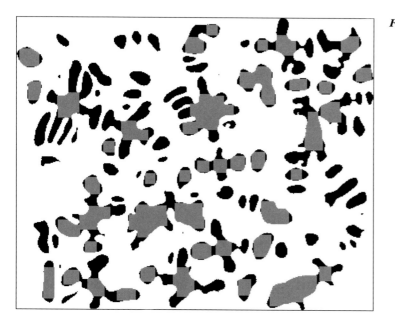

Figure 77. Opening produced by classic erosion/dilation to a depth of six. Dark pixels are those removed. The image is the same as in Figures 75 and 78.

It relies on the fact that eroding the binary image will usually cause touching features to separate before they disappear.

The classical method for accomplishing this separation (Jernot, 1982) is an iterative one. The image is repetitively eroded, and at each step those separate features that disappeared from the previous step are designated ultimate eroded points (UEPs) and saved as an image, along with the iteration number. Saving these is necessary because the features will in general be of different sizes and would not all disappear in the same number of iterations, as mentioned above in connection with **Figure 46**. The process continues until the image is erased.

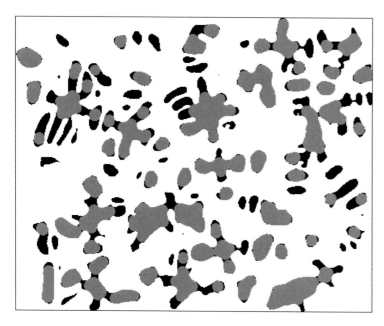

Figure 78. Opening produced by thresholding the EDM of features (erosion) and then of background (dilation) to a depth of six. Dark pixels are those removed. The image is the same as in Figures 75 and 77.

Then, beginning with the final image of UEPs, the image is dilated using classical dilation, but with the added logical constraint that no new pixel may be turned ON if it causes a connection to form between previously separate features or if it was not ON in the original image. At each stage of the dilation, the image of UEPs that corresponds to the equivalent level of erosion is added to the image using a logical OR. This process causes the features to grow back to their original boundaries, except that lines of separation appear between the touching features.

The method just described has two practical drawbacks: the iterative process is slow, requiring each pixel in the image to be processed many times, and the amount of storage required for all of the intermediate images is quite large. The same result can be obtained more efficiently using an EDM. Indeed, the name "watershed" comes directly from the EDM. Imagine that the brightness values of each pixel within features in an EDM correspond to a physical elevation. The features then appear as a mountain peak. **Figure 79** illustrates this for a circular feature.

If two features touch or overlap slightly, the EDM shows two peaks, as shown in **Figure 80**. The slope of the mountainside is the same, so the larger the feature the higher the peak. The ultimate eroded points are the peaks of the mountains, and where features touch, the flanks of the mountains intersect. The saddles or watersheds of these mountains are the lines selected as boundaries by the segmentation method. The placement of these lines according to the relative height of the mountains (size of the features) gives the best estimate of the separation lines between features. The term "watershed," often used for this segmentation procedure, can be understood by considering the mountains in **Figure 80**. Rain that falls on each mountain top will run down the sides to reach all pixels in the underlying feature. The separation lines divide the features according to the regions that belong to each mountain top.

Implementing the segmentation process using an EDM approach (Russ & Russ, 1988b) is very efficient, both in terms of speed and storage. Only a single distance map image is required, and it is constructed without iteration. The ultimate eroded points are located as a special case of local maxima (there is a further discussion of UEPs below) and the brightness value of each directly corresponds to the iteration number at which it would disappear in the iterative method. Dilating these features is fast, because the distance map supplies a constraint. Starting at the brightest value and iteratively decrementing this to 1 covers all of the brightness levels. At each one, only those pixels at the current brightness level in the distance map need to be considered. Those that do not produce a join between feature pixels are added to the image. The process continues until all of the pixels in the features, except for those along the boundary lines, have been restored.

Figure 81 shows an example of this method, applied to a binary image from a polished section through a sintered metal powder.

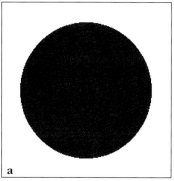 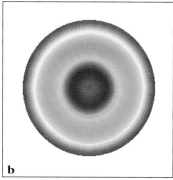 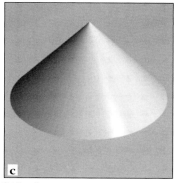

Figure 79: Interpreting the Euclidean distance map as the height of pixels:
a) *binary image of a circular feature;* *b)* *Euclidean distance map with pixels color coded to show distance from boundary;* *c)* *rendered display showing pixel heights.*

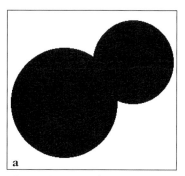 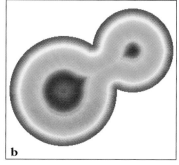 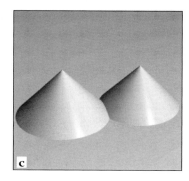

Figure 80: EDM for touching features:
a) *binary image of two touching circular features;* *b)* *Euclidean distance map with pixels color coded to show distance from boundary;* *c)* *rendered display showing pixel heights. Note the boundary between the two cones.*

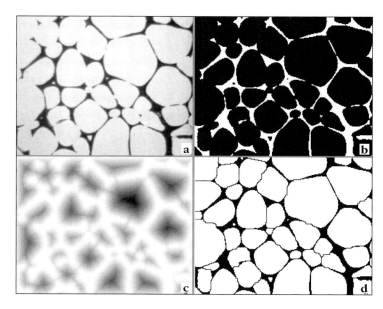

Figure 81. Watershed segmentation applied to a sintered microstructure:
a) *original grey scale image;*
b) *thresholded binary image;*
c) *Euclidean distance map;*
d) *segmentation lines produced by the algorithm.*

The original image (**Figure 81a**) shows considerable contact between the individual particles, which must be separated to measure the binary image (**Figure 81b**). The EDM (**Figure 81c**) shows the peaks rising to different heights, depending on the size of the features. Since the features are not perfectly round, the location of the peak (or UEP) within each one is asymmetric and the maximum brightness value corresponds to the shortest distance to the nearest boundary points. After the dilation process, **Figure 78d** shows the features with separation lines.

Of course, this method is not perfect. **Figure 82** illustrates the most common difficulties. The original image is an agglomerated soot particle. Watershed segmentation does not separate particles whose contact is broad enough that the ridge in the EDM has no minimum. Also, it produces multiple separation lines when the minimum is so gradual that minor variations or noise in the edge shape can cause fluctuations in the ridge value. The presence of a third feature may shift the location of the minimum, thereby displacing the separation line. All of these problems arise because finding the minimum is a local process and hence is susceptible to local noise.

Watershed segmentation also provides another tool to complete grain boundary tesselations, discussed above. **Figure 83** shows the same test image as **Figure 70**. Inverting the image so that the grains, rather than the boundaries, are features and then performing watershed segmentation reconstructs most of the boundaries. As shown in the image, it misses some boundaries and adds others, depending on the shape of the grains.

The presence of holes within features confuses the watershed algorithm and breaks the features up into many fragments. It is therefore necessary to fill holes before applying the watershed. However, there may also be holes in the image between features as well as those within them. Normal hole filling would fill them in since any region of background not connected to the edge of the image is considered a hole. This difficulty can be overcome if some difference in hole size or shape can be identified to permit filling only the holes within features and not those between them (Russ, 1995f). In the example shown in **Figure 84**, the holes within features (organelles within the cells) are both smaller and rounder than spaces between the touching cells.

Ultimate eroded points

The ultimate eroded points (UEPs) described in the watershed segmentation technique can be used as a measurement tool in their own right. The number of points gives the number of separable features in the image, while the brightness of each point gives a measure of their sizes. In addition, the location of each point can be used as a location for the feature if clustering or gradients are to be investigated.

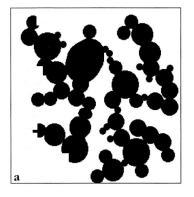

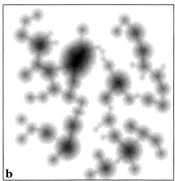

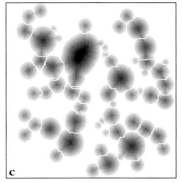

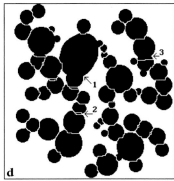

Figure 82. Example of watershed segmentation:
a) original binary image of an agglomerated soot particle;
b) Euclidean distance map of image *a*;
c) watershed segmentation lines superimposed on image *c*;
d) result, showing typical errors: 1 = features not separated because there is no minimum in ridge of EDM; 2 = multiple separation lines where ridge has a long and gradual minimum subject to noise; 3 = displaced separation line due to presence of a third feature.

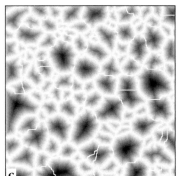

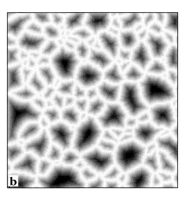

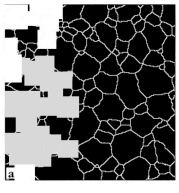

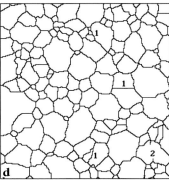

Figure 83. Watershed segmentation method for separating grains:
a) inverted image showing complete network;
b) Euclidean distance map of image *a*;
c) automatic segmentation of image *b*;
d) resulting network with some typical errors marked: 1 = extra lines drawn across grains of nonconvex shape; 2 = missing lines for pairs of squat grains.

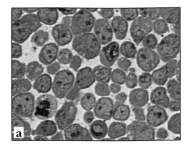

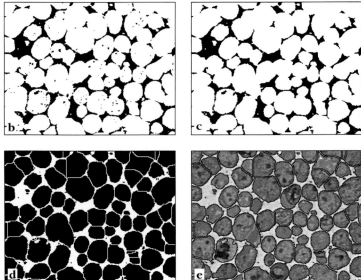

Figure 84. Selective filling of holes before a watershed:

a) *original image (light micrograph of cells);*

b) *thresholded holes;*

c) *removal of internal holes based on size and shape;*

d) *watershed applied to the inverse of figure **c**;*

e) *separation of many of the cells in the original image by the watershed.*

The formal definition of a UEP in a continuous, rather than pixel-based, image is simply a local maximum of brightness. When the image is subdivided into finite pixels, the definition must take into account the possibility that more than one pixel may have equal brightness, forming a plateau. The operating definition for finding these pixels is recursive.

$$\{U: \quad \forall \ U_j \text{ neighbors of } U_i, \ |U_j| \leq |U_i|$$
$$\text{AND} \tag{4}$$
$$\forall \ U_j \text{ neighbors of } U_i \text{ such that } |U_j| = |U_i|, \ U_i \in U\}$$

In other words, the set of pixels which are UEPs must be as bright or brighter than all neighbors; if the neighbors are equal in brightness, then they must also be part of the set.

The brightness of each pixel in the distance map is the distance to the nearest boundary. For a UEP, this must be a point that is equidistant from at least three boundary locations. Consequently, the brightness is the radius of the feature's inscribed circle. **Figure 85** applies this to the measurement of latex spheres in a

Figure 85. *Ultimate eroded points in a binary image of partially overlapped latex spheres **(a)** and the histogram **(b)** of the brightness of the points which gives a direct measure of particle sizes.*

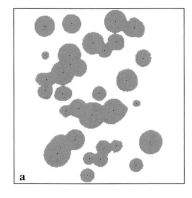

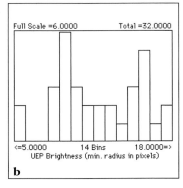

thin section imaged in a TEM. Each feature is shown marked with the location of the UEP. The figure shows a histogram of particle size as determined by the brightness of the UEPs. This is much faster than convex segmentation, since the iterative dilation is bypassed, and much faster than measurement, since no feature identification or pixel counting is required.

Fractal dimension measurement

The method described above for determining a fractal dimension from successive erosion and dilation operations has two shortcomings: it is slow and has orientational bias because of the anisotropy of the operations. The EDM offers a simple way to obtain the same information (Russ, 1988). For example, **Figure 86** shows an image containing four irregular features (paint pigment particles from an SEM image). The EDM is shown in **Figure 87**. Thresholding this image at different brightness levels selects bands of pixels having any distance from the original boundary (now defined as a line between pixels). The perimeter defined by this sausage band is simply the area (number of pixels) in the band divided by its mean width (the number of brightness levels included in the band). **Figure 88** shows examples of the bands of pixels along the boundary (called Minkowski sausages) obtained by thresholding the distance map.

Plotting this perimeter vs. the width of the sausage on a log-log Richardson plot produces slopes giving the feature fractal dimension, as illustrated in **Figure 89**. The resulting fractal dimensions for the four features are shown in **Figure 86**. The method is fast and robust, and the values vary less with feature size, position, or orientation than any of the other methods described. In fact, it is not even necessary to perform the various thresholding operations to obtain the thickened boundary lines. Instead, the brightness histogram of the distance map directly gives the number of pixels at each distance, which can be used to form the regression plot.

Medial axis transform

The skeletonization discussed above uses an iterative erosion that removes pixels from the outside edges, provided that they do not cause a disconnection that would separate a feature into two (or more) parts. The number of iterations required is proportional to the largest dimension of any feature in the image. As is usual with erosion operations, there may be directional bias.

Very similar information can be obtained much more quickly from the distance map. The ridge of locally brightest values in the EDM contains those points that are equidistant from at least two points on the boundaries of the feature. This ridge constitutes the medial axis transform (MAT). As for the UEPs, the MAT is precisely defined for a continuous image but only approximately defined for an image composed of finite pixels (Mott-Smith, 1970).

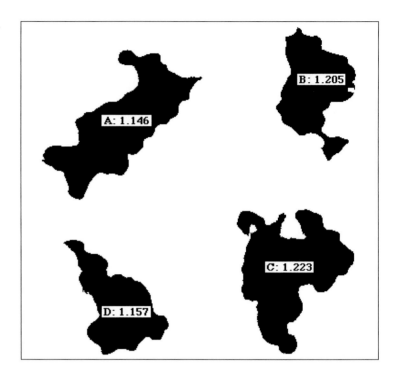

Figure 86. *Binary image of four paint pigment particles, each marked with its fractal dimension.*

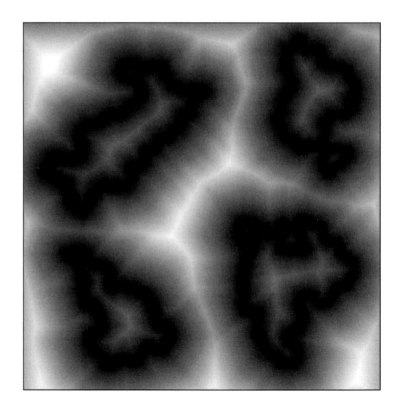

Figure 87. *Euclidean distance map of both the features and the background in Figure 86. (Plotted with inverted grey scale to show boundaries.)*

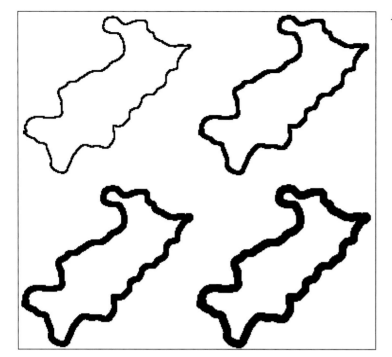

Figure 88. The results of progressively thresholding the EDM of feature A in Figure 86 at different values, to obtain the pixels within varying distances of the boundary.

In most cases, the MAT corresponds rather closely to the skeleton obtained by sequential erosion. Since it is less directionally sensitive than any erosion pattern and because of the pixel limitations in representing a line, it may differ slightly in some cases. The uses of the MAT are the same as the skeleton. End points and nodes can be counted and the branches and links measured. Because it comes from the EDM, which is constructed without iteration, the MAT can be faster to obtain. **Figure 90** shows a comparison of the skeleton and MAT of an irregular feature. The skeleton is more sensitive to minor irregularities along the feature periphery, which can produce additional branches.

A combined use of the MAT and EDM is shown in **Figure 91**. The values along the MAT represent the distance to the edge of the feature and can be used to find the maximum and minimum

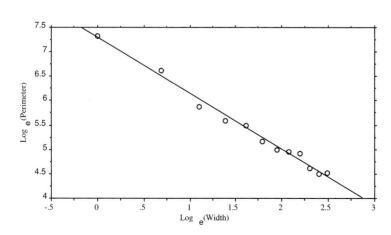

Figure 89. Richardson plot of perimeter (area of the thresholded band divided by width) vs. width for feature A in Figure 86. The slope of the plot is −0.146, giving a fractal dimension of 1.146. The area can be determined directly from the histogram of the EDM, without creating the thresholded images in Figure 86.

Figure 90. *Comparison of the skeleton (**a**) and medial axis transform (**b**) of the same feature. The skeleton is much more sensitive to irregularities along the feature periphery.*

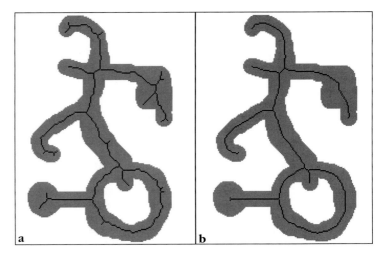

widths. A histogram of these values gives the variation in width. Interpreting these values is complicated for a feature with branch points, however.

Cluster analysis

The spatial distribution of features in an image is often interesting, but it is not simple to characterize. One method of analysis (Schwarz & Exner, 1983) uses the spatial coordinates of the centroids of features, sorts through them to locate the nearest-neighbor feature for each feature present, and then constructs a distribution

Figure 91. Use of the Euclidean distance map to measure feature width:

a) *test image consisting of two features of variable width, one with a branch point, and the skeleton of each shown superimposed;*

b) *Euclidean distance map of the features;*

c) *using the skeleton to select only the points in the distance map which lie along the axis, but retaining their values (shown here with color coding);*

d) *histogram of the values of the points in image **c** for each pixel, which characterizes the mean and variation in feature width.*

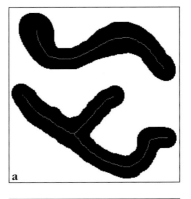

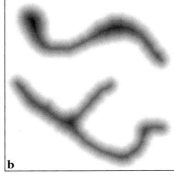

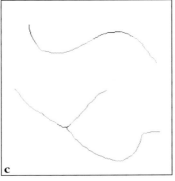

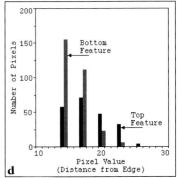

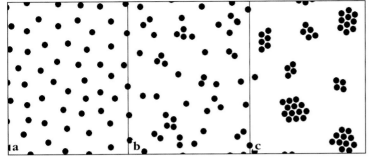

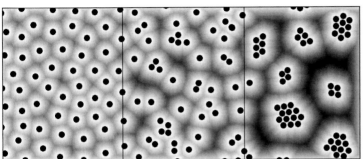

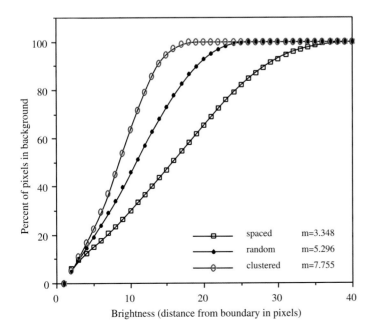

Figure 92. Example
distributions of features:
TOP: **a)** *uniformly spaced;*
      b) *randomly arranged;*
      c) *clustered;*
BOTTOM: Euclidean distance
   *map of the background
   around features.*

plot of the frequency of nearest-neighbor distances. This requires measuring individual features. It is also based on center-to-center distances, and not the distance between feature boundaries. The histogram of brightness values for the EDM of the background between features also contains information on feature clustering.

Figure 92 shows an example of distributions that are clustered, spaced, and random, with the EDM of the background surrounding them. The cumulative histograms of these images are shown in **Figure 93**; the curves are significantly different for the

*Figure 93. Cumulative brightness
   histograms for the EDM of the
   background pixels in each
   region of Figure 91, with the
   least-squares slope for the
   central 80% of each
   distribution.*

spaced	m=3.348
random	m=5.296
clustered	m=7.755

three cases. For tightly clustered feature distributions, the curve rises steeply because there are few points far from a feature boundary. Conversely, for a well-spaced arrangement of features, the curve rises slowly. The slopes, fitted to the straight line portions of the data in the central 80% of the values, are shown.

The axes of these plots are a fraction of the background vertically and brightness horizontally. Brightness values are just distances from the nearest feature boundary, so the slopes of the lines have units of 1/length. The length characterized by these slopes is a measure of how far from a feature boundary a randomly placed point on the image is expected to lie. This method can be applied to images without measuring individual features. It is sensitive to the clustering of etch pits marking dislocations in silicon; to inclusions in metals; oxides or other defects in coatings; and so forth.

Edge effects are present for the center-to-center method (since it cannot be known if the nearest feature to one near the edge is actually within the field of view). To overcome this problem, the distance map can be constructed with brightness values that increase toward the edge of the image, so that the edge will form a ridge. This procedure is equivalent to surrounding the image with repetitions of the same distribution, with each of the four sides forming a mirror image as shown schematically in **Figure 94**. This approximation will be satisfactory if the region covered by the image is a statistically representative sample of the complete population of features, the usual requirement for stereological measurements.

A different approach to detecting clusters is shown in **Figure 95**. The figure could represent the clustering of cell nuclei in tumors or of pores in a ceramic, for example. The skeleton of the background surrounding the points, or the skiz, is obtained first. Then the EDM of the regions inside the skiz lines is calculated and the original points used as a mask. This assigns the values from the distance map to the points. These are not distances from any physical feature in the original specimen, such as cell walls or grain boundaries, but simply distances from the lines in the skiz.

Figure 94. *Features in an image with mirror reflections on all four sides, with their EDM showing the straight ridges formed at the image boundary lines.*

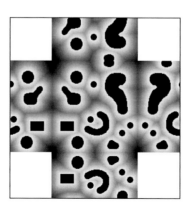

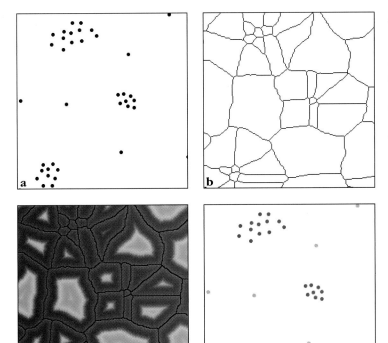

Figure 95. Measurement of clustering using the skiz and EDM:
a) *diagram of features;*
b) *skiz (skeleton of the background);*
c) *Euclidean distance map of the regions delineated by the skiz;*
d) *values from the EDM assigned to the original features (using it as a mask). The clustered features can now be selected by thresholding.*

However, the skiz represents the loci of points equidistant from the boundary lines, so the brightness values are proportional to the distance from each point to its nearest neighbor. This allows the points that are clustered together to be selected by simple brightness thresholding.

Because the distance map encodes each pixel with the straight line distance to the nearest background point, it can also be used to measure the distance of many points or features from irregular boundaries. In the example shown in **Figure 96** the image is first separated into R, G, B planes and thresholded to define the boundary lines (which might represent grain boundaries, cell membranes, etc.) and points (particles, organelles, etc.). The image of the thresholded points of features is then combined with the Euclidean distance map of the interior so that all pixels in the features have the color coding from the distance map. Measuring the color or brightness of the features gives the distance of each feature from the boundary.

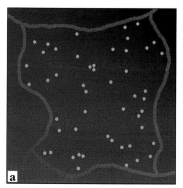

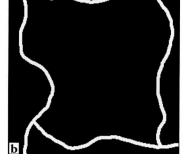

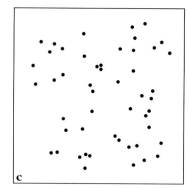

Figure 96. Measurement of distance from a boundary:

a) example image;

b) thresholded interior region;

c) thresholded features;

d) Euclidean distance map of the interior (color coded);

e) distance value assigned to features.

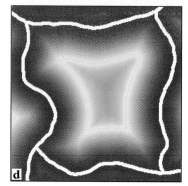

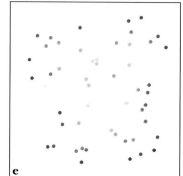

Image Measurements

The distinction between image processing, which has occupied most of the preceding chapters, and image analysis lies in the extraction of information from the image. Image processing, like word processing (or food processing) is the science of rearrangement. Pixel values may be altered according to neighboring pixel brightnesses, or shifted to another place in the array by image warping, but the sheer quantity of pixels is unchanged. So in word processing it is possible to cut and paste paragraphs, perform spell-checking, or alter type styles without reducing the volume of text. And food processing is also an effort at rearrangement of ingredients to produce a more palatable mixture, not to boil it down to the essence of the ingredients. Image analysis, by contrast, attempts to find those descriptive parameters, usually numeric, that succinctly represent the information of importance in the image.

The processing steps considered in earlier chapters are in many cases quite essential to carrying out this task. Defining the features to be measured frequently requires image processing to correct acquisition defects, enhance the visibility of particular structures, threshold them from the background, and perform further steps to separate touching objects or select those to be measured. And we have seen in several of the earlier chapters opportunities to use these processing methods themselves to obtain numeric information.

Measurements that can be performed on features in images can be grouped into four classes: brightness, location, size and shape.

For each class, quite a variety of different specific measurements can be made, and there are a variety of different ways to perform the operations. Most image analysis systems offer at least a few measures in each class. Users find themselves at some time or another having to deal with several different measurement parameters. As noted above, most of these techniques produce a numeric output suitable for statistical analysis or presentation graphics. Frequently, the interpretation of the data is left to a separate program, either a simple spreadsheet relying on the user's programming ability, or a dedicated statistics package. In a few cases, the numbers are converted to go/no go decisions. Examples might include quality control testing of the size and placement of holes in a part, or medical pathology decisions based on the identification of the presence of cancerous cells.

Brightness measurements

Normally in the kinds of images we have been discussing here, each pixel records a numeric value that is often the brightness of the corresponding point in the original scene. Several such values can be combined to represent color information. The most typical range of brightness values is from 0 to 255 (8 bit range), but depending on the type of camera, scanner or other acquisition device a large range of 10 or more bits, up to perhaps 16 (0 to 65,535) may be encountered. Rarely, the stored values may be real numbers rather than integers (for instance, elevation data). However, in most cases these images are still stored with a set of discrete integer "grey" values because it is easier to manipulate such arrays and convert them to displays. In such cases a calibration table or function is maintained to convert the integer values to meaningful real numbers when needed.

The process of creating such a calibration function for a particular imaging device, or indeed for a particular image, is far from trivial (Inoue, 1986; Chieco et al., 1994; Swing, 1997). Many of the cameras and other devices that have been mentioned for acquiring images are neither perfectly linear (or logarithmic), nor completely consistent in the relationship between the pixel's numeric value and the input signal (e.g., photon intensity). Many video cameras have an output function that varies with the overall illumination level. The presence of automatic gain circuits, or user-adjustable gamma controls, makes it more difficult to establish and maintain any kind of calibration. In general, any kind of automatic gain or dark level circuitry, automatic color balancing, etc., will serve to frustrate calibration of the camera. With consumer-level video and still cameras, it is not always possible to turn such "features" off.

For color imaging cameras may incorporate automatic white balance adjustments (which are intended for a type of scene much different than the majority of scientific images). Control of the color temperature of the light source and maintaining consistency

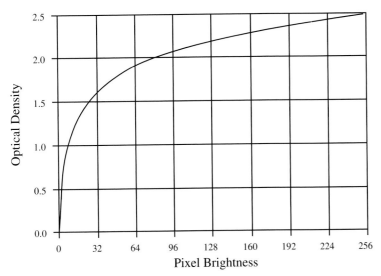

Figure 1. *Calibration of optical density vs. pixel brightness if the latter is adjusted to linearly span the range from 0.1 (fog level) to 2.5 (exposed film).*

of the camera response to perform meaningful color measurement is rarely possible with video type cameras.

Even when the use of a stable light source and consistent camera settings can be assured, the problem of calibration remains. Some standards are reasonably accessible, for example, density standards in the form of a step-wedge of film. Measurement of the brightness of regions in such a standard can be performed as often as needed to keep a system in calibration. In scanning large area samples such as electrophoresis gels, it is practical to incorporate some density standards into every sample so that calibration can be performed directly. In other cases, separate standard samples can be introduced periodically to check calibration.

Optical density is defined as

$$O.D. = Log_{10}(\frac{I}{I_0}) \tag{1}$$

where I/I_0 is the fraction of the incident light that penetrates through the sample without being absorbed or scattered. If a camera or scanner and its light source are carefully adjusted so that the full range of linear brightness values covers the range of optical density from 0.1 (a typical value for the fog level of unexposed film) to 2.5 (a moderately dense exposed film), the resulting calibration of brightness vs. optical density would be as shown in **Figure 1**. The shape of the curve is logarithmic.

At relatively high density/dark pixel values the sensitivity is quite good. A difference of 1 pixel brightness value at the dark end of the scale is only about 0.002. But at the low density end of the scale, a difference of one pixel brightness value corresponds to an optical density change of 0.3, which is very large. This is an indication that when trying to apply a linear camera or scanner

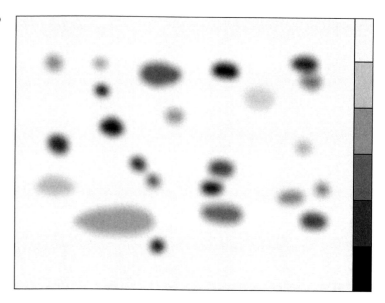

Figure 2. *Scanned image of a 2D electrophoresis separation, with a grey scale calibration wedge.*

to optical density reading, more than 8 bits of grey scale are needed. An input device with more precision can be used with a lookup table that converts the values to the logarithmic optical density scale and then stores that in an 8-bit image.

It is not uncommon to include a grey wedge in a film to be scanned for one- or two-dimensional separation of organic molecules. **Figure 2** shows an example. The grey wedge of known density values allows the construction of a calibration scale (**Figure 3**) that can then be used to measure the integrated optical density of each object (**Figure 4**).

The use of a calibration scale raises another point. It is common for features to contain some variation in pixel brightness. The average density (or whatever other quantity is calibrated against pixel brightness) is not usually recorded linearly. It thus becomes important to take this into account when determining an average value for the density, or an integrated total dose, or any other

Figure 3. *Calibration plot from the grey scale wedge in Figure 2, showing the relationship between optical density and pixel brightness for this particular scanner.*

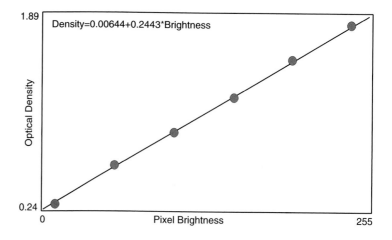

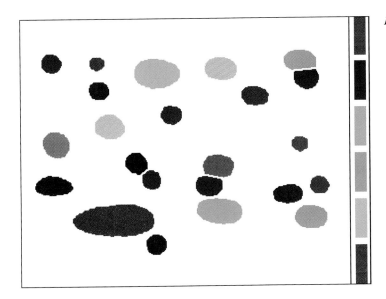

Figure 4. Measured data from Figure 2, using the calibration plot from Figure 3 to compute the integrated optical density of each spot.

calibrated quantity. If all of the pixels within the feature are simply averaged in brightness, and then that value is converted using the calibration scale, the wrong answer will be obtained. It is instead necessary to convert the value from each pixel to the calibrated values, and then sum or average those. It is also important not to include adjacent background pixels that are not part of the feature, which means that the delineation must be exact and not some arbitrary shape (a circle or square) imposed by system limitations. Nor is reliance on manual outlining usually acceptable, since humans usually draw outlines larger than the boundaries around features. The solution is to use the same routines that threshold and segment the image into discrete features. The pixels in that binary image define the features and can be used as a measurement mask to locate the corresponding pixels in the grey scale array.

For one-dimensional measurements of density, the procedure is the same. **Figure 5** shows an example of a film exposed in a Debye-Scherer X-ray camera. The total density of each line, and its position, are used to measure the crystal structure of materials. Knowing that the lines extend vertically, it is reasonable to average the values in the vertical direction to reduce noise and obtain

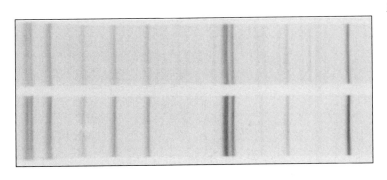

Figure 5. Two Debye-Scherer X-ray films. The vertical lines occur at angles that are related to the atomic spacing in the lattice structure of the target material. Small differences in intensity and the presence of additional lines indicate the presence of trace amounts of additional compounds.

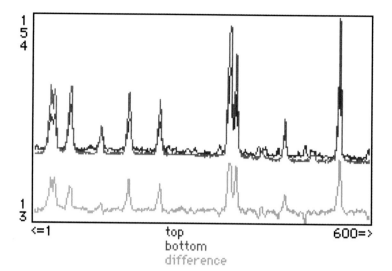

Figure 6. Integrated intensity plots along the Debye films from Figure 5, with the difference between them.

a more precise plot of the density variations along the film (**Figure 6**). Converting the individual pixel values to density before summing them is the correct procedure that gives the proper values for the relative line intensities. The linear plots of intensity values may be subtracted to find differences or used with statistical routines to detect peaks.

Figure 7 shows a similar procedure for tracks in an electrophoresis separation. Using the brightness profile measured between the tracks allows a simple correction to be made for background variations. The brightness values are averaged across the center of the tracks, avoiding the edges.

Of course, not all images have this convenient relationship between intensity and a property of the sample being imaged, such as density. In microscope images, phase differences can also produce contrast, and diffraction effects or polarization effects may also be present. In real-world images, the surface orientation and characteristics of objects influence the brightness, as does the interplay between the light source color and the surface color. In most of these cases, the brightness cannot

Figure 7. A one-dimensional electrophoresis separation. Intensity scans along the center of each track are leveled by subtracting scans between the tracks (the example shows the top track).

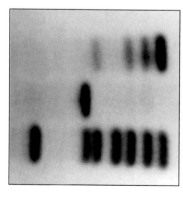

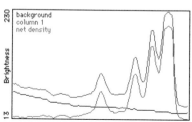

be measured to provide information about the sample. It is difficult enough to use the relative brightness values to delineate regions that are to be grouped together or separated from each other.

When color images are digitized, the problem of having enough bits to give enough precision for each of the color planes is amplified. Many of the higher-end scanners acquire more than 8 bits, sometimes as many as 12, for each of the RGB planes, use these to determine the color information, and then create an optimized 8-bit representation to send to the computer. But even with this increase in precision, it is difficult to achieve accurate color representation. As pointed out in Chapter 1, the digitization of color requires far greater control of camera settings and lighting than can normally be achieved with a video camera. Even a flat bed scanner, which offers greater consistency of illumination and typically uses a single CCD linear array with various filters to obtain the RGB information, is not a good choice for measurement of actual color information. However, such scanners can be calibrated to reproduce colors adequately on particular printers.

The pixel brightness value need not be optical density or color component information, of course. Images are so useful to communicate information to humans that they are used for all kinds of data. Even within the most conventional use of the idea of imaging, pixel values can be related to the concentration of dyes and stains introduced into a specimen. In an X-ray image from the SEM, the brightness values are approximately proportional to elemental concentration. These relationships are not necessarily linear nor easy to calibrate. X-ray emission intensities are affected by the presence of other elements. Fluorescence intensities depend not only on staining techniques and tissue characteristics, but also on time, since bleaching is a common phenomenon.

In infrared imaging, brightness is a measure of temperature. Backscattered electron images from the scanning electron microscope have brightness values that increase with the average atomic number, so that they can be used to determine chemical composition of small regions on the sample. In a range image, the pixel brightness values represent the elevation of points on the surface and are usually calibrated in appropriate units.

These examples are at best a tiny sample of the possible uses of pixel values. But the measurement of the stored values and conversion to some calibrated scale is a broadly useful technique. Statistical analysis of the data provides mean values and standard deviations, trends with position, comparisons between locations, within or between images, and so forth. For such procedures to work, it is important to establish useful calibration curves, which requires standards and/or fundamental knowledge and is properly a subject beyond the scope of this text.

Determining location

In several of the examples for measuring brightness values, the location of features was also needed for interpretation of the results. For a typical irregular feature extending over several pixels, there can be several different definitions of location, some easier to calculate than others. For instance, the x, y coordinates of the midpoint of a feature may be determined simply as halfway between the minimum and maximum limits of the pixels comprising the feature. Normally, the pixel addresses themselves are just integer counts of position, most often starting from the top left corner of the array. This convention arises from the way that most computer displays work, using a raster scan from the top left corner. There may be some global coordinate system of which the individual image is just a part, and these values may also be integers, or real number values that calibrate the pixel dimensions to some real world units such as latitude and longitude, or millimeters from the surface of a microscope sample.

Establishing a real-world calibration for pixel dimensions is often quite difficult, and maintaining them while shifting the specimen or the camera (by moving the microscope stage or the satellite, for instance) presents a variety of challenges. Often, locating a few known features in the image itself can serve to establish fiduciary marks that allow this sort of calibration, so that all of the other features in the image can be accurately located. Shifting the sample, stage or camera so that successive viewing frames overlap allows position calibration to be transferred from one field to the next, but the errors are cumulative and may grow rapidly due to the difficulty of accurately locating the same feature(s) in each field to a fraction of a pixel. This also assumes that there are no distortions or scan nonlinearities in the images.

The feature's minimum and maximum limits are easy to determine by finding the pixels with the largest and smallest coordinates in the horizontal and vertical directions. These limiting coordinates define a bounding rectangle around the feature, and the midpoint of the box is then taken as a location for the feature. However, the midpoint is not a preferred representation of location, because it is too easily biased by just a few pixels (for instance a whisker sticking out from the rest of the feature). One application in which these box coordinates are used, however, is in computer drawing programs. Many such programs allow the user to select a number of drawn objects and then move them into alignment automatically. The options are typically to align the objects vertically by their top, center or bottom, and horizontally by their left, center or right edges. These are exactly the box coordinates and midpoint discussed.

For irregularly shaped features, it would seem preferable to take into account the actual feature shape and location of all the pixels present. This approach defines the centroid of the feature, a unique x, y point that would serve to balance the feature on a

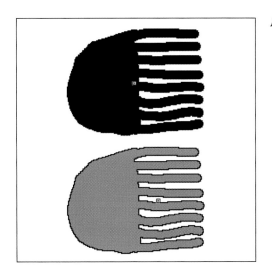

Figure 8. Centroid location of an irregular feature is calculated correctly using all of the pixels (top). Using just the boundary pixels displaces the location (bottom).

pinpoint if it were cut out of a rigid, uniform sheet of cardboard. The coordinates of this point can be determined by averaging the coordinates of each pixel in the object.

$$C.G._x = \frac{\sum_i x_i}{Area} \qquad C.G._y = \frac{\sum_i y_i}{Area} \tag{2}$$

where the *Area* is just the total number of pixels present. Notice that this equation provides a set of coordinates that are not, in general, integers. The center of gravity or centroid of an object can be determined to subpixel accuracy, which can be very important for locating features accurately in a scene.

If the feature has been encoded as discussed in Chapter 6 on segmentation, only the boundary pixels are available to the program performing the calculation. If the centroid is calculated according to **Equation 2** using these boundary pixels only, the result is quite wrong. The calculated point will be biased toward whichever part of the boundary is most complex and contains the most pixels (**Figure 8**). This bias can even vary with the orientation of the boundary with respect to the pixel array because square pixels are larger in the diagonal direction than in their horizontal and vertical dimension.

The correct centroid location can be calculated from a boundary representation such as chain code. The correct calculation uses the pairs of coordinates x_i, y_i for each point in the boundary, where x_0, y_0 and x_n, y_n are the same point (i.e., the boundary representation is a closed loop with the two ends at the same place).

$$C.G._x = \frac{\sum_i (x_i + x_{i-1})^2 \cdot (y_i - y_{i-1})}{Area} \qquad C.G._y = \frac{\sum_i (y_i + y_{i-1})^2 \cdot (x_i - x_{i-1})}{Area} \tag{3}$$

and it is now necessary to calculate the area as

$$Area = \frac{\sum_i (x_i + x_{i-1}) \cdot (y_i - y_{i-1})}{2} \tag{4}$$

Parenthetically, it is worth noting here that some of the attractiveness of chain code or boundary representation as a compact way to describe a feature is lost when you try to use that data to calculate simple things like the area or centroid of the feature.

The definition of centroid or center of gravity just given treats each pixel within the feature equally. For some purposes, the pixel brightness, or a value calculated from it using a calibration curve, makes some pixels more important than others. For example, the accurate location of the spots and lines in the densitometric examples shown earlier would benefit from this kind of weighting. That modification is quite easy to introduce by including the brightness-derived value in the summations in **Equation 2**.

$$C.G._x = \frac{\sum_i Value_i \cdot x_i}{\sum_i Value_i} \qquad C.G._y = \frac{\sum_i Value_i \cdot y_i}{\sum_i Value_i} \tag{5}$$

The denominator is now the integrated density (or whatever the parameter related to brightness may be). Of course, this kind of calculation requires access to the individual pixel brightness values, and so cannot be used with a boundary representation of the feature.

Orientation

Closely related to the location of the centroid of a feature is the idea of determining its orientation. There are a number of different parameters that are used, including the orientation of the longest dimension in the feature (the line between the two points on the periphery that are farthest apart, also known as the maximum Feret's diameter), and the orientation of the major axis of an ellipse fitted to the feature boundary. But just as the centroid is a more robust descriptor of the feature's location than is the midpoint, an orientation defined by all of the pixels in the image is often better than any of these because it is less influenced by the presence or absence of a single pixel around the periphery where accidents of acquisition or noise may make slight alterations in the boundary.

The moment axis of a feature is the line around which the feature, if it were cut from rigid, uniform cardboard, would have the lowest moment of rotation. It can also be described as the axis which best fits all of the pixels in the sense that the sum of the squares of their individual distances from the axis is minimized. This is the same criterion used, for example, to fit lines to data points when constructing graphs. Determining this axis and its orientation angle is straightforward, and just involves summing pixel coordinates and the products of pixel coordinates for all of the pixels in the image. As for the example in **Equation 5**, it is possible to weight each pixel with some value, instead of letting each one vote equally. The most convenient procedure for the calculation is to add up a set of summations as listed in **Equation 6**.

$$
\begin{aligned}
S_x &= \sum x_i \\
S_y &= \sum y_i \\
S_{xx} &= \sum x_i^2 \\
S_{yy} &= \sum y_i^2 \\
S_{xy} &= \sum x_i \cdot y_i
\end{aligned}
\tag{6}
$$

Once these sums have been accumulated for the feature, the net moments about the x and y axes, and the angle of the minimum moment are calculated as shown in **Equation 7**.

$$
\begin{aligned}
M_{xx} &= S_{xx} - \frac{S_x^2}{Area} \\
M_{yy} &= S_{yy} - \frac{S_y^2}{Area} \\
M_{xy} &= S_{xy} - \frac{S_x \cdot S_y}{Area} \\
\Theta &= \tan^{-1}\left\{ \frac{M_{xx} - M_{yy} + \sqrt{(M_{xx} - M_{yy})^2 + 4 \cdot M_{xy}^2}}{2 \cdot M_{xy}} \right\}
\end{aligned}
\tag{7}
$$

Neighbor relationships

The location of individual features may be less important in some applications than the relationships between neighboring features. For instance, **Figure 9** shows several distributions of points that can be considered as the centroids of the original features present. How can such distributions be compactly described to reveal the extent to which they are random, regularly spaced, or clustered?

Schwarz and Exner (1983) showed that a histogram of the distribution of the distances between nearest neighbors can provide an answer. Actually, the distance between any pair of neighbors, second nearest, etc., can be used instead, but in most cases the nearest-neighbor pairs are the easiest to identify. Once the coordinates of the centroid points representing each feature have been determined, sorting through the resulting table to locate the nearest neighbor for each point is a straightforward task (best left to the computer). The straight line distances

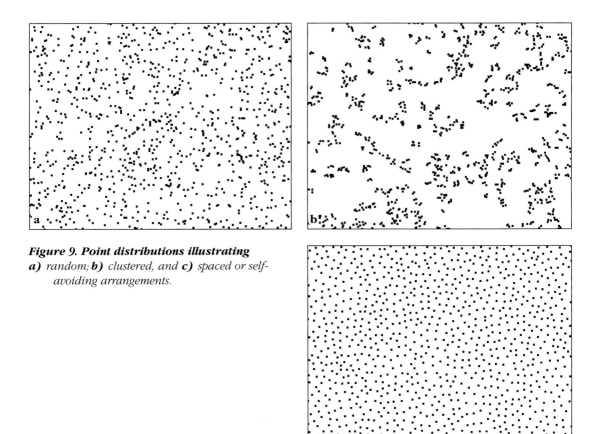

Figure 9. Point distributions illustrating
a) random; b) *clustered, and* *c)* *spaced or self-avoiding arrangements.*

between these points are calculated and used to construct the histogram. This in turn can be characterized by the mean and variance (or standard deviation) of the distribution. A word of caution is needed in dealing with feature points located adjacent to the edge of the field of view (Reed & Howard, 1997): if the distance to the edge is less than the distance found to the nearest neighbor within the field of view, the distance should not be used in the distribution, because it may cause bias. It is possible that another feature outside the field of view would actually be closer. For large images (fields of view) containing many features, this problem is only a minor concern. The nearest-neighbor distance method also generalizes to three dimensions, in the case of 3D imaging; the method has been used with a confocal microscope (Baddeley et al. 1987; Russ et al. 1989; Reed et al. 1997). A related statistical test on all neighbor pairs can also be used (Shapiro et al., 1985).

Consider now the particular distributions shown in **Figure 9**. The image in **Figure 9a** is actually a random distribution of points, often called a Poisson random distribution because the histogram of nearest-neighbor distances is in fact a Poisson distribution (**Figure 10**). This is the sort of point distribution you might observe if you just sprinkled salt on the table. Each point is

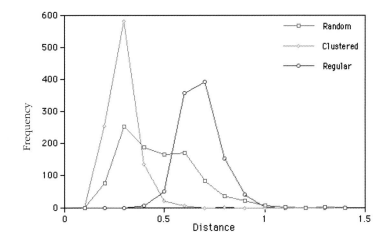

Figure 10. *Histogram of nearest-neighbor distances for each of the point distributions in Figure 9. The mean value of the clustered distribution is less than, and that for the self-avoiding distribution is greater than, that for the random one.*

entirely independent of the others, hence "random." For such a distribution, the mean distance between nearest neighbors is just

$$Mean = \frac{0.5}{\sqrt{\dfrac{N}{Area}}}$$ (8

where N is the number of points within the area of the field of view. And for a Poisson distribution, the variance is equal to the mean (the standard deviation is equal to the square root of the mean). The consequence is that for a random distribution of points, the number of points per unit area of the surface is all that is needed to determine the mean and variance of the histogram of nearest-neighbor distances.

When clustering is present in the point distribution, most points have at least one neighbor that is quite close by. Consequently, the nearest-neighbor distance is greatly reduced. In most cases, the variance also becomes less, as a measure of the uniformity of the spacing between the clustered points. As shown in the image in **Figure 9b**, this clustering produces a histogram (**Figure 10**) that is much narrower and has a much smaller mean value than the Poisson distribution obtained for the random case. Examination of stars in the heavens indicates that they strongly cluster (into galaxies and clusters of galaxies). People also cluster, gathering together in towns and cities.

Likewise, when the points are self-avoiding as shown in **Figure 9c**, the nearest-neighbor distances are also affected. The mean value of the histogram increases to a larger value than for the random case. The variance also usually drops, as a measure of the uniformity of the spacings between points. Self-avoiding or regular distributions are common in nature, whether you look at the arrangement of mitochondria in muscle tissue or precipitate particles in metals, because the physics of diffusion plays a role in determining the arrangement. The mitochondria are distributed to provide energy as uniformly as practical to the fibers. Forming one precipitate particle depletes the surrounding matrix of that element. Even the location of shopping centers is to some degree self-avoiding, in order to attract a fresh market of customers.

The ratio of the mean value of the nearest-neighbor distance distribution to that which would be obtained if the same number of points were randomly distributed in the same area provides a useful measure of the tendency toward clustering or self-avoidance for the features, and the variance of the distribution provides a measure of the uniformity of the tendency. This method has one important limitation of using the distances between the center points of the features. If the features are small compared to the distances between them, this is fine. If the individual features occupy a significant fraction of the total image area, then it might be more interesting to study the edge-to-edge distances between features, which is somewhat harder to calculate.

The Euclidean distance map (EDM) introduced in Chapter 7 on binary images can be used to determine those edge-to-edge distances. The local minimum points (pixels that have a smaller value than any of their neighbors) in the EDM of the background locate midpoints between feature boundaries. The pixel value is one-half of the distance (the radius of the inscribed circle) between the feature boundaries. A histogram of these values can be used to study the feature spacings, but not just the spacing between nearest neighbors. It is very difficult to isolate individual particle spacings this way because there may be multiple local minima between features, depending on the shapes of the boundaries.

Finding nearest-neighbor pairs using the centroid coordinates of features can also be used to characterize anisotropy in feature distributions. Instead of the distance between nearest neighbors, we can measure the direction from each feature to its nearest neighbor. For an isotropic arrangement of features, the nearest-neighbor directions should be a uniform function of angle. Plotting the histogram as a rose plot shows any deviations from this uniform function and indicates the degree of anisotropy.

For instance, if the regularly spaced distribution of feature points in **Figure 9c** is measured, the rose plot is reasonably circular and indicates that the distribution is isotropic. If the image is stretched 10% in the horizontal direction and shrunk 10% in the vertical direction, the total number of features per unit area is unchanged. The visual appearance of the image (**Figure 11**) does not reveal the anisotropy to a casual observer. But a plot of the rose of nearest-neighbor directions (**Figure 12**) shows that most of the features now have a nearest neighbor that is situated above or below. The elongation of the rose plot is a sensitive indicator of this type of anisotropy.

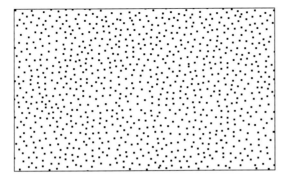

Figure 11. *Stretching the point distribution in Figure 9c horizontally and compressing it vertically introduces nonuniformity in the nearest neighbor directions.*

Alignment

One thing that people are very good at seeing in images that is not so easy to find by computer algorithm is alignment and arrangement of features. We are so good at it that we sometimes find such alignments and arrangements when they don't really exist. Constellations in the sky are a good example of this tendency to bring order to disorder.

There are many image analysis situations in which an algorithmic procedure for determining an alignment or arrangement is needed. One of the most common is completing broken lines, especially straight lines. Such a procedure is useful at all magnifications, from trying to locate electric transmission lines in reconnaissance photos (which show the towers but not the wires) to trying to delineate atomic lattices in transmission electron microscopy. In general, the points along the line are not spaced with perfect regularity (whether they are transmission towers or atoms). This irregularity, and the sensitivity to noise in the form of other points of features near but not part of the line, make

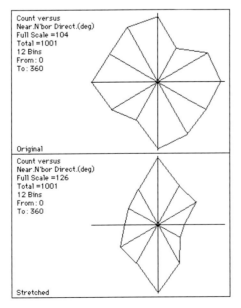

Figure 12. *Rose plot of nearest neighbor directions for the point distributions in Figure 9c and Figure 11.*

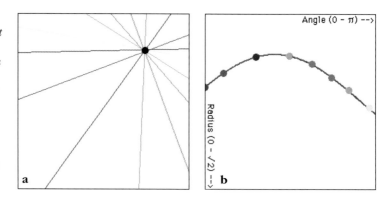

Figure 13. *Principle of the Hough transform. Each point in the real space image* **(a)** *produces a sinusoidal line in Hough space* **(b)** *representing all possible lines that can be drawn through it. Each point in Hough space* **(b)** *corresponds to a line in real space. The real space lines* **(a)** *corresponding to a few of the points along the sinusoid are shown, with color coding to match them to the points.*

frequency-domain techniques difficult to apply and poor in resulting precision.

Instead of Fourier space, another image transformation into Hough space can be used to find these alignments (Hough, 1962; Duda & Hart, 1972; Ballard, 1981). Different Hough spaces are used to fit different kinds of shapes, and it is necessary in most cases to have a pretty good idea of the type of line or other arrangement that is to be fit to the data. We will start with the straight line, since it is the simplest case. The conventional way to fit a line to data points on a graph is the so-called "least squares" method where the sum of the squares of the vertical deviations of each point from the line is minimized. The Hough method is superior to this because it minimizes the deviations of points from the line in a direction perpendicular to the line, and it deals correctly with the case of the points not being uniformly distributed along the line.

Two parameters are required to define a straight line. In Cartesian coordinates, the equation of a straight line is

$$y = m \cdot x + b \qquad (9$$

where m is the slope and b the intercept. Because m becomes infinitely large for lines that are nearly parallel to the y axis, this representation is not usually used in the Hough transform. Instead, the polar coordinate representation of a line is used. This consists of a radius ρ and angle φ, which define the line as shown schematically in **Figure 13**. It is possible either to allow the angle to vary from 0 to 2π and to keep ρ positive, or to allow ρ to be either positive or negative and to restrict the angle φ to a range of 0 to π. The latter convention is used in the examples that follow. The black point shown in **Figure 13a** generates the sinusoid in Hough space shown in **Figure 13b**. Each point along this sinusoid corresponds to the ρ-φ values for a single line passing through the original point. Several of these are shown in color, where the color of the point in Hough space matches the corresponding line in real space.

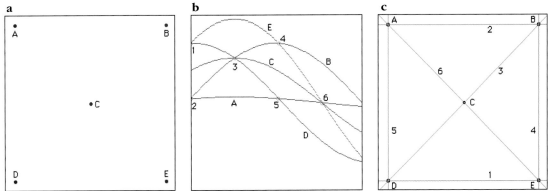

Figure 14. Duality of lines and points in Hough and real space. *Each of the labeled points in **a** generates a sinusoidal line in the Hough space shown in **b**. The numbered crossing points in this space generate the lines in the real space image shown in **c**.*

Hough space is an accumulator space. This means that it sums up the votes of many pixels in the image, and points in Hough space that have a large total vote are then interpreted as indicating the corresponding alignment in the real-space image. For the linear Hough transform, used to fit straight lines to data, the space is an array of cells (pixels, since this is another image) with coordinates of angle and radius. Every point in Hough space defines a single straight line with the corresponding angle φ and radius ρ that can be drawn in the real-space image.

To construct the Hough transform, every point present in the real-space image casts its votes into the Hough space for each of the lines that can possibly pass through it. As shown in **Figure 13**, this means that each point in the real-space image generates a sinusoid in Hough space. Each point along the sinusoid in Hough space gets one vote added to it for each point in the real-space image. The superposition of the sinusoids from several points in real space causes the votes to add together where they cross. These crossing points, as shown in **Figure 14**, occur at values of ρ and φ that identify the lines that go through the points in the real-space image.

In this example, the duality of lines and points in real and Hough space is emphasized. Each of the five original points (labeled *A...E*) in real space produces a sinusoid (similarly labeled) in Hough space. Where these sinusoids cross, they identify points in Hough space (labeled *1...6*). These points correspond to lines back in real space (similarly labeled) that pass through the same points. Notice for instance that three lines pass through point *A* in real space, and that the sinusoid labeled *A* in Hough space passes through the points for each of those three lines.

If there are several such alignments of points in the real-space image, then there will be several locations in the Hough transform that receive numerous votes. It is possible to find these points either by thresholding (which is equivalent to finding lines

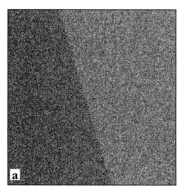

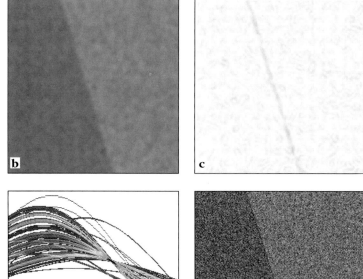

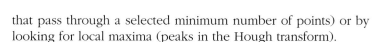

Figure 15. Fitting a line to a noisy edge using the Hough transform:

a) *the original noisy image;*

b) *smoothing to reduce the noise;*

c) *application of a Sobel gradient filter;*

d) *Hough transform produced from the gradient image;*

e) *line defined by the maximum point in the Hough transform.*

that pass through a selected minimum number of points) or by looking for local maxima (peaks in the Hough transform).

If the original real-space image contains a step in brightness, and an image-processing operation such as a gradient (e.g., Sobel filter) has been applied, then an improved detection and fit of a line to the edge can be achieved by letting each point in the image vote according to the magnitude of the gradient. This means that some points have more votes than others, according to how certain it is that they lie on the line. The only drawback to this approach is that the accumulator space must be able to handle much larger values or real numbers when this type of voting is used, than in the simpler case where pixels in a binary image of feature points either have one vote or none. **Figure 15** shows an example of fitting a line to a noisy edge using a gradient operator and the Hough transform. Notice that the location of the maximum point in Hough space involves the same requirements for using the pixel values to interpolate a location to subpixel dimensions as discussed at the start of this chapter.

This proportional voting system is useful when there are many points to be fit, with some points being more important than others. Summing the votes according to brightness (or some value obtained from brightness) allows some points to be weighted more and produces an improved fit. **Figure 16** shows a Hough transform of a convergent beam electron diffraction pattern. The

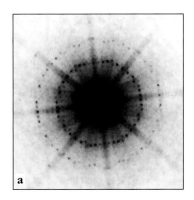

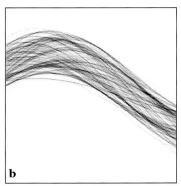

most intense spots in the Hough transform identify each of the spot alignments in the pattern.

The Hough transform can be adapted straightforwardly to other shapes, but the size and dimensionality of the Hough space used to accumulate the votes increases with the complexity of the shape. Fitting a circle to a series of points is used to measure electron diffraction patterns and to locate holes in machined parts. A generalized circular Hough transform requires a three-dimensional space, since three parameters are required to define a circle (the x, y coordinates of the center and the radius). Each point in the real-space image produces a cone of votes into the Hough space, corresponding to all of the circles of various radii and center positions that could be drawn through the point.

But if one or two of these values are known (for instance, the center of the electron diffraction pattern is known, or the radius of the drilled hole) or at least can vary over only a small range of possible values, then the dimensionality and/or size of the Hough space is reduced and the entire procedure becomes quite rapid. Accurately fitting a circle to an irregularly spaced set of points of varying brightness is a good example of the power that the Hough approach brings to image measurement. Since the brightness of the point in Hough space that defines the circle is also the summation of the votes from all of the points on the corresponding circle in real space, this approach offers a useful way to integrate the total brightness of points in the electron diffraction pattern as well.

Figure 17 shows an example of using a circular Hough transform to locate the "best fit" circles in a selected area diffraction pattern. The pattern itself has bright spots with irregular locations around each circle. A human has little difficulty in estimating where the circles lie, but this is generally a difficult thing for computer algorithms that examine only local pixel regions to accomplish. The Hough transform locates the circles and also provides a measure of the integrated brightness around each circle. This approach has been used to identify asbestos fibers from the very spotty electron diffraction patterns from a few fibers.

Figure 17. Selected area electron diffraction pattern with principal circles located by a circular Hough transform, and the integrated circular density of the pattern.

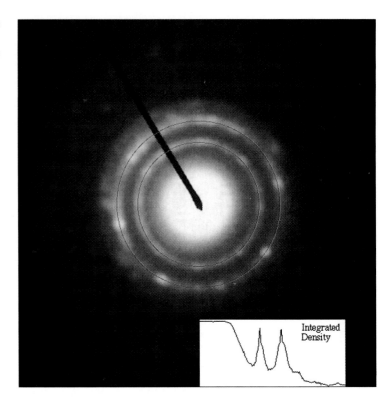

Integrated Density

Figure 18 shows an example from machine vision used to locate edges and holes accurately for quality control purposes or robotics guidance. In spite of overall noise in the image, the fit is quite rapid and robust. A separate region of interest (ROI) is set up covering the area where each feature is expected. In each ROI, a gradient operator is applied to identify pixels on the edge. These are then used to perform a Hough transform, one for a straight line and one for a circle. The resulting feature boundaries are shown, along with the measured distance between them. Since many pixels have contributed to each feature, the accuracy of location is much smaller than the pixel dimensions.

The Hough transform approach can be used to fit other alignment models to data as well. The limitation is that as the algebraic form of the model changes, each of the adjustable con-

Figure 18. Use of the Hough transform to locate an edge and a circle in a machined part, in order to measure the distance between them to subpixel accuracy.

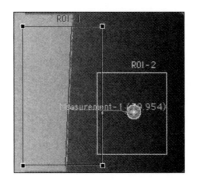

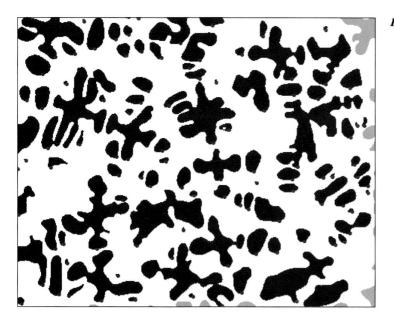

Figure 19. *Counting features by a unique point. The red dots mark the right end of the lowest line of pixels in each feature. Features that touch the upper and left boundaries are counted, but those that touch the bottom and right edges are not.*

stants requires another dimension in Hough space. Constructing the transform and then finding the maximum points becomes time-consuming.

Counting features

Counting the number of features present in an image or field of view is one of the most common procedures in image analysis. The concept seems entirely straightforward, and it is surprising how many systems get it wrong. The problem has to do with the finite bounds of the field of view. In the case in which the entire field of interest is within the image, there is little difficulty. Each feature has simply to be defined by some unique point, and those points counted. Depending on how features are recognized, some algorithms may ignore features that are entirely contained within holes in other features. This problem most often arises when boundary representation is used to define the feature boundaries in the binary image. Determining whether it is appropriate to count features that lie inside other features is a function of the application, and consequently must be left up to the user.

When the field of view is a sample of the entire structure or universe to be counted, the result for the number of features is generally given as number-per-unit-area. When features intersect the edge of the field of view, it is not proper to count all features that can be seen. The most common solution to produce an unbiased result is to count those features that touch two edges, for instance the top and left, and to ignore those that touch the other two edges, for instance the right and bottom. This is equivalent to counting each feature by its lower right corner. Since each feature has one and only one lower right corner, counting those points is equivalent to counting the features. (**Figure 19**).

Figure 20. *Edge-touching features. Counting all of the red and black features gives the correct total number of features per unit area, but only the black features (non-edge-touching) can be measured, and they include a disproportionate number of small features.*

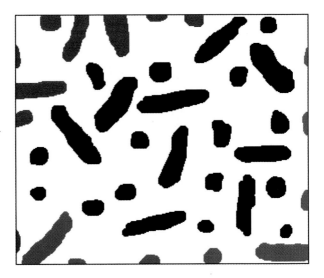

This method is the same as determining the number of people in a room by counting noses. Since each person has one nose, the nose count is the same as the people count. If a smaller region was marked within the room, so that people might happen to straddle the boundary, counting the noses would still work. Anyone whose nose was inside the region would be counted, regardless of how much of the person lay outside the region. Conversely, any person whose nose was outside would not be counted, no matter how much of the person lay inside the region. It is important to note that in this example, we can see the portions of the people that are outside the region, but in the case of the features in the image, we can not. Any part of the feature outside the field of view is by definition not visible, and we can't know anything about the amount or shape of the feature outside the field of view. That is why it is important to define a unique point for each feature to use in counting.

The convention of counting features that touch two edges only is not implemented in all systems. Some software packages offer a choice of counting all features regardless of edge touching, or counting only those features that do not touch any edge. Note that when measuring features, as opposed to counting them, a more complicated procedure will be needed. Any feature that touches any edge cannot be measured, because it is not all imaged and therefore no size, shape or position information can be correctly obtained. If only the features in **Figure 20** that did not touch any edge were counted, the proportions of large and small features would be wrong. It is more likely that a large feature will touch an edge, and so a disproportionate fraction of the large features intersect an edge of the field of view and cannot be measured.

There are two ways to correct for this bias. They produce the same result, but are implemented differently. The older method

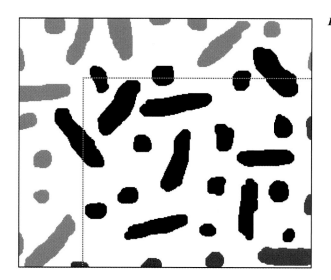

Figure 21. Use of a guard frame for unbiased feature measurements. Measuring all of the black features whose lower-right corners lie within the guard frame area gives a correct result. Features that touch an edge or lie outside the guard frame are not measured.

is to set up a "guard frame" around the image, as shown in **Figure 21**. In this case, features that touch the lower and right edges of the field of view are not counted or measured, as before. Features that cross the top and left edges of the guard frame are counted and measured in their entirety. Features that lie only within the guard frame are not counted, whether they touch the actual edge of the field of view or not. The number of features counted is then an accurate and unbiased measure of the number per unit area, but the area (the denominator in the fraction) is the area within the guard frame, not the entire area of the image. Since it is necessary for the guard region to be wide enough that no feature can extend from within the active region across the guard region to the edge of the field, the active region may be reduced to as little as one-quarter of the total image area.

The second method uses the entire image area and measures all of those features that do not touch any of the edges. In order to compensate for the bias arising from the fact that larger features are more likely to touch the edge and be bypassed in the measurement process, features are counted in proportion to the likelihood that a feature of that particular size and shape would be likely to touch the edge of a randomly placed image frame. The so-called adjusted count for each feature is calculated as shown in **Figure 22**.

$$\text{Count} = \frac{W_x \cdot W_y}{(W_x - F_x) \cdot (W_y - F_y)} \tag{10}$$

where W_x and W_y are the dimensions of the image in the x and y directions (in pixels), and F_x and F_y are the maximum projected dimensions of the feature in those directions. These are simply the same bounding-box coordinates as discussed above in connection with finding a feature's location. When the feature

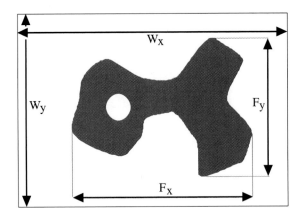

Figure 22. *Adjusting the count for each measured feature, according to its individual dimensions.*

dimensions are small compared to the dimensions of the field of view, the fraction is nearly 1.0 and simple counting is unaffected. This is the case for counting small features. When the feature extends across a larger fraction of the field of view in either direction, it is more likely that a random placement of the field of view on the sample will cause it to intersect an edge; thus the features that can be measured must be counted more than once to correct for those that have been overlooked. The adjusted count factor makes that compensation.

Special counting procedures

The examples of counting in the previous section make the tacit assumption that the features are separate and distinct. In earlier chapters, procedures for processing images in either the grey scale or binary format were shown whose goal was to accomplish the separate delineation of features to permit counting and measurement. However, there are numerous situations in which these methods are not successful, or at least very difficult. Sometimes, if there is enough separate knowledge about the specimen, counting can be accomplished even in these difficult cases.

As an example, **Figure 23** shows a collection of crossing fibers. Such structures are common in biological samples, wood fibers used in paper production, food technology, textiles, and many more situations. Since the fibers cross, from the point of view of the image analysis algorithms there is only a single feature present, and it touches all sides of the field of view. However, it is possible to estimate the number of fibers per unit area, and the average fiber length. By thresholding the fibers and skeletonizing the resulting binary image, a series of crossing midlines is revealed. In this image, the end points of fibers can be counted as those pixels that have exactly one touching neighbor. This is not a perfect method, as there may be some ends of real fibers that are hidden because they lie exactly on another fiber, but in principle it is possible to detect these occurrences as well because they produce pixels with exactly three neighbors, and

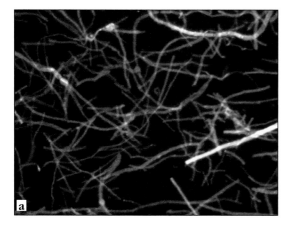

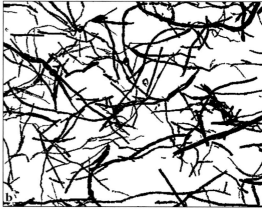

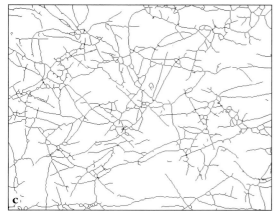

Figure 23. *Image of crossing wood fibers* **(a)**. *The number of fibers per unit area can be estimated by thresholding* **(b)** *and skeletonizing the fibers* **(c)**, *and counting the number of ends, which in this image number 279.*

one of the angles at the junction will be about 180 degrees. However, even without this refinement, the end point count gives a useful approximation for the number of fibers.

Recall that in the preceding section we decided to count each feature by one unique point. Counting the end points of fibers uses two unique points per fiber. It is a little like the old joke about how to count the number of cows in a field ("Count the number of hooves and divide by four."). In this case, we count the number of end points and divide by two, to get the number of fibers. Dividing by the image area gives the number of fibers per unit area. If the total length of fiber (the total length of the skeletonized midline) is divided by the number of fibers (one half the number of ends), the result is the average fiber length.

In the earlier chapter on binary image processing, several techniques for separating touching features were discussed. One of the more powerful, known as watershed segmentation, utilizes the Euclidean distance map. This operation assigns a grey scale value to each pixel within a feature proportional to the distance from that pixel to the nearest background point. The valleys, or points that lie between two higher pixels in this distance map, then are used to locate boundaries that are ultimately drawn

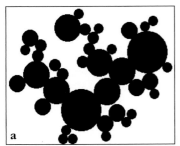 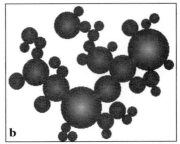 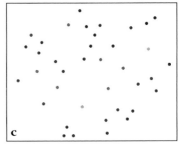

Figure 24. Counting and sizing touching particles: a) binary image of touching circles; *b)* Euclidean distance map (color indicates distance of pixel from nearest background point); *c)* ultimate points (local maxima in the Euclidean distance map), whose color gives the radius.

between features in order to separate them. Because there is a built-in assumption in this method that any indentation around the periphery of the feature cluster indicates a separation point, this technique is also known as convex segmentation.

If the purpose of the processing and segmentation is to count the features, there is a short-cut method that saves much of the computation. In the Euclidean distance map (EDM), every local maximum point (pixels equal to or greater than all eight of their neighbors) is a unique point that represents one feature that will eventually be separated from its touching companions. Finding these so-called ultimate eroded points provides another rapid way to count the features present. In addition, the grey scale value of that point in the EDM is a measure of the size of the feature, since it corresponds to the radius of the circle that can be inscribed within it. **Figure 24** shows a simple example of some touching circles, with the ultimate points found from the Euclidean distance map.

Counting touching particles presents many difficulties for image analysis algorithms. If the particles are not simple convex shapes that lie in a single plane and happen to touch at their boundaries, watershed segmentation is not usually able to separate them successfully. A typical example of a more difficult problem is shown in **Figure 25**. The clay particles that coat this paper sample form a layer that is essentially one particle thick, but the overlaps are quite extensive. In order to obtain a useful estimate of the number of particles per unit area of the paper, it is again necessary to use the idea of finding one unique point per particle.

In this case, the way the image is formed by the scanning electron microscope provides an answer. Most of the particles are somewhat angular and have a single highest point that appears bright in the secondary electron image. These points can be isolated using a top hat filter, as shown in the figure. These are simply points that are brighter by a selected amount than the brightest of their neighbors. The top hat filter is just the difference between two rank filters with different diameters. The analogy is to the shape of a top hat, with a crown and brim. If the grey

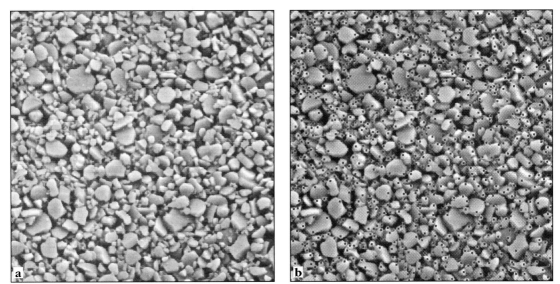

Figure 25. *Counting overlapping particles:* **a)** *SEM image of clay particles on paper with* **b)** *superimposed points from a top hat filter used to locate a local brightest point, which can be used to estimate the number of particles.*

scale values of the pixels are imagined to represent elevations, then placing the top hat on the surface so that the brim rests on the ground corresponds to the larger rank neighborhood. If a local peak rises through the crown of the hat (the smaller rank neighborhood), then the filter is considered to have found a peak. The height of the crown can be adjusted to select peaks of a certain size. Obviously, a similar strategy could be used with dark points to count pits, in which case the filter is sometimes called a rolling ball filter, invoking the idea that a ball placed on the grey scale surface would come to rest on one of the pits.

In the clay coating example, the top hat filter finds one unique point with a local maximum in brightness for most of the clay particles. A few are missed altogether because they have a shape or orientation that does not produce a characteristic bright point, and a few particles have sufficiently irregular shapes that they produce more than a single characteristic point. This means that counting the points gives only an estimate of the particle density on the paper, but for many quality control purposes this sort of estimate is sufficient to spot changes.

Another approach to counting particles in clusters is shown in **Figure 26**. This is a TEM image of carbon black particles. There are a few instances of isolated particles, but most of them are present in the form of clusters of varying sizes. If it can be assumed that the particles in the clusters are similar in size and density to the isolated ones, then it becomes possible to estimate the number of particles in a cluster from the integrated density of the cluster. Measuring the average integrated density of an isolated particle, and dividing that value into the integrated density

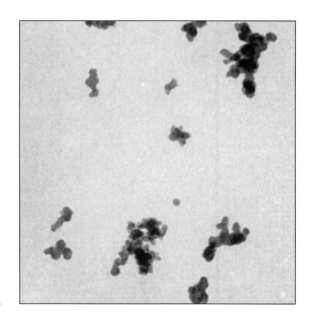

Figure 26. *Clusters of carbon-black particles viewed in the transmission electron microscope. Dividing the integrated density of each cluster by the mean integrated density for a single particle provides an estimate of the number of particles in each cluster.*

of each cluster, provides a number that is an estimate of the number of particles present.

Feature size

The most basic measure of the size of features in images is simply the area. For a pixel-based representation, this is the number of pixels within the feature, which is straightforwardly determined by counting. For boundary representation, the area can be calculated as discussed above (**Equation 4**). Of course, it must be remembered that the size of a feature in a two-dimensional image may be related to the size of the corresponding object in three-dimensional space in various ways depending on how the image was obtained. The most common type of images is a projection, in which the features are basically shadows of the objects, or planar sections, in which the features are slices across the objects. In each case, if enough objects are viewed in random or known directions, it is possible to estimate the volume of the objects from the projections. The rules for these estimates, which are heavily based on geometric probability, are provided by the science of stereology. The estimates are statistical in nature, meaning that the volume of an individual object is not determined exactly, but the distribution of sizes of many objects can be described.

Figure 27 shows a projected image of spherical particles dispersed on a flat substrate. The diameters can be measured straightforwardly from such an image subject to the usual restriction that there must be enough pixels in each feature to give a precise measure of its size. When the particles cover a large size range, as they do in this image, this creates a problem. With the resolution of a typical video camera, the smallest features are only one or a few pixels in size, and are not well defined (in fact

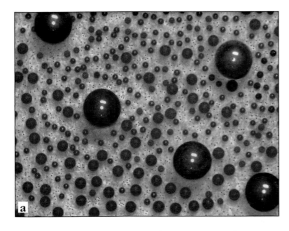

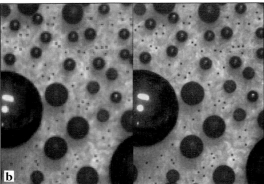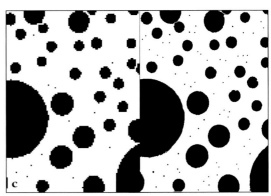

Figure 27. Image of spherical particles dispersed on a flat surface:

a) *overall image, acquired with a high resolution 1600×1200 pixel digital camera;*

b) *enlarged portions or images obtained at video camera resolution and digital camera resolution;*

c) *same regions after thresholding, hole filling and watershed segmentation.*

many are not even thresholded). A high resolution digital camera provides superior results. The alternative would be to increase the optical magnification to enlarge the small particles, but then the large ones would be likely to intersect the edges of the screen and could not be measured. Multiple sets of data taken at several magnifications would be required, unless a high resolution camera can be used.

As an example of a classical stereological calculation based on shape unfolding, consider the image shown in **Figure 28**. These are graphite nodules in cast iron that are approximately spherical in shape. Similar arguments can be made for the pores present in enamel (see **Figure 89** in Chapter 1), the gas bubbles in a loaf of bread, or grapefruit packed into a carton. Sections through such a structure show circles. Measurement of the size distribution of the circles does not directly give the size distribution of the spheres, because with a random section the plane may pass through the sphere at the equator, near one of the poles, or anywhere in between.

For a sphere, the probability of getting a circle of a particular size by random sectioning can be calculated. The largest size circle is, of course, the same as the equatorial diameter of the sphere. Smaller size circles appear with a definite and calculable frequency distribution. A superposition of spheres produces a

Figure 28. *Light microscope image of graphite nodules in cast iron, with graphs showing histograms of the size distribution of circles, and the calculated distribution of the sizes of spheres that would produce the observed circle distribution.*

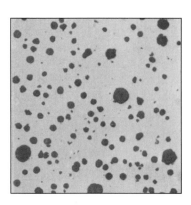

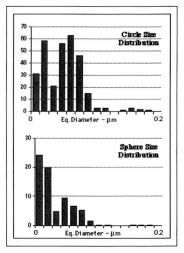

mixture of circle sizes in which the largest circles can only come from the largest spheres, while all of the spheres may contribute to the smaller circles. Unfolding the distribution of the circles produced by each sphere size produces a distribution of sphere sizes, as shown in the figure.

A similar procedure could be employed for any shape object, by determining the size distribution of the intersections produced by random sectioning. This classic method has a rich history, but also an important limitation. Knowledge of the shape of the three-dimensional object is critical to its success, since the distribution of intersection sizes varies considerably with shape (**Figure 29** shows an example of cubes vs. spheres). If the shapes are unknown or variable, or worse if they vary with feature size, the method fails. Also, all unfolding methods are expressly statistical in nature, and so they require good sampling and enough data. The counting errors (or measurement errors) made in obtaining the data from the two-dimensional slices are magnified in the prediction of the three-dimensional size distribution.

In spite of these limitations (or perhaps because their magnitude and effect are not appreciated), unfolding of size distributions is commonly performed. When the shape of the three-dimensional objects is not known, it is common to assume they are simple spheres, even when the observed features are clearly not circles. The argument that this gives some data that can be compared from one sample to another, even if it is not really accurate, is actually quite wrong and simply betrays the general level of ignorance about the rules and application of stereological procedures.

Even for such a simple idea as counting pixels to determine feature area, some decisions must be made. For instance, consider the object shown in **Figure 30**. Should the pixels within internal holes be included in the area or not? Of course, this depends on the intended use of the data. If the hole is a section through an

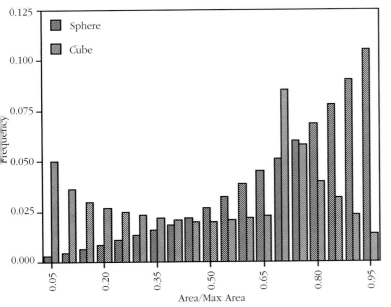

Figure 29. *Size distribution of intercept areas produced by random sectioning of a sphere and a cube.*

internal void in an object, then it should be included if the area of the feature is to be related to the object volume. But it is hard to know whether the hole may be a section through a surface indentation in that object, in which case it would be more consistent to also include in the area those pixels in fjords around the feature boundary. As shown in the figure, this produces three different possible area measurements, which we may call the net area, the filled area, and the convex area.

Measuring the first two is basically a counting exercise. In the process of labeling the pixels that touch each other and comprise the feature, it is common to also detect the presence of internal holes and count the pixels within them. Alternately, a hole-filling operation can be used to deal with internal holes. This operation was mentioned in the chapter on binary image processing. Basically, it is done by taking the inverse of the image and identifying

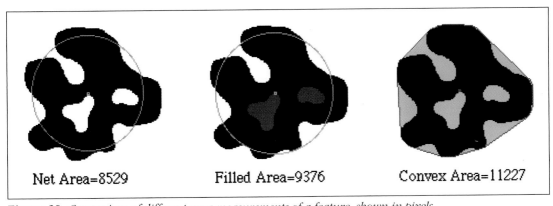

Figure 30. *Comparison of different area measurements of a feature, shown in pixels.*

all features that do not intersect the boundary of the image. These are holes, and the pixels can be added back to the original image to fill in the holes. Determining whether to include those pixels in the area then becomes a user decision.

The convex area is a slightly more difficult proposition. In some cases, a combination of dilation and erosion steps can be used to construct a convex hull for the feature and fill any boundary irregularities, so that pixel counting can be used to determine the area. However, on a square pixel grid these methods can cause some other distortions of the feature shape, as was shown in Chapter 7. Another approach that constructs an n-sided polygon around the feature is shown in the next section. This method is sometimes called the taut-string or rubber-band boundary of the feature, since it effectively defines the minimum area for a convex shape that will cover the original feature pixels.

However the area is defined and determined, it of course requires that a conversion factor between the size of the pixels and the dimensions of the real-world structures be established. Calibration of dimension is usually done by capturing an image of a known standard feature and measuring it with the same algorithms as later used for unknown features. For macroscopic or microscopic images, a measurement scale may be used. Of course, it is assumed that the imaging geometry and optics will not vary. For some remote sensing operations, the position and characteristics of the camera are known and the magnification is calculated geometrically.

Most modern systems use square pixels that have the same vertical and horizontal dimensions, but for distances to be the same in any direction on the image it is also necessary that the viewing direction be normal to the surface. If it is not, then image warping as discussed in Chapter 3 is required. Some systems, particularly those that do not have square pixels, allow different spatial calibrations to be established for the horizontal and vertical directions. For area measurements based on pixel counting, this does not matter. But for length measurements and the shape parameters discussed below, this discrepancy creates serious difficulties.

Once the area has been determined, it is often convenient to express it as the equivalent circular diameter. This is linear measure, calculated simply from the area as

$$Eq.\,Diam.= \sqrt{\frac{4}{\pi}Area} \qquad (11$$

Figure 31 shows several features of different sizes and shapes with the equivalent circle diameter shown based on the net feature area (pixel count). Features of different shape or orientation can fool the eye and make it difficult to judge relative size, and the area values tend to overemphasize large features. The equiv-

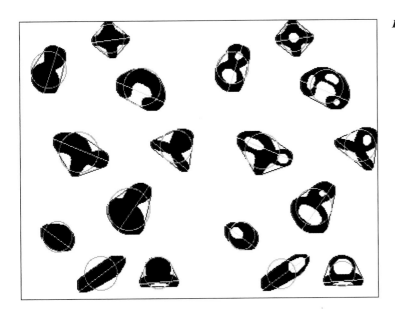

Figure 31. An assortment of features with their equivalent circular diameter (green), convex bounding polygon (red) and longest chord (yellow). Some parameters are not affected by the presence of internal holes in the feature set on the right.

alent diameter values offer a simple and easily compared parameter to characterize size.

It is not always necessary to measure the individual areas of features to determine the important characteristics of a structure. For images that are sections through a solid, one of the rules of stereology is that the volume fraction of a phase (where phase is a generic name for any identifiable structure or component) is exactly equal to the area fraction shown on a random section. Whether this is the amount of a mineral in an ore body, the extent of porosity in a ceramic, or the volume of nuclei in a group of cells, the method is the same. A count of the total number of pixels in the features divided by the total number of pixels in the image, or in some larger structure of interest, is all that is required, without regard to how the pixels may be arranged.

In some cases, this area fraction can be determined from the histogram of the original or processed grey scale image, without any need even to threshold it or deal with the actual pixel array. **Figure 32** shows an example. The area fraction of the image occupied by each phase in the dendritic metal alloy is simply given by the size of each corresponding peak in the histogram.

In **Figure 33**, the volume fraction of dark shot particles in each of two cylinders must be determined by measuring both the total area of dark pixels and also the area of the circular cross section of the cylinder. This idea of a reference area is particularly common in biological microscopy, where an organ, cell or nucleus is typically measured to define a denominator for calculating the area fraction. **Figure 34** shows an example, a light micrograph of a microtomed section through a rat lung. Thresholding the lung tissue and measuring its area gives the net value. Filling the holes and measuring again gives the total area. The ratio of the two

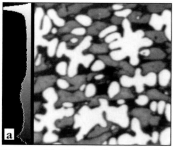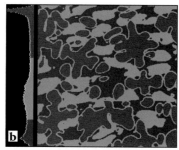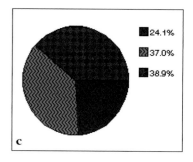

Figure 32. Measuring area fraction from the histogram:
a) grey scale image of a metal alloy with its histogram, showing three
phases (white, grey, dark); **b)** the same image with colors assigned to ranges of grey values
corresponding to each of the peaks in the histogram; **c)** the volume fractions of the three phases.

gives the area fraction (and hence the volume fraction) of the
lung that is tissue (the balance is air space).

When the reference area is irregular and possibly not free from
holes or not continuous, as the case of the galvanized coating
(zinc on steel) shown in **Figure 35**, measuring both the region of
interest and the reference area can be complicated. In this exam-

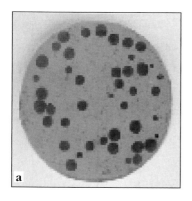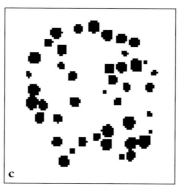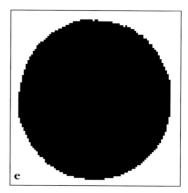

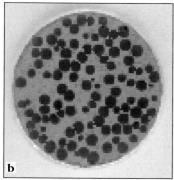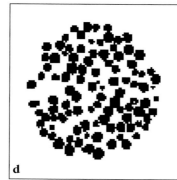

**Figure 33. Two images of cross-sections through shot particles embedded in a cylinder, showing
the use of a reference area:**
a & b) grey scale images of the entire cylinder cross section; **c & d)** thresholded images of the shot; **e & f)**
thresholded images of the cylinder. The area fractions of the cylinder occupied by the shot are 17.4 and
43.1%, respectively.

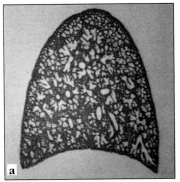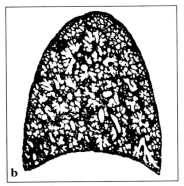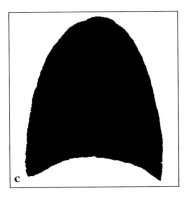

Figure 34. An example of an irregular reference area:
a) light micrograph of a section through rat lung; b) thresholded to provide the net area of lung tissue; c) filled to give the total cross-section area. The ratio of the two values gives the volume fraction.

ple, image processing is needed to delineate the structure of the iron-zinc intermetallic phase within the coating to allow its measurement. In addition, separation of the coating from the metal substrate and the mounting medium is needed to define the entire coating cross-sectional area.

Caliper dimensions

As shown in **Figure 22**, a caliper dimension represents another measurement of feature size. A projected or shadow dimension in the horizontal or vertical direction, also known as a Feret's diameter, can be determined simply by sorting through the pixels or the boundary points to find the smallest and largest coordinates, and then taking the difference. These dimensions were introduced before in terms of the bounding box around the feature, used to correct for its probability of intersecting the edge of a randomly placed image field.

By rotating the coordinate axes, it is similarly possible to locate the minimum and maximum points in any direction. For purposes of constructing the convex or taut-string outline mentioned

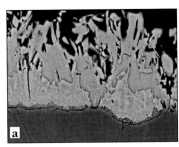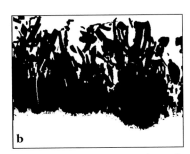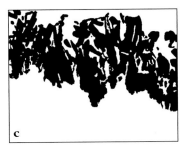

Figure 35. Reference area method applied to a cross section of a zinc coating on steel:
a) SEM image of a polished cross-section through the coating; b) thresholding of the entire coating as the reference area; c) segmentation of the zinc-rich area after sharpening edges. The net area fraction of the zinc-rich phase in the coating is 76.5%.

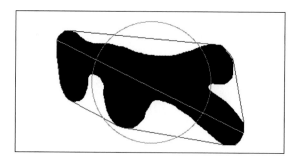

Figure 36. An irregular feature with its equivalent circular diameter (green), longest chord (yellow) and the convex boundary produced by a 32-sided polygon formed from the caliper dimensions (red).

above in connection with feature area, using a modest number of rotation steps will produce a useful result. For instance, with 16 steps (rotating the axes in 180/16=11.25 degree steps) a bounding polygon with 32 corners and sides is obtained. **Figure 36** shows an example, and since this is just the polygon used to determine the convex area, additional examples appear in **Figure 24**. Actually, it would be just as easy to use 18 steps of 10 degrees, but for historic reasons the use of powers of two ($16=2^4$) in computer programs is common. It is only for extremely long and narrow features that more sides than this might be required to produce a bounding polygon that is a good approximation to the outer boundary.

With such a polygon, the minimum and maximum caliper diameters can be found by sorting through the pairs of corner points. The maximum caliper or maximum Feret's diameter is another very common measure of feature size. It is also sometimes called the feature length, since it corresponds closely to the longest distance between any two points on the periphery.

When boundary representation is used, it is possible to search directly for the maximum chord by sorting through the points to find the two with maximum separation. There are various ways to speed up this search, which would otherwise have to calculate the sum of squares of the x- and y- coordinate differences between all pairs of boundary points. One is to consider only those points that lie outside the equivalent circle. Determining the area by pixel counting (in this case, the area including any internal holes) and converting it to the equivalent diameter with **Equation 11**, provides a circle size. Locating that circle with its center on the feature centroid will cover any points inside the circle, and leave just those points that lie farther away. These are candidates for the most widely separated pair.

An even more restrictive selection of the points to be searched can be obtained from the dimensions of the bounding rectangle. As shown in **Figure 37**, arcs drawn tangent to each side with their center in the middle of the opposite side will enclose most of the boundary of the feature. Only points that lie on or outside the arcs need to be used in the search, and points lying outside

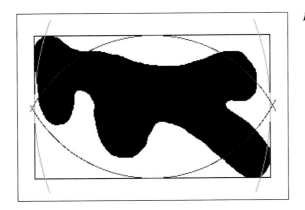

Figure 37. *Construction used to limit the search for boundary points giving the maximum chord. The blue arcs are drawn with centers in the middle of the horizontal edges of the bounding box, and the green arcs are drawn with centers in the middle of the vertical edges. Only the red points along the perimeter, which lie outside those arcs, are candidates for endpoints of the longest chord.*

one arc need only to be combined with those that lie outside the opposite arc. For a reasonably complex feature whose boundary may contain thousands of points, these selection algorithms offer enough advantage to be worth their computational overhead when the actual maximum dimension is needed.

The procedure of rotating the coordinate system, calculating new x', y' values for the points along the feature boundary, and searching for the minimum and maximum values, is much simpler and more efficient. For any particular angle of rotation α, the sine and cosine values are needed. In most cases these are simply stored in a short table corresponding to the specific angles used in the program. Then the new coordinates are calculated as

$$x' = x \cdot \cos \alpha - y \cdot \sin \alpha$$
$$y' = y \cdot \sin \alpha - x \cdot \cos \alpha \tag{12}$$

When this process is carried out at a series of rotational angles, the points with the largest difference in each rotated coordinate system form the vertices of the bounding polygon discussed above. The pair with the greatest separation distance is a close approximation to the actual maximum dimension of the feature. The worst-case error occurs when the actual maximum chord is exactly halfway between the angle steps, and in that case the measured length is short by

$$Meas.Value = TrueValue \cdot \cos\left(\frac{\alpha}{2}\right) \tag{13}$$

For the example mentioned above of 11.25 degree steps, the cosine of 5.625 degrees is 0.9952. This means that the measurement is less than one-half percent low. For a feature whose actual maximum dimension is 200 pixels, the value obtained by the rotation of coordinate axes would be one pixel short.

If the same method is used to determine a minimum caliper dimension for the feature (sometimes called the breadth), this is

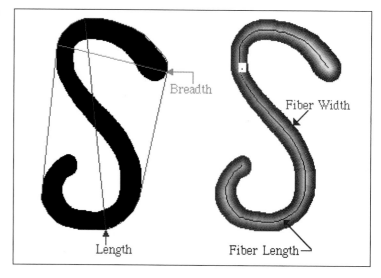

Figure 38. *Comparison of caliper dimensions (Length and Breadth) with values determined from the skeleton and Euclidean distance map (Fiber Length and Fiber Width).*

equivalent to finding the pair of opposite vertices on the bounding polygon that are closest together. The error here can be much greater than for the maximum caliper dimension, because it depends on the sine of the angle and on the length of the feature rather than its actual breadth. A narrow feature of length L and actual width W oriented at an angle the same 5.625 degrees away from the nearest rotation step would have its breadth estimated as $L \cdot \sin(5.625) = 0.098 \cdot L$. This doesn't even depend on W, and if the actual length L is large and the width W is small, the potential error is very great.

Consider a feature shaped like the letter "S" shown in **Figure 38**. If this is a rigid body, say a cast-iron hook for use in a chain, the length and breadth as defined by the minimum and maximum caliper dimensions may have some useful meaning. On the other hand, if the object is really a worm or noodle that is flexible, and the overall shape is an accident of placement, it would be much more meaningful to measure the length along the fiber axis and the width across it. To distinguish these from the maximum and minimum caliper dimensions, these are sometimes called the fiber length and fiber width.

There are two quite different approaches to measuring these dimensions. Of course, it is still up to the user to determine which set of parameters offers the most useful values for describing the features in a particular situation. One approach goes back to the binary image processing discussed in Chapter 7. If the feature is skeletonized, the skeleton or medial axis transform is obtained. These are very similar structures in most cases, the distinction depending on whether an iterative erosion is used to produce the skeleton, or the Euclidean distance map is used to find the medial axis transform. In either case, the length of the midline offers a measure of the length of the fiber, except for the details of the fiber ends. **Figure 39** shows an example of

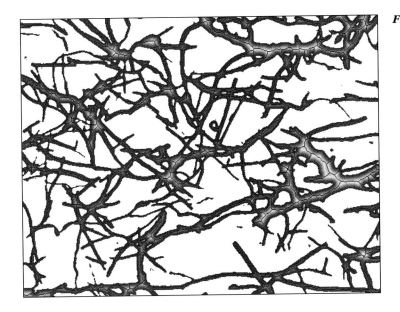

Figure 39. The image of wood fibers from Figure 23, with the skeleton superimposed on the Euclidean distance map. The histogram of pixel values along the fiber centers gives the distribution of fiber widths in the image.

the use of this technique, which can even be used for overlapping fibers.

Determining the length of the midline accurately requires more than just counting the number of pixels in it, because on a square pixel grid the distance between pixels that touch diagonally is greater by √2 than the distance orthogonally. Counting the touching pairs as a function of direction and calculating the dimension accordingly produces a slight overestimate of the length. Instead of using the strictly geometric distances of 1.0 and 1.414, Smeulders (1989) has shown that calculating the length as

$$Length = 0.948 \cdot (num.\ of\ orthogonal\ neighbors)$$
$$+ 1.340 \cdot (num.\ of\ diagonal\ neighbors) \qquad (14$$

gives a mean error of only 2.5% for lines that run in all directions across the square pixel grid.

When the Euclidean distance map is used to find the medial axis transform, the grey scale values assigned to the pixels along the midline represent the radius of the inscribed circle centered at that point. Averaging these values for all of the points in the midline gives a useful estimate of the fiber width.

Figure 40 shows an example of this type of measurement. The image shows a network of nerve axons. The variation in contrast from side to side, and of different diameter fibers, can be dealt with by subtracting a ranked background, as shown. Then the thresholded fibers are reduced to their midlines (as shown in blue). Branch and crossing points are erased by removing pixels in the midline that have more than two neighbors. This leaves the branches, which are measured using **Equation 14** to obtain a histogram showing the distribution of lengths.

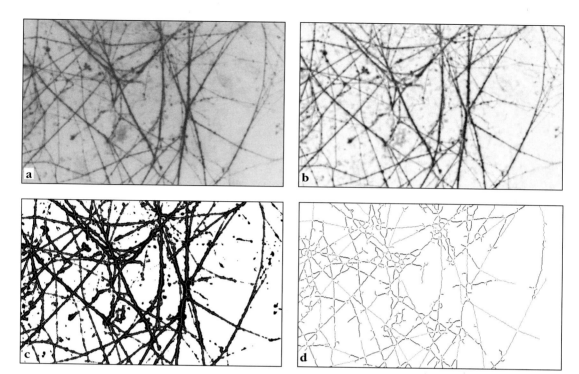

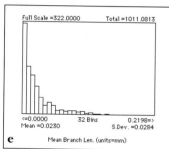

Figure 40. Measurement of length of the skeleton:
a) *micrograph of nerve axons;*
b) *contrast leveled by subtracting ranked background;*
c) *thresholded fibers, with the medial axis transform marked in blue;*
d) *separated branches of the skeleton, color coded according to length;*
e) *distribution of measured lengths.*

A second approach to estimating values for the length and width of a fiber is based on making a geometric assumption about the fiber shape. If the feature is assumed to be a uniform-width ribbon of dimensions F (Fiber Length) and W (Fiber Width), then the area (A) and perimeter (P) of the feature will be $A = F \cdot W$ and $P = 2 \cdot (F + W)$. These parameters can both be measured. As we will see below, the perimeter is one of the more troublesome values to determine. But for a ribbon with smooth boundaries as assumed here, the perimeter can be measured with reasonable accuracy. Then the fiber length and width can be calculated from the measured perimeter and area as

$$F = \frac{P - \sqrt{P^2 - 16 \cdot A}}{4}$$

$$W = \frac{A}{F}$$

(15

Minor modifications to this model can be made, for example by assuming that the ends of the ribbon are rounded instead of

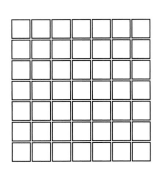

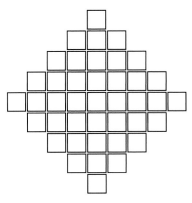

Sum of Edges = 28 units
Chain code perimeter = 28.0 units

Sum of Edges = 36 units
Chain code perimeter = $20\sqrt{2}$ = 28.28

Figure 41. *Comparison of perimeter estimation by chain code vs. summation of pixel edge lengths, as a function of orientation.*

square, but the principle remains the same. The difficulty with this approach is its sensitivity to the shape model used. If the feature is not of uniform width or is branched, for instance, the average value of the inscribed circle radius still produces a consistent and meaningful result, while the calculation in **Equation 15** may not.

Perimeter

The perimeter of a feature seems to be a well-defined and familiar geometrical parameter. Measuring a numerical value that really describes the object turns out to be less than simple, however. Some systems estimate the length of the boundary around the object by counting the pixels that touch the background. Of course, this underestimates the actual perimeter because, as noted above for the measurement of skeleton length, the distance between corner-touching pixels is greater than it is for edge-touching pixels. Furthermore, this error depends on orientation, and the perimeter of a simple object like a square will change as it is rotated under the camera. **Figure 41** compares the variation in perimeter that is obtained by counting the edges of pixels to the more accurate value obtained from the chain code, as a square is rotated. The sensitivity of measurement values to orientation is often used as a test of system performance.

If boundary representation is used to represent the feature, then the Pythagorean distance between successive points can be summed to estimate the perimeter, as

$$Perim = \sum_i \sqrt{(x_i - x_{i-1})^2 + (y_i - y_{i-1})^2} \qquad (16$$

In the limiting case of chain code, the links in the chain used for boundary representation are either 1.0 or $\sqrt{2}$ pixels long, and can be used to estimate the perimeter. It is only necessary to count the number of odd chain code values and the number of even chain code values, since these distinguish the orthogonal or diagonal directions. The same argument as used above for the irregularity of the pixel representation of the midline applies to the boundary line, and using the modified values from **Equation 14** may be applied to reduce this source of error.

The basic difficulty with perimeter measurements is that for most objects they are very magnification-dependent. Higher image magnification reveals more boundary irregularities and hence a larger value for the perimeter. This is not the case for area, length, or the other size dimensions discussed above. As the imaging scale is changed so that the size of individual pixels becomes smaller compared to the size of the features, measurement of these other parameters will of course change, but the results will tend to converge toward a single best estimate. For perimeter, the value increases.

In many cases, plotting the measured perimeter against the size of the pixels, or a similar index of the resolution of the measurement, produces a plot that is linear on logarithmic axes. This kind of self-similarity is an indication of fractal behavior, and the slope of the line gives the fractal dimension of the boundary. Fractal behavior has been investigated for large and small objects, ranging from maps or aerial photographs of islands (**Figure 42**) to roughness viewed with the scanning tunneling microscope. Many natural shapes and phenomena are observed to follow this pattern.

However, even if the feature boundary is not strictly fractal (implying the self-similarity expressed by the linear log-log plot of perimeter vs. measurement scale), there is still some increase in measured perimeter with increased imaging magnification. This makes the perimeter values suspect as real descriptors of the object, and at least partially an artefact of the imaging method and scale used. Further, any noise in the image may be expected to cause a roughening of the boundary and increase the apparent perimeter.

Figure 42. *Richardson plots constructed for three of the Hawaiian islands. The variation of measured coastline perimeter using different stride lengths gives the fractal dimensions shown.*

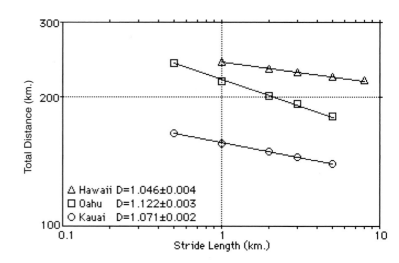

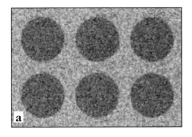

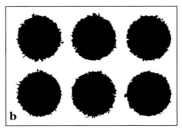

Circle	Area	Perimeter
1	5027	358
2	5042	338
3	4988	343
4	5065	391
5	5020	372
6	5030	313
average	5028.7	352.5
std.dev.	25.4 (0.5%)	27.4 (8%)
original	5024	254

Figure 43 shows a simple example. Random grey scale noise is superimposed on six circles. The original circles were drawn with a diameter of 80 pixels, and had a measured area of 5024 pixels and perimeter (by the chain-code method) of 254 pixels, close to the exact values for a circle. Measuring a series of noisy images will produce a value for the area that averages to the correct mean, as pixels are added to or removed from the feature. But the perimeter is always increased as shown by the results in **Figure 43**. The variation in area measurements is only 0.5%, while that for the perimeter measurements is 8%, and the mean value is far too high. This bias introduced by the imaging procedure is another cause for concern in perimeter measurements.

If perimeter is measured, there is still the need to choose among the same three alternatives discussed for area measurements. The total perimeter includes the length of boundaries around any internal holes in the feature. The net perimeter excludes internal holes and just measures the exterior perimeter. The convex perimeter is the length of the convex hull or bounding polygon, and bridges over indentations around the periphery of the feature. The same considerations as mentioned in connection with area measurement apply to selecting whichever of these measures describes the aspect of the feature that is important in any particular application.

Ellipse fitting

Since most real features have quite irregular shapes, it is not easy to find size measures that compactly and robustly describe them and allow for their classification and comparison. The use of equivalent circular diameter (based on feature area) is one attempt. Recognizing that not all features are equiaxed or evenly approximately round, many systems also provide for the use of an ellipse to describe the feature. The fact that the ellipse has two axes seems to allow describing both a size, a degree of departure from circularity, and even an orientation.

The major and minor axes of the ellipse are determined in several different ways, however. These actually represent some quite different aspects of the feature size and shape, and may be more misleading than helpful unless the user is fully aware of (and careful with) their various biases.

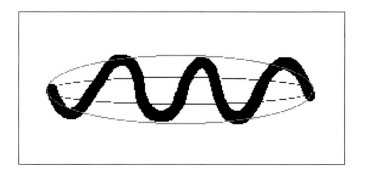

Figure 44. *An irregular feature with two superimposed ellipses. The major axis of both is the feature length (maximum caliper dimension), but one has the minor axis equal to the feature width (minimum caliper dimension) and the other has the same area as the feature.*

One definition of the ellipse axes can be taken from the minimum and maximum caliper dimensions of the feature, discussed above. The maximum caliper dimension does a good job of representing a maximum dimension, and indicates the feature orientation at least within the step size of the search (typically between 10 and 15 degrees). If this is taken as the major dimension of the ellipse, then the minor axis could be assigned to the minimum caliper dimension. This approach can lead to several difficulties. First, as pointed out above, this value may seriously overestimate the actual minimum dimension for a long, narrow feature. Second, the direction of the minimum dimension is not, in general, perpendicular to the maximum dimension. Third, the resulting ellipse area is not the same as the area of the feature. **Figure 44** shows an example of these drawbacks for a simple square feature in which the maximum dimension is the diagonal, and the minimum is the edge length (at an angle of 45 degrees). The ellipse defined by the caliper dimensions does not capture the important size properties of the feature.

Since the breadth as defined by the minimum caliper dimension is suspect, a modification of this approach uses the maximum caliper dimension as the ellipse major axis, and determines the minor axis in order to make the ellipse area agree with the feature area. Since the area of an ellipse is $(\pi/4) \cdot a \cdot b$ where a and b are the axes, once the major axis has been determined the minor axis can be adjusted to agree with the feature area. The orientation angle can be either the approximate value determined from the steps used in the maximum caliper dimension search, or the orientation angle determined from the moment calculation shown earlier (**Equation 7**). As shown in **Figure 44**, this tends to produce ellipses that have a longer and narrower shape than our visual perception of the feature.

The moments from **Equation 7** can be used directly to produce a fitted ellipse. This is perhaps the most robust measure, although it requires the most calculation. Surprisingly, it seems to be little used. Instead, many systems fit an ellipse not to all of the pixels in the feature area, but instead to the pixels along the feature boundary. This procedure is very hard to justify. Irregularities along one portion of the feature's boundary will significantly bias the ellipse (**Figure 45**).

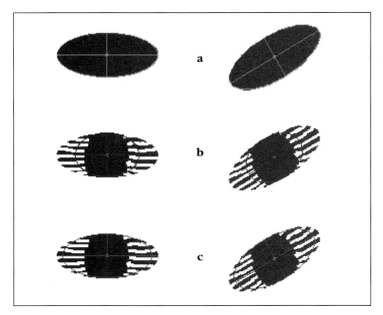

Figure 45. Fitting an ellipse to a feature:
a) the major and minor axes fit to the feature length and breadth;
b) fit to the moments of all pixels in an irregular feature;
c) fit to the boundary pixels of the same feature.

Describing shape

Shape is not something that human languages are well equipped to deal with. We have few adjectives that describe shape, even in an approximate way (e.g., rough vs. smooth, or fat vs. skinny). In most conversational discussion of shapes, it is common to use a prototypical object instead ("shaped like a ..."). Of course, this assumes we all agree about the important aspects of shape found in the selected prototype. Finding numerical descriptors of shape is difficult because the correspondence between them and our everyday experience is slight, and the parameters all have a "made-up" character.

The oldest class of shape descriptors are simply combinations of size parameters, arranged so that the dimensions cancel out. Length/Breadth, for example, gives us Aspect Ratio, and changing the size of the feature does not change the numerical value of aspect ratio. Of course, this assumes we have correctly measured a meaningful value for length and breadth, but this was discussed in the previous section.

Since there are dozens of possible size parameters, there are hundreds of ways that these can be combined into a formally dimensionless expression that might be used as a shape descriptor. In fact, there are only a few relatively common combinations, but even these are plagued by an absolute inconsistency in naming conventions. **Table 1** summarizes some of the most widely used shape parameters calculated as combinations of size measurements. Note that in any particular system the same parameter may be called by some quite different name, or the name shown for a different parameter in the table. Also, some systems define the parameters as the inverse of the formula shown, or add (or remove) constant multipliers such as π.

Table 1. Representative shape descriptors

$$Formfactor = \frac{4\pi \cdot Area}{Perimeter^2}$$

$$Roundness = \frac{4 \cdot Area}{\pi \cdot Max\ Diameter^2}$$

$$Aspect\ Ratio = \frac{Max\ Diameter}{Min\ Diameter}$$

$$Elongation = \frac{Fiber\ Length}{Fiber\ Width}$$

$$Curl = \frac{Length}{Fiber\ Length}$$

$$Convexity = \frac{Convex\ Perimeter}{Perimeter}$$

$$Solidity = \frac{Area}{Convex\ Area}$$

$$Compactness = \frac{\sqrt{\left(\frac{4}{\pi}\right) Area}}{Max\ Diameter}$$

$$Modification\ Ratio = \frac{Inscribed\ Diameter}{Maximum\ Diameter}$$

$$Extent = \frac{Net\ Area}{Bounding\ Rectangle}$$

The burden placed on the user, of course, is to be sure that the meaning of any particular shape descriptor is clearly understood and that it is selected because it bears some relationship to the observed changes in shape of features, since it is presumably being measured in order to facilitate or quantify some comparison. **Figures 46** through **49** illustrate several of these parameters which distinguish between features. In general, each of them captures some aspect of shape, but of course none of them is unique. An unlimited number of visually quite different shapes can be created with identical values for any of these dimensionless shape parameters.

Figure 46 shows four variations on one basic shape, which is stretched and smoothed by erosion and dilation. Notice that formfactor varies with surface irregularities, but not with overall elongation, while aspect ratio has the opposite behavior. **Figure 47** shows four variations on one basic shape with the values of several shape parameters. Examination of the values shows that the parameters vary quite differently from one shape to another. **Figure 48** shows several shapes with the values of their curl.

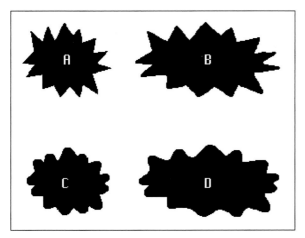

Figure 46. *Variations on a shape produced by erosion/dilation and by horizontal stretching. The numeric values for formfactor and aspect ratio (listed below) show that stretching changes the aspect ratio and not the formfactor, and vice versa for smoothing the boundary.*

Shape	Formfactor	Aspect Ratio
A	0.257	1.339
B	0.256	2.005
C	0.459	1.294
D	0.457	2.017

Figure 49 illustrates the differences between these parameters in a different way. The "features" are simply the 26 capital letters, printed in a font with a serif (Times Roman). In each horizontal row, the colors code the value of a different measured shape parameter. The variation in each set is from red (largest numeric value) to magenta (smallest numeric value). The independent variation of each of the shape factors is remarkable. This suggests on the one hand that shape factors are a powerful tool for feature identification. However, the large variety of such factors, and the inability of human vision to categorize or estimate them, suggests that people do not use these parameters to recognize letters.

Fractal dimension

Quite a few of the shape parameters discussed above and summarized in **Table 1** include the perimeter of the feature. As was pointed out in an earlier section, this is often a problematic size parameter to measure, with a value that is an artefact of image magnification. In fact, the concept of perimeter may be fundamentally

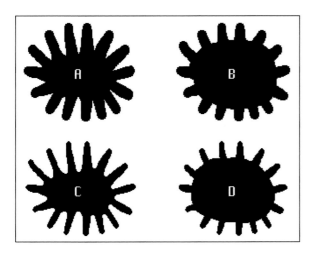

Figure 47. *Another set of four related shapes with the numeric values for their measured shape parameters.*

Shape	Roundness	Convexity	Solidity	Compactness
A	0.587	0.351	0.731	0.766
B	0.584	0.483	0.782	0.764
C	0.447	0.349	0.592	0.668
D	0.589	0.497	0.714	0.768

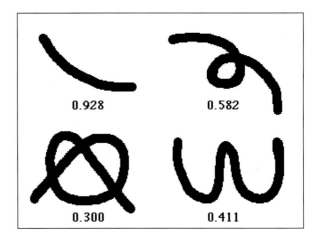

Figure 48. *Four features with different values of curl, indicating the degree to which they are "curled up."*

0.928   0.582

0.300   0.411

flawed when it is applied to many real objects. If a real-world object is actually fractal in shape, the perimeter is undefined. Measuring the object boundary at higher magnification will always produce a larger value of perimeter. Consider a cloud, for example. What is the length of the boundary around the projected image of the cloud? Measurements covering many orders of magnitude, from a single small cloud in the sky observed by visible light, up to entire storm systems viewed by radar or from weather satellites, show that the perimeter of clouds obeys fractal geometry. Presumably this trend would continue at smaller and smaller scales, at least down to the dimensions of the water molecules. What, then, does the perimeter really mean?

Objects that are fractal seem to be the norm rather than the exception in nature. Euclidean geometry with its well-defined and mathematically tractable planes and surfaces is usually only found as an approximation over a narrow range of dimensions,

Figure 49. *Measurement of a series of shapes (letters of the alphabet). In each row, the colors of the features code the relative numeric value (red=high, magenta=low) of a different shape parameter, corresponding to the labels.*

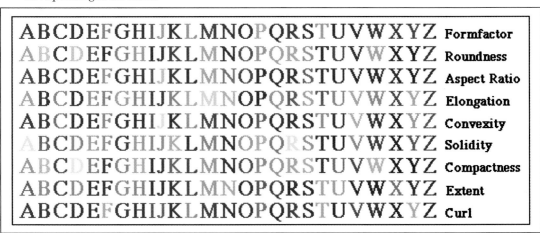

where mankind has imposed it. Roads, buildings, and the surface of the paper on which this book is printed are flat, straight and Euclidean, but only in the dimension or scale where humans are concerned. Magnify the paper surface and it becomes rough. Look at the roads from space and they cease to be straight. The use of fractal dimensions to describe these departures from Euclidean lines and planes is a relatively new conceptual breakthrough that promises a new tool for describing roughness.

Briefly, the fractal dimension is the rate at which the perimeter (or surface area) of an object increases as the measurement scale is reduced. There are a variety of ways to measure it. Some are physical, such as the number of gas molecules that can adhere to the surface in a monolayer, as a function of the size of the molecule (smaller molecules probe more of the small surface irregularities and indicate a larger surface area). Some are most easily applied in frequency space, by examining the power spectrum from a two-dimensional Fourier transform as discussed in Chapter 5. Others are relatively easily measured on a thresholded binary image of features.

Perhaps the most widely used fractal measurement tool is the so-called Richardson plot. This was originally introduced as a procedure applied manually to the measurement of maps. Setting a pair of dividers to a known distance, the user starts at some point on the boundary and strides around the perimeter. The number of steps multiplied by the stride length produces a perimeter measurement. As the stride length is reduced, the path follows more of the local irregularities of the boundary and the measured perimeter increases. The result, plotted on log-log axes, is a straight line whose slope gives the fractal dimension. Deviations from linearity occur at each end: at long stride lengths, the step may miss the boundary altogether, while at short stride lengths the finite resolution of the map limits the measurement.

When boundary representation is used for a feature, a Richardson plot can be constructed from the points by calculating the perimeter using the expression shown above, and then repeating the same procedure using every second point in the list, every third point, and so forth. As points are skipped, the average stride length increases and the perimeter decreases, and a Richardson plot can be constructed. When every nth point in the list is used to estimate the perimeter, there are n possible starting positions. Calculating the perimeter using each of them, and averaging the result, gives the best estimate. The stride length for a particular value of n is usually obtained by dividing the total perimeter length by the number of strides. In all these procedures, it is recognized that there may be a partial stride needed at the end of the circuit, and this is included in the process.

The variability of the stride length in this procedure is made worse by the fact that the x, y coordinates of the boundary points are digitized in a grid. Unlike the manual process of walking along a map boundary, there may not be a point recorded at the location one stride length away from the last point, and so it is necessary either to interpolate from the actual data or to use some other point and alter the stride length. Interpolation makes the tacit assumption that the boundary is locally straight, which is in conflict with the entire fractal model. Altering the stride length may bias the plot. Combined with the general difficulties inherent in the perimeter measurement procedure, the Richardson method is usually a poor choice for measuring digitized pixel images.

A second technique was shown in the chapter on binary image processing. Dilating the boundary line by various amounts is equivalent to sweeping a circle along it. The area of the circle does not increase directly with the radius, because of the irregularities of the boundary. Plotting the area swept out by the circle (sometimes called the sausage) vs. the radius (again on log-log axes) produces a line whose slope gives the fractal dimension. This Minkowski technique is actually older than the Richardson method. It works well on pixel-based images, particularly when the Euclidean distance map is used to perform the dilation. This method is both faster than the iterative dilation method, since it assigns to each pixel a grey scale value equal to the distance from the boundary, and less directionally biased. Examples of this method were shown in Chapter 7. The Minkowski method produces a dimension that is not identical to the Richardson method (or to the other fractal dimension procedures discussed), and so it is important when comparing values obtained from different specimens to use only one of these methods.

A third approach to fractal dimension measurement produces another dimension, similar in meaning but generally different in value to the others discussed. The Kolmogorov dimension is often determined manually by grid counting. A mesh of lines is drawn on the image and the number of grid squares through which the boundary passes is counted. When this number is plotted on log-log axes vs. the size of the grid, the slope of the line again gives the fractal dimension. Automatic implementation and application to a pixel image can be performed by progressively coarsening the image into 2×2, 3×3, etc. blocks of pixels, and is sometimes called mosaic amalgamation. This is perhaps the fastest method, but has the least numeric precision because it has the fewest possible steps and hence the fewest points to establish the line. **Figure 50** compares the three methods.

However it is determined, the fractal dimension produces a single numeric value that summarizes the irregularity of "roughness" of the feature boundary (**Figure 51**). The relationship between this boundary and what it may represent in three dimensions is not simple. For the case of a section through an isotropic surface, the boundary fractal dimension is smaller than the surface fractal dimension by exactly 1.0, the topological dimension of the sectioning plane. However, few real surfaces are perfectly isotropic,

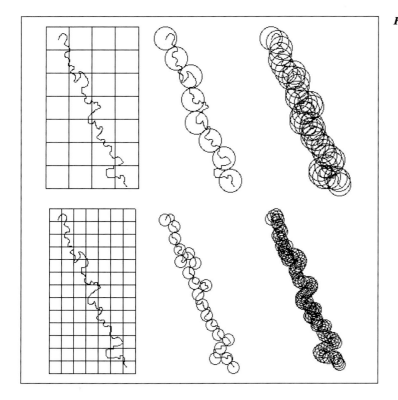

*Figure 50. The principle of three common fractal measurement techniques: (**left**) counting the number of grid squares through which the boundary passes as a function of grid size (Kolmogorov dimension); (**center**) counting the number of strides needed to walk along the boundary, as a function of stride length (Richardson dimension); (**right**) area swept out by continuously moving a circle along the boundary, as a function of circle size (Minkowski dimension).*

and in the presence of preferred orientations this simple relationship breaks down. Even more serious, if the boundary measured is a projected outline of a particle, the boundary irregularities will be partially hidden by other surface protrusions, and the measured fractal dimension will be too small by an amount that depends on the size of the particle and on its roughness. There is no general correction for this, and in spite of the fact that this procedure is very commonly used, the data obtained (and their subsequent interpretation) remain very open to question.

Harmonic analysis

The fractal dimension attempts to condense all of the details of the boundary shape into a single number that describes the

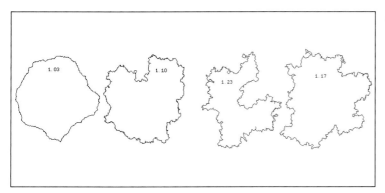

Figure 51. Several fractal outlines with varying fractal dimensions.

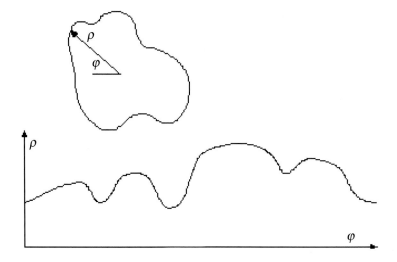

Figure 52. *Illustration of the procedure for unrolling a feature profile.*

roughness in one particular way. There can, of course, be an unlimited number of visually different boundaries with the same fractal dimension. At the other extreme it is possible to use a few numbers to preserve all of the boundary information in enough detail to effectively reconstruct the details of its appearance.

Harmonic analysis is also known as spectral analysis, or shape unrolling (Schwartz & Shane, 1969; Ehrlich & Weinberg, 1970; Zahn & Roskies, 1972; Beddow et al., 1977; Flook, 1982; Kuhl & Giardina, 1982; Kaye et al., 1983; Rohlf & Archie, 1984; Barth & Sun, 1985; Ferson et al., 1985; Bird et al., 1986; Diaz et al., 1989; Rohlf, 1990; Diaz et al, 1990; Verscheulen et al., 1993). It begins by converting the boundary to a function of the form Radius (Angle) or $\rho(\varphi)$. As shown in **Figure 52**, a radius drawn from the feature centroid is drawn as a function of angle, and plotted to unroll the shape. This plot obviously repeats every 2π, and as a periodic or repeating function is straightforwardly subjected to Fourier analysis. This allows the determination of the a and b terms in the series expansion

$$\rho(\varphi) = a_0 + a_1 \cos(\varphi) + b_1 \sin(\varphi) + a_2 \cos(2\varphi) + b_2 \sin(2\varphi) + \dots \quad (17$$

This series is endless, or at least continues up to as many terms as there are points along the periphery. However, it is a characteristic of Fourier analysis that only the first few terms are needed to preserve most of the details of feature shape. As shown in **Figure 53**, with only 10–25 terms in the series, the original shape can be redrawn to as good a precision as the original pixel representation. In most cases, the phase information δ_i for each term in the series can be discarded without much effect, and a single coefficient c_i used for each frequency.

$$c_i = \sqrt{a_i^2 + b_i^2}$$
$$\rho(\varphi) = \sum c_i \cdot \sin(2\pi i \varphi - \delta_i) \quad (18$$

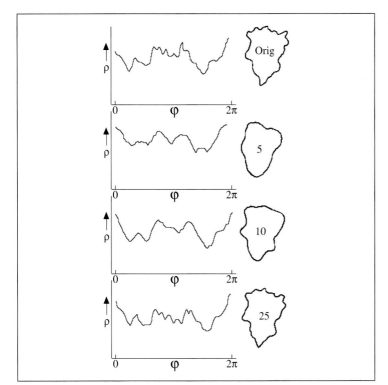

Figure 53. *Reconstruction of a real feature outline from the first 5, 10 and 25 terms in the Fourier expansion (Kaye, 1983).*

The first few values of c in the harmonic or Fourier expansion of the unrolled boundary thus contain a great deal of information about the feature shape.

Of course, this method has serious problems if the shape is re-entrant so that the radial vector is multivalued. In order to avoid that problem, an alternative approach to shape unrolling plots the slope of the line as a function of the distance along the line. This plot is also a repeating function, and can be analyzed in exactly the same way.

The chain code boundary representation of a feature already contains the slope vs. position information along the boundary, with the single exception that the data are not uniformly spaced (the diagonal links being longer than the horizontal and vertical ones). An effective way to deal with this is to replace each horizontal link with five shorter conceptual sublinks, each in the same direction, and each diagonal line with seven shorter sublinks. The ratio of 7:5 is close enough to $\sqrt{2}$ for practical purposes, and the total number of sublinks along the boundary is still reasonably short. A plot of the link value vs. position now gives the unrolled feature shape. Remember from Chapter 7 that the links are typically numbered to indicate direction.

Performing a Fourier analysis of the sequence of values along the chain code for the feature produces a list of c_i values that contain the shape information. These can be compared between classes of objects using standard statistical tests such as stepwise regression or principal components analysis, to determine which of the terms may be useful for feature classification or recognition. In a surprising number of cases, this approach proves to be successful. The identification of particles in sediments with the rivers that deposited them, the correlation of the shape of foraminifera with the water temperature in which they grew, and the discrimination of healthy from cancerous cells in Pap smears, are but a few of the successes of this approach.

In spite of its successes, the harmonic analysis approach has been little used outside of the field of sedimentation studies. In part this neglect is due to the rather significant amount of computing needed to determine the parameters, and the need to apply extensive statistical analysis to interpret them. However, as computer power has continued to increase and cost to decrease, this cannot be the major reason any longer. The probable cause is that the frequency terms have no obvious counterpart in human vision. The shape information that we extract visually from images does not reveal these numeric factors. The distinction between two sediments based on the 7th harmonic coefficient can be understood to somehow represent the presence of that frequency in the boundary irregularities of the object, but to a human observer that is masked by other variables. The success of the approach illustrates the power of computer-based measurement algorithms to surpass human skills not only quantitatively (in terms of accuracy and precision) but even qualitatively (in terms of the types of things that can be measured). But that doesn't mean that humans feel comfortable using such tools.

Topology

Harmonic analysis uses characteristics of feature shape that are quite different from those that human vision selects. On the other hand, topological parameters are those which seem most obvious to most observers. When asked to differentiate the stars on the U.S., Australian, and Israeli flags we don't discuss dimension or angles, but the number of points. The most obvious difference between a disk and the letter "O" is not the slight ellipticity of the latter, but the presence of the central hole. Topological properties are quite different from metric ones. If the feature were drawn onto a sheet of rubber, stretching it to any size and with any distortion will not change the topology.

Some topological properties of features can be determined directly, such as the number of internal holes. Finding holes within features can be done either directly as the areas are measured and the features labeled, or by inverting the image and finding the features that do not touch the image boundaries, as discussed earlier. Most algorithms that identify features sum the total area from the pixel array and compare each line of pixels to the preceding line, to assign the same label or feature number to

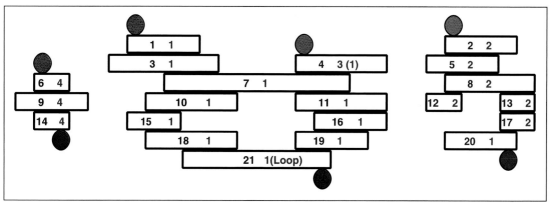

Figure 54. *The logic of feature counting. Each horizontal line of pixels (for instance as produced by run-length encoding) is compared to the preceding line. The line segments are numbered in red, in sequential order. If no touching line is found (magenta circles) it signals the start of a new feature identification, which is assigned to the line segment (green labels). If two (or more) touching line segments on the preceding scan line are found with different numbers, it is an indicator that two previously separate features have merged, and one of the label numbers is changed to match the other (see the example where feature 3 is recognized to be part of feature 1). If two touching line segments on the preceding scan line have the same number, it indicates that a loop has been formed and there is an internal hole in the feature (see the example at the bottom of feature 1). If no line segment is found on the next scan line, it indicates that the feature has ended and can be counted.*

line segments that touch a segment in the previous line. When one segment in a line touches two segments in the previous line that already carry the same identifying number, then it indicates the closure of a boundary around an internal hole as shown schematically in **Figure 54**.

Other properties, such as the number of sharp corners along the periphery, may be obtained from a boundary representation. For instance, the presence of a sharp corner is detected as a sequence of increasing (or decreasing) values in chain code values along the boundary. Similarly, straight segments are represented by chain code values that do not vary significantly over a selected length. In both cases, the decision as to how much variation is important, and over what distance, becomes an arbitrary definition. Chain code for a boundary or skeleton line is inherently noisy since the pixel-to-pixel neighbor distances can vary in only 45-degree steps. Placing a "straight" line or a ninety-degree corner on a pixel grid will produce quite different chain code sequences depending on small variations in overall orientation.

A third category of topological properties, such as the number of points on the stars mentioned above, are most readily determined using the skeleton or medial axis transform. As pointed out in Chapter 7, the skeleton consists of pixels along the midline of the features. Pixels with only a single touching neighbor are end points, while those with more than two neighbors are branch points. Counting the branch and end points, and the number of loops (holes), provides a compact topological representation of

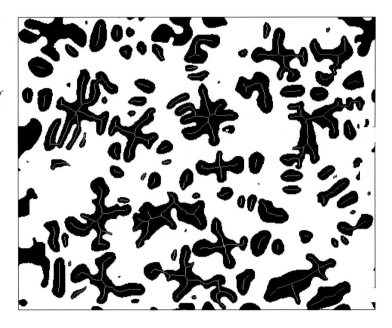

Figure 55. *Features (thresholded from the dendrites image in Figure 32) with their skeletons superimposed. The number of ends, branches and loops give the topology of the features, and can also be measured to obtain size information. Features that intersect the edge of the field cannot be measured and so are not coded.*

feature characteristics. **Figure 55** shows several features with their medial axis transforms superimposed. Counting the number of end points allows color-coding the features according to this topological property (**Figure 56**).

These characteristics of features are important to visual classification and recognition, as can be easily shown by considering our ability to recognize the printed letters in the alphabet regardless of size and modest changes in font or style. Many character recognition programs that convert images of text to letters stored in a file make heavy use of topological rules.

Figure 56. *The features from Figure 55 color coded according to the number of end points in the skeleton. Features that are the same color share this particular topological characteristic.*

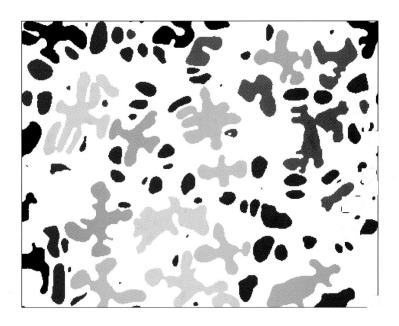

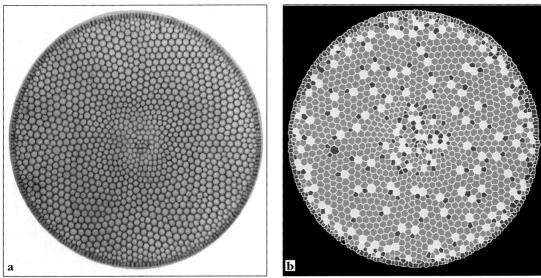

Figure 57. *An image of a diatom* **(a)** *with the holes in the structure color-coded according to the number of sides* **(b)**. *The predominant shape is six-sided, but there are some 5- and 7-sided holes that generally lie adjacent to each other.*

Another topological property of a feature is its number of sides. In the case of a space-filling structure such as cells in tissue, grains in a metal, or fields in an aerial survey, the number of sides each feature has is the number of other features it adjoins. Since the features are separate, there must be a line of background pixels that separate them. In many cases, this line is produced by image processing, by skeletonizing the original thresholded image of the boundaries and then inverting it to define the pixels. Counting the number of neighbors for each feature can be accomplished by checking the feature identification number of pixels that touch each of the background pixels in the boundaries. Building a table of the features that abut each other feature allows counting the number of such neighbors. Labeling the features according to the number of neighbors can reveal some interesting properties of the structure. **Figure 57** shows the labeling of the number of neighbors in a diatom, an essentially two-dimensional structure. **Figure 58** shows a similar labeling for grains in a three-dimensional metal structure, as revealed on a two-dimensional section.

The number of sides that a feature has can also be described in another way. If corner points are defined as above, then counting the number of sides is accomplished directly from the chain code. A second approach that is less sensitive to minor irregularities in the boundary pixels uses the convex or bounding polygon. As described above, this polygon is usually constructed with some fixed and relatively large number of sides. For instance, performing rotation of axes in 16 steps would form a 32-sided polygon. But as shown in **Figure 59**, many of the vertices in this polygon may be close together if the feature shape

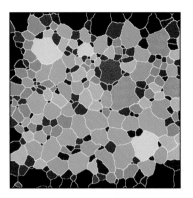
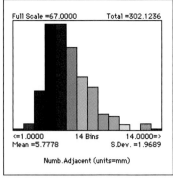

Figure 58. *Grains in a copper-beryllium metal alloy, color coded according to the number of nearest neighbors. The plot of the frequency distribution of number of neighbors is log-normal in an ideal grain structure (fully recrystallized). This is also true for the number of neighbors in three dimensions.*

has a relatively sharp corner. Setting an arbitrary limit on the distance between vertices that can be merged (usually expressed as a percentage of the total polygon perimeter) allows collecting nearby vertices together. Of course, counting the vertices is equivalent to counting the sides. Setting a threshold for the minimum length of the polygon side (again, usually as a percentage of the total perimeter) to consider it as a representation of a side of the feature can be used to count sides.

Feature identification

The recognition or identification of features in images is a very rich and complicated topic. Implementations that utilize fuzzy logic or neural nets to combine input information all start with the same kind of measurements discussed here. Such methods are used to recognize faces, military targets in surveillance photos, fingerprints, and everyday tasks such as reading printed or handwritten text. This chapter will not delve into the algorithms used to perform these operations. However, many systems offer a rudimentary feature classification capability based either on user-entered limit value or data measured on training sets of features. Most of these can utilize many different parameters, and so operate in a high-dimensionality space where the classes are described geometrically, usually as either boxes or ellipsoids.

Figure 59. *Fitting a 32-sided bounding polygon to a feature. The polygon vertices are marked in green and show clustering around each of the five major corners of the feature.*

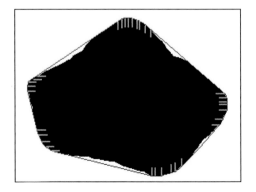

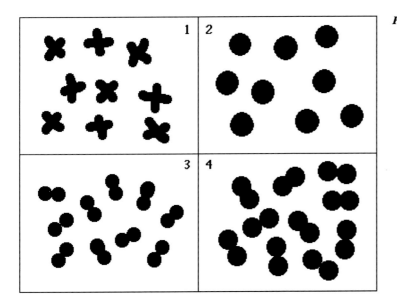

Figure 60. An example of four small training classes of different groups of features. Two of these are the same shape but have different sizes, while the others have an intermediate size and different shapes. No single measurement parameter uniquely discriminates them.

Figures 60 to **62** show an illustrative example. Four training classes of objects are imaged (**Figure 60**) and measured. There is no single size or shape parameter that can distinguish all four classes, but a combination of two parameters (area and formfactor) can. The individual measurements are plotted in **Figure 61** to show the clusters of points. Some programs can locate clusters of points to find classifications, but here we work on the assumption that the training objects are already known and the four classes established. In this two-dimensional example, it would be possible to describe the classes by breaking the space up into regions with simple boundaries (e.g., rectangles or polygons). However, a more flexible approach that is even easier to

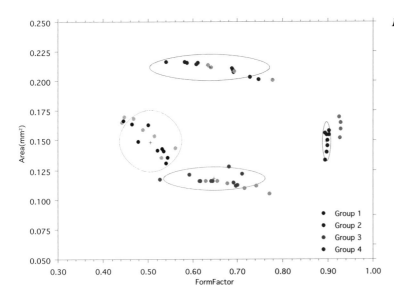

Figure 61. A plot of the measured values of area and formfactor for the features in Figure 60, color coded according to identity. The outlined points are unknowns from Figure 62, and not part of the training population. For each group, the mean value is shown, and an ellipse drawn with major and minor axes equal to two standard deviations of each measured parameter.

Figure 62. An example of unknown features to be identified using the plot in Figure 61. The color codes identify the class whose mean is closest to the measured area and formfactor of the unknown. A black outline indicates that the feature does not lie within the two-standard-deviation ellipse.

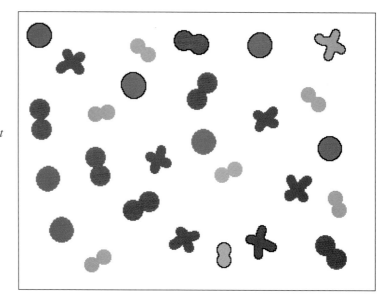

compute is to determine the mean and standard deviation values for the parameters measured from each training group, and use these to draw an ellipse. The ones shown in the figure have major and minor axes equal to 2 times the standard deviation of the data, so it is expected that a few percent of the observations will fall outside the ellipses. Obviously, other criteria could be used.

New unknown objects are then imaged and measured as shown in **Figure 62**. The measurement values for the same parameters are plotted on the graph, and the distance from the center of each ellipse measured. The nearest class is reported as the identification (in this example by color-coding the feature in the image). If the point does not lie within the ellipse then the identification is marked to indicate a lower degree of confidence (the dark outlines on the features in the figure).

This approach is extremely rapid to apply, scales up easily to higher dimensions (more measurement parameters), and allows new classes to be added simply by measuring a new training population of objects, but it also has many limitations. For one thing, selecting the best measurement parameters to distinguish the various classes is far from simple. Here it has been left to human judgment. Statistical methods such as stepwise regression or principal components analysis are better able to sort through a large number of measurement parameters to find the most economical set to use.

Another limitation is the inherent assumption that the clustering of points in each class is described by mean and standard deviation. In fact, this is often observed for size measurements (or sometimes for the logarithm of size values) but rarely for shape parameters or color and density values. It is possible to make "non-parametric" models for the classes, for instance by constructing an n-dimensional histogram of the observations, but this gets closer to a fuzzy logic implementation of the identification technique, and requires many more observations in the training sets.

A third limitation is, of course, the training set requirement. Selecting a population of representatives from each class that are statistically balanced and include all of the important variations is very difficult. Using a large training population can become time-consuming or expensive, and a small one may be quite biased. Unlike some other approaches to classification, this method cannot learn from its mistakes or improve with experience.

Fourth, the calculation of the distance from the measured point for an unknown to the center of each class amounts to an assumption that the measurement space is orthogonal and all of the distance axes have the same meaning. This limitation is by no means necessary. For instance, why should a difference of 0.1 in shape factor have the same importance as a difference of 0.1 in size? And if the shape parameter happens to use the size parameter (for instance if length and roundness were our two axes in the preceding example), it is equivalent to having graph axes that are not Cartesian, or an ellipse whose major and minor axes are not necessarily parallel to the parameter axes.

It is quite easy to list the weaknesses of this simple and direct approach, but it is also true that many of the automatic classification problems for which image analysis is actually used are simple enough that simple methods like this work. Implementing a more rigorous method based on more exact statistical techniques is always an option when needed.

Three-dimensional measurements

Many of the measurement procedures discussed above for two-dimensional images generalize directly into three dimensions. Images acquired by confocal light microscopy, seismic imaging, medical or industrial tomography, and even in some cases serial sectioning can be represented in many different ways, as discussed in the next chapters. But for image processing and measurement purposes, an array of cubic voxels (volume elements, the three dimensional analog to pixels) is the most useful. Image processing in these arrays uses neighborhoods just as in two dimensions, although these contain many more neighbors and consequently take longer to apply (in addition to the fact that there are many more voxels present in the image).

Image measurements still require identifying those pixels that are connected to each other. In two dimensions, it is necessary to decide between an 8-connected and a 4-connected interpretation of touching pixels. In three dimensions, voxels can touch on a face, edge or corner, and again the rules for features and background cannot be the same. It is more difficult to identify internal holes in features, since the entire array must be tested to see if there is any connection to the outside. However, the logic remains the same.

This consistency of principle applies to most of the measurements discussed in this chapter. Summing up the numeric values of voxels (or something calculated from them) to obtain the total density, or water content, or whatever property has been calibrated, is straightforward. So are location measurements using the voxel moments. Orientations in three dimensional space require two angles instead of one. Neighbor relationships (distance and direction) have the same meaning and interpretation as in two dimensions.

The three-dimensional analog to feature area is feature volume, obtained by counting voxels. The caliper dimensions in many directions and the bounding polyhedron can be determined by rotation of coordinate axes and searching for minimum and maximum points. Of course, getting enough rotations in three dimensions to fit the polyhedron adequately to the sample is much more work than in two dimensions. In fact, everything done in three-dimensional voxel arrays taxes the current limits of small computers: their speed, memory (to hold all of the voxels), displays (to present the data using volumetric or surface rendering), and the human interface. For instance, with a mouse, trackball, or other pointing device it is easy to select a location in a two-dimensional image. How do you accomplish this in three dimensions? Various schemes have been tried, none with wide acceptance.

It was noted above that perimeter is a somewhat troublesome concept and a difficult measurement in two dimensions. The analog to perimeter in three dimensions is the surface area of the feature, and it has all of the problems of perimeter plus some more. The idea that the surface area may be an artefact of voxel resolution remains, and is exacerbated by the somewhat coarser resolution usually available in three dimensional images. Measuring the length of the perimeter came down to using boundary representation or chain code. For a three-dimensional surface, boundary representation is the list of coordinates of vertices of a polyhedron with triangular facets. Calculating the area of a triangle from its three corners is straightforward, but knowing which three points to use for any particular triangle is not. As a very simple example, consider four points as shown in **Figure 63**. There are two different ways the surface can be constructed between them, with different surface areas.

Chain code in two dimensions relies on the fact that there is only one path around any feature, no matter how complicated. This is not true in three dimensions. There is no unique order in which triangular facets between boundary voxels must be followed. In fact for objects that are topologically shaped like a torus (have at least one open hole through them), there is no guarantee that a

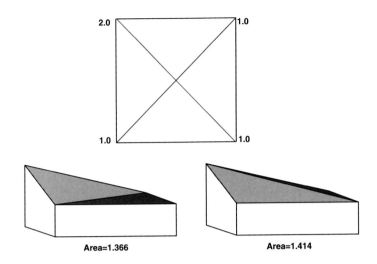

Figure 63. *Tiling a surface with triangular facets has two different solutions. In this simple example, the elevation of the four corners of a square are shown. Triangles can be constructed using either diagonal as the common line. As shown, this produces a surface that is either convex or concave, with a surface area of either 1.366 or 1.414 square units.*

continuous surface path will completely cover the surface and reach all points on it. This means that there is no convenient analog to chain code, and many of the two-dimensional measurements that were based on it are difficult to perform in three dimensions.

Likewise, the three-dimensional skeleton is harder to obtain. There are actually two "kinds" of skeleton that can be calculated for voxel arrays. One is the set of midlines, and the other is a set of planes. The latter is formed by connecting the skeleton lines in each plane section, while the former is a connection between the junction points of the skeletons in each plane section. This set of midlines can also be obtained as a medial axis transform, by using the three-dimensional analog of the Euclidean distance map to find the centers of inscribed spheres. Neither type of skeleton by itself captures all of the topological properties of the feature. The planes can show twists and protrusions not visible in the line skeleton, for example.

Measuring the length of a voxel line is similar to a pixel line. Since there are three ways the voxels can touch, the rule shown earlier in **Equation 14** must be extended, to become:

$$
\begin{aligned}
Length = \ & 0.877 \cdot (num.\ of\ face\ touching\ neighbors) \\
& +1.342 \cdot (num.\ of\ edge\ touching\ neighbors) \qquad (19 \\
& +1.647 \cdot (num.\ of\ corner\ touching\ neighbors)
\end{aligned}
$$

But deciding what voxel patterns to count to identify the important topological properties of the structure is not entirely clear.

Most of the shape parameters calculated as ratios of dimensions have simple (although equally limited) generalizations to three dimensions. Harmonic analysis can also be performed in three dimensions, by expressing the radius as a function of two angles and performing the Fourier expansion in two dimensions. As noted above, there is no analog to the chain code description of slope as a function of position, so the method is restricted to shapes that are not reentrant or otherwise multiple-valued (only one radius value at each angle). Fractal dimensions are very important for dealing with three-dimensional surfaces and networks, although in most cases it remains easier to measure them in two dimensions.

In fact, this generalization holds for most image measurement tasks. The practical difficulties of working with three-dimensional voxel arrays are considerable. The size of the array and the amount of computing needed to obtain results are significant. Because of memory restriction, or limitations in the resolution of the 3D imaging techniques, the voxel resolution is usually much poorer than the available pixel resolution in a two-dimensional image of the structure. Consequently, to the extent that the needed information can be obtained from two-dimensional images and related by stereology to the three-dimensional structure, that is the preferred technique. It is faster and often more precise.

This approach does not work for all purposes. Strongly anisotropic materials require so much effort to section in enough carefully controlled orientations, and are still so difficult to describe quantitatively, that three-dimensional imaging may be preferred. And above all, topological properties of the structure such as the number of objects per unit volume, or the connectivity of a network, are simply not accessible on two-dimensional sections. These can only be studied in three dimensions, and consequently require three dimensional imaging, processing and measurement.

Figure 64 shows an example in which twelve equally spaced sections have been cut through a three-dimensional structure. The shapes of the slices are primarily elliptical, and suggest that the structure is probably a cylindrical one. But the overall shape remains hard to construct in the mind. **Figure 65** shows the actual object, an overhand knot.

This shows another aspect of three-dimensional measurements. Most of the discussion of two-dimensional images was based on an array of pixels, and so far all of the discussion of 3D images has assumed they consist of voxels. But as will be discussed in Chapter 10, many three-dimensional structures are studied by obtaining a set of parallel section planes that are relatively widely spaced. This is generally described as a "serial section" technique, although physical sectioning is not always required. Constructing the object(s) from the sections is discussed in Chapter 10.

Measuring the features from the sections is computationally straightforward. The volume is estimated as the summation of section area times section spacing, and the surface area can be estimated as the summation of the section perimeter times section

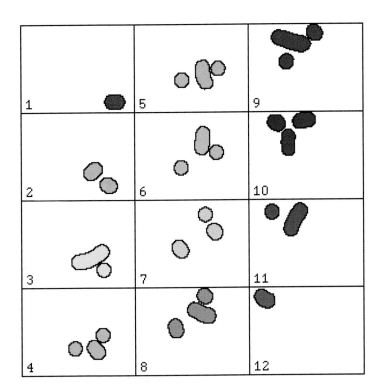

Figure 64. *Twelve serial sections through a three-dimensional structure (the color codes represent the section elevation).*

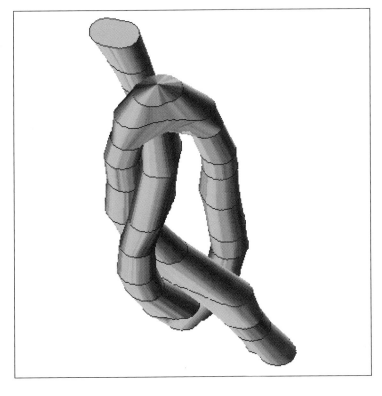

Figure 65. *The reconstructed object from the sections in Figure 64 (an overhand knot). The topology is very difficult to recognize from the sections.*

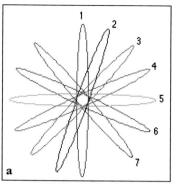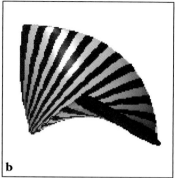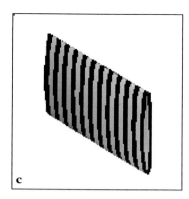

Figure 66. Reconstruction of a spiral structure:
a) the individual section outlines; b) the correct reconstruction of the surfaces; c) the incorrect reconstruction that results if the outlines are rotated for a "best fit."

spacing. But few objects have perfectly smooth surfaces. The section perimeter will reveal the roughness in the plane of the section. But the reconstruction technique generally connects the section profiles together with planes that are perfectly smooth, which underestimates the surface area. Even if the surface is smooth, the volume and surface area will be underestimated if it is curved as the fiber is in the knot.

Aligning the sections correctly is vital both to correctly understand the topology of the structure, and to measure the volume and surface. In the simple example shown in **Figure 66**, the actual structure is a spiral. If the serial sections are rotated to achieve a "best fit" from one section to the next, the result is a straight, untwisted structure with less volume and surface area than the actual structure.

Only when the sections are very closely spaced do these problems go away. In the limit when the section spacing becomes the same as the resolution within the individual section images, it is equivalent to a voxel array. This is generally preferred for measurement purposes.

9

3D Image Acquisition

Volume imaging vs. sections

Studying the three-dimensional structures of solid objects is often a goal of imaging. Many of the two-dimensional images used in the preceding chapters have been sections through three-dimensional structures. This is especially true in the various types of microscopy, where either polished flat planes or cut thin sections are needed in order to form the images in the first place. But the specimens thus sampled are three-dimensional, and the goal of the microscopist is to understand the three-dimensional structure.

There are quantitative tools of great power and utility that can convert measurements on two-dimensional (2D) images to three-dimensional (3D) values (Underwood, 1970; Weibel, 1979; Kurzydlowski & Ralph, 1995; Reed & Howard, 1997). These enable the measurement of volume fraction of phases, surface area of interfaces, mean thickness of membranes, and even the size distribution of particles seen only in a random section. But there are many aspects of structure, both quantitative and qualitative, that are not accessible from two-dimensional section images. Topological properties comprise a major category of such information, including such "simple" properties as the number of separate objects in a volume. Features visible in a single two-dimensional section do not reveal the actual three-dimensional structure present, as shown in **Figure 1**. In the preceding chapter, a method was shown for unfolding the distribution of circles to determine the size distribution and total number of spheres in a sample. However, this procedure requires making a critical assumption that the objects are all spheres. If the shape of

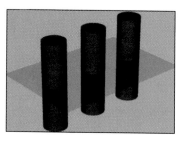
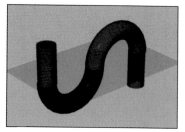
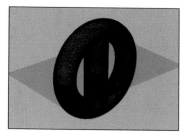

Figure 1. Examples of sections through three different structures that produce the same 2D sections: a) *three discrete objects;* **b)** *one object with simple connectivity;* **c)** *one object with multiple connectivity.*

features is unknown, can vary, or is a function of size, then this method fails.

Furthermore, as valuable as measurement data may be, they cannot provide the typical viewer with a real sense of the structure. As pointed out in the first chapter, we are overwhelmingly visual creatures—we need to *see* the 3D structure. Furthermore, our world is 3D. We are accustomed to looking at external surfaces, or occasionally through transparent media, not at thin sections or polished cut surfaces. Try to imagine (again the need to resort to a word with its connotation of vision) standing by a busy street in which an imaginary plane exists transverse to traffic flow, and that you can see that plane but nothing else. What do cars and people look like as they pass through that plane?

If you have a well-developed geometric sense, or experience as a radiologist or draftsman, you may be able to accurately visualize the appearance of that plane as portions of torsos, engine blocks, even simple shapes like tires, are cut by the plane. Most people will have difficulty imagining such collections of sections, and when asked to sketch the sections of even simple shapes will produce wildly inaccurate results.

If you doubt this, give yourself a simple test. Get some Cheerios, or rotini noodles, or some other simple food object that has a well defined shape (**Figure 2**). Then mix up an opaque matrix (fudge is good) and stir in the objects. While it is hardening, try to draw what various representative random slices through the structure might look like. After it has hardened, cut slices through the sample and compare the actual results to your sketches. My experience with students is that they have a strong tendency to imagine sections through the object that are parallel to principal axes, and ones that pass through the geometrical center of the objects. For the Cheerios (little tori), few actual sections consist of two side-by-side circles or one annulus. For the rotini, most people do not realize that sections through the curved surfaces actually produce straight lines.

As difficult as this particular visualization task may be, even fewer people can make the transition in the opposite direction: given a collection of section data, to reconstruct in the mind a correct representation of the three-dimensional structure. This is true even of those who feel quite comfortable with the 2D images themselves. Within the world of the two-dimensional images, recognition and understanding can be learned as a separate knowledge base that need not relate to the 3D world. Observing the characteristic appearance of dendrites in polished metal samples, or that of mitochondria in thin electron microscope sections of cells, does not necessarily mean that the complex 3D shapes of these objects become familiar. In fact, both of these examples are good illustrations of erroneous three-dimensional interpretations that have persistently been made from two-dimensional section images.

Because of this difficulty in using 2D images to study 3D structure, there is interest in 3D imaging. It may be performed directly, as discussed in this chapter, by actually collecting a three-dimensional set of information all at once, or indirectly by gathering a sequence of 2D (slice) images and then combining them, as discussed in the next chapter. There are a variety of ways to acquire essentially 2D images to assemble the data needed for 3D imaging, and also a great variety of ways to present the information to the user. Many of each are discussed in Chapter 10. The large number of approaches suggests that no one way is best, either for most viewers or for most applications.

Any method that reconstructs internal structural information within an object by mathematically reconstructing it from a series

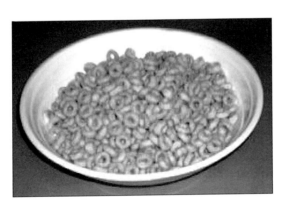

Figure 2. *Food objects (Cheerios and rotini noodles) that are useful for experimenting with the relationship between three-dimensional shapes and two-dimensional section images. These are somewhat simpler and much more consistent than many natural structures we would like to understand.*

of projections is generally referred to as tomography. It may be used to obtain true three-dimensional arrays of voxels (the 3D analog of the pixel in a 2D image), or to obtain a two-dimensional image from a series of one-dimensional line projections. The latter method is used in most medical imaging, which is by far the most common application of CT (computed tomography) at the present time. However, the same basic techniques are used for 3D imaging and for other imaging signals.

Medical tomography primarily uses X-ray absorption, magnetic resonance (MRI), positron emission (PET), and sound waves (ultrasound). Other fields of application and research use many different frequencies of electromagnetic radiation, from X- and gamma rays (nm wavelengths), through visible light and even microwave radiation (wavelengths from cm up). Besides photons, tomography is regularly performed using electrons and neutrons. In addition to absorption of the particles or radiation, tomography can be based on the scattering or emission of radiation as well.

Sound waves produced by small intentional explosions or by "ground thumpers" are used to image underground strata for prospecting, while naturally occurring noise sources such as earthquakes are used to perform seismic tomography, imaging underground faults, rock density beneath volcanoes, and locating discontinuities between the mantle and core of the earth. There are also devices listening for moon- and mars-quakes, which will reveal their internal structure, and active studies of the seismic structure of the sun.

Basics of reconstruction

X-ray absorption tomography is one of the oldest, most widely used methods and will be used here to illustrate the various parameters, artefacts, and performance possibilities. Images produced by Computer Assisted Tomography (CAT scans) and similar methods using magnetic resonance, sound waves, isotope emission, X-ray scattering or electron beams, deserve special attention. They are formed by computer processing of information from many individual pieces of projection information obtained nondestructively through the body of an object, which must be unfolded to see the internal structure. The mathematical description of the process presented here is that of X-ray absorption tomography, as it is used both in medical applications and in industrial testing (Herman, 1980; Kak & Slaney, 1988). Similar sets of equations and methods of solution apply to the other signal modalities.

Absorption tomography is based on physical processes that reduce intensity as radiation or particles pass through the sample in straight lines. In some other kinds of tomography, the paths are not straight and the reconstruction takes place along curved lines (e.g., magnetic resonance imaging and X-ray scattering tomography), or even along many lines at once (seismic tomography). This makes the equations and graphics slightly more confusing, but does not affect the basic principles involved.

X-rays pass through material but are absorbed along the way according to the composition and density which they encounter. The intensity (number of photons per second) is reduced according to a linear attenuation coefficient μ, which for an interesting specimen is not uniform but has some spatial variation so that we can write $\mu(x,y,z)$, or for a two-dimensional plane through the object, $\mu(x,y)$. The linear attenuation coefficient is the product of the mass absorption coefficient, which depends on the local elemental composition and the density. In medical tomography, the composition varies only slightly, and density variations are primarily responsible for producing images. For industrial applications, significant variations in composition are also usually present. The measured intensity along a straight line path through this distribution is given by

$$\int \mu(x,y)\, dS = \log_e \frac{I_o}{I_d} \tag{1}$$

where I_o is the incident intensity (from an X-ray tube or radioisotope) that is known and generally held constant, and I_d is the detected intensity. This is called the ray integral equation and describes the result along one projection through the object.

If a series of parallel lines are measured, either one at a time by scanning the source and detector, or all at once using many detectors, a profile of intensity is obtained which is called a view. As shown schematically in **Figure 3**, this function is usually plotted as the inverse of the intensity, or the summation of absorption along each of the lines. The function is written as $P(\phi,t)$ to indicate that it varies with position along the direction t as rays

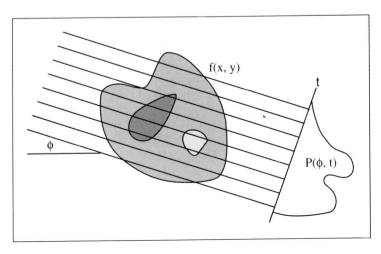

f(x, y)

t

ϕ

P(ϕ, t)

Figure 3. Illustration of a set of projections through an object at a viewing angle ϕ forming the function P.

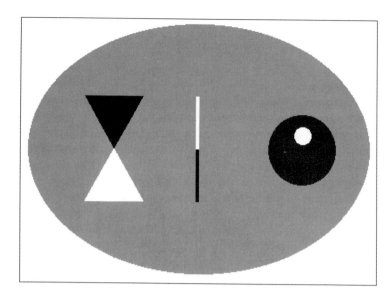

Figure 4. *A phantom (test object with geometrical shapes of known density).*

sample different portions of the object, and also with angle φ as the mechanism is rotated around the object to view it from different directions (or equivalently as the object is rotated).

Each of the views is a one-dimensional profile of measured attenuation as a function of position, corresponding to a particular angle. The collection of many such views can be presented as a two-dimensional plot or image in which one axis is position *t* and the other is angle φ. This image is called a sinogram or the Radon transform of the two-dimensional slice. **Figures 4** and **5** show a simple example. The construction of a planar figure as shown in **Figure 4** is called a phantom, and is used to evaluate the important variables and different methods for reconstructing the object slice from the projection information. The individual

Figure 5. *Sixteen attenuation profiles for the phantom in Figure 4 **(a)** and the sinogram or Radon transform **(b)** produced by plotting 180 such profiles (each as one horizontal line).*

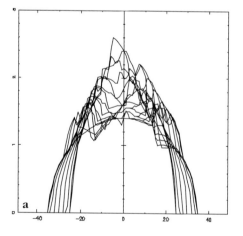

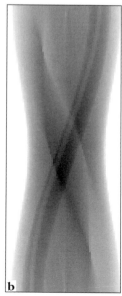

projection profiles shown in **Figure 5** show some variation as the angle is changed, but this presentation is difficult to interpret. The sinogram in **Figure 5** organizes the data so that it can be examined more readily.

The name sinogram comes from the sinusoidal variation of position of projections through the various structures within the phantom as a function of rotation, which is evident in the example. The name Radon transform acknowledges the fact that the principles of this method of imaging were published in 1917 by Radon. However, the equations he presented did not provide a practical way to implement a reconstruction since they required a continuous array of projections, and it was not until Hounsfield and Cormack developed a practical reconstruction algorithm and hardware that CAT scans became a routine medical possibility. A. M. Cormack developed a mathematically manageable reconstruction method at Tufts University in 1963–64, and G. N. Hounsfield designed a working instrument at EMI, Ltd. in England in 1972. They shared the Nobel prize in 1979.

The Fourier transform of the set of projection data in one view direction can be written as

$$S(\phi\omega) = \int P(\phi,t)\, e^{-j2\pi\omega t} dt \qquad (2$$

Radon showed that this could also be written as

$$S(\phi\omega) = \iint f(x,y)\, e^{-j2\pi\omega(x\cos\phi + y\sin\phi)} dx\, dy \qquad (3$$

which is simply the two-dimensional Fourier transform $F(u,v)$ for the function $f(x,y)$ with the constraints that $u = \omega \cos \phi$ and $v = \omega \sin \phi$. This is simply the equation of the line for the projection.

What this relationship means is that starting with the original image of the phantom, forming its two-dimensional Fourier transform as discussed in Chapter 5, and then looking at the information in that image along a radial direction from the origin normal to the direction ϕ would give the function S, which is just the one-dimensional Fourier transform of the projection data in direction ϕ in real space. The way this is useful in practice is to measure the projections P in many directions, calculate the one-dimensional transforms S, plot the complex coefficients of S into a two-dimensional transform image in the corresponding direction, and after enough directions have been measured, perform an inverse 2D Fourier transform to recover the spatial domain image for the slice. This permits a reconstruction of the slice image from the projection data, so that a nondestructive internal image can be obtained. It is the principle behind tomographic imaging.

Figure 6. Reconstruction in frequency space. The (complex) one-dimensional Fourier transforms of projection sets or views at different angles are plotted into a two-dimensional frequency domain image, which is then reconstructed:
a) *8 views in frequency space;*
b) *180 views in frequency space;*
c) *reconstruction from image a;*
d) *reconstruction from image b.*

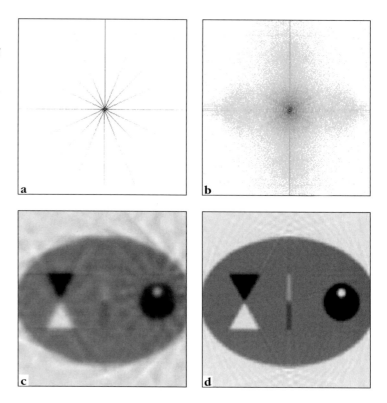

Figure 6 shows an example. Eight views or sets of projections are taken at equal angle steps, the Fourier transform of each is calculated and plotted into a 2D complex image, which is then reconstructed. The image quality is only fair, because of the limited number of views. When 180 views at one degree intervals are used, the result is quite good. The artefacts which are still present arise because of the gaps in the frequency space image. This missing information is especially evident at high frequencies (far from the origin) where the lines from the individual views become more widely spaced. All tomographic reconstruction procedures are sensitive to the number of views, as we will see.

By collecting enough views and performing this Fourier space reconstruction, it is possible to perform real tomographic imaging. In practice, few systems actually work this way. An exactly equivalent procedure that requires less computation is also available, known as filtered backprojection. This is the method used in most medical scanners and some industrial applications.

The principle behind backprojection is simple to demonstrate. The attenuation plotted in each projection in a view is due to the structure of the sample along the individual lines, or ray integrals. It is not possible to know from one projection just where along the line the attenuation occurs, but it is possible to distribute the measured attenuation evenly along the line. If this is done for only a single view, the result is not very interesting. But if it is done along projections from several views, the superposi-

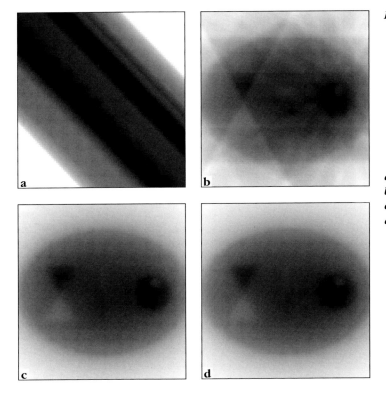

tion of the density or attenuation values should correspond to the features present in the structure.

Figure 7 illustrates this result for the same phantom. It is possible to see the dense (dark) cylinder with its hollow (light) core in the projections. Data from several views overlap to delineate the cylinder in the reconstructed image. There is a problem with this result, however. The attenuation or density of uniform regions in the original phantom is not constant, but increases toward the center of the section. Also, edges are blurred.

The cause of this problem can be described in several different but equivalent ways. The projections from all of the views contribute too much to the center of the image, where all projections overlap. The effect is the same as if the image was viewed through an out-of-focus optical system whose blur or point spread function is proportional to $1/r$ where r is the frequency, or the distance from the center of the frequency transform.

We saw in Chapter 5 how to remove a known blur from an image: multiply the frequency space transform by the inverse function before retransforming. Based on the Fourier approach, and writing the reverse transformation in terms of polar coordinates, this gives

$$f(x,y) = \int_0^\pi \int_{-\infty}^\infty S(\phi\varpi)\, |\varpi|\, e^{j2\pi\varpi t} d\varpi d\phi \qquad (4$$

or, in terms of x and y,

$$f(x,y) = \int\limits_{0}^{\pi}\int\limits_{-\infty}^{\infty} Q_\phi(x \cos\phi + y\sin\phi)d\phi \qquad (5$$

where

$$Q_\phi = \int\limits_{-\infty}^{+\infty} S(\phi,\varpi) |\varpi| \, e^{j2\pi\varpi t}d\varpi \qquad (6$$

This is just the convolution of S, the Fourier transform of the projection, by $|\omega|$ the absolute value of frequency. In frequency space, this is an ideal inverse filter which is shaped as shown in **Figure 8**. But, as was pointed out in Chapter 5, convolutions can also be applied in the spatial domain. The inverse transform of this ideal filter is also shown in **Figure 8**. Note its similarity to the shape of a Laplacian or difference of Gaussians as discussed in Chapter 4.

As a one-dimensional kernel or set of weights, this function can be multiplied by the projection P just as kernels were applied to two-dimensional images in Chapters 3 and 4. The weights are multiplied by the values, and the sum is saved as one point in the filtered projection. This is repeated for each line in the projection set or view. **Figure 9** shows the result for the projection data, presented in the form of a sinogram. Edges (high frequencies) are strongly enhanced, and low-frequency information is suppressed.

The filtered data are then projected back, and the blurring is corrected as shown in **Figure 10**. Filtered backprojection using an ideal or inverse filter produces results identical to the inverse Fourier transform method described above. The practical implementation of filtered backprojection is easier because the projec-

Figure 8. An ideal inverse filter, which selectively removes low frequencies, and its spatial domain equivalent kernel.

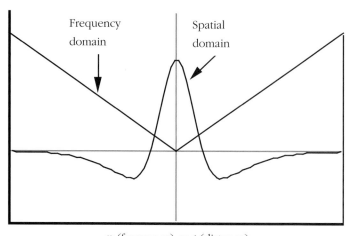

ω (frequency) or t (distance)

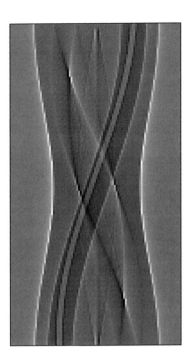

Figure 9. *The filtered projection data from Figure 5, shown as a sinogram.*

tion data from each view can be filtered by convolution (a one-dimensional operation) and the data spread back across the image as it is acquired, with no need to store the complex (i.e., real and imaginary values) frequency space image needed for the Fourier method, or retransforming it afterwards.

Notice in **Figure 10** that the quality of the image, and the effect of number of views on the artefacts, is identical to that shown for the frequency space method in **Figure 6**. In the absence of noise in the data and other effects which will be discussed below, these two methods are exactly equivalent.

Algebraic reconstruction methods

The problem of solving for the density (actually, for the linear attenuation coefficient) of each location in the image can also be viewed as a set of simultaneous equations. Each ray integral (or summation, in the finite case we are dealing with here) provides one equation. The sum of the attenuation coefficients for the pixels (or voxels) along the ray, each multiplied by a weighting factor that takes into account the actual path length of that ray through the pixel, is equal to the measured absorption. **Figure 11** illustrates the relationship between the pixels and the ray integral equations.

The number of unknowns in this set of equations is the number of pixels in the image of the slice through the specimen. The number of equations is the number of ray integrals, which is generally the number of detectors used along each projection profile times the number of view angles. This is a very large number of

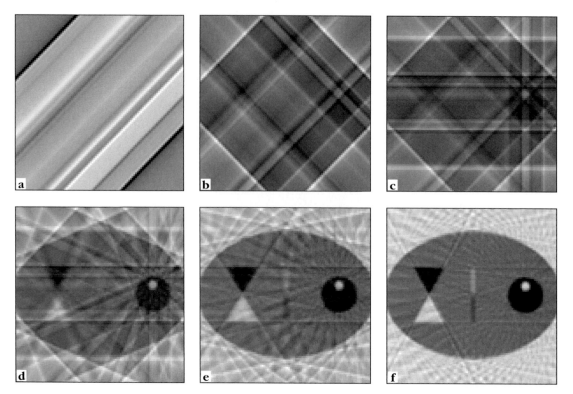

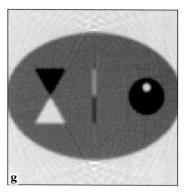

Figure 10. Filtered backprojection. The method is the same as in Figure 7, except that the values for each view have been filtered by convolution with the function in Figure 8:
a) 1 view;
b) 2 views;
c) 4 views;
d) 8 views;
e) 16 views;
f) 32 views;
g) 180 views.

equations, but fortunately many of the weights are zero (most pixels are not involved in any one particular ray integral equation). Furthermore, the number of equations rarely equals the number of unknowns. But fortunately there are a number of practical and well-tested computer methods for solving such sets of sparse equations when they are under- or overdetermined.

It is not our purpose here to compare the various solution methods. A suitable understanding of the method can be attained using the simplest of the methods, known as the algebraic reconstruction technique or ART (Gordon, 1974). In this approach, the equations are solved iteratively. The set of equations can be written as

$$\mathbf{A}^{m \cdot n}\, \mathbf{x}^{n} = \mathbf{b}^{m} \qquad (7$$

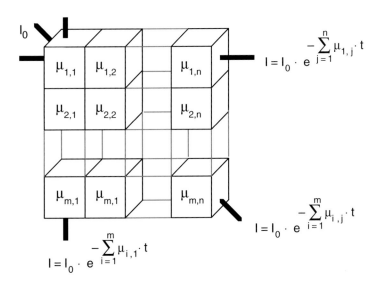

$$I = I_0 \cdot e^{-\sum\limits_{j=1}^{n} \mu_{1,j} \cdot t}$$

$$I = I_0 \cdot e^{-\sum\limits_{i=1}^{m} \mu_{i,j} \cdot t}$$

$$I = I_0 \cdot e^{-\sum\limits_{i=1}^{m} \mu_{i,1} \cdot t}$$

Figure 11. *Schematic drawing of pixels (or voxels, since they have depth) in a plane section of the specimen, and the ray integral equations that sum up the attenuation.*

where n is the number of voxels, m is the number of projections, and $\mathbf{A}$ is the matrix of weights that correspond to the contribution of each voxel to each ray path. The voxel values are the $\mathbf{x}$ values and the projection measurements are the $\mathbf{b}$ values. The classic ART method calculates each iterative set of $\mathbf{x}$ values from the preceding ones as

$$\mathbf{x}^{k+1} = \mathbf{x}^k + A_i (b_i - A_i^{\lambda} \mathbf{x}^k) \| A_i \|^2 \tag{8}$$

The value of λ, the relaxation coefficient, generally lies between 0 and 2, and controls the speed of convergence. When λ is very small, this becomes equivalent to a conventional least squares solution. Practical considerations, including the order in which the various equations are applied, are dealt with in detail in the literature (Censor, 1983, 1984).

Figure 12 shows a simple example of this approach. The 16×16 array of voxels has been given density values from 0 to 20 as shown in **Figure 12b**, and three projection sets at view angles of 0, 90 and 180 degrees calculated for the fan beam geometry shown in **Figure 12a**. For an array of 25 detectors, this gives a total of 75 equations in 256 unknowns. Starting with an initial guess of uniform voxels (with density 10), the results after one, five and fifty iterations are shown. The void areas and internal square appear rather quickly, and the definition of boundaries gradually improves. The errors, particularly in the corners of the image where fewer ray equations contain any information, and at the corners of the internal dense square, where the attenuation value changes abruptly, are evident. Still, considering the extent to which the system is underdetermined, the results are rather good.

Figure 12. Example of the application of an iterative solution. Three projection sets were calculated for an array of 25 detectors, with view directions of 0, 90, and 180° (a). *The simulated specimen **(b)** contains a 16 × 16 array of voxels. The calculation results after*

c) *one,*

d) *five, and*

e) *fifty iterations are shown.*

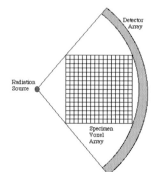

a *schematic diagram showing one set of projections through specimen*

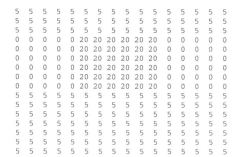

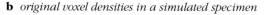

b *original voxel densities in a simulated specimen*

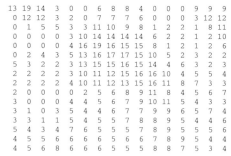

c *reconstruction after one iteration*

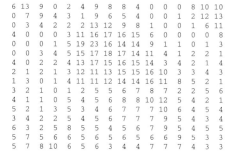

d *reconstruction after five iterations*

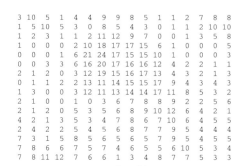

e *reconstruction after fifty iterations*

Kacmarz' method for this solution is illustrated in **Figure 13**, for the very modest case of three equations and two unknowns, and λ=1. Beginning at some initial guess, for instance that all of the pixels have the same attenuation value, one of the equations is applied. This is equivalent to moving perpendicular to the line representing the equation. This new point is then used as a starting point to apply the next equation, and so on. Since in the real case, the equations do not all meet in a perfect point, because of finite precision in the various measurements, counting statistics, machine variation, etc., there is no single point that represents a stable answer. Instead, the solution converges toward a region that is mostly within the region between the various lines, and then oscillates there. However, in a high-dimensionality space

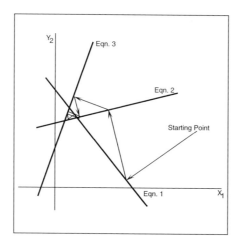

Figure 13. *Schematic diagram of Kacmarz' method for iteratively solving a set of equations, shown here for the case of two unknowns.*

with some noisy equations, it is possible for the solution to leave this region and wander away after many iterations.

In real cases with many dimensions, the convergence may not be very fast. The greatest difficulty in using the iterative algebraic technique is deciding when to stop. Logically, we would like to continue until the answer is as good as it can get, but without knowing the "truth" this stopping point is not possible to judge exactly. Some methods examine the change in the calculated image after each iteration and attempt to judge from that when to stop (for instance, when the normalized total variation in pixel values falls below some arbitrary limit, or when it increases from the previous iteration). This method is prone to serious errors in some cases, but is used nonetheless. It should be noted that the penalty for continuing the iteration is not simply the computational cost, but also the possibility that for some sets of data, the answer may start to diverge (leave the bounded region near the crossover point). This condition is, of course, highly undesirable.

Given the drawbacks to the algebraic approach, and the relative simplicity and straightforward approach of the filtered backprojection method, why would we use this method? There are several potential advantages of algebraic methods such as ART. First, the filtered backprojection method, and the Fourier transform method which it embodies, require that the number of views be rather large, and that they be equally spaced so that frequency space is well filled with data. Missing angles, or entire sets of angles which may be unattainable due to physical limitations, present problems for filtered backprojection and introduce significant artefacts. ART methods can still produce an acceptable reconstruction. There may still be lack of detail in portions of the reconstructed image which are undersampled by the projections, but the artefacts do not spread throughout the entire image. In fact, acceptable reconstructions are often obtained with only a very few views as shown in **Figure 12**.

Another advantage to ART is the ability to apply constraints. For instance, it is possible in a filtered backprojection or Fourier transform method to calculate negative values of density (attenuation) for some voxels, because of the finite measurement precision. Such values have no physical meaning. In the iterative algebraic method, any such values can be restricted to zero. In the schematic diagram of **Figure 13**, this amounts to restricting the solution to the quadrant of the graph with positive values.

In fact, any other prior knowledge can also be applied. If it is known that the only possible values of density and attenuation in the specimen correspond to specific materials, then the values can be easily constrained to correspond. Any geometric information, such as the outside dimensions of the object, can also be included (in this case, by forcing the voxels outside the object boundaries to zero).

It is even possible to set up a grid of voxels that are not all of the same size and spacing. This setup might allow, for instance, the use of a fine voxel spacing in the interior of an object where great detail is desired, but a much coarser grid outside (or vice versa). This would still allow the calculation of the contribution of the outside material to the ray integrals, but would reduce the number of unknowns to produce a better solution for any given number of views and projections. Sets of nonsquare pixels or noncubic voxels can also be used when necessary to conform to specific object shapes and symmetries.

The flexibility of the algebraic method and its particular abilities to use *a priori* information often available in an industrial tomography setting compensates for its slowness and requirements for large amounts of computation. The calculation of voxel weights (the **A** matrix) can be tedious, especially for fan beam or other complex geometries, but no more so than backprojection in such cases, and it is a one-time calculation. The use of solution methods other than the iterative approach described here can provide improved stability and convergence.

Maximum entropy

There are other ways to solve these huge sets of sparse equations. One is the so-called maximum entropy approach. Maximum entropy was mentioned as an image processing tool to remove noise from a two-dimensional image in Chapter 3. Bayes' theorem is the cornerstone for the maximum entropy approach, given that we have relevant prior information which can be used as constraints. In the case where no prior information is available but noise is a dominant factor, Bayes' theorem leads to the classical or "least squares" approximation method. It is the use of prior information that permits a different approach.

The philosophical justification for the maximum entropy approach comes from Bayesian statistics and information theory.

It has also been derived from Gibbs' concept of statistical thermodynamics (Jaynes, 1967). For the nonspecialist, it can be described as follows: find the result (distribution of brightnesses in pixels of the image, distribution of density values in a voxel array, or practically anything else) that is feasible (consistent with the known constraints, such as the total number of photons, the non-negativity of brightness or density at any point, the physics involved in the detector or measurement process, etc.) and has the configuration of values which is most probable.

This probability is defined as being able to be formed in the most ways. For an image formed by photons, all photons are considered indistinguishable, and the order in which they arrive is unimportant, so the distribution of photons to the various pixels can be carried out in many ways. For some brightness patterns (images) the number of ways to form the pattern is much greater than others. We say that these images with greater multiplicity have a higher entropy. Nature can form them in more ways, so they are more likely. The entropy is defined as $S = -\sum p_i \log p_i$, where p_i is the fraction of pixels with brightness value i.

The most likely image (from a simple statistical point of view) is for all of the pixels to get the same average number of photons, producing a uniform grey scene. However, this result may not be permitted by our constraints, one of which is the measured brightness pattern actually recorded. The difference between the calculated scene and the measured one can only be allowed to have a set upper limit, usually based on the estimated noise characteristics of the detector, the number of photons, etc. Finding the feasible scene which has the highest multiplicity is the maximum entropy method.

For instance, in solving for the tomographic reconstruction of an object from the set of ray integral equations obtained from various view angles, we have a large set of simultaneous equations in many unknowns. Instead of formally solving the set of simultaneous equations, for instance by a traditional Gauss-Jordan elimination scheme which would take far too many steps to be practical, the maximum entropy approach recasts the problem. Start with any initial guess (in most "well-behaved" cases, the quality of that guess matters little in the end result) and then iteratively, starting at that point, find another solution (within the class of feasible solutions as defined by the constraints) that has a higher entropy. Deciding which way to move in the space defined by the parameters (the values of all the voxels) is usually done with LaGrange multipliers by taking partial derivatives and trying always to move "uphill" where the objective function used to evaluate each set of values is the entropy.

It is usually found that the solution having the maximum feasible entropy (i.e., permitted by the constraints) is hard against the boundary formed by those constraints, and if they were relaxed the solution would move higher (to a more uniform image).

Knowing or assuming that the solution lies along the constraint boundaries allows use of more efficient schemes for finding the best solution. For the noise removal problem discussed in Chapter 3, the constraint is commonly the chi-squared value of the smoothed image as compared to the measured one. This is generally assumed to be due to classical noise, and so should have an upper limit and a known distribution.

For tomographic reconstruction, the constraints are based on satisfying the ray integral equations. These are not all consistent, so a weighting scheme must be imposed on the error; linear weighting is the simplest and most often used. It turns out that in most cases, the cluster of solutions with high entropies, all permitted by the constraints, are virtually indistinguishable. In other words, the maximum entropy method does lead to a useful and robust solution. While the solution is still iterative, the method is quite efficient as compared to other solution techniques.

Defects in reconstructed images

The reconstructed example shown above was calculated using simulated projection data with no noise or any other defects. In real tomography, a variety of defects may be present in the projection sets that propagate errors back into the reconstructed image. Using the same phantom, several of the more common ones can be demonstrated.

Ideally, a large number of view angles and enough detector positions along each projection set will be used to provide enough information for the reconstruction. In the event that fewer projections in a set or fewer views are used, the image has more reconstruction artefacts and poorer resolution, definition of boundaries, and precision and uniformity of voxel values. **Figure 14** shows the effect of fewer projections in each set but still uses 180 view angles. The reconstructed images are displayed with 100×100 pixels. This ideally requires a number of ray integrals in each projection set equal to at least $\sqrt{2}$ times the width, or 141 pixels. With fewer, the resolution of the reconstruction degrades.

If fewer view angles are used (but the angular spacing is still uniform), the artefacts in the reconstruction increase as was shown above in **Figure 10**. If the view angles are not uniformly spaced, the results are much worse as shown in **Figure 15**.

In real images, the number of X-ray photons detected at each point in the projection set is subject to fluctuations due to counting statistics. In many cases, both in medical and industrial tomography, the number of photons is limited. In medical applications, it is important to limit the total exposure to the subject. In industrial applications, the limitation is due to the finite source strength of either the X-ray tube or radioisotope source, and the need to acquire as many views as possible within a reasonable

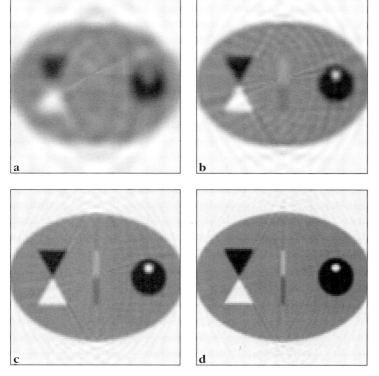

Figure 14. Effect of number of ray integrals in projection set on reconstructed image quality. Each image is reconstructed with 100×100 pixels and is calculated from 180 view angles. The images show the use of

a) *25,*
b) *49,*
c) *75,*
d) *99 ray projections, respectively.*

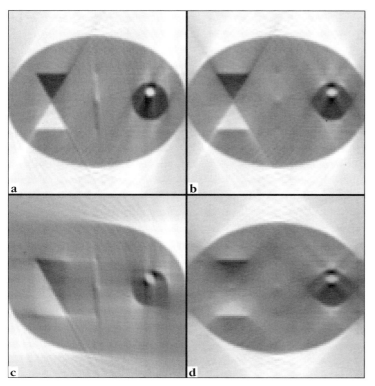

Figure 15. Effect of using a set of view angles that do not uniformly fill the angular range:

a) *150° coverage;*
b) *120° coverage;*
c) *90° coverage;*
d) *a different 90° range.*

time. In either case, the variation in the number of detected X-rays varies in a Gaussian or normal distribution whose standard deviation is the square root of the number counted. Counting an average of 100 X-rays produces a variation whose standard deviation is 10% ($\sqrt{100} = 10$), while an average of 10,000 X-rays is needed to reduce the variation to 1% ($\sqrt{10^4} = 10^2$).

The process of reconstruction amplifies the effect of noise in the projections. The filtering process suppresses the low frequencies and keeps the high frequencies, and the counting fluctuations vary randomly from point to point and so are represented in the highest frequency data. **Figure 16** shows the result. Adding a statistical or counting fluctuation of a few percent to the simulated projection data produces a much greater noise in the reconstructed image. Although the density differences in the three regions of the phantom vary by 100%, some of the regions disappear altogether when 10% or 20% noise is added to the projection data.

Suppression of the high-frequency noise in the projection data by the filtering process can reduce the effect of the noise somewhat, as shown in **Figure 17**. Notice that the noise variations in the reconstructed images are reduced, but that the high frequency data needed to produce sharp edges and reveal the smaller structures are gone as well.

Several different filter shapes are used for this purpose. **Figure 18** shows representative examples, in comparison to the shape of the ideal inverse filter that was discussed above. The plots are in terms of frequency. All of the filters reduce the low frequency values, which is required in order to prevent blurring, and all of the noise reduction filters also attenuate the high frequencies in order to suppress the noise.

Another important source of errors in the reconstruction of images is imprecise knowledge of the location of the center of rotation, or variation in that center due to imperfect mechanical mechanisms (Barnes et al., 1990). As shown in **Figure 19**, this variation also produces an effect in the reconstructed image which is magnified. The characteristic "U" shaped arcs result from an off-center rotation, because view angles in a range of 180 degrees were used. If 360-degree rotation is used, a complete circular arc is present (**Figure 20**) that also distorts the reconstruction but is more difficult to recognize. Note that it is not common to collect data over a complete 360-degree set of angles, because in the absence of off-center rotation or beam hardening the second half of the data is redundant. The effect of a variable center is equal in magnitude with 360-degree rotation, but harder to recognize. In general, it is required that the location of the center of rotation and its constancy must be less than about one-tenth of the expected spatial resolution in the reconstructed images.

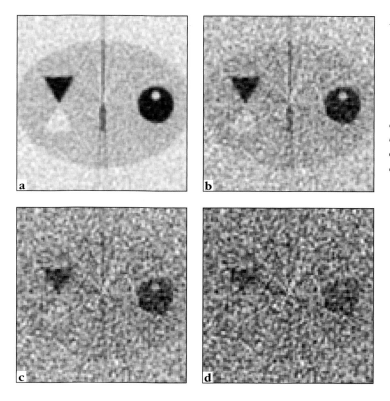

Figure 16. Effect of counting statistics on reconstruction. The images were reconstructed from simulated projection data to which Gaussian random fluctuations were added:
a) 2%;
b) 5%;
c) 10%;
d) 20%.

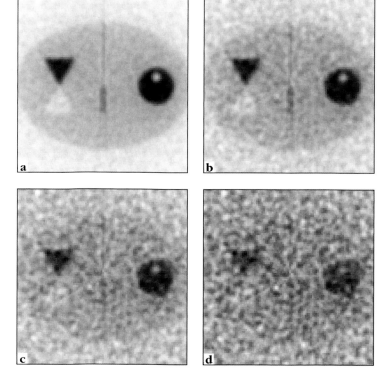

Figure 17. Reconstructions from the same projection data with superimposed counting statistics variations as in Figure 16, but using a Hann filter instead of an ideal inverse filter to reduce the high-frequency noise.

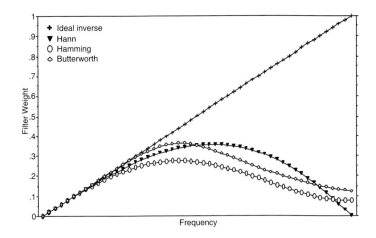

Figure 18. Filter profiles for noise reduction in filtered backprojection:

Ideal inverse: Weight = $|f|$

Hann: Weight = $|f| \cdot \{0.5 + 0.5 \cos [(\pi/2) (f/f_m)]\}$

Hamming: Weight = $|f| \cdot \{0.54 + 0.46 \cos (\pi \, f/f_m)\}$

Butterworth ($n = 3$): Weight = $|f| \cdot 1/ (1+(f/2f_m)^{2n})$

The plot legend reads:
+ Ideal inverse
▼ Hann
○ Hamming
◇ Butterworth

with the y-axis labeled "Filter Weight" (0 to 1) and the x-axis labeled "Frequency".

Beam hardening is the name used to describe the effect in which the lower energy or "softer" X-rays from a polychromatic source such as a conventional X-ray tube are preferentially absorbed in a sample. The consequence is that the effective attenuation coefficient of a voxel is different depending on whether it is on the side of the specimen near the source or farther away. This variation along the path is indicated schematically in **Figure 21**. Beam hardening is not a major problem in medical tomography because the variation in composition of the various parts of the human body is only slight. Everything is mostly water with some addition of carbon, a trace of other elements, and for bones, some calcium. The density is variable, and is in fact what the reconstructed image shows, but the range of variation is small. This uniformity makes X-ray tubes an acceptable source, and simple backprojection a suitable reconstruction method.

Industrial applications commonly encounter samples with a much greater variation in composition, ranging across the entire periodic table and with physical densities that vary from zero (voids) to more than ten times the density of biological tissue. This large range of variation makes beam hardening an important problem. One solution is to use a monochromatic source such as a radioisotope or a filtered X-ray tube. Another is to use two different energies (Schneberk et al., 1991) or a combination of absorption and X-ray scattering data (Prettyman et al., 1991) and to use the two projection sets to correct for the change in composition in the reconstruction process. However, this method increases the complexity significantly and requires an algebraic method rather than backprojection or Fourier techniques.

Figure 22 shows a representative example of the beam hardening effect in the same phantom used above. In this case, the sample composition is specified as void (the lightest region and the surroundings), titanium (the medium grey region of the elliptical object), and iron (the dark region). The total width is 1 cm, and the X-ray tube is assumed to be operating at 100 kV. This is in

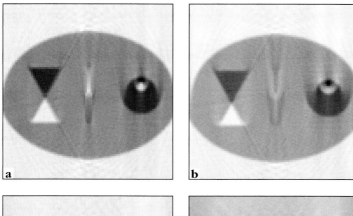

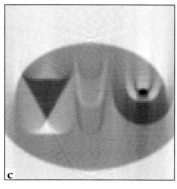
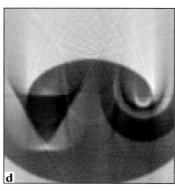

Figure 19. Effect of errors in the center of rotation on the reconstructed image. In each of these images, the center is consistent, but displaced from the location assumed in the rotation by a fraction of the image width:
a) 0.5%
b) 1.0%
c) 2.5%
d) 5.0%

Figure 20. Repeating the reconstructions of Figure 19 using the same number of views (180) but spread over 360° instead of 180°, with the center of rotation displaced from the assumed location by a fraction of the image width:
a) 0.5%
b) 1.0%
c) 2.5%
d) 5.0%

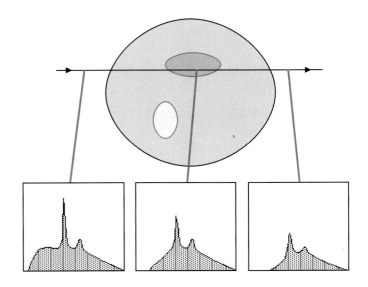

Figure 21. Schematic diagram of beam hardening. *The energy spectrum of X-rays from an X-ray tube is shown at the beginning, middle, and end of the path through the specimen. As the lower energy X-rays are absorbed, the attenuation coefficient of the sample changes independent of any actual change in composition or density.*

fact a very modest amount of beam hardening. A larger specimen, a lower tube voltage, higher atomic number elements, or a greater variation in atomic number of density, would produce a much greater effect.

Figure 23 shows reconstructions of the image using view angles which cover 180 degrees and 360 degrees, respectively. In most tomography, 180 degrees is adequate since the projections are expected to be the same regardless of direction along a ray path. This assumption is not true in the case of beam hardening (as it was not for the case of off-center rotation), and so better results

Figure 22. *Example of beam hardening effect on the sinogram or Radon transform (a) and the inverse filtered data (b). Notice that the contrast of each feature changes according to where it lies within the rotated object.*

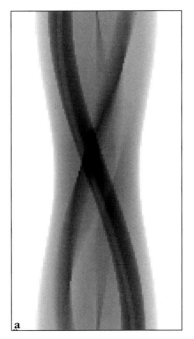

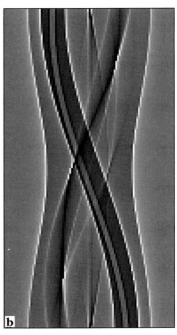

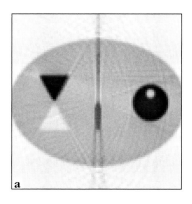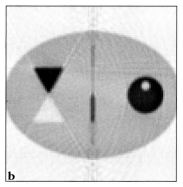

Figure 23. Reconstruction of the beam hardened data from Figure 22:

a) *180 views covering 180°;*

b) *180 views covering 360°.*

are obtained with a full 360 degrees of data. Notice though that artefacts are still present. This is particularly true of the central feature, in which the narrow void is hardly visible. **Figure 24** shows the same phantom with no beam hardening, produced by specifying a monochromatic X-ray source.

When X-rays pass through material, the attenuation coefficient that reduces the transmitted intensity consists of two principal parts: the absorption of the X-rays by the excitation of a bound electron, and the scattering of the X-rays either coherently or incoherently into a different direction. In either case, the photons are lost from the direct ray path, and the measured intensity decreases. However, in the case of scattering, the X-rays may be redirected to another location in the detector array (see the discussion of the geometries of various generations of instrument designs, below).

When this scattering happens, the measured projection profiles contain additional background on which the attenuation data are superimposed. The presence of the background also produces artefacts in the reconstruction as shown in **Figure 25**. The effect is visually similar to that produced by beam hardening.

In addition, the uniform regions in the object are reconstructed with a variable density due to the background. **Figure 26** shows this reconstruction for a simple annular object, and **Figure 27** shows plots across the center of the reconstructions. The deviation

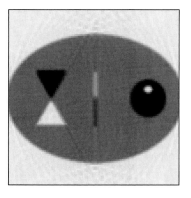

Figure 24. *Reconstruction of the same phantom as in Figure 23 but using a monochromatic 50-kV X-ray source. Notice particularly the void in the center of the object, which is not visible in Figure 23.*

Figure 25. Reconstruction of the phantom in Figure 24 when the measured projection sets include scattered background radiation of

a) 5,

b) 10,

c) 20, and

d) 40% of the average intensity. The effect on the image is similar to beam hardening. Small features are obscured by artefacts, and the overall contrast changes.

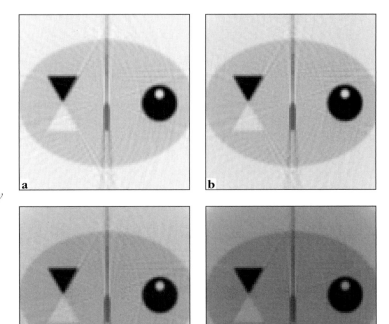

from a uniform density in the reconstruction is called cupping. Note that this example uses materials similar to those in the human body. However, medical tomography is not usually required to produce a quantitatively accurate measure of density, but only to show the location of internal structures and boundaries. Industrial tomography is often called upon to measure densities accurately so as to quantify gradients in parts due to processing, and this source of error is therefore of concern.

Although medical applications rarely need to measure densities exactly, they do require the ability to show small variations in density. A test phantom often used to demonstrate and evaluate performance in this category is the Shepp and Logan (1974) head phantom. Composed of ellipses with densities close to 1.0, it

Figure 26. Reconstruction of a simple annulus with outer composition of calcium carbonate (an approximation to bone) and an inner composition of water (an approximation to tissue):

a) no scattered background;

b) 10% scattered background in projection data.

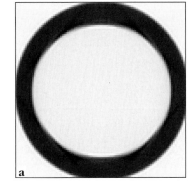
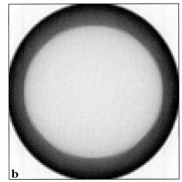

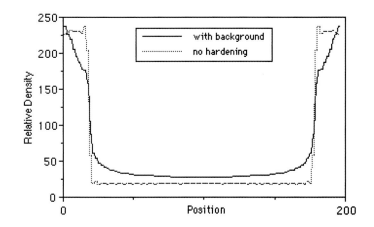

Figure 27. Line profiles of the density in the images in Figure 26.

mimics in simplified form the human head, surrounded by a much denser skull, and containing regions slightly lower or higher in density that model the brain structure and the presence of tumors. The ability to image these areas is critical to the detection of anomalies in real head scans.

Figure 28 shows a reconstruction of this phantom. Using the full dynamic range of the display (values from 0 to 255) linearly to represent the image does not reveal the internal detail within the phantom. Applying histogram equalization (as discussed in Chapter 4) expands the contrast in the center of the histogram so that the different regions become visible. The figure shows the cumulative histograms of display brightness for the original and histogram-equalized images. In the former, the steps show the principal density values; after equalization the values more closely approximate a straight line, and the steps show the distinction between similar regions. A profile plot across the central region shows the different regions with quite uniform density values (**Figure 29**).

Tomography can be performed using other modalities than X-ray absorption. One is emission tomography, in which a radioactive isotope is placed inside the object and then reveals its location by emitting gamma ray photons. Detectors around the object can specify the lines along which the source of the photons lie, producing data functionally equivalent to the attenuation profiles of the conventional case. **Figure 30** shows an example of emission tomography using real data, in which another artefact is evident.

The bright areas in the reconstruction are cavities within a machined part that contain a radioactive isotope. The sinogram shows the detected emission profiles as a function of view angle. Notice that the width of the regions varies with angle. This variation is due to the finite width of the collimators on the detectors, which cover a wider dimension on the far side of the object as indicated schematically in **Figure 31**. This effect is also present

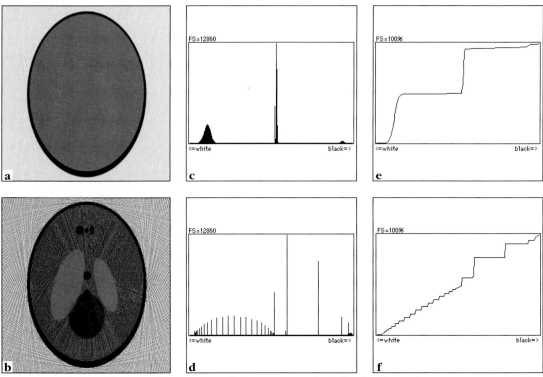

Figure 28. Shepp and Logan phantom, intended to represent the difficulty of visualizing a tumor inside the human head. The regions of varying density inside the "brain" range in relative densities from 1.0 to 1.04, while the "skull" has a density of 2.0. They are not visible in the reconstructed image unless some contrast expansion is used. Here, histogram equalization (bottom) is used to spread the grey scale nonlinearly to show the various ellipses and their overlaps (and also to increase the visibility of artefacts in the reconstruction). The graphs show the brightness histograms and their cumulative plots. In the latter, the effect of the equalization is especially evident.

in X-ray absorption tomography, due to the finite size of apertures on the source and the detectors. If the angle of the collimators is known, this effect can be included in the reconstruction, either by progressively spreading the data as the filtered

Figure 29. Brightness profiles across the images in Figure 28, showing the uniformity and sharpness of transitions for the regions and the effect of histogram equalization.

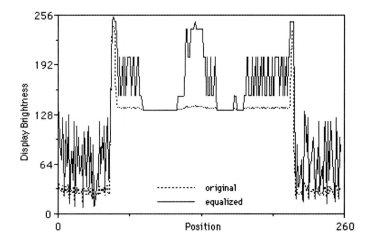

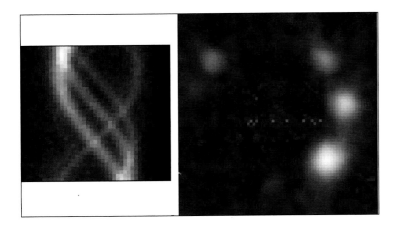

profile is spread back across the voxel array, or by adjusting the voxel weights in the algebraic reconstruction technique.

Imaging geometries

First-generation tomographic systems collected projection sets at a variety of view angles by moving a source and detector just as shown in **Figure 3**. **Figure 32** shows the procedure used to collect a complete set of projection data. This is called a pencil-beam or parallel-beam geometry, in which each ray integral is parallel and the projection set can be directly backprojected. It is not very efficient, since only a small solid angle of the generated X-rays can be used, and only a single detector is in use.

Second-generation instruments added a set of detectors so that a fan beam of X-rays could be detected and attenuation measured along several lines at the same time, as shown in **Figure 33**. This procedure requires fewer view angles to collect the same amount of data, but the attenuation measurements from each detector are actually for different angles and there is some reordering of the data needed before it can be used.

The so-called fan-beam geometry is appealing in its efficiency, and the next logical step, in so-called third-generation instru-

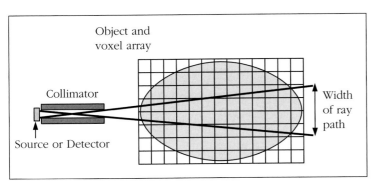

Figure 31. Schematic diagram showing the effect of a finite collimator angle on the dimensions and voxels covered in different parts of the object.

Figure 32. *First-generation geometry. The detector and source move together to collect each projection set, and rotate to many view angles to collect all of the required data.*

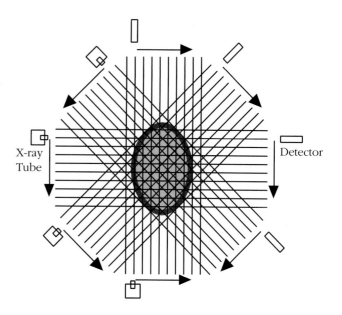

X-ray Tube

Detector

ments used for medical imaging, was to use a larger array of detectors (and to arrange them on an arc so that each covered the same solid angle and had normal X-ray incidence) and a single X-ray tube. The detectors and tube rotate together about the object as the X-ray tube is pulsed to produce the series of views (**Figure 34**). In fourth-generation systems, a complete ring of detectors is installed and only the source rotates (**Figure 35**). Notice that the X-rays are no longer normally incident on the detectors in this case. There is a fifth-generation design in which even less hardware motion is required: the X-rays are generated

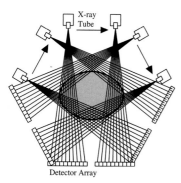

X-ray Tube

Detector Array

Figure 33. *Second-generation geometry. The detector array simultaneously measures attenuations in a fan beam, requiring fewer view angles than first-generation systems to collect the data.*

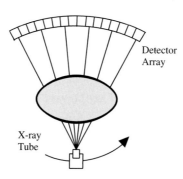

Detector Array

X-ray Tube

Figure 34. *Third-generation geometry. The X-ray tube and detector array rotate together around the object being imaged, as the tube is rapidly pulsed to produce each view.*

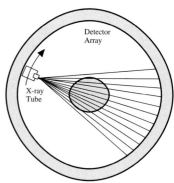

Detector Array

X-ray Tube

Figure 35. *Fourth-generation geometry. The detector array forms a complete ring and is fixed. The X-ray tube rotates around the object and is pulsed. Data from the detectors are sorted out to produce the projection sets.*

by magnetically deflecting an electron beam against a fixed target ring, rotating the source of X-rays to produce the same effective geometry as in fourth-generation systems.

These latter types of geometry are less used in industrial tomography, since they are primarily intended for imaging speed, to minimize exposure and acquire all of the projections before anything can move in the person being imaged. First- or second-generation (pencil or fan beam) methods in which a series of discrete views are collected provide greater flexibility in dealing with industrial problems. However, all of the methods are equivalent if the various ray integrals using individual detectors in the fan-beam geometry are sorted out according to angle, and either backprojected, used in a Fourier transform method, or used to calculate an algebraic reconstruction with appropriate weights.

Three-dimensional tomography

While the most common application of tomography is to form images of planar sections through objects without physical sectioning, the method can be directly extended to generate complete three-dimensional images. Chapter 10 shows several examples of 3D displays of volume data. Most of these, including many of the tomographic images, are actually serial section images. Whether formed by physical sectioning, optical sectioning (for instance, using the confocal light microscope), or conventional tomographic reconstruction, these methods are not true 3D data sets.

The distinction is that the pixels in each image plane are square, but as they are extended into the third dimension as voxels, they do not necessarily become cubes. The distance between the planes, or the depth resolution, is not inherently the same as the pixel size or resolution within the plane. In fact, few of these methods have depth resolution that is even close to the lateral resolution. Some techniques such as physical or optical sectioning have much poorer depth resolution. Others such as the secondary ion mass spectrometer have depth resolution that is far better than the lateral resolution of images. This has profound effects for three-dimensional image presentation, for image processing, and especially for three-dimensional structural measurement.

True three-dimensional imaging is possible with tomographic reconstruction. The object is represented by a three-dimensional array of cubic voxels, and the individual projection sets become two-dimensional arrays (projection images). Each projection is from a point, and is referred to as a cone-beam geometry (by analogy to the fan-beam method used for single slice projections). The set of view directions must include orientations that move out of the plane and into three dimensions, described by two polar angles. This does not necessarily require rotating the object with two different polar angles, since using a cone-beam imaging geometry provides different angles for the projection lines, just as

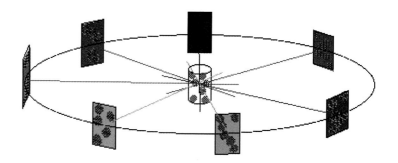

Figure 36. *Geometry for volume imaging using radial projections obtained by rotating the sample about a single axis.*

a fan beam geometry does in two dimensions. However, the best reconstructions are obtained with a series of view angles that cover the three-dimensional orientations as uniformly as possible.

Several geometries are possible. One of the simplest is to rotate the sample about a single axis as shown in **Figure 36**. This method offers the advantage of precise rotation, since as seen before, the quality of the reconstruction depends on the consistency of the center of rotation. On the other hand, artefacts in the reconstructed voxels can be significant, especially in the direction parallel to the axis and near the north and south poles of the sample. The single-axis rotation method is most often used with X-ray, neutron or gamma ray tomography, because the samples may be rather large and are relatively equiaxed so that the distance that the radiation must pass through the sample is the same in each direction.

For electron tomography, most samples are not cylindrical, and few transmission electron microscope stages permit complete movement of the sample about its axis. For a sample that is essentially slab-like, the geometry that is usually adopted is a series of tilt angles that project along the limbs of a cone, as shown in **Figure 37**. Collecting these projections by controlling

Figure 37. *Tilting the sample in a conical pattern produces a series of projections used for reconstruction in transmission electron microscopy. The spacing along the cone trace is generally not uniform.*

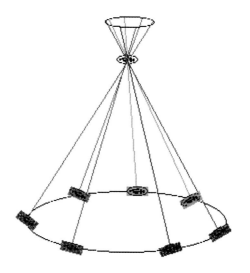

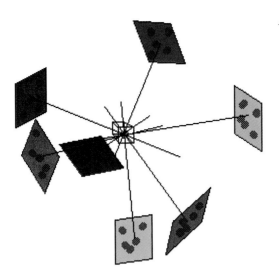

Figure 38. *Optimum 3D reconstruction is possible when a series of 3D projections is used, by rotating the sample about two axes.*

the tilt and rotation of the sample in its holder with enough precision to allow good reconstructions is very difficult. Some TEM samples consist of many repeating structures (macromolecules, virus particles, etc.), and a simple tilt of the sample can collect enough different views to be used for reconstruction. Because of the use of many different individual objects with various orientations, this method is called random-conical, as compared to the use of equal angular increments. The very small aperture angle of the beam in the TEM produces essentially parallel rather than cone-beam projections, which does simplify the reconstruction and makes backprojection possible. But the use of a limited set of views arranged in a cone produces artefacts because little information is available in the axial direction (sometimes referred to as the missing cone of information). Frank (1992) presents a thorough review of the current state of the art in electron microscope tomography.

From a theoretical viewpoint, the best reconstruction for any given number of projections is obtained when they are uniformly distributed in three-dimensional space (**Figure 38**). Constructing a mechanism to achieve accurate rotations about two precisely centered axes is difficult and not widely used. A compromise approach that is better than simple axial rotation and easier to achieve than full three-dimensional rotation uses a helical rotation of the sample (Wang et al., 1991).

The reconstruction can be performed with any of the methods used in two dimensions. For Fourier inversion, the frequency space is also a three-dimensional array, and the two-dimensional images produced by each projection are transformed and the complex values plotted on planes in the array. As for the two-dimensional case, filling the space as completely and uniformly as possible is desirable. The Fourier inversion is performed in three dimensions, but this is a direct extension of methods in

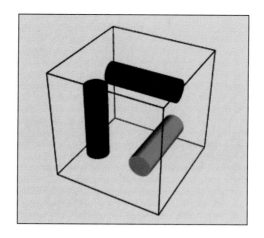

Figure 39. *Geometry of a test sample. Three cylindrical inserts of different metals (Cr, Mn and Fe) are placed in a plastic block (2 cm. on a side).*

lower dimensions and in fact the inversion can be performed in one dimension at a time (successively along rows in the *u, v,* and *w* directions).

Backprojection can also be used for 3D reconstruction, and as in the two-dimensional case is simply an implementation of the Fourier transform mathematics. The filtering of the two-dimensional images must be performed with a two-dimensional convolution, which can be carried out either by kernel operation in the spatial domain or by multiplication in the Fourier domain. The principal difficulty with the backprojection method is that calculation of the matrix of weights can be quite tricky for cone-beam geometry. These values represent the attenuation path length along each of the ray integrals through each of the voxels. The use of backprojection requires a large number of views to avoid artefacts and is most commonly used with single-axis rotation or with helical scans about a single rotational axis, with either cone-beam or parallel-beam projections (Feldkamp et al., 1984; Smith, 1990). It is difficult to apply to a full three-dimensional set of cone beams because they are spaced at relatively large angles.

Algebraic reconstruction (ART) methods are also applicable to voxel arrays. The difficulty in obtaining a uniform set of view angles, which is particularly the case for electron microscopy, can make ART particularly attractive. In fact, when using an iterative technique such as ART, the best results are often obtained with a surprisingly small number of views. **Figures 39** and **40** show an example. The specimen (about 2 cm on a side) consists of three different metal cylinders in a plastic block. Chromium, manganese and iron are consecutive elements in the periodic table, with similar densities. Tomographic reconstruction from only 12 views with 3D rotations, using a low power industrial X-ray source, shows the inserts quite well (Ham, 1993).

Of course, more views should produce a better reconstruction. But in most tomography situations, the total dose is a fixed con-

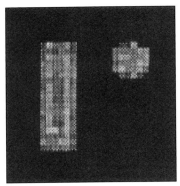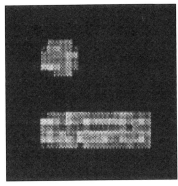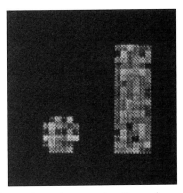

Figure 40. *Tomographic reconstruction of three planes in the xy, yz and zx orientations passing through the metal inserts in the plastic block shown in Figure 39, reconstructed using just 12 cone-beam projections with rotations in 3D.*

straint. In some cases, this can be because of concerns about radiation damage to the sample. Dosage to the sample is a concern for medical X-ray tomography, of course. But it also creates problems for electron tomography. The amount of energy deposited in each cubic nanometer of the sample from a focused electron beam is great enough to cook biological tissue, disrupt molecules, and change the structure we want to image. But even for industrial tomography, the total flux of radiation that can be generated and the time spent acquiring the images usually is limited. There is a necessary tradeoff between the number of projections and the time spent acquiring each one. More time on each projection improves the statistical quality of the image, so acquiring more projections makes each one noisier, and vice versa. In some experiments with a limited total photon budget, the best quality reconstructions with full three-dimensional rotation were obtained with only 12 projections (Ham, 1993). This small number of views requires an iterative method rather than backprojection.

The limited number of photons becomes particularly critical when low-intensity sources are used. Synchrotrons are excellent sources of X-rays with high brightness and the ability to select a specific monochromatic energy, but are not usually conveniently available for tomographic work. Radioactive sources of gamma rays present handling difficulties and have low intensities as well. X-ray tubes are a convenient source for tomography, with adjustable voltage and a variety of target materials that emit different X-ray spectra. Such a source is not monochromatic, which would cause significant beam hardening effects for many specimens, as discussed above.

Absorption filters can be used to select just a single band of energies from a polychromatic source. For each view angle, two projection images are collected using filters whose absorption edge energies are different. The ratio of the two images yields the attenuation information for the elements whose absorption edges lie

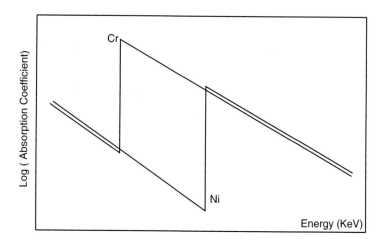

Figure 41. Diagram of the use of balanced absorption edge filters to isolate a single energy band. The plots show the absorption coefficient as a function of energy for two different filters containing the elements chromium and nickel. Elements in the sample with absorption edges between these two energies, such as manganese, iron, and cobalt, will be imaged in the ratio of the two intensities.

between the two filter energies, as indicated in **Figure 41**. A series of such image pairs can provide separate information on the spatial distribution of many elements. **Figure 42** shows an example in which the use of filters has selected two of the three metal inserts in the sample. The use of the filters reduces the already low intensity from the X-ray tube, and the use of the ratio of the two images presents a further limitation on the statistical quality of the projections. It is therefore important to use a small number of views to obtain the best possible projection images. In this example, twelve projections with full 3D rotation of axes were obtained. **Figure 43** shows the artefacts present in the reconstruction when the same number of views is obtained with single axis rotation.

The electron microscope produces images in which contrast is due to attenuation, and a series of views at different angles can be reconstructed to show three-dimensional structure. The use of an arbitrary series of angles is quite difficult to do for materials specimens because of diffraction of the electrons from planes of atoms in the crystal structure. This source of contrast is not easily modeled by the usual attenuation calculation since one voxel may have

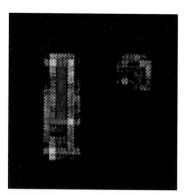
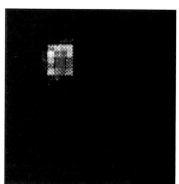

Figure 42. Reconstruction of the same three planes as shown in Figure 40, but using images obtained as a difference between two projections through different filters (Cr and Fe metal foils), which form a bandpass filter to select a narrow band of X-ray energies. Note that one of the inserts (Cr) is missing but the Mn and Fe inserts are visible. Reconstructed using 12 cone-beam projections with rotations in 3D.

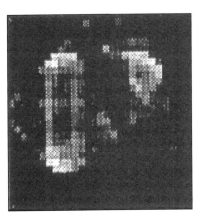

Figure 43. Reconstruction of the same plane as shown in Figure 42, reconstructed in the same way using two filters, but using 12 radial projections (rotating the sample about one axis only). Note the artefacts between and within the inserts.

quite different values in different directions. However, for non-crystalline materials such as biological specimens, the reconstruction is straightforward (Engel & Massalski, 1984; Hegerl, 1989).

Even more efficient than collecting a series of different views using multiple orientations of a single specimen is using images of many different but identical specimens that happen to have different orientations, as mentioned above. **Figure 44** shows an example. The two-dimensional image is an electron micrograph of a single virus particle. The specimen is an adenovirus that causes respiratory ailments.

The low dose of electrons required to prevent damage to the specimen makes the image very noisy. However, in a typical specimen there are many such particles, each in a different, essentially random orientation. Collecting the various images, indexing the orientation of each image by referring to the location of the triangular facets on the virus surface, and performing a reconstruction produces a 3D reconstruction of the particle in which each voxel value is the electron density. Modeling the surface of the outer protein coat of the virus produces the surface-rendered image shown in **Figure 45** (Stewart & Burnett, 1991).

At a very different scale, tomography has also been performed on the earth itself using seismography. Seismic waves are created by earthquakes or large explosions such as nuclear weapons

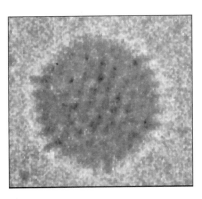

Figure 44. Transmission electron microscope image of single adenovirus particle.

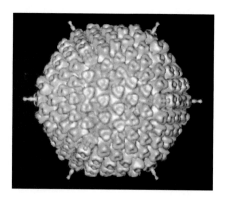

Figure 45. Reconstruction of the adenovirus particle from many transmission images.

tests. Such large-magnitude events generate two types of waves that propagate through the earth to receivers (seismographs) at many different locations. P-waves (pressure waves) are compressional pulses which can penetrate through every part of the earth's interior, while S-waves (shear waves) are transverse deformations that cannot propagate through the liquid core. In fact, the presence of a liquid core was deduced in 1906 by the British seismologist R. D. Oldham by the shadow cast by the core in seismic S-wave patterns.

The paths of seismic waves are not straight (**Figure 46**), but bend because of the variations in temperature, pressure and composition within the earth which affect the speed of transmission just as the index of refraction of glass affects light and causes it to bend in a lens system. Also similar to the behavior of light, the seismic waves may reflect at interfaces where the speed of propagation varies abruptly. This happens at the core-mantle boundary and the surface of the inner core. The propagation velocities of the P- and S-waves are different, and respond differently to composition.

Collecting many seismograms from different events creates a set of ray paths that do not uniformly cover the earth, but rather depend on the chance (and nonuniform) distribution of earthquakes and the distribution of seismographs. Nevertheless, analysis of the travel times of waves that have taken different paths through the earth permits forming a tomographic reconstruction.

Figure 46. Diagram of paths taken by pressure and shear waves from earthquakes, which reveal information about the density along the paths through the core and mantle, and the location of discontinuities.

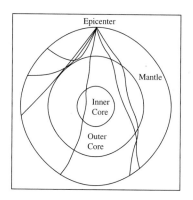

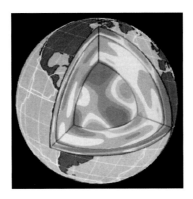

Figure 47. *Computed tomogram of the mantle, showing rock densities (light shades are hot, light rocks that are rising, and conversely).*

The density of the material (shown by shading in **Figure 47**) indicates the temperature and the direction of motion (cool, dense material is sinking through the mantle toward the core, while hot, light material is rising). Convection in the mantle is the driving force behind volcanism and continental drift.

Also of great utility are waves that have reflected (one or more times) from the various surfaces. For instance, the difference in travel times of S-waves that arrive directly vs. those which have reflected from the core-mantle boundary permit mapping the elevation of that boundary with a resolution better than 1 kilometer, and reveal that the boundary is not a smooth spherical surface. Since the relatively viscous mantle is floating on a low viscosity liquid core, and it is the relatively fast motion of the latter that produces the earth's magnetic field, the study of this interface is important in understanding the earth's dynamics.

Global tomographic reconstruction is generally insensitive to the small details of structure such as faults, but another current program to perform high resolution tomography under the state of California (where there are many faults of more than casual interest to the surface-dwelling humans) employs an array of high sensitivity seismographs, and uses the very frequent minor earthquakes there to map out the faults through the reflections that they produce.

High-resolution tomography

Medical tomography has a typical resolution of about 1 mm, which is adequate for its purpose, and radiologists generally feel comfortable with a series of planar section images. But there is considerable interest in applying true three-dimensional tomographic imaging to study the microstructure of various materials including metals, ceramics, composites and polymers, as well as larger industrial components. Some of the structural features cannot be determined from conventional two-dimensional microscopy of cross section surfaces. This includes determining the number of particles of arbitrary or variable shape in a volume, and the topology of networks or pore structures, which control the permeability of materials to fluids.

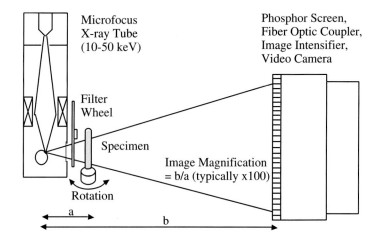

Figure 48. *Diagram of a cone-beam imaging system. The projection image magnification is the ratio of b:a. The attainable resolution is limited by the spot size of the X-ray source.*

Microfocus X-ray Tube (10-50 keV)

Phosphor Screen, Fiber Optic Coupler, Image Intensifier, Video Camera

Filter Wheel

Specimen

Image Magnification = b/a (typically x100)

Rotation

a

b

This information can only be determined by having the full three-dimensional data set, with adequate resolution, and ideally with cubic voxels. Resolution of the order of 1 μm has been demonstrated using a synchrotron as a very bright point source of X rays. Resolution of about 10 μm is possible using more readily available sources such as microfocus X-ray tubes. Filtering such sources to produce element-specific imaging is also possible, as illustrated above.

Cone-beam geometry is well suited to this type of microstructural imaging, since it provides magnification of the structure (Johnson et al., 1986; Russ, 1988; Kinney et al., 1989, 1990; Deckman, 1989). **Figure 48** shows this schematically. The magnification is strictly geometric, since X-rays are not refracted by lenses, but can amount to as much as 100:1. The projected images can be collected using conventional video technology, after conversion to visible light by a phosphor or channel plate and suitable intensification. Since the intensity of conventional small-spot X-ray sources is very low, the use of high-brightness sources such as are available at a synchrotron is particularly desirable for high-resolution imaging. So is image averaging, which may be done by using the same cooled CCD cameras used for astronomical imaging.

As will be discussed in Chapter 10, three-dimensional imaging requires many voxels, and the reconstruction process is very computer intensive. The time required to perform the reconstruction is, however, still shorter than that required to collect the various projection images. These images are generally photon-limited, with considerable noise affecting the reconstruction as indicated above. In order to collect reasonable-quality projections from a finite intensity source, the number of view angles is limited. The views should be ideally arranged to cover the polar angles optimally in three-dimensional space. This arrangement of course places demands on the quality of the mechanism used to perform the rotations and tilts, because the center of rotation must be constant and located within a few micrometers to preserve the image quality as discussed above.

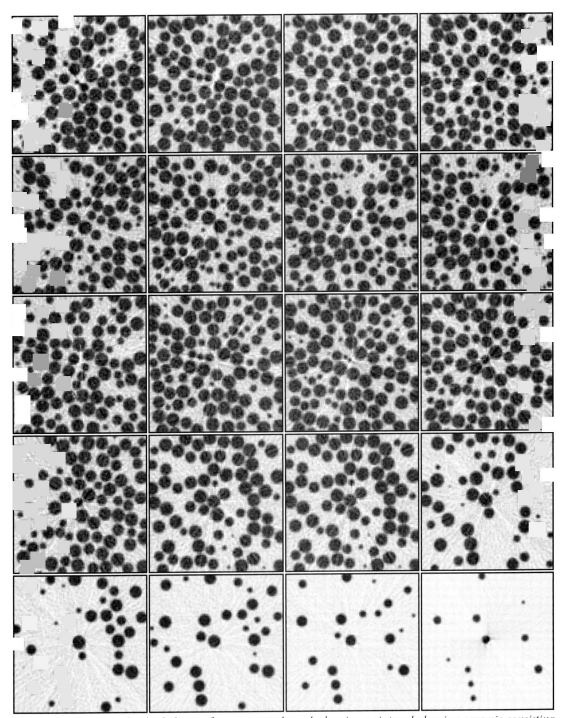

Figure 49. *Twenty individual planes of reconstructed voxels showing a sintered alumina ceramic consisting of 100-μm-diameter spheres.*

The presentation of three-dimensional information requires extensive use of computer graphics methods as will be shown in Chapter 10. **Figure 49** shows a simple series of planes of voxels from a 3D tomographic reconstruction of a porous alumina ceramic.

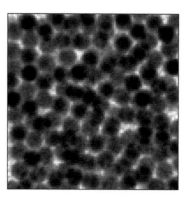

Figure 50. *A single two-dimensional projection set through the structure shown in Figure 49.*

The individual particles are approximately 100 μm diameter spheres that fill about 60% of the volume of the sample. The voxels are 10 μm cubes. **Figure 50** shows one of the projection sets through this specimen, a two-dimensional image in which the spherical particles overlap along the lines of sight and are partially transparent. A three-dimensional presentation of the data is shown in **Figure 51**.

Figure 51. *Three-dimensional presentation of the data from Figure 49.*

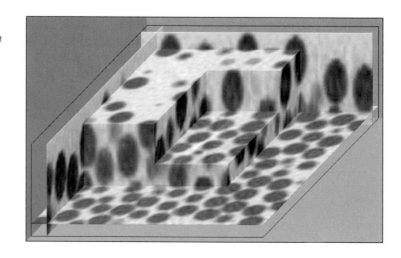

10

3D Image Visualization

Sources of 3D data

True three-dimensional imaging is becoming more accessible with the continued development of instrumentation. Just as the pixel is the unit of brightness measurement for a two-dimensional image, the voxel (volume element, the three-dimensional analog of the pixel or picture element) is the unit for three-dimensional imaging. And just as processing and analysis is much simpler if the pixels are square, so the use of cubic voxels is preferred for three dimensions, although it is not as often achieved.

There are several basic approaches to volume imaging. In Chapter 9, 3D imaging by tomographic reconstruction was described. This is perhaps the premier method for measuring the density and even in some cases the elemental composition of solid specimens. It can produce a set of cubic voxels. This is not the only or even the most common way that tomography is presently used. Most medical and industrial applications produce one or a series of two-dimensional section planes, which are spaced farther apart than the pixel resolution within the plane (Baba et al., 1984, 1988; Briarty & Jenkins, 1984; Johnson & Capowski, 1985; Kriete, 1992).

Tomography can be performed using a variety of different signals, including seismic waves, ultrasound, magnetic resonance, conventional X-rays, gamma rays, neutron beams, and electron microscopy, as well as other even less familiar methods. The resolution may vary from kilometers (seismic tomography), to centimeters (most conventional medical scans), millimeters (typical industrial applications), micrometers (current experimental work with synchrotron sources), and even nanometers (electron microscope reconstructions of viruses and atomic lattices). The same basic presentation tools are available regardless of the imaging modality or the dimensional scale.

The most important variable in tomographic imaging, as for all of the other 3D methods discussed here, is whether the data set is planes of pixels, or true voxels. As discussed in Chapter 9, it is possible to set up an array of cubic voxels, collect projection data from a series of views in three dimensions, and solve (either algebraically or by backprojection) for the density of each voxel. However, the most common way to perform tomography is to define one plane at a time as an array of square pixels, collect a series of views in two dimensions, solve for the densities in that plane, and then proceed to the next plane. When used in this way, tomography shares many similarities (and problems) with other essentially two-dimensional imaging methods that we will collectively define as serial imaging or serial section techniques.

A radiologist viewing an array of such images is expected to combine them in the mind to "see" the three-dimensional structures present. (This process is aided enormously by the fact that the radiologist already knows what the structure is, and is generally looking for things that differ from the familiar.) Only a few current-generation systems use the techniques discussed in this chapter to present three-dimensional views directly. In industrial tomography, the greater diversity of structure (and correspondingly lesser ability to predict what is expected), and the greater amount of time available for study and interpretation, has encouraged the use of computer graphics. But such displays are still the exception rather than the rule, and an array of two-dimensional planar images is more commonly used for volume imaging. This chapter concentrates on methods that use a series of two-dimensional images.

These images are obtained by dissecting the sample into a series of planar sections, which are then piled up as a stack of voxels. Sometimes the sectioning is physical. Blocks of embedded biological materials, textiles, and even some metals, can be sliced with a microtome, and each slice imaged (just as individual slices are normally viewed). Collecting and aligning the images produces a three-dimensional data set in which the voxels are typically very elongated in the "z" direction because the slices are much thicker than the lateral resolution.

At the other extreme, the secondary ion mass spectrometer uses an incident ion beam to remove one layer of atoms at a time from the sample surface. These pass through a mass spectrometer to select atoms from a single element, which is then imaged on a fluorescent screen. Collecting a series of images from many elements can produce a complete three-dimensional map of the sample. One difference from the imaging of slices is that there is no alignment problem, because the sample block is held in place as the surface layers are removed. On the other hand, the erosion rate through different structures can vary so that the surface does not remain planar, and this roughening is very difficult to account for. Also, the voxel height can be very small (essentially atomic dimensions) while the lateral dimension is many times larger.

Serial sections

Most physical sectioning approaches are similar to one or the other of these examples. They are known collectively as serial section methods. The name serial section comes from the use of light microscopy imaging of biological tissue, in which blocks of tissue embedded in resin are cut using a microtome into a series of individual slices. Collecting these slices (or at least some of them) for viewing in the microscope enables researchers to assemble a set of photographs which can then be used to reconstruct the 3D structure.

This technique illustrates most of the problems that may be encountered with any 3D imaging method based on a series of individual slices. First, the individual images must be aligned. The microtomed slices are collected on slides and viewed in arbitrary orientations. So, even if the same structures can be located in the different sections (not always an easy task, given that some variation in structure with depth must be present or there would be no incentive to do this kind of work), the pictures do not line up.

Using the details of structure visible in each section provides only a coarse guide to alignment. As shown in **Figures 1**, **2** and **3**, shifting or rotating each image to visually align the structures in one section with the next can completely alter the reconstructed 3D structure. It is generally assumed that given enough detail present in the images, some kind of average alignment will avoid these major errors. However, it is far from certain that a best visual alignment is the correct one, nor that automated methods that overlap sequential images produce the proper alignment.

The automatic methods generally seek to minimize the mismatch between sections either by aligning the centroids of features in

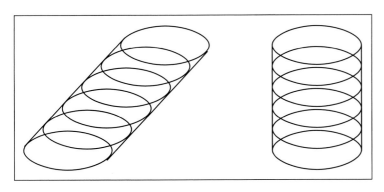

Figure 1. Alignment of serial sections with translation: sections through an inclined circular cylinder may be misconstrued as a vertical elliptical cylinder.

Figure 2. Alignment of serial sections with rotation:
a) *actual outlines in 3D serial section stack;*
b) *surface modeling applied to outlines, showing twisted structure;*
c) *erroneous result without twist when outlines are aligned to each other.*

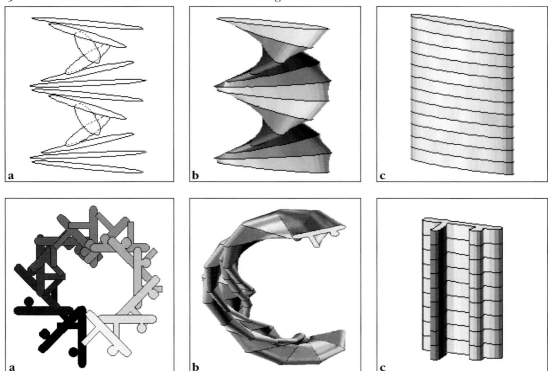

Figure 3. Loss of combined rotation and translation by aligning serial sections:
a) *example data viewed normally, using shading to mark slices at different depths;*
b) *surface modeling of data from image **a**;*
c) *incorrect result if sequential slices are aligned for best match with each other.*

the planes so that the sum of squares of distances is minimized, or by overlaying binary images from the two sections and shifting or rotating to minimize the area resulting from combining them with an Ex-OR (exclusive OR) operation, discussed in Chapter 7. This procedure is illustrated in **Figure 4**. There are two problems with this approach: solving for the minimum in either quantity as a function of three variables (x and y shift and angular orientation) is difficult and must usually proceed iteratively and slowly; plus there is no reason to expect the minimum point to really represent the true alignment, as discussed above.

One approach that improves on the use of internal image detail for alignment is to incorporate fiducial marks in the block before sectioning. These could take the form of holes drilled by a laser, threads or fibers placed in the resin before it hardens, or grooves machined down the edges of the block, for example. With several such marks that can reasonably be expected to maintain their shape from section to section and continue in some known direction through the stack of images, much better alignment is

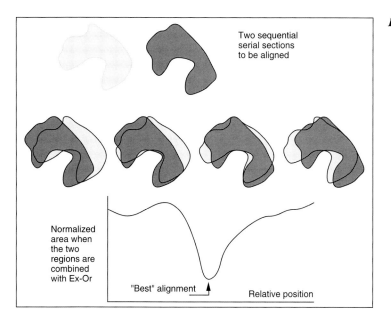

Figure 4. *Alignment of serial sections by "best fit" of features seeks to minimize mismatched area, measured by Ex-OR function, as a function of translation and rotation.*

Within the figure:

Two sequential serial sections to be aligned

Normalized area when the two regions are combined with Ex-Or

"Best" alignment

Relative position

possible. Placing and finding fiducial marks in the close vicinity of the structures of interest is often difficult. In practice, if the sections are not contiguous there may still be difficulties, and alignment errors may propagate through the stack of images.

Most fiducial marks are large enough to cover several pixels in each image. As discussed in Chapter 8, this size allows locating the centroid to a fraction of one pixel accuracy, although not all systems take advantage of this capability. Once the alignment points are identified (either from fiducial marks or internal image detail), the rotation and translation of one image to line up with the next is performed as discussed in Chapter 2. Resampling of the pixel array and interpolation to prevent aliasing produces a new image. This process takes some computational time, but this is a minor problem in comparison to the difficulty of obtaining the images in the first place.

Unfortunately, for classic serial sectioning the result of this rotation and translation is not a true representation of the original 3D structure. The act of sectioning using a microtome generally produces some distortion in the block. This 5–20% compression in one direction is the same for all sections (since they are cut in the same direction). If the fiducial marks have known absolute coordinates, then stretching of the images to correct for the distortion is possible. It is usually assumed that the entire section is compressed uniformly, although for some samples this may not be true.

Otherwise, it may be possible to use internal information to estimate the distortion. For example, if there is no reason to expect cell nuclei to be elongated in any preferred direction in the tissue, then measurement of the dimensions of many nuclei may be used to determine an average amount of compression. Obviously, this approach includes some assumptions and can only be used in particular circumstances.

Another difficulty with serial sections is calibration of dimension in the depth direction. The thickness of the individual sections is only known approximately (for example, by judging the color of the light produced by interference from the top and bottom surfaces). It may vary from section to section, and even from place to place within the section, depending on the local hardness of the material being cut. Constructing an accurate depth scale is quite difficult, and dimensions in the depth direction will be much less accurate than those measured within one section plane.

If only some sections are used, such as every second or fifth, then this error becomes much worse. It also becomes difficult to follow structures from one image to the next with confidence. However, before computer reconstruction methods became common, this kind of skipping was often necessary simply to reduce the amount of data that the human observer had to juggle and interpret.

Using only a fraction of the sections is particularly common when ultra-thin sections are cut for viewing in an electron microscope instead of the light microscope. As the sections become thinner, they increase in number, and are more prone to distortion. Some may be lost (for instance due to folding) or intentionally skipped. Portions of each section are obscured by the

Figure 5. *Four serial section images from a stack (Courtesy Dr. C. D. Bucana, Univ. of Texas M. D. Anderson Cancer Center, Houston, TX), which have already been rotated for alignment. The membranes at the upper left corner of the images are thresholded and displayed for the entire stack of images in Figure 6.*

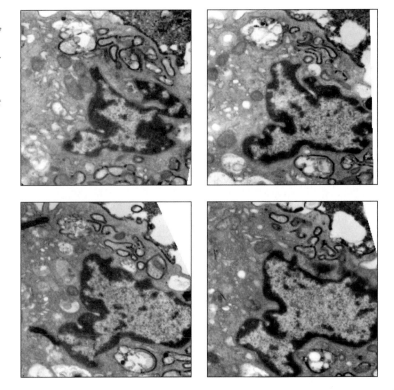

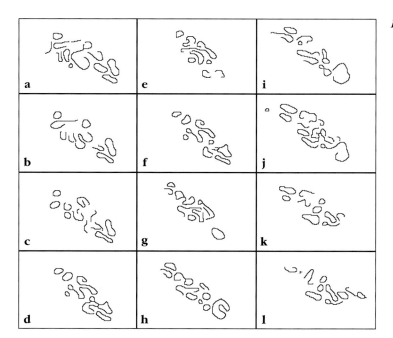

Figure 6. *Membranes from the sequential images illustrated in Figure 5, showing the changes from section to section. Because of the separation distance between the planes, these variations are too great to interpolate a model of the shape of the surfaces in 3D.*

support grid, which also prevents some from being used. At higher magnification, the fiducial marks become larger, less precisely defined, and above all more widely spaced so that they may not be in close proximity to the structure of interest.

Figure 5 shows a portion of a series of TEM images of tissue in which the 3D configuration of the membranes (dark stained lines) is of interest. The details of the edges of cells and organelles have been used to approximately align pairs of sections through the stack, but different details must be used for different pairs as there is no continuity of detail through the entire stack. The membranes can be isolated in these images by thresholding (**Figure 6**), but the sections are too far apart to link the lines together to reconstruct the 3D shape of the surface. This problem is common with conventional serial section images.

Metallographic imaging typically uses reflected rather than transmitted light. As discussed below, serial sectioning in this context is accomplished by removing layers of materials sequentially by physical polishing. The need to locate the same sample position after polishing, and to monitor the depth of polishing, can be met by placing hardness indentations on the sample, or by laser ablation of pits. These serve as fiduciary marks for alignment, and the change in size of the mark reveals the depth. In archaeological excavation the fiduciary marks may be a network of strings and a transit, and the removal tool may be a shovel. In some mining and quarrying examples it may be a bulldozer.

In most of these methods, the sequential 2D images represent the sample along planes that are separated in the z direction. The intervening material that has been removed must be inferred or interpolated from the planes. In these cases, the voxel value is not really an average over its extent, as most pixel values are. Nor is the voxel truly a discrete point value in space, since it does represent an average in the section plane. Interpolation between sections that are too far apart (in terms of the scale of the structure) can lead to some serious errors and misinterpretation. For the serial sectioning method in which slices are viewed in transmission the voxel value is a volume average, which is easier to interpret. In most cases, the voxel value is a measure of density of the material. Depending on what the radiation is (visible light, X-rays, electrons, neutrons, sound, and so forth), the value may represent the local concentration of some element or compound. In some cases, emitted radiation from voxels also gives concentration information (examples include fluorescence light microscopy and positron-emission tomography).

Optical sectioning

Physical sectioning on any scale is a difficult technique that destroys the sample. Controlling and measuring the section thickness and aligning the sections or at least locating the same position on the sample can become a major source of error. In some cases, it is possible to image sections through a sample without performing physical sectioning. The confocal scanning light microscope (CSLM) offers one way to accomplish this.

The normal operation of the transmission light microscope does not lend itself to optical sectioning. The depth of field of high numerical aperture optics is small (just a few times the lateral resolution), so that only a small "slice" of the image will be sharply focused. However, light from locations above and below the plane of focus is also transmitted to the image, out of focus, and this both blurs the image and includes information from an extended distance in the z direction. An example shown below under stereo imaging shows that it is possible to process the images to remove some of the artefacts that result from the passage of light through the sample above and below the plane of focus. The confocal microscope eliminates this extraneous light, and so produces useful optical section images without the need for processing.

This is possible because the sample is imaged one point at a time (hence the presence of "scanning" in the name). The principle was introduced in Chapter 4 (Image Enhancement), in conjunction with some of the ways that images of light reflected from surfaces can be processed. **Figure 82** in Chapter 4 showed the principle of the confocal microscope. Light from a point source (often a laser) is focused on a single point in the specimen and collected by an identical set of optics, reaching a pinhole detector.

Any portion of the specimen away from the focal point, and particularly out of the focal plane, cannot scatter light to interfere with the formation of the image. Scanning the beam with respect to the specimen (by moving the light source, the specimen, or using scanning elements in the optical path) builds up a complete image of the focal plane. If the numerical aperture of the lenses is high, the depth of field of this microscope is very small, although still several times the lateral resolution within individual image planes. Even more important, the portion of the specimen that is away from the focal plane contributes very little to the image. This makes it possible to image a plane within a bulk specimen, even one that would ordinarily be considered translucent because of light scattering.

This method of isolating a single plane within a bulk sample, called optical sectioning, works because the confocal light microscope has a very shallow depth of field. Translating the specimen in the z direction and collecting a series of images makes it possible to build up a three-dimensional data set for viewing, using the methods shown further on in this chapter.

Several imaging modalities are possible with the confocal light microscope. The most common is reflected light, in which the light reflected from the sample returns through the same objective lens as used to focus the incident light, and is then diverted by a mirror to a detector. This geometry is shown in **Figure 7**. It permits acquiring transmitted light images for focal plane sectioning of bulk translucent or transparent materials. **Figure 8** shows an example of a transmitted light focal plane section.

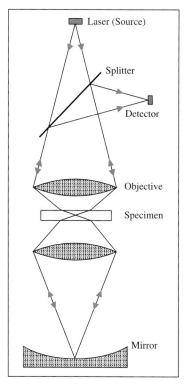

Figure 7. *Transmission confocal scanning light microscopy can be performed by passing the light through the specimen twice. Light is not imaged from points away from the in-focus point, which gives good lateral and excellent depth resolution compared to a conventional light microscope. (Figure 72, Chapter 4 shows the more common reflected light confocal microscope.)*

Figure 8. *CSLM image showing a 1/30-second image of a paramecium swimming in a droplet of water, as it passed through the focal plane of the microscope.*

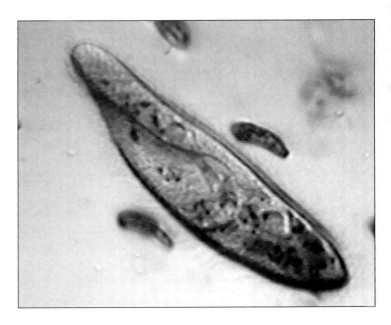

Both transmitted and reflected-light images of focal plane sections can be used in 3D imaging for different types of specimens. The characteristic of reflected-light confocal images is that the intensity of light reflected to the detector drops off very rapidly as points are shifted above or below the focal plane. Therefore for structures in a transparent medium, only the surfaces will reflect light. For any single image plane, only the portion of the field of view where some structure passes through the plane will appear bright, and the rest of the image will be dark. This characteristic permits some rather straightforward reconstruction algorithms, as will be shown.

Another widely used imaging method for the confocal microscope is emission or fluorescence, in which the wavelength of the incident light is able to cause excitation of a dye or other fluorescing probe introduced to the specimen. The lower-energy (longer wavelength) light emitted by this probe is separated from the incident light, for instance by a dichroic mirror, and used to form an image in which the location of the probe or dye appears bright. Building up a series of images in depth allows the structure labeled by the probe to be reconstructed.

The transmitted-light mode, while it is the most straightforward in terms of optical sectioning, is actually little used as yet. This situation is partly due to the difficulties in constructing the microscope with matched optics above and below the specimen, as compared to the reflection and emission modes in which the optics are only above it. However, the use of a lens and mirror beneath the specimen (shown in **Figure 7**) to return the light to the same detector as present in the more standard microscope design can produce most of the same imaging advantages (the only loss is that in passing through the specimen twice, some intensity is lost).

The principal advantages of optical sectioning are avoiding physical distortion of the specimen due to cutting, and having alignment of images from the various imaging planes. The depth resolution, while inferior to the lateral resolution in each plane by about a factor of two to three times, is still useful for many applications. However, this difference in resolution does raise some difficulties for 3D image processing, even if the distance between planes is made smaller than the resolution so that the stored voxels are cubic (which is by no means common).

Sequential removal

Many materials are opaque and therefore cannot be imaged by any transmission method, preventing any type of optical sectioning. Indeed, metals, composites, and ceramics are usually examined in the reflected light microscope. However, it is still possible to collect a series of depth images for 3D reconstruction by sequential polishing of such materials, as mentioned above.

The means of removal of material from the surface depends strongly on the hardness of the material. For some soft metals, polymers and textiles, the microtome can be used just as it was for the block of biological material, except that instead of examining the slice of material removed, the surface left behind is imaged. This approach avoids most problems of alignment and distortion, especially if the cutting can be done *in situ* without removing the specimen from the viewing position in the microscope. It is still difficult to determine precisely the thickness of material removed in each cut and to assure its uniformity.

For harder materials, the grinding or polishing operations used to produce conventional sections for 2D images can be used. Such operations generally require removing and replacing the specimen, so again fiducial marks are needed to locate the same region. Probably the most common approach to this marking is the use of hardness indentations. Several pyramid-shaped impressions are made in the surface of the specimen so that after additional abrasion or polishing, the deepest parts of the indentations are still visible. These can be accurately aligned with the marks in the original image. In addition, the reduction in size of the impression, whose shape is known, gives a measure of the depth of polish and hence of the spacing between the two images. With several such indentations, the overall uniformity of polish can also be judged, although local variations due to the hardness of particular phases may be present.

For still harder materials or ones in which conventional polishing might cause surface damage, other methods may be used. Electrolytic or chemical etching is generally difficult to control and little used. Ion beam erosion is slow, but is already in use in many laboratories for the thinning of transmission electron microscope specimens, and may be utilized for this purpose. Controlling the erosion to obtain uniformity and avoid surface roughening presents challenges for many specimens.

In situ ion beam erosion is used in the scanning electron microscope and scanning Auger microscope, for instance to allow the removal of surface contamination. This capability can be used to produce a series of images in depth in these microscopes, which generally have resolution far better than the light microscope. However, the time involved in performing the erosion may be quite long (and hence costly), and the uniformity of eroding through complex structures (the most interesting kind for imaging) may be poor.

One kind of microscope performs this type of erosion automatically as part of its imaging process. The ion microscope or secondary ion mass spectrometer (SIMS) uses a beam of heavy ions to erode a layer of atoms from the specimen surface. The secondary ions are then separated according to element in a mass spectrometer and recorded, for example using a channel plate multiplier and more-or-less conventional video camera, to form an image of one plane in the specimen for one element at a time. The depth of erosion is usually calibrated for these instruments by measuring the signal profile of a known standard, such as may be produced by the same methods used to produce modern microelectronics.

The rate of surface removal is highly controllable (if somewhat slow) and capable of essentially atomic resolution in depth. The lateral resolution, by contrast, is of about the same level as in the conventional light microscope, so in this case instead of having voxels which are high in resolution in the plane but poorer in the depth direction, the situation is reversed. The noncubic voxels create problems for processing and measurement.

Furthermore, the erosion rate for ion beam bombardment in the ion microscope or SIMS may vary from place to place in the specimen as a function of composition, structure, or even crystallographic orientation. This variation does not necessarily show up in the reconstruction, since each set of data is assumed to represent a plane, but can cause significant distortion in the final interpretation. In principle, stretching of the data in 3D can be performed just as images can be corrected for deformation in 2D. However, without fiducial marks or accurate quantitative data on local erosion rates, it is hard to accomplish this with real data.

The ability to image many different elements with the SIMS creates a rich data set for 3D display. A true-color 2D image has three bands (whether it is saved as RGB or HSI, as discussed in Chapter 1), and satellite 2D images may have as many as seven bands including infrared. The SIMS may have practically any number, with four or more being quite common. The ability of the instrument to detect trace levels (typically ppm or better) of every element in the periodic table means that even for relatively simple specimens the multiband data will present a challenge to store, display and interpret.

Another type of microscope that removes layers of atoms as it images them is the atom probe ion microscope. In this instrument, a strong electrical field between a sharply curved sample tip and a display screen causes atoms to be desorbed from the surface and accelerated toward the screen where they are imaged. The screen may include an electron channel plate to amplify the signal so that individual atoms can be seen, or may be used as a time-of-flight mass spectrometer with pulsed application of the high voltage so that the different atom species can be distinguished. With any of the instrument variations, the result is a highly magnified image of atoms from the sample, showing atom arrangements in 3D as layer after layer is removed.

Stereo

There remains another way to see three-dimensional structures. It is the same way that humans see depth in some real-world situations. Having two eyes which face forward so that their fields of view overlap permits us to use stereoscopic vision to judge the relative distance to objects. In humans, this is done point-by-point, by moving our eyes in their sockets to bring each subject to the fovea, the portion of the retina with the densest packing of cones. The muscles in turn tell the brain what motion was needed to achieve convergence, and so we know whether one object is closer or farther than another.

Further in this section, we will see stereo vision used as a means to transmit 3D data to the human viewer. It would be wrong to think that all human depth perception relies on stereoscopy. In fact, much of our judgment about the 3D world around us comes from other cues such as shading, relative size, precedence, and so on that work just fine with one eye and are used in some computer-based measurement methods (Roberts, 1965; Horn, 1970; Carlsen, 1985; Pentland, 1986). But for the moment, let us see how stereoscopy can be used to determine depth information to put information into a 3D computer data base.

The light microscope has a rather shallow depth of field, which is made even less in the confocal scanning light microscope discussed above. Consequently, looking at a specimen with deep relief is not very satisfactory. However, the electron microscope has lenses with very small aperture angles, and hence has very great depth of field. Stereoscopy is most commonly used with the scanning electron microscope (SEM) to produce in-focus images of rough surfaces. Tilting the specimen, or electromagnetically deflecting the scanning beam, can produce a pair of images from different points of view that form a stereo pair. Looking at one picture with each eye fools the brain into seeing the original rough surface.

Measuring the relief of surfaces from such images is the same in principle and in practice as using stereo pair images taken from aircraft or satellites to measure the elevation of topographic features on the earth or another planet. The richer detail in the satellite photos makes it easier to find matching points practically anywhere in the images, but by the same token requires more matching points to define the surface than the simpler geometry of typical specimens observed in the SEM. The mathematical relationship between the measured parallax (the apparent displacement of points in the left and right eye image) and the relative elevation of the two points on the surface was presented in Chapter 1.

Automatic matching of points from stereo pairs is a difficult task for computer-based image analysis (Marr & Poggio, 1976; Medioni & Nevatia, 1985; Kayaalp & Jain, 1987). It is usually performed by using the pattern of brightness values in one image, for instance the left one, as a template to search for the most nearly identical pattern in the right image. The area of search is restricted by the possible displacement, which depends on the angle between the two views and the maximum roughness of the surface. Some points will not be matched by this process because they may not be visible in both images. Other points will match poorly because the local pattern of brightness values in the pixels includes some noise, and several parts of the image may have similar noise levels.

Matching many points produces a new image in which each pixel can be given a value based on the parallax or elevation of the surface. This range image will contain many false matches, but operations such as a median filter usually do a good job of removing the outlier points to produce an overall range image of the surface. We will see later on in this chapter how range images can be displayed.

A second approach to matching stereo pairs is based on the realization that many of the points in each image will not match well because they are just part of the overall surface or structure and not the "interesting" points where surfaces meet or other discontinuities are present. This approach is presumably related to human vision, which usually spends most of its time on only the few points in each scene where discontinuities are found. Locating these interesting points based on some local property such as the variance produces a comparatively short list of points to be matched between the two images (Moravec, 1977; Quam & Hannah, 1974). A typical case may have only thousands of points, instead of the million or so pixels in the original images.

These points are then matched in the same way as above, by correlation of their neighborhood brightness patterns. Additionally, for most surfaces the order of points is preserved. This, and the limits on possible parallax for a given pair of images, reduces the typical candidate list for matching to ten or less, and produces a

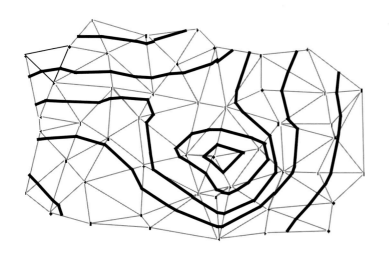

Figure 9. Drawing contour lines (isoelevation lines) on the triangular facets joining an arbitrary arrangement of points whose elevations have been determined by stereoscopy.

list of surface points and their elevations. It is then assumed that the surface between these points is well behaved and can be treated as consisting of planar facets. If the facets are small enough, it is still possible to generate a contour map of the surface as shown in **Figure 9**. A complete display of elevation, called a range image, can be produced by interpolation as shown in **Figure 10**. Other displays of these surfaces are shown below.

The transmission electron microscope (TEM) also has a very large depth of field. In most cases, the specimens observed in the TEM are very thin (in order to permit electron penetration), and the

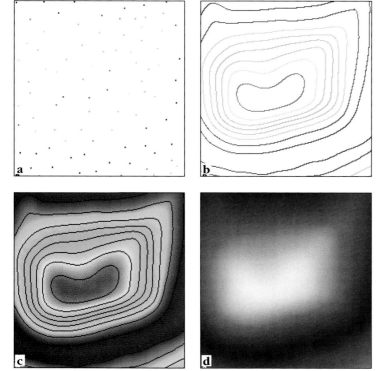

Figure 10. Interpolation of a range image:
a) isolated, randomly arranged points with measured elevation (color coded);
b) contour lines drawn through the tesselation;
c) smooth interpolation between contour lines;
d) the constructed range image (grey scale).

optical depth of field is unimportant. However, with the newest generation of high voltage microscopes, comparatively thick samples (of the order of one micrometer) may be imaged. This thickness is enough to contain a considerable amount of three-dimensional structure at the resolution of the TEM (of the order of a few nanometers). Hence, using the same approach of tilting the specimen to acquire stereo pair images, it is possible to obtain information about the depth of points and the 3D structure.

Presenting the images to a human viewer's eyes so that two pictures acquired at different times can be fused in the mind and examined in depth is not difficult. It has been accomplished for years photographically, and is now often done with modest tradeoff in lateral resolution using a computer to record and display the images. The methods discussed below for using stereo pair displays to communicate 3D information from generated images are equally applicable here.

However, it is far more difficult to have the computer determine the depth of features in the structure and construct a 3D database of points and their relationship to each other. Part of the problem is that there is so much background detail from the (mostly) transparent medium surrounding the features of interest that it may dominate the local pixel brightnesses and make matching impossible. Another part of the problem is that it is no longer possible to assume that points maintain their order from left to right. In a three-dimensional structure, points may change their order as they pass in front or in back of each other.

The consequence of these limitations has been that only in a very few, highly idealized cases has automatic fusion of stereo pair images from the TEM been attempted. Simplification of the problem using very high contrast markers, such as small gold particles bound to selected surfaces using antibodies, or some other highly selective stain, helps. In this case only the markers are considered. There are only a few dozen of these, and like the interesting points mentioned above for mapping surfaces, they are easily detected (being usually far darker than anything else in the image) and only a few could possibly match.

Even with these markers, a human may still be needed to identify the matches. Given the matching points in the two images, the computer can construct a series of lines that describe the surface which the markers define, but this surface may be only a small part of the total structure. **Figure 11** shows an example of this method in which human matching was performed. Similar methods can be applied to stained networks (Huang et al., 1994), or the distribution of precipitate particles in materials, for example.

In most matching procedures, the points in left and right images are defined in terms of pixel addresses. The error in the vertical dimension determined by stereoscopy is typically an order of magnitude greater than the precision of measurement of the

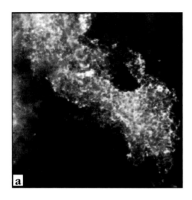

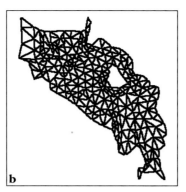

Figure 11. Example of decorating a surface with metal particles (Golgi stain) shown in this transmission electron micrograph *(a)* whose elevations are measured stereoscopically to form a network describing the surface *(b)*. (L.D. Peachey & J.P. Heath, 1989. "Reconstruction from stereo and multiple electron microscope images of thick sections of embedded biological specimens using computer graphics methods." J. Microscopy, *153: 193-204)*

parallax. Improving the measurement of parallax between features to subpixel accuracy is therefore of considerable interest. Such improvement is possible in some cases, particularly when information from many pixels can be combined. As described in Chapter 8, the centroids of features or the location of lines can be specified to accuracy of 1/10th pixel or better.

3D data sets

In the case of matching of points between two stereo pair images, the database is a list of a few dozens or perhaps hundreds of coordinates that usually define either a surface or perhaps nodes in a network structure. If these points are to be used for measurement, the coordinates and perhaps some information on which are connected to which are all that is required. If image reconstruction is intended, it will be necessary to interpolate additional points between them to complete a display. This is somewhat parallel to the use of boundary representation in two dimensions. It may offer a very compact record of the essential (or at least of the the selected) information in the image. But it requires expansion to be visually useful to the human observer.

The most common way to store 3D data sets is as a series of 2D images. Each single image, which we have previously described as an array of pixels, is now seen to have depth. This depth is present either because the plane is truly an average over some depth of the sample (as in looking through a thin section in the light microscope) or based on the spacing between that plane and the next (as for instance a series of polished planes observed by reflected light). Because of the depth associated with the planes, we refer to the individual elements as voxels (volume elements) rather than pixels (pixel elements).

For viewing, processing and measurement, the voxels will ideally be regular and uniformly spaced. This goal is often accomplished with a cubic array of voxels, which is easiest to address in computer memory and corresponds to the way that many image acquisition devices function. Other arrangements of voxels in space offer some advantages. In a simple cubic arrangement, the

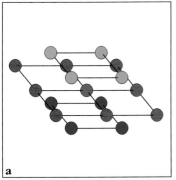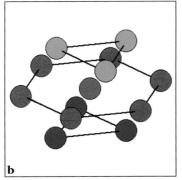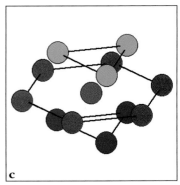

Figure 12. Lattice arrangements of atoms or voxels in which all neighbors are equidistant:
a) body-centered cubic (BCC); *b)* face-centered cubic (FCC); *c)* hexagonal close-packed (HCP).
Lines join the points which lie in each plane, indicated by color.

neighboring voxels are at different distances from the central voxel. More symmetrical arrangements are possible. The arrangements of atoms in metal crystals typically occupy sites in one of three lattice configurations: body-centered cubic (BCC), face-centered cubic (FCC), or hexagonal close packed (HCP). The first of these surrounds each atom (or voxel) with eight touching neighbors at the same distance, and the other two have twelve equidistant neighbors. **Figure 12** shows these arrangements, drawn to emphasize the planes of lattice points.

The advantage of these voxel-stacking arrangements is that processing of images can treat each of the neighbors identically, and that measurements are less biased as a function of direction. Of course, in order to fill space, the shapes of the voxels in these cases are not simple. Storing and addressing the voxel array is difficult, as is acquiring images or displaying them. Usually the acquired image must be resampled by interpolation to obtain voxels in one of these patterns, and a reverse interpolation is needed for display. For most purposes, these disadvantages outweigh the theoretical advantages, just as the use of a hexagonal pixel array is rarely used for two-dimensional images. Cubic arrays are the most common three-dimensional arrangement of voxels.

If the voxels are not cubic because the spacing between planes is different from the resolution within each plane, it may be possible to adjust things so that they are. In the discussion that follows, we will assume that the depth spacing is greater than the spacing within the plane, but an analogous situation could be described for the reverse case. This adjustment could be done by interpolating additional planes of voxels between those which have been measured. Unfortunately, doing this will not help much with image processing operations, since the assumption is that all of the neighbors are equal in importance, and with interpolation they are clearly redundant.

The alternative approach is to reduce the resolution within the plane by sampling every nth pixel, or perhaps by averaging pixels together in blocks, so that a new image is formed with cubic voxels. This resolution reduction also reduces the amount of storage that will be required, since many fewer voxels remain. However, it seems unnatural to give up resolution. In a few cases where cubic voxels are required for analysis, this is done.

A variety of different formats are available for storing 3D data sets, either as a stack of individual images or effectively as an array of voxel values with x,y,z indices. Such arrays become very large, very fast. A 512×512 or 640×480 pixel 2D image, which represents a very common image size for digitizing video images, occupies 250 or 300K bytes of storage, using one byte per pixel (256 grey values). This is easily handled in the memory of a desktop computer, or recorded on a floppy disk. A 512×512×512 3D image would occupy 128 megabytes of memory! This size is too large for any but a few computers, and presents difficulties just in storing or transmitting from place to place, let alone processing. Most of the data sets in this chapter are much smaller, for instance 256×256×50 (3.2 megabytes). The same operations shown here can be used for larger data sets, given time, computer power, or both.

Some compression in the size of the storage requirements can be achieved. The individual 2D images can be compressed either using run-length encoding (especially useful for binary images), or by the JPEG (Joint Photographers Expert Group) compression algorithms based on a discrete cosine transform, discussed in Chapter 2. There is not yet a standardized algorithm extending to three-dimensional images, but there are emerging standards for time sequences of images. One, the MPEG (Moving Pictures Expert Group) approach, is based on the fact that in a time series of images, most of the pixels do not change much in successive frames. Similar assumptions have been used to transmit video conferences over telephone lines; only the changing pixels must be transmitted for each frame. This high correlation from frame to frame should also be true for a series of planes in 3D, and may lead to standardized algorithms for compacting such images. They will still require unpacking for display, processing and measurement.

It is instructive to compare this situation to that of computer-aided drafting. For manmade objects with comparatively simple surfaces, only a tiny number of point coordinates are required to define the entire 3D structure. This kind of boundary representation is very compact, but it often takes many minutes to render a drawing with realistic surfaces from such a data set. For a voxel image, the storage requirements are great but information is immediately available without computation for each location, and the various display images shown in this chapter can usually be produced very quickly (sometimes even at interactive speeds) by modest computers.

For instance, given a series of surfaces defined by boundary representation or a few coordinates, the generation of a display may proceed by first constructing all of the points for one plane, calculating the local angles of the plane with respect to the viewer and light source, using those to determine a brightness value, and plotting that value on the screen. At the same time, another image memory is used to store the actual depth (z-value) of the surface at that point. After one plane is complete, the next one is similarly drawn except that the depth value is compared point by point to the values in the z-buffer to determine whether the plane is in front of or behind the previous values. Of course, each point is only drawn if it lies in front. This procedure permits multiple intersecting planes to be drawn on the screen correctly. (For more information on graphic presentation of 3D data, see Foley & Van Dam, 1984 or Hearn & Baker, 1986.)

Additional logic is needed to clip the edges of the planes to the stored boundaries, to change the reflectivity rules used to calculate brightness depending on the surface characteristics, and so forth. Standard texts on computer graphics describe algorithms for accomplishing these tasks and devote considerable space to the relative efficiency of various methods because the time involved can be significant. By comparison, looking up the value in a large array, or even running through a column in the array to add densities or find the maximum value, is very fast.

Slicing the data set

Since most 3D image data sets are actually stored as a series of 2D images, it is very easy to access any of the individual image planes, usually called slices. Playing the series of slices back in order to create an animation or "movie" is perhaps the most common tool available to let the user view the data. It is often quite effective in letting the viewer perform the 3D integration, and as it recapitulates the way the images may have been acquired (but with a much compressed time base), most viewers can understand images presented in this way. A simple user interface need only allow the viewer to vary the speed of the animation, change direction or stop at a chosen slice, for example.

One problem with presenting the original images as slices of the data is that the orientation of some features in the three-dimensional structure may not show up very well in the slices. It is useful to be able to change the orientation of the slices to look at any plane through the data, either in still or animated playback. This change in orientation is quite easy to do as long as the orientation of the slices is parallel to the x, y, or z axes in the data set. If the depth direction is understood as the z axis, then the x and y axes are the horizontal and vertical edges of the individual images. If the data are stored as discrete voxels, then accessing the data to form an image on planes parallel to these directions is just a matter of calculating the addresses of voxels using offsets to the start of each row and column in the array. This addressing can be done at real-time speeds if the data are

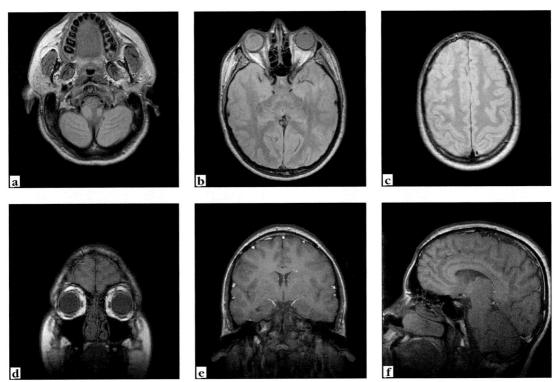

Figure 13. A few slices from a complete set of MRI head scan data. *Images **a** through **c** show transaxial sections (3 from a set of 46), images **d** and **e** are coronal sections (2 from a set of 42), and **f** is a sagittal section (1 from a set of 30).*

held in memory, but is somewhat slower if the data are stored on a disk drive because the voxels that are adjacent along scan lines in the original slice images are stored contiguously on disk and can be read as a group in a single pass. However, when a different orientation is required the voxels must be located at widely separated places in the file, and it takes time to move the head and wait for the disk to rotate.

Displaying an image in planes parallel to the x, y, and z axes was shown in Chapter 9, **Figure 51**, and **Figure 49** showed the collection of individual slice images (x, y planes) through the data set. **Figure 13** shows another example of orthogonal slices. The images are magnetic resonance images (MRI) of a human head. The views are generally described as transaxial (perpendicular to the subject's spine), sagittal (parallel to the spine and to the major axis of symmetry), and coronal (parallel to the spine and perpendicular to the "straight ahead" line of sight). Several individual sections are shown in each orientation.

It is actually not too common to perform this kind of resectioning with MRI data (or most other kinds of medical images) because the spacing of the planes is greater than the resolution in the plane, and the result is a visible loss of resolution in one direction in the resectioned slices due to interpolation in the z

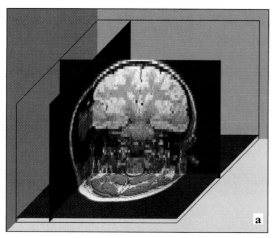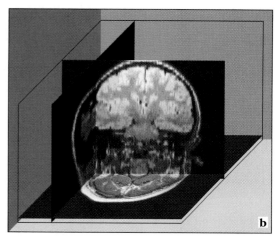

Figure 14. Comparison of two vertical slices through the 3D MRI data set from Figure 13: a) *slices extended vertically;* **b)** *linear interpolation between slices.*

direction. The alternative to interpolation is to extend the voxels in space; in most cases, this is even more distracting to the eye, as shown in **Figure 14**. Interpolation between planes of pixels can be done linearly, or using higher order fits to more than two planes, or more than just the two pixels immediately above and below. But while interpolation produces a visually acceptable image, it can ignore real structure or create apparent structure. **Figure 15** shows an example of interpolation which creates an impression of structure which is not actually present.

In Chapter 9, **Figure 51**, the data were obtained with cubic voxels, for which this interpolation is not a problem. In several of the figures later in this chapter, much greater loss of resolution in the z direction will be evident when plane images are reconstructed by sampling and interpolation of the original data. In the case of **Figure 13**, the MRI images were actually obtained as three complete sets of parallel slice images, in each of the three directions.

Combining several views at once using orthogonal planes adds to the feeling of three-dimensionality of the data. **Figure 16**

Figure 15. Interpolation in a 3D array. In this example, only two images of the top and bottom of a woven fabric are used. The points between the two surfaces are linearly interpolated and bear no relationship to the actual 3D structure of the textile.

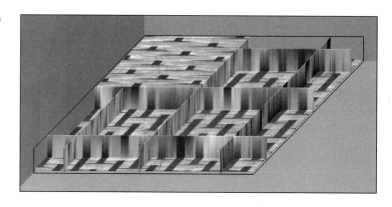

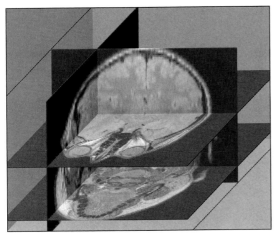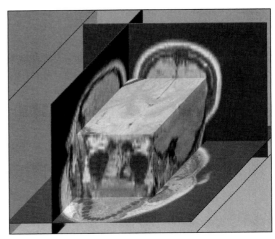

Figure 16. Several views of the MRI head data from Figure 13 along section planes normal to the axes of the voxel array. The voxels were taken from the transaxial slices, so the resolution is poorer in the direction normal to the planes than in the planes.

shows several examples of this using the same MRI head data based on plane images obtained in the transaxial direction. The poorer resolution in the z direction is evident, but still the overall impression of 3D structure is quite good. These views can also be animated, by moving one (or several) of the planes through the data set while keeping the other orthogonal planes fixed to act as a visual reference.

Unfortunately, there is no good way to demonstrate this time-based animation in a print medium. Once upon a time, children's cartoon books used a "flip" mode with animation printed on a series of pages that the viewer could literally flip or riffle through at a fast enough rate to cause flicker-fusion in the eye and see motion. That form of animation takes a lot of pages and is really only good for very simple images such as cartoons. It is unlikely to appeal to the publishers of books and technical journals. All that can really be done here is to show a few of the still images from such a sequence and appeal to the reader's imagination to supply a necessarily weak impression of the effect of a live animation.

Figure 17 shows a series of images that can be used to show "moving pictures" of this kind. They are actually a portion of the series of images which Eadweard Muybridge recorded of a running horse by setting up a row of cameras that were tripped in order as the moving horse broke threads attached to the shutter releases. His purpose was to show that the horse's feet were not always in contact with the ground (in order to win a wager for Leland Stanford, Jr.). The individual still pictures show that. Once it was realized that such images could be viewed to recreate the impression of smooth motion, our modern motion picture industry (as well as television) became possible.

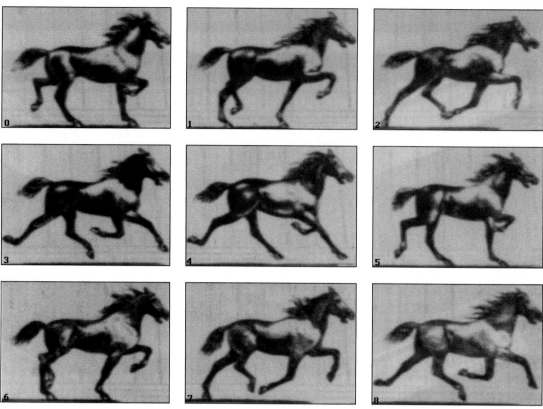

Figure 17. A few of the series of historic photographs taken by
Eadweard Muybridge to show the motion of a running horse.
Viewed rapidly in succession, these create the illusion of continuous
motion.

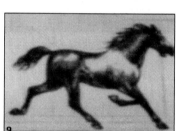

It is difficult to show motion using printed images in books.
There is current interest in the use of videotape or compact disk
(CD-ROM) for the distribution of technical papers, which will
perhaps offer a medium that can use time as a third axis to substitute for a spatial axis and show 3D structure through motion.
The possibilities will be mentioned again in connection with
rotation and other time-based display methods.

Motion, or sequences of images, is used to show multidimensional data in many cases. "Flipping" through a series of planes
provides a crude method of showing data sets that occupy three
spatial dimensions. Another effective animation shows a view of
an entire three-dimensional data set while varying the opacity of
the voxels. Even for a data set that occupies two spatial dimensions, transitions between many kinds of information may be
used effectively. **Figure 18** shows this multiplicity with weather

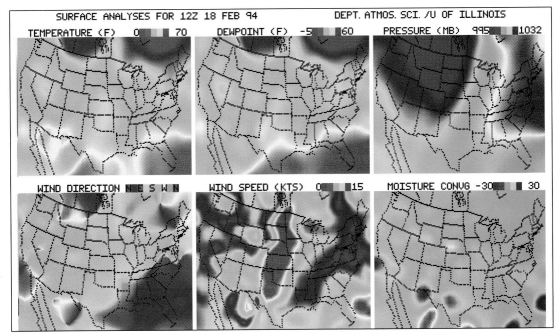

Figure 18. *Weather data for the United States.*

data, showing temperature, wind velocity and other parameters displayed onto a map of the United States. In general, displays that utilize a two-dimensional map as an organizing basis for multidimensional data such as road networks, geological formations, and so on, are called geographic information systems (GIS).

Of course, time itself is also a valid third dimension and the acquisition of a series of images in rapid succession to study changes in structure or composition with time can employ many of the same analytical and visualization tools as images covering three space dimensions. **Figure 19** shows a series of images recorded at video rate (30 frames per second) from a confocal light microscope. Such data sets can be assembled into a cube in which the Z direction is time, and changes studied by sectioning this volume in planes along the Z direction, or viewed volumetrically, or as a time sequence.

Arbitrary section planes

Restricting the section planes to those perpendicular to the x, y or z axes is obviously limiting for the viewer. It is done for convenience in accessing the voxels in storage and creating the display. If some arbitrary planar orientation is selected, the voxels must be found that lie closest to the plane. As for the case of image warping, stretching and rotating discussed in Chapter 2, these voxels will not generally lie exactly in the plane, nor will they have a regular grid-like spacing that lends itself to forming an image. **Figure 20** shows an example of a plane section

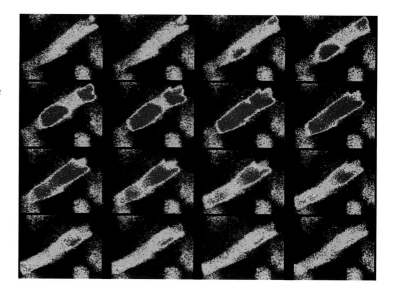

Figure 19. *A series of images of adult rat atrial myocytes loaded with the calcium indicator fluo-3. The images were recorded at video rate (30 frames per second) from a confocal light microscope. (Images courtesy of Dr. William T. Mason and Dr. John Hoyland, Department of Neurobiology, Babraham Institute, Babraham, Cambridge, U.K.).*

through an array of cubic voxels, in which portions of various size and shape are revealed. These variations complicate displaying the voxel contents on the plane.

The available solutions are either to use the voxels that are closest to the section plane, plot them where they land, and spread them out to fill any gaps that develop, or to establish a grid of points in the section plane and then interpolate values from the nearest voxels, which may be up to 8 in number. As for the case of rotation and stretching, these two solutions have different shortcomings. Using the nearest voxel preserves brightness values (or whatever the voxel value represents) but may distort boundaries and produce stair-stepping or aliasing. Interpolation makes the boundaries appear straight and smooth, but also smooths the brightness values by averaging so that steps are blurred. It is also slower, because more voxels must be located in the array and the interpolation performed.

Producing an animation by continuously moving a section plane at an arbitrary orientation requires a significant amount of

Figure 20. *Intersection of a plane with an array of cubic voxels. The plane is viewed perpendicularly, showing the different areas and shapes of the intersection regions.*

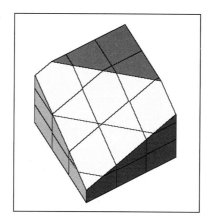

computation, even if it is essentially simple calculation of addresses and linear interpolation of values. Instead of doing this calculation in real time, many systems instead create new images of each of the plane positions, store them, and then create the animation by playing them back. This procedure is fine for demonstrating something that the user has already found, but because of the time delay is not a particularly good tool for exploring the 3D data set to discover the unexpected.

The ultimate use of planar resectioning would be to change the location and orientation of the section plane dynamically in real time, allowing instant response to the scene. Chapter 1 pointed out that humans study things by turning them over, either in the hand or in the mind. This kind of turning-over is a natural way to study objects, but requires a fairly large computer memory (to hold all of the voxel data), a fairly speedy processor and display, and a user interface that provides the required number of degrees of freedom.

Positioning an arbitrary plane can be done in two different ways, which of course produce the same results but feel quite different to the user. One is to move the plane with respect to a fixed 3D voxel array. This can be done, for example, by dragging the corners of the plane along the x, y, z axes. A different method is to keep the section plane fixed perpendicular to the direction of view while allowing the data set to be rotated in space. Combined with the ability to shift the section plane toward or away from the viewer (or equivalently to shift the data set), this method allows exactly the same information to be obtained.

The principal difference between these approaches is that in the latter case the image is seen with perspective or foreshortening, so that size comparisons or measurements can be made. Obtaining such data may be important in some applications. On the other hand, keeping the data set fixed and moving the section plane seems to aid the user in maintaining orientation within the structure.

Figure 21 shows the voxels revealed by an arbitrary section plane through the 3D data set from the MRI image series. The appearance of the voxels as a series of steps is rather distracting, so it is more common to show the value of the nearest voxels to the plane, or to interpolate among the voxels to obtain brightness values for each point on the plane as shown in **Figure 22**.

Also useful is the ability to make some of the pixels in section planes transparent, allowing the viewing of other planes behind the first, and making the 3D structure of the data more apparent. **Figure 23** shows an example of this for the spherical particle data shown in **Figures 49-51** of Chapter 9. The series of parallel slices are not contiguous planes of voxels, and the separation of the planes has been increased by a factor of two in the z direction. The voxels whose density falls below a threshold that

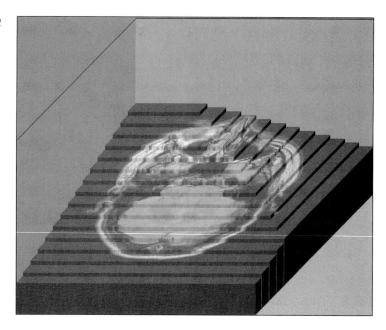

Figure 21. *Sampling voxels along inclined planes in a 3D array. Showing the entire voxel is visually distracting and does not produce a smooth image.*

roughly corresponds to that of the particles have been made transparent. This allows seeing voxels which are part of particles in other section planes behind the first.

Figure 24 shows a similar treatment for the MRI data set of the human head. The threshold for choosing which voxels to make transparent is more arbitrary than for the spheres, since there are void and low density regions inside as well as outside the head. However, the overall impression of 3D structure is clearly enhanced by this treatment.

Figure 22. *Smooth interpolation of image pixels on arbitrary planes positioned in a voxel array.*

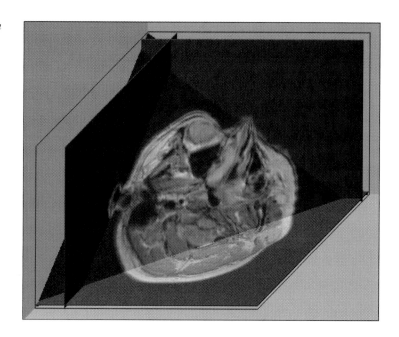

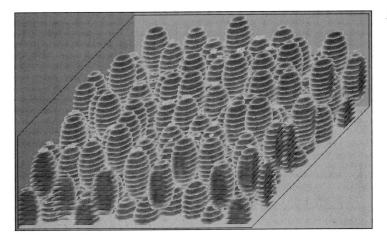

Figure 23. *"Exploded" view of voxel layers in the tomographic reconstruction of spherical particles (Figures 49-51, Chapter 9). The low-density region surrounding the particles is shown as transparent.*

The use of color

Assignment of pseudo-colors to grey scale 2D images was discussed in earlier chapters. It sometimes permits distinguishing subtle variations which are imperceptible in brightness in the original. But, as noted before, it more often breaks up the overall continuity and gestalt of the image so that the image is more difficult to interpret. Of course, the same display tricks can be used with three-dimensional sets of images, with the same consequences.

A subtle use of color or shading is to apply slightly different shading to different planar orientations shown in **Figures 16** and **22** to increase the impression of three-dimensionality. In this example, a grey scale difference between the x, y, and z orientations is evident. Light tints of red, green, and blue can be used for this as well.

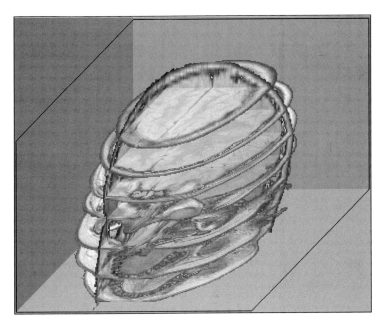

Figure 24. *View of several orthogonal slices of the MRI head data with transparency for the low-density regions in the planes.*

It is more useful to employ different color scales to distinguish different structures, as was also demonstrated for 2D images. It requires separate processing or measurement operations to distinguish the different structures. When applied to 3D data sets, the colored scales assist in seeing the continuity from one image to another, while providing ranges of brightness values for each object.

One of the most common ways that multiple colors can be used to advantage in 3D image data is to code multiband data such as the elemental concentrations measured from the secondary ion mass spectrometer. This use of pseudo-color is analogous to similar coding in 2D images, very frequently used for X-ray maps from the SEM and (of course) for remotely sensed satellite images, in which the colors may either be "true" or used to represent colors beyond the range of human vision, particularly infrared. Of course, the other tools for working with multiband images in 2D, such as calculating ratios, can also be applied in 3D.

Figure 25 shows example images for the SIMS depth imaging of elements implanted in a silicon wafer. Comparing the spatial location of the different elements is made easier by superimposing the separate images and using colors to distinguish the elements. This is done by assigning red, green, and blue to each of three elements and then combining the image planes, with the result shown in **Figure 26**.

Volumetric display

Sectioning the data set, even if some regions are made transparent, obscures much of the voxel array. Only the selected planes are seen and much of the information in the data set is not used. The volumetric display method shows all of the 3D voxel information. For simple structures displaying everything can be an advantage, while for very complex ones the overlapping features and boundaries can become confusing.

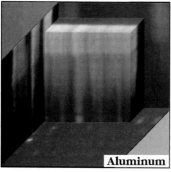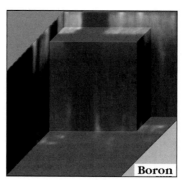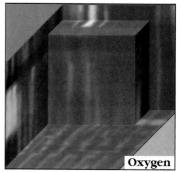

Figure 25. Views of plane sections for the elements aluminum, boron, and oxygen in a silicon wafer, imaged by secondary ion mass spectrometry. Figure 26 shows a full color image of all three elements on another orthogonal set of planes.

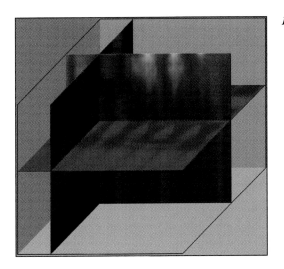

Figure 26. *Color coding of elementary intensity from SIMS images in Figure 25. The multiband 3D data set is sectioned on x, y, and z planes, and the 256-level (8-bit) brightness scale for the elements aluminum, boron, and oxygen are assigned to red, green, and blue, respectively.*

A volumetric display is produced by ray tracing. In the simplest model used, a uniform light source is placed behind the voxel array. For each straight line ray from the light source to a point on the display screen, the density value of each voxel that lies along the path is used to calculate a reduction in the light intensity following the usual absorption rule: $I/I_0 = \exp(-\Sigma\rho)$. Performing this calculation for rays reaching each point on the display generates an image. The total contrast range may be adjusted to the range of the display by introducing an arbitrary scaling constant. This scaling can be important because the calculated intensities may be quite small for large voxel arrays.

Notice that this model assumes that the voxel values actually correspond to density, or to some other property that may be adequately modeled by the absorption of light. The image shown in Chapter 9, **Figure 50**, in fact corresponds closely to this model, since it shows the projected view through a specimen using X-rays. In fact, X-ray tomographic reconstruction, discussed in the preceding chapter, proceeds from such views to a calculation of the voxel array. Having the array of voxel values then permits generating many kinds of displays to examine the data. It seems counter-productive to calculate the projection view again, and indeed in such a view as shown in the figure, the ability to distinguish the individual particles and see their relationship is poor.

One of the advantages of this mode is that the direction of view can be changed rather easily. For each, it is necessary to calculate the addresses of voxels which lie along each ray. When the view direction is not parallel to one of the axes, this addressing can be done efficiently using integer arithmetic to approximate the sine/cosine values. Also in this case, an improved display quality is obtained by calculating the length of the line segment along each ray through each pixel. The absorption rule then becomes $I/I_0 = \exp(-\Sigma\rho t)$.

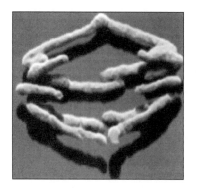

Figure 27. *Reconstruction of chromosomes in a dividing cell from CSLM 3D data. The chromosomes are opaque and the matrix around them transparent, and shadows have been ray cast on the rear plane to enhance the 3D appearance.*

This method is far short of a complete ray tracing, although it is sometimes described as one. In a true ray-traced image, refraction and reflection of the light is included along with the absorption. **Figure 27** shows an example in which the inclusion of shadows greatly increases the 3D impression. More complex shading, in which features cast shadows on themselves and each other, requires calculations which are simply too time-consuming for routine use in this application. With the simple absorption-only method, it is possible to achieve display speeds capable of rotating the array (changing the view direction) interactively with high-end desktop computers.

Of course, it is always possible to generate and save a series of projection images that can then be played back as an animation or movie. But these are primarily useful for communicating some information already known to another viewer, while interactive displays may assist in discovering the structural relationships in the first place.

These types of volumetric displays are practically always isometric rather than perspective-corrected. In other words, the dimension of a voxel or feature does not change with distance. This is equivalent to looking at the scene through a long focal length lens, and given the inherent strangeness of data in most 3D image sets does not generally cause significant discomfort to viewers. True perspective correction requires that x, y dimensions on the screen be adjusted for depth. Particularly for rotated views, perspective adds a significant amount of computation.

Much faster generation of projection images is possible if the addressing can be simplified and the variation in distance through different voxels can be ignored. **Figure 28** shows an approximation that facilitates these changes. Each plane of voxels is shifted laterally by an integral number of voxel spaces, which makes the address calculation particularly simple. The planes remain normal to the view direction, so that all distances through pixels are the same. This kind of shifting can give the impression of rotation for small angles. Beyond about 25–30 degrees, the distortion of the 3D structure due to stretching may

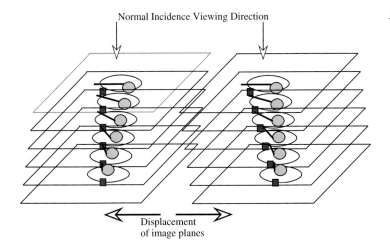

Normal Incidence Viewing Direction

Displacement
of image planes

Figure 28. Schematic diagram of shifting image planes laterally to create illusion of rotation or to produce stereo pair images for viewing.

become visually objectionable. However, this method provides a fast way to cause some relative displacement of features to better understand the structure.

Figure 29 shows such a view through a joint in the leg of a head louse. The original series of images were obtained with a transmission confocal light microscope, with nearly cubic voxels (the spacing between sequential focal planes was 0.2 μm in depth). The individual muscle fibers are visible but overlapped. Shifting the stack to approximate rotation gives the viewer the ability to distinguish the various muscle groups. Again, a time sequence (hard to show in print media) is used as a third dimension to display 3D data as the planes are shifted, and since no complex arithmetic is needed to run this sequence it is practical to create such animations in a small computer.

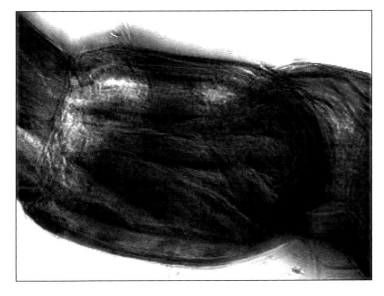

Figure 29. Volumetric projection image through a stack of 60 CSLM images of a joint in the leg of a head louse. Each plane is displaced by one voxel dimension to produce a view at 45°.

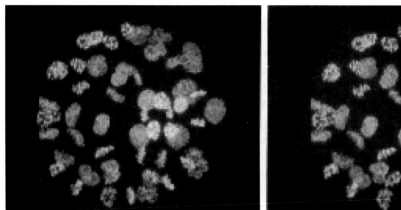
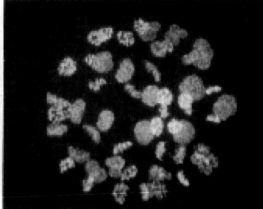

Figure 30. *Stereo pair presentation of Feulgen-stained DNA in a sea urchin embryo. The cells form a hollow sphere, evident in the stereo images, with some cells in the act of cell division. This image shows a volumetric image that is "ray cast" or "ray traced," using an emission model, with different offsets for the individual optical sections to produce a stereo effect. See also Figure 31 for a surface image of the same data. (Image courtesy R. G. Summers, C.E. Musial, P-C. Cheng, A. Leith, M. Marko, "The use of confocal microscopy and stereocon reconstructions in the analysis of sea urchin embryonic cell division,"* J. Electron Microscope Tech. *1991; 18: 24-30).*

Stereo viewing

In many of the images in this chapter, two adjacent images in a rotation or pseudo-rotation sequence can be viewed as a stereo pair. For some readers looking at them will require an inexpensive viewer which allows one to focus on the separate images while keeping the eyes looking straight ahead (which the brain expects to correspond to objects at a great distance). Other readers may have mastered the trick of fusing such printed stereo views without assistance. Some, unfortunately, will not be able to see them at all. A significant portion of the population seems not to actually use stereo vision, due for instance to uncorrected amblyopia ("lazy eye") in childhood.

Stereo views are so useful to a reasonable fraction of people that it may be useful to display them directly on the viewing screen. Of course, with a large screen, it is possible to draw the two views side by side. **Figures 30** and **31** show examples of stereo pair presentation of 3D images using both the volumetric display method discussed above and the surface-rendered method discussed below, for the same specimen (derived from confocal light microscope images of a sea urchin embryo). **Figure 32** shows another stereo pair presentation of skeletonized data (skeletonization is also discussed below) obtained from neurons imaged in the confocal light microscope. For many people this mode requires a viewer and presents some problems of alignment.

A more direct stereo display method uses color planes in the display for the left- and right-eye views. For instance, **Figure 33** shows a stereo pair of blood vessels in the skin of a hamster, imaged live using a confocal light microscope in fluorescence

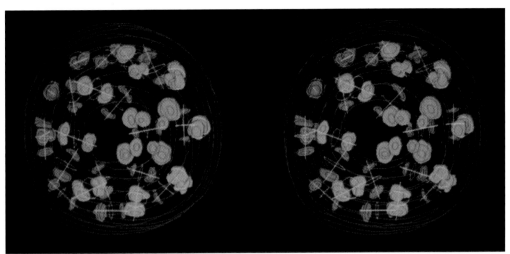

Figure 31. *Stereo view of the data set from Figure 30, but surface rendered and color coded. The surface image shows contours within each section that render the surfaces of the chromosomal masses but obscure any internal detail or structures to the rear. Contour lines for the embryo are also shown.*

mode. The 3D reconstruction method used pseudo-rotation by shifting of the focal section planes with the emission rules discussed below. Combining these images using red and green to display two views of the same 3D data set is shown in **Figure 34**. The images are overlapped, and the viewer (equipped with glasses having appropriate red and green filters) can easily look at the combined images. Of course, this method cannot be used for color images, as discussed below.

These stereo views were constructed from multiple sections by projecting or ray tracing through a stack of images as shown in **Figure 28**. The individual sections were obtained by confocal

Figure 32. *Stereo images of skeletonized lines (manually entered from serial section data) from two neurons in hippocampus of 10-day-old rat, showing branching and 3-D relationships. (J.N. Turner, D.H. Szaeowski, K.L. Smith, M. Marko, A. Leith, J.W. Swann, "Confocal Microscopy and Three-Dimensional Reconstruction of Electrophysically Identified Neurons in Thick Brain Slices,"* J. Electron Microscope Tech. *1991: 18: 11-23).*

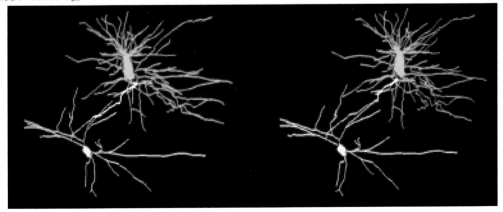

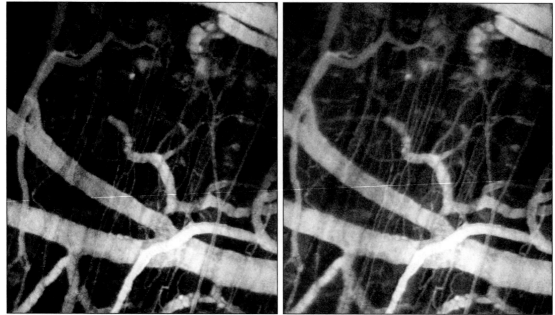

Figure 33. *Stereo view of multiple focal plane images from a CSLM showing light emitted from fluorescent dye injected into the vasculature of a hamster and viewed live in the skin. This image is also shown in Figure 34.*

microscopy, which has very shallow depth of field and can be used to obtain a continuous set of voxel planes. Other techniques that produce continuous arrays of thin sections can also be used, of course. But it is even possible to perform this type of reconstruction using a conventional optical microscope, in spite of the blurring of the images due to the large depth of field and the effect of light passing through the specimen above and below

Figure 34. *Stereo pair of the same image pair shown in Figure 33, using red and cyan for different eye views. This allows viewing the image with normal eye vergence, using glasses (red lens on left eye, green or blue on right). See an additional example in the Introduction.*

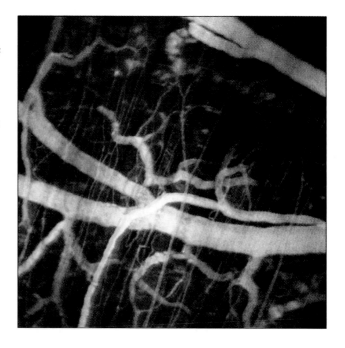

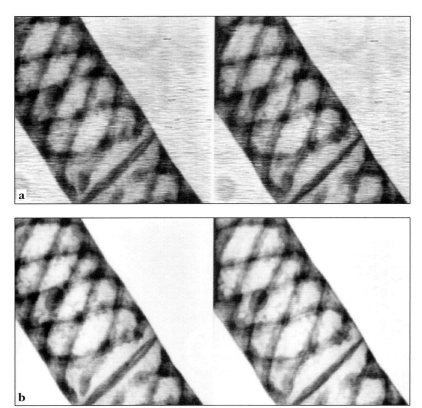

Figure 35. *Sharpening of focal sections by Wiener filtering. The images are produced by ray tracing two projections at angles of about ±2.4 degrees through 90 serial optical sections in a 50 μm thick section. The sample is Spirogyra. **a)** uncorrected images; **b)** Wiener inverse filtered (Lin et al., 1994).*

the image planes. Removing artefacts such as blur from images by processing in frequency space was discussed in Chapter 5. **Figure 35** shows an example of using Wiener inverse filtering to accomplish this deblurring in the creation of a stereo pair. The images were reconstructed from 90 optical sections spaced through a 50 μm thick section, which is much closer than the depth of field of the optics. The use of the inverse filter removes most of the artefacts from the images and produces a clear stereo pair image (Lin et al., 1994).

Another approach to the same kind of sharpening is to apply an iterative procedure that uses neighboring images to estimate the artefacts in each plane. This so-called Van Cittert filter requires using neighbor planes on each side out to about twice the dimension of the point spread function, which is in this case the depth of optical focus (Jain, 1989).

For projection of stereo pair images, it is possible to use two slide projectors equipped with polarizing filters that orient the light polarization at right angles (usually 45 degrees to the right and left of vertical). Viewers wearing polarized glasses can then see the stereo effect, and color can still be used. This display method requires special specular projection screens that reflect the light without losing the polarization, and works best for viewers in line with the center of the screen. However, it has become a rather popular method of displaying 3D data. Of course, it is not as practical for interactive exploration of a data set since photographic slides must be made first. Polarization can also be used with live computer displays, as discussed below.

The difference in viewing angle for the two images can be adjusted somewhat arbitrarily to control the visual impression of depth. The angle can be made to correspond to the typical vergence angle of human vision for normal viewing. Using a typical interocular distance of 7.5 cm, and a viewing distance of 1 meter, the actual vergence angle is 4.3 degrees. For closer viewing, larger angles are appropriate. The judgment of depth thus depends on our brain's interpretation of the viewing distance, which in some cases is apparently based on the focus distance to the image. If the angle is varied, the impression of depth can be adjusted to expand or compress the z dimension, as shown in **Figure 36**.

Special display hardware

Other specialized display hardware for 3D image analysis may be useful in some cases. Holography offers the promise of realistic three-dimensional display that can be viewed from different directions (Blackie et al., 1987). Attempts to generate such displays by calculating the holograms have been experimentally successful, although they are too slow for interactive use. At present, the best holograms are displayed using coherent light from a laser and high resolution film. In order to produce live displays from a computer, a screen such as an LCD can be used in place of the film. However, the resolution and control of the light modulation (relative intensity) is not really adequate.

Another custom approach is called a varifocal mirror (Fuchs et al., 1982). Each plane of voxels in the 3D array is drawn one at a time on the display CRT. The screen is not viewed directly by the user, but is reflected from a mirror. The mirror is mounted on a speaker voice coil so that it can be moved. As each different plane of voxels is drawn, the mirror is displaced slightly as shown schematically in **Figure 37**. This movement changes the distance from the viewer's eye to the screen, and gives the impression of depth. In order to achieve high drawing speeds (so that the entire set of planes can be redrawn at least 30 times per second), this technique is usually restricted to simple outline drawings rather than the entire voxel data set.

The mirror technique also suffers from a slowdown if the planes are not normal to the x, y, z axes so that trigonometric calculations are required to access the data. The alternative approach is to continue to draw outlines in the major orthogonal planes, but to move the mirror during the drawing of each outline to corre-

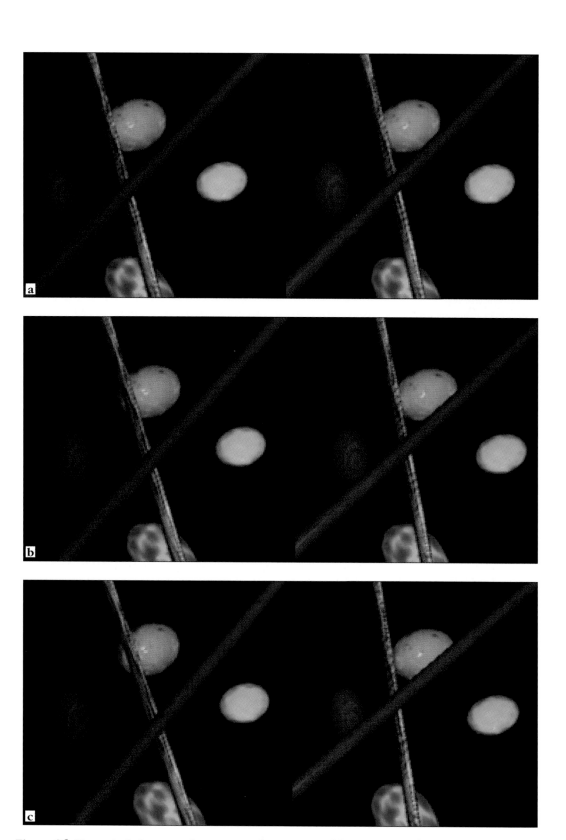

Figure 36. Stereo pair images of a generated structure with varying angles to control the apparent depth of the structure in the z direction: a) ±1 degree; b) ±3 degrees; c) ±5 degrees.

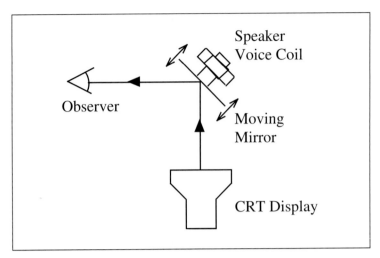

Figure 37. *Diagram of the operation of a varifocal mirror to show depth in images. The speaker voice coil rapidly varies the position of the mirror, which changes the distance from the viewer's eye to the cathode ray tube display as it draws information from different depths in the data set.*

Speaker
Voice Coil

Observer

Moving
Mirror

CRT Display

spond to the tilting of the plane. This requires a much higher and more complex frequency response from the mechanical devices used to control the mirror.

Another, more recent development for real-time viewing of 3D computer graphics displays uses stereo images. The computer calculates two display images for slightly different orientations of the data set or viewing positions. These are displayed alternately using high-speed display hardware which typically shows 120 images per second. Special hardware is then used to allow each eye to see only the correct images, at a rate of 60 times per second, fast enough to eliminate flicker (the minimum rate for flicker fusion is usually at least 16 frames per second; commercial moving pictures typically use 24 frames, and television uses 25 for European and 30 in U.S. systems).

The visual switching may be done by installing a liquid crystal device on the display monitor that can rapidly switch the polarization direction of the transmitted light, so that viewers can watch through glasses containing polarizing film. A second approach is to wear special glasses containing active liquid crystal devices which can rapidly turn clear or opaque. Synchronizing pulses from the computer cause the glasses to switch as the images are displayed, so that each eye sees the proper view.

Such devices have been used primarily for graphics design, in which substantial computer resources are used to model three-dimensional objects, generate rendered surface views, and allow the user to freely rotate and zoom. With the number of disciplines interested in using 3D computer graphics, it seems assured that new hardware (and the required corresponding software) will continue to evolve for this purpose. These tools will surely be adapted to the display of 3D image data and used at scales ranging from nanometers (electron and ion microscopy) to kilometers (seismic exploration). It is possible to imagine using other senses than visual to deal with multiband data (e.g., sound which changes pitch and volume to reveal density and composition as you move a cursor over the display of a voxel array). However, since vision is our primary sense it seems likely that most methods will be primarily visual, and the researcher who is color blind or cannot see stereo will remain disadvantaged.

There is also no consensus on the best input and control devices for complex computer graphics displays. Rotating or shifting the viewpoint in response to horizontal or vertical motion of the now ubiquitous mouse gives a rather crude control. For moving points, lines and planes in 3D, some more flexible device will be required. Simply locating a specific voxel location in the array can be done in several different ways. One is to use an x,y input device (mouse, trackball, etc.) for two axes and periodically shift to a different control, which may be a scroll bar on the screen, to adjust the distance along the third axis. Another is to move two cursors, one on an x-y projection and one on an x-z projection, for example. Such approaches usually feel rather clumsy because of the need to move back and forth between two areas of the screen and two modalities of interaction. Appropriate color-coding of the cursor to report depth can help.

Three-axis joysticks and sonic digitizers that allow the user to point in space (multiple sensors triangulate the position) exist but are hardly standard. The dataglove, an instrumented glove or framework that fits on the hand and reports all motion of joints to the computer, has been used to move molecules around each other to study enzyme action. Supplemented by force feedback, this method gives the researcher rich information about the ways that molecules can best fit together. Perhaps the ultimate virtual reality is using such gloves while wearing a helmet that reports head position, with built-in displays for each eye, so that the computer can create appropriate stereo displays as you move around inside your data set. However, such tools remain inaccessible to the typical user of image analysis computers at this writing.

At the other extreme, it is important to remember the history of 3D visualization (Cookson, 1994), which began with physical models constructed of wood, plastic or plaster. Building such a model from a series of section planes was very difficult and time-consuming, and still could not reveal all of the internal detail. Computer modeling has progressed from simple outlines to hidden line removal, surface construction, shading and rendering, and full volumetric or ray-traced methods.

Ray tracing

The example of volumetric display shown in **Figure 29** performed a simplified ray tracing to sum the density values of voxels and calculate a brightness based on light being absorbed as it propagated from back to front through the 3D data set. While this model does correspond to some imaging situations such as the transmission light or electron microscope and tomography, there are many other situations in which different rules are appropriate.

In the process of traversing a voxel array, following a particular line of sight that will end in one pixel of a ray-traced image, the variables which are available include:

a) The brightness and perhaps color of the original light source placed behind the array. This illumination source will control the contribution that transmission makes to the final image.

b) The location of the first and/or last voxels with a density above some arbitrary threshold taken to represent transparency. These voxels will define surfaces that can be rendered using reflected light. Additional rules for surface reflectivity, the location and brightness of the light sources, and so forth, must be added.

c) The location of the maximum or minimum values, which may define the location of some internal surface for rendering.

d) The rule for combining voxel values along a path. This may be multiplication of fractional values, which models simple absorption according to Beer's law for photons provided that the voxel values are linear absorption values. In some cases density is proportional to attenuation, so this rule can produce interpretable images. There are other convolution rules available as well, including linear summation and retention of maximum or minimum values. While these may also correspond to some physical situations, their greatest value is that they produce images which can delineate internal structure.

e) The relationship between the voxel values and the intensity (and perhaps color) of light originating in each voxel, which represents fluorescence or other emission processes.

The combining rules mentioned briefly in part **d** of the above list correspond to the various image processing tools described in Chapters 2 and 3 for combining pixels from two or more images. They include arithmetic (multiplication, addition), rank ordering (minimum or maximum value) and Boolean logic. It is also possible to include lateral scattering so that point sources of light spread or blur as they pass through the voxel array, or even to combine several modes. This approach to realism through computation is rarely justified since the measured voxel values are not generally directly related to light transmission or scattering.

A software package for 3D visualization may make any or all of these parameters accessible to the user, along with others. For example, we will see that control of the surface reflectivity and roughness, and the location of the incident light source(s), affects the appearance of rendered surfaces. In performing a convolution of transmitted light along ray paths from a light source behind the voxel array, the relationship between the voxel values

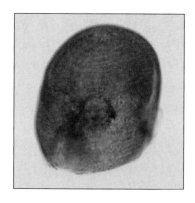
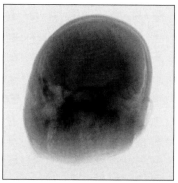
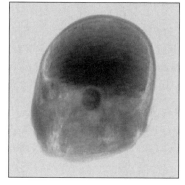
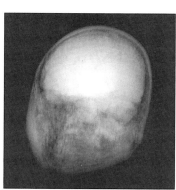

Figure 38. *Volumetric imaging of the MRI head data from Figure 13. Varying the relationship between voxel values and the opacity used to absorb light transmitted along each ray through the structure allows selection of which structures are revealed.*

and the absorption of the light is another parameter that offers control. By varying the relationship between voxel value and opacity (linear attenuation coefficient), it is possible to make some structures appear or to remove them, allowing others to be seen.

Figure 38 shows an example of this presentation. The data set is the same as used in **Figures 13**, **16** and others. The voxel values come from the MRI measurement technique and approximately correspond to the amount of water present. Not enough information is given to fully describe the structures actually present in a human head, so there is no "correct" relationship between voxel value and light absorption for the volumetric rendering. Using different, arbitrary curves, it is possible to selectively view the outer skin, bone structure, or brain.

Using color permits even more distinctions to be made. **Figure 39** shows images of a hog heart reconstructed using different relationships for opacity vs. voxel value that emphasize the heart muscle or the blood vessels. In this example, each voxel is assumed both to absorb the light from the source placed behind the voxel array and to contribute its own light along the ray in proportion to its value and with color taken from an arbitrary table. The result allows structures with different measured values to appear in different colors.

Of course, with only a single value for each voxel it is not possible to model absorption and emission separately. By performing dual-energy tomography in which the average atomic number

Figure 39. *Volumetric rendering of MRI data. Specimen is a hog heart. (Data courtesy B. Knosp, R. Frank, M. Marcus, R. Weiss, Univ. of Iowa Image Analysis Facility and Dept. of Internal Medicine). Changing the arbitrary relationship between voxel value and display opacity for the voxels allows selectively showing the heart muscle or blood vessels.*

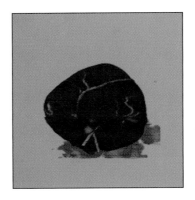 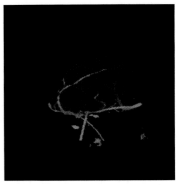

and average density are both determined, or multienergy tomography in which the concentration of various elements in each voxel is measured, such techniques become possible. They represent straightforward implementation of several of the multiband and color imaging methods discussed in earlier chapters, but are not yet common as neither the imaging instrumentation nor the computer routines are yet widely available. It is consequently usually necessary to adopt some arbitrary relationship between the single measured set of voxel values and the displayed rendering that corresponds to the major voxel property measured by the original imaging process.

For example, in fluorescence light microscopy, or X-ray images from the SEM, or ion microscopy (as shown in **Figure 25**), the voxel value is a measure of emitted brightness that is generally proportional to elemental concentration. These 3D data sets can also be shown volumetrically by a simplified ray tracing. Instead of absorbing light from an external light source, the rule is to sum the voxel values as brightnesses along each path.

Figure 33 showed an application using the fluorescence confocal light microscope. A dye was injected into the blood vessel of a hamster, which was excited by the incident light from the microscope. The emitted light was collected to form a series of 2D images at different focal depths, and these were then arranged in a stack to produce a 3D data set. In this case the spacing between the planes is much greater than the resolution within each image plane. Sliding the image stack laterally as discussed above produces an approximation of rotation and impression of depth. The brightness values for each voxel are then summed along vertical columns to produce each image.

This emission model is very easy to calculate but does not take into account any possible absorption of the emitted light intensity by other voxels along the ray path. Generally, simple 3D data sets have only one piece of data per voxel and there is no separate information on density and emission brightness, so no such correction is even possible. Sometimes a simple reduction in intensity in proportion to the total number of voxels traversed, known as a "distance fade", may be used to approximate this

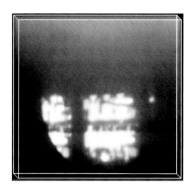 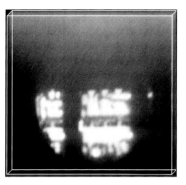

Figure 40. *Stereo pair display of emission rule volumetric images of boron concentration in a silicon wafer, imaged by a secondary ion mass spectrometer.*

absorption effect. Usually, it is assumed that the emission intensity is sufficiently high and the structure sufficiently transparent that no such correction is needed, or that it would not change the interpretation of the structure.

When multiband data are available, as for instance in the SIMS data set used in **Figures 25** and **26**, emission rules can be used with the assignment of different colors (at least up to three) to different signals. **Figures 40** and **41** show a volumetric view of these data using emission rules, presented as a stereo pair. The monochrome figure shows a single element (boron) while in the color image, multiple elements are combined. The use of color in the images forces the use of two side-by-side images for viewing, and the density of information in the images that results from overlaying the 8-bit (256 grey level) values from each element at every point makes it quite difficult to fuse these images for satisfactory stereo viewing.

Using the same data set, it is possible to use the location of the frontmost voxel along each line of sight whose value is above an arbitrary threshold to define the location of an internal boundary. If this resulting surface is then rendered as a solid surface with incident reflected light, another representation of the data is obtained as shown in **Figure 42**.

This figure illustrates some of the different ways that an internal surface can be revealed. **Figure 43** shows several views of the spiral cochlear structure from the ear of a bat (Keating, 1993).

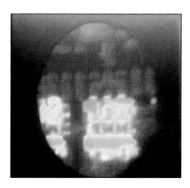 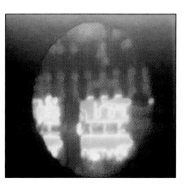

Figure 41. *Stereo pair of volumetric images from the SIMS data set. Colors assigned to the different elements are Red=Aluminum, Green=Boron, and Blue=Oxygen, with 256 brightness levels of each. The use of color for elemental information precludes color coding of views as in Figure 31. The density of information in this display is so great that fusing the images to see the depth is quite difficult.*

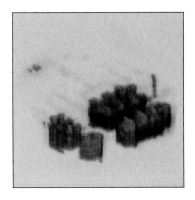

Figure 42. Surface-rendered display of the same data as in Figure 41. The internal surface of the boron-rich region is determined by arbitrary thresholding, and then rendered using an arbitrarily placed light source.

Slices through the 3D voxel array do not show that the structure is connected. Thresholding to show all of the voxels within the structure reveals the topology of the spiral. A series of section images can be shown as either wire frame outlines, or with the surface rendered. The outlines are more convenient for rotating to view the structure from different directions.

Reflection

Another important imaging modality is reflection. The conventional CSLM, seismic reflection mapping, acoustic microscopy, and so forth, acquire a 3D image set whose voxel values record

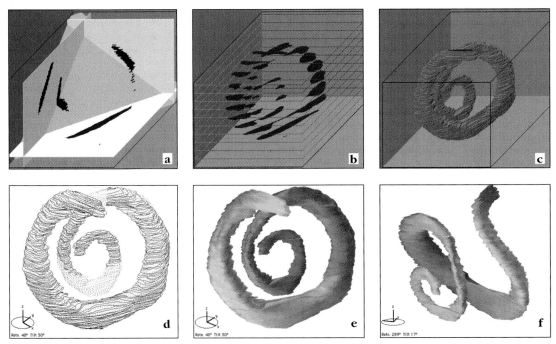

*Figure 43. Cochlear structure from the ear of a bat (Keating, 1993): **a)** arbitrary planar slices through the voxel array; **b)** array of parallel slices through the array; **c)** surface revealed by thresholding the voxels; **d)** outlines delineating the structure in all voxel planes; **e)** surface reconstructed from the outlines in **d**; **f)** the same structure as shown in **e**, rotated to a different point of view.*

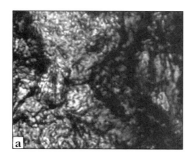

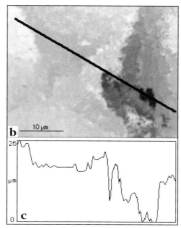

Figure 44. Depth measurement using the confocal scanning light microscope:

a) *extended focus image of an alumina fracture surface obtained by keeping the brightest value from many focal planes at each pixel location;*

b) *range image obtained by assigning a grey scale value to each pixel according to the focal plane image in which the brightest (in focus) reflectance is measured;*

c) *elevation profile along the traverse line shown in figure b.*

the reflection of the signal from that location. This voxel array is generally used to locate boundaries where strong reflections occur, within a matrix that may be otherwise opaque. In the CSLM the matrix is transparent (either air or liquid) and the strongest reflection at each x, y point is where the specimen surface is in focus. This means that recording a set of images as a 3D data array makes it possible to locate the surface in three dimensions. Most systems use the processing methods discussed in Chapter 6 to find the brightest value at each pixel, and thus construct the surface range image.

One way to generate such a display is to go down columns of the data array (just as in volumetric ray tracing), looking for the maximum voxel value. Keeping only that value produces an image of the entire surface in focus, as was shown in Chapter 4. Since the same methods for rotating or shifting the data array to alter the viewing direction can be used, it is also possible to find the maxima along any viewing direction and display the surface as an animation sequence or to construct a stereo pair. In principle, fitting a curve based on the known depth-of-field characteristics of the optics to the brightness values along a vertical column of voxels can locate the surface with subpixel accuracy. **Figure 44** shows the alumina fracture (from Chapter 1, **Figures 64** and **65**) both as an extended-focus image and as a range image (in which pixel brightness is proportional to elevation). Several presentation modes for range images are available to assist in visualizing the three-dimensional shape of the surface. One, shown in **Figure 44**, is simply to plot the brightness profile along any line across the image, which gives the elevation profile directly.

Figure 45 shows several of the presentation modes for range images. The specimen is a microelectronics chip imaged by reflection CSLM, so both an extended-focus image and a range image can be obtained from the series of focal plane sections. From the range image data, plotting contour maps, grid or mesh plots, or shaded isometric displays is a straightforward exercise in computer graphics.

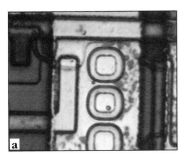 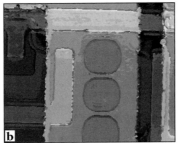 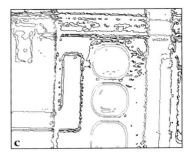

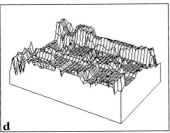 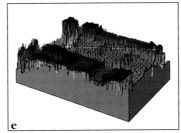 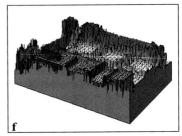

Figure 45. Presentation modes for surface information from the CSLM (specimen is a microelectronics chip):

a) *the in-focus image of the surface reflectance obtained by keeping the brightest value at each pixel address from all of the multiple focal plane images;*

b) *the elevation or range image produced by grey scale encoding the depth at which the brightest pixel was measured for each pixel address;*

c) *contour map of the surface elevation with grey scale coding for the height values;*

d) *isometric grid drawing of the elevation data, with grid spacing equal to 6 pixels;*

e) *the same grid as in figure d with shading to show the elevation values;*

f) *the grid from figure d with the reflectance data from figure a superimposed.*

One of the classic ways to show surface elevation is a contour map (**Figure 45c**), in which isoelevation lines are drawn, usually at uniform increments of altitude. These lines are of course continuous and closed. This is the way topographic maps are drawn, and the same methods are useful at any scale. Since the contour map reduces the pixel data from the original range image to boundary representation, the method for forming the boundaries is the same as discussed in Chapter 5 for segmentation. The lines may be labeled or color-coded to assist in distinguishing elevations.

A shortcut way to draw contour lines on a range image is to present the data as a shaded isometric view, as in **Figure 46**, which shows the elevation data for the alumina fracture surface of **Figure 45**. In this image, a 3D representation (without perspective) is used to draw a vertical line for each pixel in the range image to a height proportional to the value. The image is also shaded so that each point has its grey scale value. Replacing the grey scale values with a pseudo-color table allows communication of the elevations in a particularly easy-to-interpret way, and in fact many topographic maps use similar methods to show elevations.

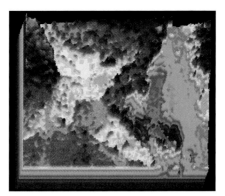

Figure 46. Isometric view of elevation data for the alumina fracture surface shown in Figure 44. A rapidly varying color palette is used to facilitate comparison.

Constructing a contour map can be either simple or complex. The simplest method merely locates those pixels that have neighbors that are above and below the threshold level. But, as shown in **Figure 47**, this produces a very coarse approximation. Interpolating between pixel addresses produces a much better map, as shown in the figure.

Figure 48 shows an example that looks broadly similar to **Figure 46**, but represents data at a very different scale. This is a three-dimensional view of Ishtar Terra on Venus. The data come from the spacecraft Magellan's side-looking mapping radar. This synthetic-aperture radar bounces 12.5-cm-wavelength radar waves off the surface, using the echo time delay for range, and the Doppler shift to collect signals from points ahead of and

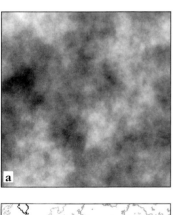
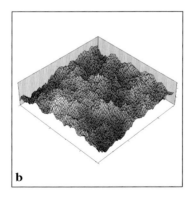
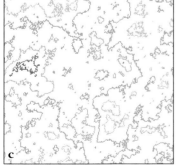
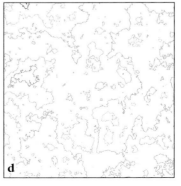

*Figure 47. **Surface of a metal fracture:***

a) range image (grey scale proportional to elevation);

b) shaded grid;

c) contour map produced by selecting pixels with neighbors above and below each of five thresholds;

d) contour map produced by linear interpolation.

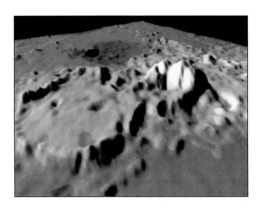

Figure 48. *Reconstructed surface image of Ishtar Terra on Venus, looking northeast across Lakshmi Panum toward Maxwell Montes with an exaggerated vertical scale.* (S. Saunders [1991] "Magellan: the Geologic Exploration of Venus" Engineering and Science, *Spring 1991: 15-27*).

behind the direct line of sight. The two-dimensional images obtained by processing the signals are similar in appearance to aerial photographs.

Rendering of a surface defined by a range image produces a realistic image of surface appearance, as compared to grid or isometric contour map displays that are more abstract and more difficult for visual interpretation, as shown in **Figure 49**. However, the quantitative interpretation of the surface data is more readily accessible in the range image. Also, it is difficult to select realistic surface colors and textures to be applied. It is possible to apply brightness values to an isometric display of range data that come from another image of the same area, such as the original reflectivity or texture information. When multiband images are

Figure 49. Display modes for surface information:
a) *range image;*
b) *grid mesh;*
c) *isometric view;*
d) *rendered terrain.*

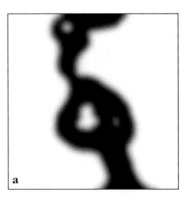

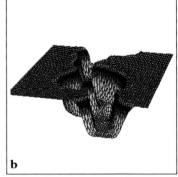

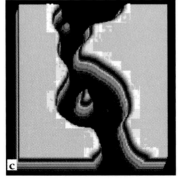

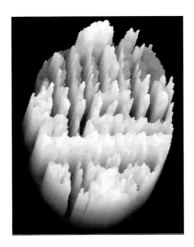

Figure 50. *Isometric display of elevation data within a volume: the height of the maximum concentration of Si in the SIMS voxel array in Figure 40.*

recorded, this combination is particularly effective. **Figure 44f** shows an example of this display mode.

The surfaces discussed in the preceding section are in fact external physical surfaces of the specimen. Internal surfaces may be defined as boundaries between distinct regions, or in more subtle ways. For instance, **Figure 50** shows the data from the SIMS example used above, in which the depth of the voxel having the maximum concentration of silicon at any location is shown. This surface isolation provides a visualization of the shape of the implanted region. The image is shown as a shaded isometric display, as discussed above.

Surfaces

Surfaces to be examined may be either physical surfaces revealed directly by reflection of light, electrons or sound waves, or surfaces internal to the sample and revealed only indirectly after the entire 3D data set has been acquired. The use of computer graphics to display them is closely related to other graphics display modes used in computer assisted design (CAD), for example. However, the typical CAD object has only a few numbers to describe it, such as the coordinates of corners. Generating the interpolated surfaces and calculating the local orientation and hence the brightness of the image at many points requires a significant amount of computing.

In contrast, the image data discussed here is typically a complete 3D data set, or at least a complete 2D range image derived from the 3D set. Consequently, there is elevation data at every pixel location in the display image, which allows for an extremely rapid image generation. Rendering the surface images shown here took only a few seconds on a desktop computer. Doing the same for a typical CAD object would take many minutes.

Some instruments produce range images directly. Large-scale examples include radar mapping, elevation measurement from stereo pair calculations, and sonar depth ranging. At a finer scale, a standard tool for measuring precision machined surfaces is interferometry, which produces images as shown in **Figure 51a**. The brightness is a direct measure of elevation, and the image can be comprehended more easily in an isometric display as shown in **Figure 51c**. Notice that the lens artefact (the faint ring structure at the left side of the image) is not true elevation data and when presented as such looks quite strange.

Displays of surface images (more formally of range images, since real surfaces may be complex and multivalued, but range images are well behaved and single valued) can use any of the techniques described above. These include wire mesh or line profile displays, contour maps, and shaded isometric displays, all compared for the same image data in **Figure 51**. These all involve a certain level of abstraction. Chapter 11 provides greater detail on the visualization and analysis of these images.

The simple set of line profiles (**Figure 51b**) gives an impression of surface elevation and requires no computation, although the need to space the lines apart loses some detail. Consequently, it is sometimes used as a direct display mode on instruments such as the SEM or STM. Unfortunately, the signal that is displayed in this way may not actually be the elevation, and in this case the pseudo-topographic display can be quite misleading. Adding grid or mesh lines in both directions (**Figures 51d** and **51e**) not only requires additional computation, but also increases the effective spacing and decreases the lateral resolution of the display.

Generating an image of a surface that approximates the appearance of a real, physical surface is known generically as rendering and requires more computational effort. Examples are shown in **Figures 51g** and **51h**. The physical rules that govern the way real surfaces look are simple and are summarized in **Figure 52**. The important variables are the intensity and location of the light source and the location of the viewer. Both are usually given in terms of the angles between the normal vector of the surface and the vectors to the source and viewer. The absolute reflectivity of the surface (or albedo) must be known; if this varies with wavelength we say that the surface is colored because some colors will be reflected more than others.

Finally, the local roughness of the surface controls the degree of variation in the angle of reflection. A very narrow angle for this spread corresponds to a smooth surface that reflects specularly. A broader angle corresponds to a more diffuse reflection. One of the very common tricks in graphic arts, which can be seen any evening in television advertising, is the addition of bright specular reflections to objects to make them appear metallic and hopefully more interesting.

For a typical surface defined by a few points, as in CAD drawings, the surface is broken into facets, often triangular, and the

Figure 51. Presentation modes for the surface elevation data from an optical interferometer (specimen is the machined surface of nickel):

a) original image, in which the grey scale brightness encodes height;

b) isometric view produced by drawing multiple line profiles across the surface;

c) isometric view with superimposed grey scale values from image *a*;

d) isometric view with a full grid drawn at a spacing of 8 pixels;

e) the same grid with shading from figure *a*;

f) a contour map with grey scale shading to indicate the height of lines;

g) the surface data rendered as it would appear with a diffuse material;

h) the surface data rendered as it would appear with a specular material.

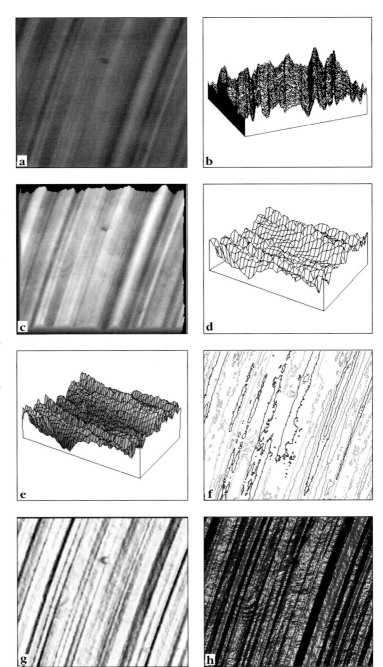

orientation of each facet is calculated with respect to the viewer and light source. The reflected light intensity is then calculated, and the result plotted on the display screen or other output device to build the image. This would seem to be a rather fast process with only a small number of facets, but the problem is that such images do not look natural. The large flat facets and the abrupt angles between them do not correspond to the continuous surfaces we encounter in most real objects.

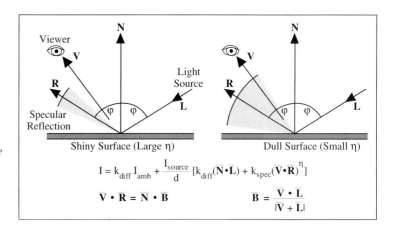

Shading the brightness values between facets (Gouraud shading) can eliminate these abrupt edges and improve the appearance of the image, but requires much interpolation. Better smoothing can be achieved (particularly when there are specular reflections present) by interpolating not the brightness values but the angles between the centers of the facets. The interpolated angles are then used to generate the brightness values, which vary nonlinearly with angle. This Phong shading is even more computer-intensive.

For continuous pixel images, each set of three pixels can be considered to define a triangular facet as shown schematically in **Figure 53**. The difference in value (elevation) of the neighboring pixels gives the angles of the local surface normal directly. A pre-calculated lookup table (LUT) of the image brightness values for a given light source location and surface characteristics completes the solution with minimum calculations. Since this is done at the pixel level in the display, no interpolation of shading is needed. **Figure 54** includes displays of a rendered surface with different light source locations and surface characteristics.

The examples of display modes in **Figure 54** show the reconstruction of a surface from the rather sparse information in a contour map. The map is converted to a range image by applying smoothing to interpolate values between the contour lines. This map can then be shown as an isometric or perspective-corrected grid, with or without superimposed shading. Finally, the facets can be rendered using the relationships of **Figure 52**.

Figure 53. *Diagram showing the construction of a triangular tesselation on a surface formed by discrete height values for an array of pixels.*

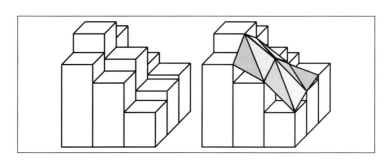

Figure 54. Presentation modes derived from data in an elevation contour map:

a) *the original map, with uniform grey levels shown between the contours to indicate relative height;*

b) *continuous elevation values interpolated between the contour lines by smoothing the grey scale values in figure **a**;*

c) *perspective view of the surface shown with a shaded grid;*

d) *image **c** from a different point of view;*

e) *perspective display showing each pixel elevation, shading and a superimposed grid;*

f) *perspective display with a different grey scale image of the same surface superimposed;*

g) *the surface rendered as a diffuse surface;*

h) *the surface rendered as a specular surface with a different location for the light source.*

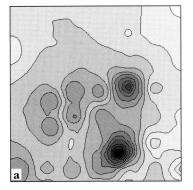

a

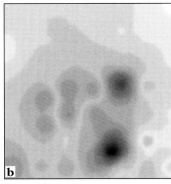

b

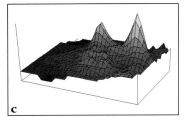

c

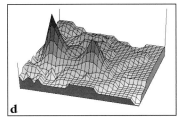

d

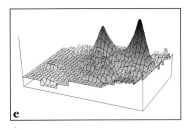

e

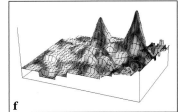

f

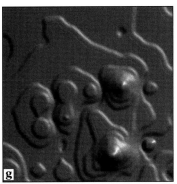

g

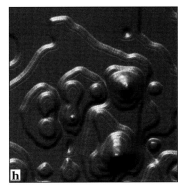

h

Applying image processing operations beforehand to range image data is often used to improve the resulting surface image. Smoothing with kernels that calculate a weighted average corresponds to Phong shading. Applying a median filter removes noise that would show up as local spikes or holes in the surface. The names of filters such as the rolling ball operator discussed in Chapter 3 come directly from their use on range images. This particular operator tests the difference between the minimum value in two neighborhood regions of different sizes and eliminates points that are too low. The analogy is that depressions which a ball of defined radius cannot touch as it rolls across the surface are filled in.

Rendering a surface (calculating its brightness according to its orientation relative to the viewer and light source) using the lookup table approach is fast, provided that the appropriate tables for different light source locations and surface characteristics have been calculated beforehand. The tables are not large and can be stored for a reasonable number of cases. The tables permit a nearly real-time animation of a rendered surface with a moving light source (see **Figure 55**), which is another way to use the dimension of time to reveal three-dimensional spatial information. Changing the surface characteristics, from diffuse to specular or from white reflection to colored, can be used to show multiband data. Obviously additional surface images are needed to specify these characteristics.

Rendered surfaces from range images have the appearance of real, physical objects and so communicate easily to the viewer. However, they obscure much of the information present in the original 3D image data set from which they have been extracted. More complex displays, which require real ray tracing, can make surfaces that are partially reflecting and partially transmitting so that the surface can be combined with volumetric information in the display. This presentation has somewhat the appearance of embedding the solid surface in a partially transparent medium, like fruit in Jell-O. Such displays can be dramatic in appearance

Figure 55. *Rendered surface from Figure 54 with moving light source (four frames from an animation sequence). Notice that when viewed alone, lighting from below (figure**d**) causes the peaks to appear as valleys.*

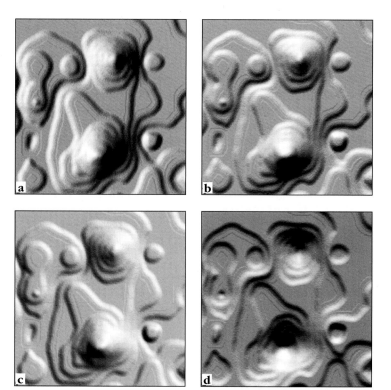

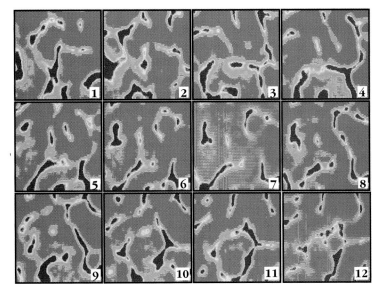

Figure 56. *Sequential images from an ion microscope, showing two-phase structure in an Fe-45% Cr alloy aged 192 hours at 540°C (M. K. Miller, Oak Ridge National Laboratories, Oak Ridge, TN).*

and useful for communicating complex three-dimensional information, but are too slow to generate to be used to explore complex data sets interactively.

Multiply connected surfaces

Rendering techniques are not restricted, of course, to simple range images. Indeed, it is for complex, multiply connected surfaces that 3D image data is most needed, since the topology of such surfaces cannot be studied in 2D images. Rendering more complex surfaces is also possible but takes a little longer. **Figure 56** shows a series of 2D planes in a 3D data set from an ion microscope. The sample, a two-phase metal alloy, shows many regions in each image. It is only in the full 3D data set that the connection between all of the regions is evident. In fact, each of the two phase regions in this specimen is a single, continuous network intimately intertwined with the other. This cannot be seen well even by using resectioning in various directions (**Figure 57**).

Volumetric displays of this data set can show some of the intricacy, especially when the live animation can be viewed as the

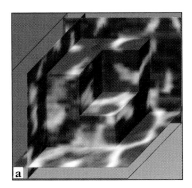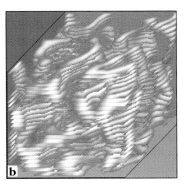

Figure 57. Section views of the 3D voxel array formed from the images in Figure 56:

a) *stored brightness values along several arbitrary orthogonal planes;*

b) *stored values on a series of parallel planes with dark voxels made transparent.*

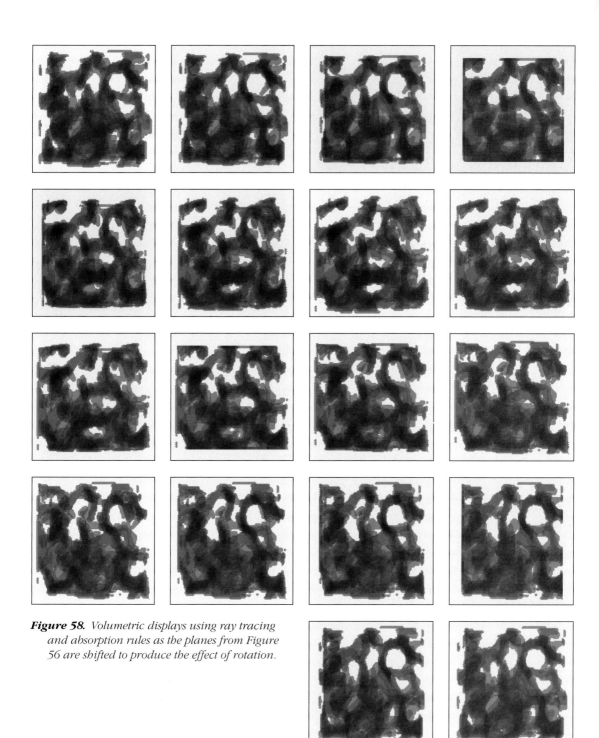

Figure 58. *Volumetric displays using ray tracing and absorption rules as the planes from Figure 56 are shifted to produce the effect of rotation.*

rotation is carried out. **Figure 58** shows a few orientations of the data set using ray tracing to produce a volumetric display; viewed rapidly in sequence, these produce the visual effect of rotation. However, the complexity of this structure and the precedence in which features lie in front and in back of others limits

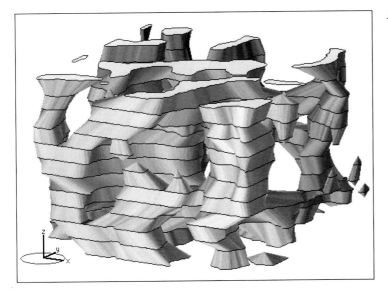

Figure 59. *Simple rendering of the boundary surface between the two phases in the specimen from Figure 56, by interpolating planar facets between the planes.*

the usefulness of this approach. Isolating the boundary between the two phases allows a rendered surface to be constructed as shown in **Figure 59**. With the faceting shown, this display can be drawn quickly enough (a few seconds on a desktop computer) to be useful as an analysis tool. A complete smoothed rendering (**Figure 60**) takes much longer (about one-half hour on the same computer) or requires access to graphics supercomputers.

The rendering of the surface follows the determination of the various surface facets. The simplest kind of facet is a triangle. In the example shown in **Figure 59**, a series of narrow rectangles or trapezoids are used to connect together points along each section outline. For features in which the sections are similar in shape and size, this faceting is fairly straightforward. When the shapes change considerably from section to section, the resulting facets offer a less realistic view of the surface shape.

The greatest difficulty is dealing with splits and merges in the structure. This means that the number of outlines in one section is greater than in the next, and so the surface must somehow divide. **Figure 61** shows two ways to do this. In one, the junction actually lies in one of the planes. It may either be drawn by hand or located by various algorithms, such as dividing the feature normal to its moment axis at a point which gives area ratios equal to those of the two features in the next section. The result is fairly easy to draw, since no surface facets intersect.

The second method constructs surface facets from sets of points along the feature boundaries from the single feature in one section to both of the features in the next section plane. This technique moves the junction into the space between planes, and produces a fairly realistic picture, but requires more calculation. The intersecting planes must be drawn with a z-buffer, a computer graphics technique that records the depth (in the viewing

Figure 60. *Two high-resolution rendered views of the boundary surface between the two phases in the specimen from Figures 56 to 59.*

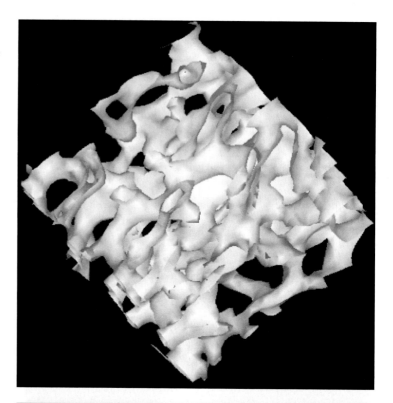

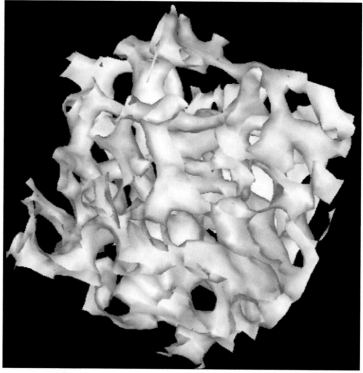

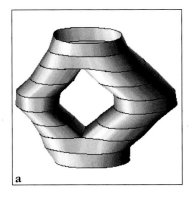 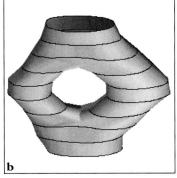

Figure 61. Two ways to render the surface between serial section outlines where splits or merges occur:

a) *dividing one plane into arbitrary regions that correspond to each branch;*

b) *continuous surfaces from each branch to the entire next outline, with intersection between the planes.*

direction) of each image point, and only draws points on one surface where they lie in front of the other.

The major drawback to this kind of surface rendering from serial section outlines is that the surfaces hide what is behind them, and even with rotation it may not be possible to see all parts of a complex structure. Combining surface rendering with transparency (so that selective features are shown as opaque and others as partially transparent, letting other structures behind become visible) offers a partial solution. **Figure 62** shows an example in which one kind of feature (the spheres) has been given the property to show with a reduced brightness through any superimposed surface. This allows the spheres to be seen where they lie behind the columns. However, the dimming is not realistic (since the density of the columns is not known), and other structures behind the columns are completely hidden.

In the example shown in **Figures 59** and **60**, the boundary was determined by thresholding in each of the 2D image planes, since the plane spacing was not the same as the in-plane resolution. A certain amount of interpolation between the planes is required, which makes the curvature and roughness of surfaces

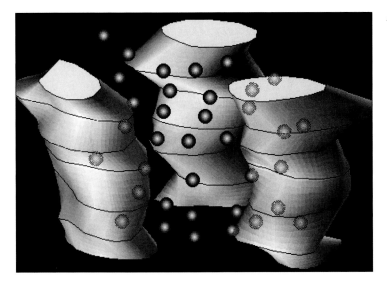

Figure 62. *Combining surface rendering with partial transparency to show structures otherwise hidden by surfaces in front. The spheres that lie behind the frontmost surfaces are dimmed or shown in a different color. Notice that this is only partial transparency in that the front vertical column is completely opaque to the rear one, and the spheres are dimmed uniformly without regard to the actual amount of material in front of them.*

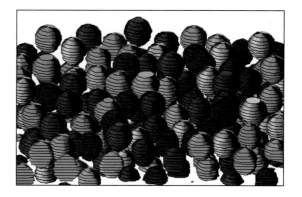

Figure 63. Rendered surface image of spherical particles from tomographic reconstruction (see Chapter 9, Figures 49-51) created by interpolating surface tiles between the slices shown in Figure 23, and assigning arbitrary colors to each feature.

different in the depth or z direction. For data sets with true cubic voxels, as for example the tomographic reconstruction shown in Chapter 9, **Figure 51**, the resolution is the same in all directions, and greater fidelity can be achieved in the surface rendering. **Figure 63** shows the surface rendered image from that data set.

Multiple colors are needed to distinguish the many features present (about 200 roughly spherical particles) in this structure. This use of pseudo-color is particularly important to identify the continuity of multiply connected surfaces. **Figure 64** shows another example in which the structural organization of the braid is much easier to see when each fiber is assigned a unique color palette.

The braided fibers in **Figure 64** emphasize that serial section reconstruction for 3D displays is certainly not restricted to microscopy and medical applications. The study of woven textiles and fibers used in composite materials uses the same methods (Gowayed et al., 1991). **Figure 65** uses color coding to identify the muscles and bones in a common everyday example of serial sectioning. The images were acquired by visiting the local supermarket and photographing each roast sliced from a side of

Figure 64. Rendered surface image of a triple braided textile reconstructed from serial section images. Colors are assigned to each fiber to make it easier to follow them through the braid. A series of shades of each color are used to indicate surface orientation.

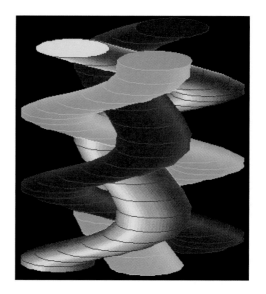

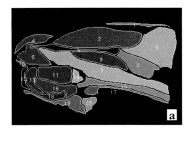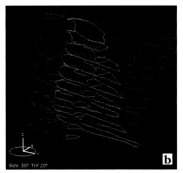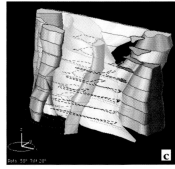

Figure 65. Serial sections through a side of beef: a) one section with features numbered; *b)* stack of slices; *c)* rendered result, showing selected muscles with solid surfaces and several bones with dashed outlines.

beef. After aligning the images and thresholding them to delineate the various structures, the stack of slices can be rendered to reveal the three-dimensional structure of the muscles and bones.

Image processing in 3D

The emphasis so far has been on the display of 3D image data, with little mention of processing. Most of the same processing tools that were described in the preceding chapters for 2D images can be applied more or less directly to 3D images for the same purposes. Arithmetic operations such as ratios in multiband data are used, for instance, in exactly the same way. Each voxel value is divided by the value of the voxel at the same location in the second image. This kind of operation does not depend on the images having cubic voxels.

However, many processing operations that use neighborhoods, e.g., for kernel multiplication, template matching, rank operations, and so forth, do require cubic voxel arrays. In a few instances, a kernel may be adapted to noncubic voxels by adjusting the weight values so that the different distance to the neighbors in the z direction is taken into account. This adjustment only works when the difference in z distance as compared to the x, y directions is small, for instance a factor of 2 or 3 as may be achieved in the confocal light microscope. It will not work well if the image planes are separated by ten times (or more) the in-plane resolution. And any departure from cubic voxel shape causes serious problems for ranking or template-matching operations.

In these cases, it is more common to perform the processing on the individual planes and then form a new 3D image set from the results. **Figure 66** shows a series of pseudo-rotation views of the MRI head images used above. Each slice image has been processed using a Frei and Chen operator to extract edges. These edges show the internal structure as well as the surface wrinkles in the brain. Furthermore, image processing was used to form a

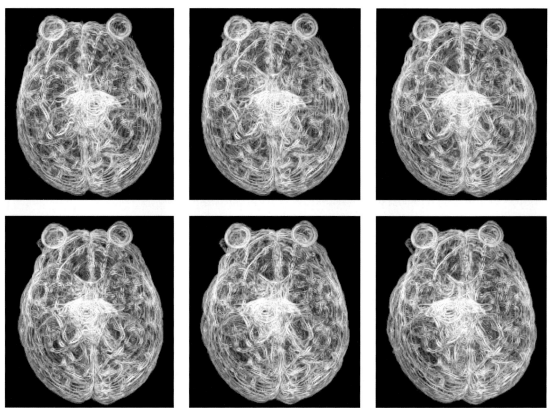

Figure 66. *Several views of the brain from the MRI data set. The skull has been eliminated, individual image planes have been processed with an edge operator, and the resulting values have been used with emission rules to create a volumetric display. Lateral shifting of the planes produces pseudo-rotation. Each pair of images can be viewed in stereo, or the entire sequence used as an animation. Structures are visible from the folds in the top of the brain to the spinal column at the bottom.*

mask to delineate the brain (defined as the central bright feature in each slice) and isolate it from other portions of the image. The result is a series of slice images which show only the brain, processed to show the internal edges.

Another display trick has been used here. It is not clear just what volumetric display mode is appropriate for such processed images. Instead of the conventional absorption mode, in which transmitted light is passed through the data array, these images use the emission mode, in which each voxel emits light in proportion to its value. That value is the edgeness of the voxel as defined by the Frei and Chen operator. In other words, we see the edges glowing in space. In a live animation, or for those readers who can use pairs of the images to view the 3D data set stereoscopically, this image creates a fairly strong impression of the 3D structure of the brain. The same type of display of lines in space can be used to display contours within a 3D data set.

This illustration may serve as an indication of the flexibility with which display rules for 3D images can be bent. Nontraditional display modes, particularly for processed images, are often quite effective for showing structural relationships. There are no guidelines here, except for the need to simplify the image by eliminating extraneous detail to reveal the structure that is important; an experimental approach is encouraged.

The use of two-dimensional processing of image planes in a 3D data set should be used with some care. It is only justified if the planes have no preferred orientation and are random with respect to the structure, or conversely if the planes have a very definite but known orientation that matches that of the structure. The latter situation applies to some situations involving coatings. When possible, 3D processing is preferred, even though it imposes a rather significant computing load. The size of neighborhoods increases as the cube of dimension. A kernel of modest size, say 7×7, may be fast enough for practical use in 2D, requiring 49 multiplications and additions for every pixel. In 3D, the same 7×7×7 kernel requires 343 multiplications and additions per voxel, and of course the number of total voxels has also increased dramatically so that processing takes much more time.

For complex neighborhood operations such as gradient or edge finding in which more than one kernel is used, the problem is increased further because the number of kernels must increase to deal with the higher dimensionality of the data. For instance, the 3D version of the Sobel gradient operator would use the square root of the sum of squares of derivatives in three directions. And since it takes two angles to define a direction in three dimensions, an image of gradient orientation would require two arrays, and it is not clear how it would be used.

The Frei and Chen operator (Frei & Chen, 1977), a very useful edge detector in 2D images, can be extended to three dimensions by adding to the size and number of the basis functions. For instance, the first basis function (which measures the gradient in one direction and corresponds to the presence of a boundary) becomes

$$
\begin{array}{ccccccccc}
-\sqrt{2/3} & -\sqrt{1/2} & -\sqrt{2/3} & & & & & & \\
-\sqrt{1/2} & -1 & -\sqrt{1/2} & 0 & 0 & 0 & & & \\
-\sqrt{2/3} & -\sqrt{1/2} & -\sqrt{2/3} & 0 & 0 & 0 & +\sqrt{2/3} & +\sqrt{1/2} & +\sqrt{2/3} \\
& & & 0 & 0 & 0 & +\sqrt{1/2} & +1 & +\sqrt{1/2} \\
& & & & & & +\sqrt{2/3} & +\sqrt{1/2} & +\sqrt{2/3}
\end{array}
$$

It should be noted that in three dimensions, it is possible to construct a set of basis functions to search for lines as well as surfaces. It remains to find good ways to display the boundaries which these operators find.

Three-dimensional processing can be used in many ways to enhance the visibility of structures. In **Figure 40**, the boron concentration was shown volumetrically using emission rules. How-

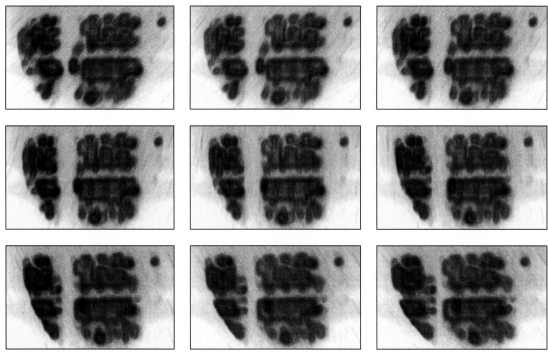

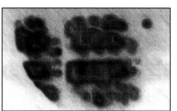

Figure 67. *Volumetric display of boron concentration from SIMS image data set. The series of images shows pseudo-rotation by shifting of planes, using the local 3D variance in pixel values to locate edges. The magnitude of the variance is used as an effective density value to absorb light along rays through the voxel array.*

ever, the overlap between front and rear portions of the structure makes it difficult to see all of the details. The surface rendering in **Figure 42** is even worse in this regard. **Figure 67** shows the same structures after 3D processing. Each voxel in the new image has a value that is proportional to the variance of voxels in a 3×3×3 neighborhood in the original image set. These values are displayed volumetrically as a transmission image. In other words, the absorption of light coming through the 3D array is a measure of the presence of edges; uniform regions appear transparent. The visibility of internal surfaces in this "cellophane" display is much better than in the original, and the surfaces do not obscure information behind them, as they would with rendering.

The time requirements for neighborhood operations are even worse for ranking operations. The time required to rank a list of values in order increases not in proportion to the number of entries, as in the kernel multiplication case, but as $N \cdot \log (N)$. This assumes a maximally efficient sorting algorithm and means that ranking operations in really large neighborhoods take quite a long time.

For template-matching operations such as those used in implementing erosion, dilation, skeletonization, and so forth, the situation is worse still. The very efficient methods possible in 2D by using a lookup or fate table based on the pattern of neighbors will no longer work. In 2D, there are 8 neighbors so a table with $2^8=256$ entries can cover all possibilities. In 3D there are 26 adjacent neighbors and $2^{26}=67$ million patterns. Consequently, either fewer neighboring voxels can be considered in determining the result, or a different algorithm must be used.

All of the morphological operations (erosion, dilation, etc.) have direct generalizations in three dimensions (Gratin & Meyer, 1992). Normally, for practical reasons, cubic voxels are used. This means that consideration must be given to the difference between face-, edge- and corner-touching neighbors. In principle, the more symmetrical arrangements of voxels shown above in **Figure 12** would allow simpler erosion/dilation rules and more uniform processing, but these are rarely used. The three-dimensional analog of a Euclidean distance map can be constructed by a direct extension of the two-dimensional method, and has the same advantages both for improving isotropy and for distance measurement from surfaces or boundaries.

Skeletonization in 3D analogous to that in 2D would remove voxels from a binary image if they touched a background or OFF voxel, unless the touching ON voxels did not all touch each other (Halford & Preston, 1984; Lobregt et al., 1980). If touching is considered to include the corner-to-corner diagonal neighbors as well as edge-to-edge touching and face-to-face touching, then a minimum skeleton can be constructed. However, if a table for the 26 possible touching neighbors cannot be used, then it is necessary to actually count the touching voxels for each neighbor, which is much slower.

It should be noted that skeletonization in 3D is entirely different from performing a series of skeletonizations in the 2D image planes and combining or connecting them. In 3D, the skeleton becomes a series of linear links and branches that correctly depict the topology of the structure. If the operation is performed in 2D image planes, the skeletons in each plane form a series of sheetlike surfaces that twist through the three-dimensional object and have a different topological relationship to the structure. This is shown schematically in **Figure 68**. The skeleton of linear links and branches in 3D has been formed by connecting the ultimate eroded points (UEPs) in each section (see Chapter 6).

Measurements on 3D images

As discussed in Chapter 8, it is clear that one of the reasons to collect and process images is to obtain quantitative data from them. This is true for 3D imaging as well as 2D, and consequently some additional comments about the kinds of measure-

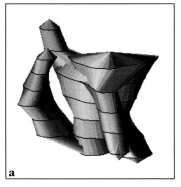 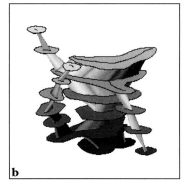 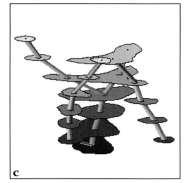

Figure 68. Skeletonization in 3D:

a) *an irregularly shaped solid object represented by planar sections;*

b) *connecting the 2D skeletons of the individual planar intersections;*

c) *3D skeleton formed by connecting the ultimate eroded points of the 2D sections.*

ments that can be performed, their practicality and the accuracy of the results seem appropriate.

Measurements are broadly classified into two categories: feature-specific and global or scene-based. The best known global measurement is the volume fraction of a selected phase or region. Assuming that the phase can be selected by thresholding (perhaps with processing as discussed in Chapter 3), then the volume fraction is determined simply by counting the voxels in the phase and dividing by the total number of voxels in the array or in some other separately defined reference volume. The result is independent of whether the voxels are cubic. In fact, the same result can be obtained by counting pixels on image planes and does not depend in any way on the arrangement of the planes into a 3D array.

A second global parameter is the surface area per unit volume of a selected boundary. There are stereological rules for determining this value from measurements on 2D images. One method counts the number of crossings that random lines (for a random structure, the scan lines can be used) make with the boundary. Another method measures the length of the boundary in the 2D image. Each of these values can be used to calculate the 3D surface area.

It might seem that directly measuring the area in the 3D data set would be a superior method without assumptions. In practice, it is not clear that this is so. First, the resolution of the boundary, particularly if it is irregular and rough, depends critically on the size of pixels or voxels. The practical limitation on the number of voxels that can be dealt with in 3D arrays may force the individual voxels to be larger than desired. It was pointed out before that a 512×512 image in 2D requires 0.25 megabytes of storage, while the same storage space can hold only a 64×64×64 3D array.

The use of smaller pixels to better define the boundary is not the only advantage of performing measurements in 2D. The summation of boundary area in a 3D array must add up the areas of triangles defined by each set of three voxels along the boundary. A table can be constructed giving the area of the triangle in terms of the position differences of the voxels, but the summation process must be assured of finding all of the parts of the boundary. There is no unique path that can be followed along a convoluted or multiply-connected surface that guarantees finding all of the parts.

For other global properties such as the length of linear features or the curvature of boundaries, similar considerations apply. The power of unbiased 2D stereological tools for measuring global parameters is such that the efficiency and precision of measurement makes them preferred in most cases.

Feature-specific measurements include measures of size, shape, position and density. Examples of size measures are volume, surface area, length (maximum dimension), and so forth. In three dimensions, these parameters can be determined by direct counting. The same difficulties for following a boundary in 3D mentioned above still apply. But in 2D images the measurements of features must be converted to 3D sizes using relationships from geometric probability. These calculations are based on shape assumptions and are mathematically ill-conditioned. This means that a small error in measurements or assumptions is magnified in the calculated size distribution.

Simple shapes such as spheres produce good results. **Figure 69** shows the result for the tomographic image of spherical particles shown in **Figure 23**. The measurement on 2D plane slices gives circle areas that must be unfolded to get a distribution of spheres. The result shows some small errors in the distribution, including negative counts for some sizes which are physically impossible. But the total number and mean size are in good agreement with the results from direct 3D measurement.

When feature shapes are more complicated or variable, 2D methods simply do not work. If information on the distribution of

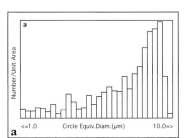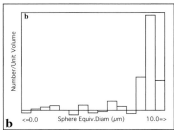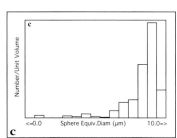

Figure 69. Comparison of 2D and 3D measurement of size of spherical particles in structure shown in Figures 23 and 63:
a) size distribution of circles in 2D plane sections;
b) estimated size distribution of spheres by unfolding the circle data in *a* (note negative values);
c) directly measured size distribution of spheres from 3D voxel array.

shapes and sizes is needed, then measurement in 3D, even with the problem of limited resolution, is the only available technique.

Position of features in 3D is not difficult to determine. Counting pixels and summing moments in three directions provides the location of the centroid and the orientation of the moment axes. Likewise, feature density can be calculated by straightforward summation. These properties can be determined accurately even if the voxels are not cubic and are affected only slightly by a reduction in voxel resolution.

Shape is a difficult concept even in two dimensions. The most common shape parameters are formally dimensionless ratios of size, such as (volume)$^{1/3}$/(surface area)$^{1/2}$ or length/breadth (length is easy to define as the longest dimension, but just as for the 2D case, the proper definition and measurement procedure for breadth is not so obvious). The selection of a parameter which has meaning in any particular situation is very ad hoc, either based on the researcher's intuition or on trial-and-error and regression. In 3D the values may be less precise because of the poorer voxel resolution, but the accuracy may be better because the size parameters used are less biased. And it may be important to the user's intuition to consider three-dimensional shape factors, which are less unfamiliar than two-dimensional ones.

The other approaches to shape in 2D are harmonic analysis (which unrolls the feature boundary and performs a Fourier analysis on the resulting plot), and fractal dimension determination; both were discussed in Chapter 8. These parameters can be determined rather efficiently in two dimensions, but only with great difficulty in three dimensions. Since the 2D results are related stereologically to 3D structure, it is preferable to perform these measurements on the individual 2D image planes.

Closely related to shape is the idea of topology. This is a non-metric description of the basic geometrical properties of the object or structure. Topological properties include the numbers of loops, nodes and branches (Aigeltinger et al., 1972). The connectivity per unit volume of a network structure is a topological property that is directly related to such physical properties as permeability. It is not possible to determine topological properties of 3D structures from 2D images, so these must be measured directly on the 3D data set, perhaps after skeletonization to simplify the structure (Russ & Russ, 1989). Another example, a reconstruction showing the topology of an overhand knot, was shown in Chapter 8.

Conclusion

There is little doubt that 3D imaging will continue to increase in capability and popularity. It offers direct visualization and measurement of complex structures and 3D relationships, which cannot be as satisfactorily studied using 2D imaging. Most of the kinds of imaging modalities that produce 3D images, especially tomographic reconstruction, are well understood, although the hardware will benefit from further development (as will the computers and software). Current display methods are barely adequate to the task of communicating the richness of 3D image data sets to the user. New display algorithms and interface control devices will surely emerge, driven not only by the field of image processing but also by other related fields such as visualization of supercomputer data. The continued increase in computer power and memory is certain. Watching and using these developments offers an exciting prospect for the future.

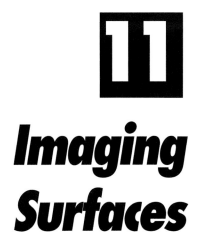

Imaging Surfaces

In many different disciplines surfaces are more important than bulk structures. Mechanical interaction between parts involves friction and wear between surfaces, many chemical interactions take place on surfaces (including catalysis) and most modern electronic devices consist of thin layers of materials laid down in intricate patterns on the surface of substrates. The appearance of objects is dominated by their surface characteristics, textures, and coatings. In all these cases and many more, scientists and engineers need to characterize surfaces and the ways in which fabrication and use modify them. Imaging plays important roles in obtaining the information as well as presenting it for human visualization and analysis.

Producing surfaces

Surfaces are produced in a wide variety of processes, some tightly controlled and some quite chaotic. One of the oldest techniques by which mankind has produced intentional surfaces is by removal of material, for instance creating a statue or a stone tool by removing chips from a larger block of stone. Modern fabrication of parts typically involves machining, grinding and polishing to remove material and to create a surface with specific macroscopic dimensions and also microscopic roughness.

Machining is a process in which a cutting tool removes chips from the material as it is moved relative to the workpiece. The shape of the tool's cutting tip or edge, its speed and the depth of cut, control the dynamics of chip formation which can be either ductile (long continuous chips) or brittle (short broken ones).

The surface typically displays long grooves in one direction whose shape is determined in large part by the shape of the tool. Grinding is a process in which many small cutting points, typically facets of hard particles cemented together into a wheel, simultaneously remove material from a surface. Polishing results when many loose hard particles slide and roll between two surfaces, removing material as the surfaces move relative to one another. Impact erosion (such as sandblasting) uses particles to produce small craters on the surface. Each of these processes involves both plastic deformation and fracture, and has many variables such as applied forces, the presence of liquids, etc., which dramatically modify the appearance and performance of the resulting surface (as well as the tools or particles doing the work). There are a wide variety of other methods, ranging from fracture to electrical spark discharges, plastic deformation of surfaces by rolling, forging or extrusion, chemical etching, and so on, which modern technology employs to produce surfaces of parts by the removal or rearrangement of material. **Figure 1** shows a few different surfaces.

There are other methods which build up surfaces by deposition. Again, this may be physical or chemical. Liquids solidify to leave solid coatings, sometimes accompanied by polymerization or formation of crystalline structures. Some liquids solidify in a mold which controls some of the surface morphology, some do not and other forces such as viscosity and surface tension are more important. Freezing of liquids or gases onto a substrate may produce either very smooth or extremely rough surfaces depending on how the particles and molecules can move on the surface (**Figure 2**). Electroplating typically produces quite smooth surfaces by deposition of atoms from chemical solution, while ballistic deposition and aggregation of particles may generate ones with porous fractal surfaces. Some deposited layers are then subjected to selective removal, either by chemical or physical processes. This is the process by which complex multilayer electronic chips and a coming generation of micromechanical devices are fabricated.

Another concern about surfaces is their cleanliness. The presence of particulates, either lying loosely on the surface or attached by electrostatic or chemical forces, can disrupt the deposition of the carefully controlled layers used in microelectronics, so elaborate clean rooms and handling methods are required. Surface defects such as pits and scratches are also of concern. Chemical modification of surfaces is called contamination, oxidation, or corrosion depending on the circumstances. This is strongly controlled by the environment. Sometimes such processes may be carried out intentionally to protect the original surface from other environmental effects (for instance, aluminum is anodized to produce a thin oxide layer that produces a chemically inert, mechanically hard surface that resists further contamination in use). Electrical and optical properties of surfaces can be modified greatly by extremely thin contamination layers.

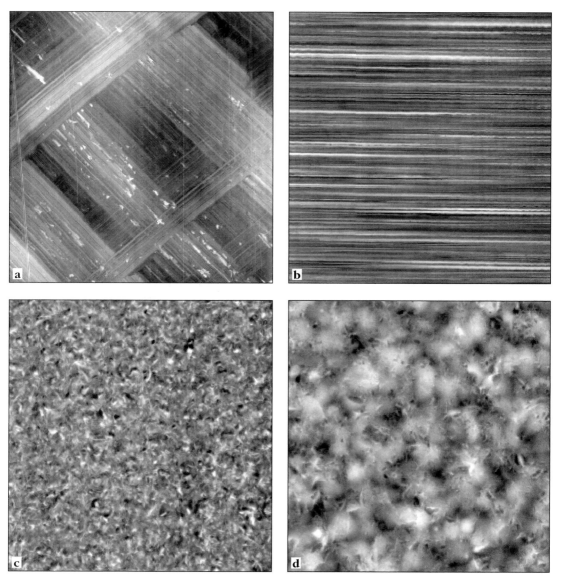

Figure 1. Range images of metal surfaces (each shows 1 square millimeter with grey scale proportional to elevation):

a) machined (flycut) surface of aluminum;

b) ground surface of stainless steel;

c) vapor-polished surface of aluminum;

d) shot-blasted surface of brass. Images courtesy Rank Taylor Hobson Ltd., obtained with a scanning probe instrument with 5 μm radius diamond stylus.

In all these cases, there is a great need to characterize the surfaces so that the topography of the surface, and perhaps other properties such as chemical composition or electrical parameters, can be determined. Some of the surface characterization data are obtained directly by imaging methods. Even when the data are obtained in other ways, visualizing the surfaces is an imaging technique, relying on the human interpretation of the

Figure 2. *Photograph of a glaze covering a ceramic pot. The glaze flows down the surface in a molten state and solidifies to an amorphous glass under the forces of surface tension. Subsequently, the atoms rearrange themselves to form crystals which nucleate and grow in the glaze, producing visually interesting patterns and also modifying the surface geometry.*

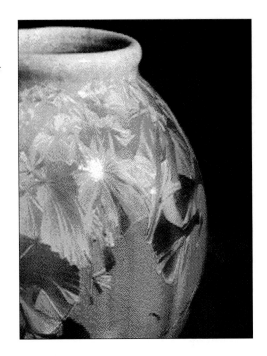

images to detect important information about the surfaces. Measurement follows to reduce the image data to a few selected numbers that can be used for process control, and to correlate the structure of the surfaces with their fabrication history on the one hand and with their performance and behavior on the other.

Devices that image surfaces by physical contact

Most of the measurement methods used to characterize surfaces are based on either some kind of microscope that provides magnified images of the surface, or scattering of radiation or particles from the surface. The methods may provide measurement of either composition or geometry, including the thickness of thin layers. Many different kinds of microscopes (and some tools that may not be conventionally thought of or named as microscopes) are used to study surfaces. Many of these require no surface preparation, or at most minimal cleaning; a few such as the SEM may require applying conductive coatings to electrical insulators. The common methods use visible light, electrons, ions, physical contact, electron tunneling, sound waves, and other signals to produce images that sometimes can be directly related to the surface geometry and in other cases are primarily influenced by the surface slope, composition, coating thickness, or microstructure. The most immediately useful imaging methods are those whose output consists of "range" values in which the elevation of the surface is directly represented in the values often shown as either profile traces or grey scale images. Although most of the examples shown here will be ones in which the grey scale directly encodes elevation, it should be understood that a similar display

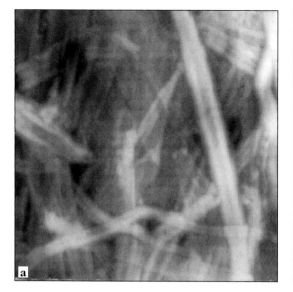

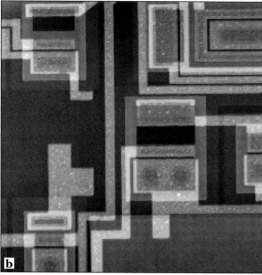

Figure 3. Range images obtained with a scanned stylus instrument:
a) paper;
b) microelectronic chip.

of chemical information or elemental concentration can be dealt with using the identical measurement and visualization tools.

One method that covers some of the newest devices such as the Atomic Force Microscope (AFM) and quite old and well established methods used in industrial manufacturing such as profilometers is the use of a mechanical stylus that is dragged across the surface. Motion of the stylus is amplified to record the elevation of the surface point by point. If a full raster scan is used, this produces an array of elevation data that can be displayed as an image, as shown by the examples in **Figure 1**. If the mass of the moving parts of the stylus assembly is kept as low as possible, forces of a few milligrams can keep the stylus in contact with the surface (at least for surfaces that have slopes up to about 45 degrees) at quite high scanning rates. The images in **Figure 1** were obtained in about 50 seconds each, as an array of 500×500 points covering a 1 mm square area.

Stylus instruments used in industry typically use diamond-tipped styli with a tip radius of about 1 micrometer, which defines the lateral resolution that the instruments can provide. Vertical motion may be sensed using inductive, capacitance or interference gauges, which are capable of subnanometer sensitivity. With suitable calibration, which is typically provided by scanning over known artefacts, these methods are routinely used to quantitatively measure surface elevations in many industrial settings to measure surface finish, the thickness of layers, etc. These instruments have primarily been used with metal and ceramic parts, but are also capable of measuring a wide variety of softer and more fragile materials as shown in **Figure 3**.

The AFM also uses a stylus but a much smaller one (Quate, 1994; Wickramasinghe, 1991). The scanning tunneling microscope (STM) stimulated a range of new microscopies which use essen-

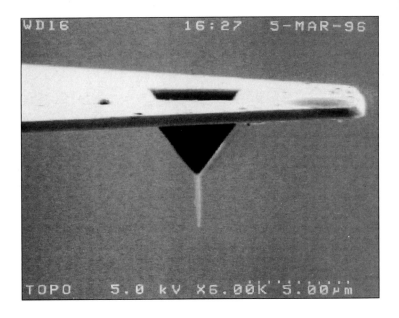

Figure 4. *Scanning electron microscope image of an ultrafine tip used for high resolution atomic force microscopy. (Image courtesy Topometrix Corp.).*

tially the same scanning and feedback principles to obtain nanometer resolution images. The atomic force microscope was introduced in 1986 as a new instrument for examining the surface of insulating crystals. There was a clear implication from the first that it would be capable of resolving single atoms, although unambiguous evidence for atomic resolution did not appear until 1993. The AFM has evolved into a flexible instrument that provides new insights in the fields of surface science, electrochemistry, biology and physics, and new adaptations of the technology continue.

By etching silicon or silicon nitride to a sharp point, or by depositing carbon in such a way that it grows into a long thin spike, a stylus can be fabricated with a tip radius of a few nanometers (**Figure 4**). This allows much greater lateral resolution than profilometer styli. But such tips are extremely fragile and easily deformed, so a variety of techniques have been devised to utilize them to probe a surface. Typically, the tip is used as a reference point and the surface is translated in the z (elevation) direction to contact it. The tip is attached to or a part of a cantilever arm whose deflection is monitored by deflection of a light beam on the rear face or sometimes by interference measurement, and vertical sensitivity below one nanometer is easily obtained. Either the sample or the stylus can be translated in an *X, Y* raster pattern to cover the entire surface to create a complete image. The translation is typically accomplished with piezoelectric devices, which limits the total range of motion.

The traditional and still most common mode of operation places the tip in sliding contact with the surface. In order to reduce the lateral and shear forces on the stylus and the surface, the stylus may be rapidly raised and lowered ("tapping mode"), or the lateral forces may be measured by the twisting of the stylus to determine the elastic modulus of the surface material, or the friction between the stylus and surface. Additional modes can be used in which physical contact is not actually required. For example, the stylus can track the surface without touching it with somewhat lower resolution by using attractive Van der Waals forces. In addition, some systems use strategies such as heating the tip and measuring the heat loss when it is close to the surface, vibrating it and measuring a change in characteristic frequency when it is close to the surface, or using it as a guide for light photons that interact with the surface and detect its presence without contact. The electric or magnetic force gradient and distribution above the sample surface can be measured using amplitude, phase or frequency shifts, while scanning capacitance microscopy measures carrier (dopant) concentration profiles on semiconductor surfaces. The original operational mode, whose development won a Nobel prize, was scanning tunneling microscopy (STM) which measures the surface electronic states in semiconducting materials. The variety of operational modes of the scanned probe microscope seems nearly unlimited as manufacturers and users experiment with them, but many of these techniques are applicable only to a particular set of materials and surface types. The same technology has been used to modify surfaces, either by pushing individual atoms around or by writing patterns into masks used for lithographic manufacture of microelectronic and micromechanical devices.

One of the problems faced by AFMs is the difficulty in making quantitative dimensional measurements. Most designs use open-loop piezoelectric ceramic devices for scanning, which suffer from hysteresis and nonlinearity. Software correction, no matter how elegant, can only go so far in correcting the resulting image distortions and measurement errors due to its inability to adapt to the topography of each individual sample. This particularly affected the use of the AFM in the metrology-intensive semiconductor industry. A few recent designs use a much more expensive approach which employs a separate interferometric measurement device in each axis to provide a closed-loop measurement of the piezo scanner's movement. These permit accurate measurements to be made on small structures such as microelectronic and micromechanical devices, magnetic storage devices, and structures such as the compact disk stamper shown in **Figure 5**.

The AFM is limited in the area that it can scan and the speed with which it can do so, and in the relief of the specimen which can be present without interfering with the cantilever arm. Special designs which attempt to alleviate one or more of these limitations are required for specific applications, as is true for all surface measurement approaches. But it is useful to have an overview of the general range of capabilities of the different techniques. **Figure 6** shows a graph (a Stedman diagram named after Margaret Stedman of the British National Physical Laboratories) that plots the range of lateral and vertical distances

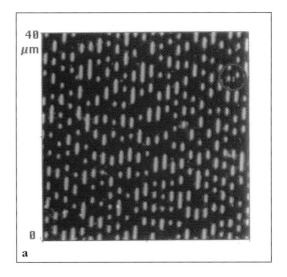

Figure 5. *AFM image of a defect on a CD stamper. The presentation modes are discussed below. (Image courtesy Topometrix Corp.).*

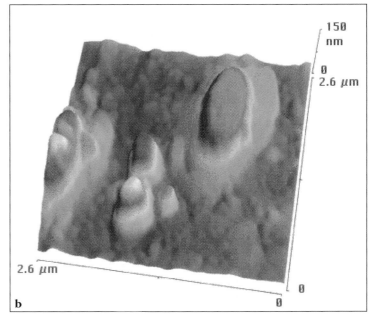

which can be accommodated by various surface measurement techniques. Notice that the minimum vertical dimensions detected by several methods is about the same, but the AFM has much better lateral resolution and the stylus instruments have a much larger range. Some of the other techniques plotted on the diagram will be discussed later in this chapter, but none of them offers a perfect combination of range and resolution in both vertical and lateral directions along with quantitative accuracy and an ability to deal with most kinds of surfaces.

Noncontacting measurements

Stylus instruments are limited in speed by the need to move a probe with finite mass across the specimen one line at a time.

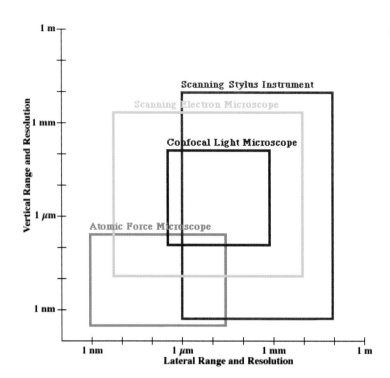

Figure 6. *Comparison of the typical range and resolution of several surface imaging technologies.*

They also touch the surface which raises concerns about specimen damage. Indeed, AFMs have been used to create surface topography as well as to image it, and industrial stylus instruments are often accused of leaving surface markings where they have been used on soft metal surfaces. For some surfaces the best solution is to make a replica that can be scanned. Plastic replicas can preserve fine detail as shown in **Figure 7**, and remove concern about damage to the original specimen.

It would seem that using light as a probe would make it possible to overcome concerns about speed or damage. Unfortunately, it also raises others. The principle concern is that the light does not interact with the same surface that the tip feels, so that the measured elevation does not agree with that from the stylus methods (which are accepted according to various international standards for surface measurement). In many materials the light waves penetrate to a small distance beneath the surface as they are reflected, and this surface impedance depends upon the dielectric properties of the material (which may be modified near the surface by contamination or oxidation layers). Very fine scale structure can also produce speckle and interference effects that alter the returned light in ways that mimic quite different surface structures and give incorrect results. Also, the presence of contaminant or oxidation films or local surface tilt angles of more than a few degrees can reduce the amount of light scattered back to the detector so that some points on the surface are not measured at all.

There are a wide variety of ways that light can be used to probe surfaces. One choice is to use a point probe of light focused to

Figure 7. Scanned stylus image of a plastic replica of human skin:
a) grey scale representation of the elevation data;
b) photorealistic visualization of the surface.

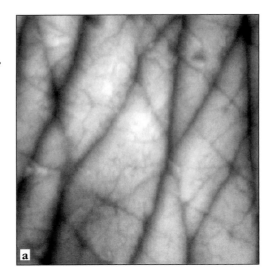

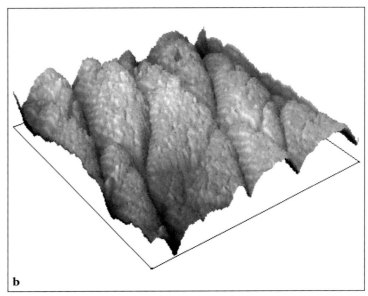

a point that is then scanned over the sample in the same way that a stylus would be, while other instruments image light from the entire area of interest at once. Point probes may use confocal optics to detect the distance to the specimen (also called focus detection), which also requires vertical scanning of either the sample or the optics. This can be done for each point, which is slow because of the need to move a finite mass, or the scan can be performed over the entire area for each Z setting as in most confocal light microscopes. In this method, the light intensity at each location is stored for each Z setting and then the peak intensity value (which may be interpolated between settings) is used to determine the surface elevation at that location. It is also possible to construct an optical point probe that uses a lens with large chromatic aberrations, and to detect the wavelength of light that is most strongly reflected. Because the lens brings each wavelength to focus at a different working distance, this provides a measure of the surface elevation. Other optical techniques such as triangulation are very sensitive to the local surface slope and have relatively poor lateral resolution.

The method which provides the greatest resolution over the greatest range is interference, and this can be done with either a point probe or for the entire surface, and with either monochromatic (usually laser) light or with white light. The classic Michelson-Morley interferometer uses mirrors to send light along two pathways, and then recombines them to produce interference patterns that show fringes corresponding to differences in dimensions that can be much smaller than the wavelength of the light. When one leg of the interferometer reflects light from the sample surface, these fringes can be used to directly measure surface elevations. The lateral resolution is only as good as the light microscope used to collect the reflected light, or about 1 μm, but the depth resolution can be 1 nm or better. However, for samples that do not reflect light well or that have steep cliffs or deep pits, there may not be enough light reflected, or the spacing of the fringes may be too close together, to provide results.

When monochromatic light is used it is possible to interpolate the elevation of a point to about 1 nm, about 1/1000th the wavelength of light. However, the fringes must be far enough apart (the surface elevation must vary gradually) that it is possible to keep track of the changes in elevation because the interference pattern repeats with every multiple of the light wavelength. Many modern systems use more than one wavelength of light or white light instead. This produces constructive interference only at one focal depth, where the path lengths are equal and all of the wavelengths are in phase. When a surface is being imaged, this means that only points along one isoelevation contour are bright. Varying the distance between the specimen and the optics allows scanning in Z to determine the elevation of points over the entire image. This takes longer than a simple monochromatic interference pattern but can handle surfaces with much more relief and steeper slopes.

Indirect interference techniques such as projection of grids to produce moiré patterns, also produce two-dimensional arrays of elevation data. Imagine light streaming through venetian blinds onto the floor of a room. If the floor is flat, the strips of light will be straight when viewed from above. If there are irregularities, they show up directly as deviations in the lines of light and shadow. Scaled down to the dimensions of interest on surfaces, or at least to distances of a few micrometers which is the resolution of the light optics used to view the stripes, this same structured light method is easily used to measure surface geometry. Image processing can be used to detect the edges of the shadows, interpolating along each scan line to accuracies much better than the pixel spacing. Depending on the geometry this can produce vertical measurement accuracy similar to the lateral resolution of the optics (typically about 1 μm), but of course for only a few locations across the sample surface unless the line pattern is scanned. Toolmakers' microscopes and quality control examination of planed surfaces of lumber (among other applications) use the same basic method.

In a modern modification of the technique, mirrors or prisms are used to deflect a beam of laser light in patterns across the work piece to produce the same type of image. This has the advantage of being able to measure in various orientations and directions. Closely related to the idea of structured light is shadowing of surfaces with evaporated or deposited metal or carbon coatings, followed by measurement of the shadows cast by features and irregularities on the surface. If the image of the grid pattern in the incident light passes through another similar grid, it produces a moiré pattern, whose dark lines can be used to reveal the shape of the object. This technique is particularly useful for revealing local strains and deviations of surfaces from ideal geometric forms. Because it is fast and noncontacting, this method is often used in medical applications, ranging from orthopedic work on curvature of the spine to measuring the curvature of the lens of the eye before and after corrective surgery.

Microscopy of surfaces

Most forms of microscopy produce images in which intensity is related to the reflection of light (or some other signal) from the surface. This is only indirectly related to the surface geometry, and includes other information such as composition. In spite of the difficulties in interpretation, this is still the most widespread procedure for surface examination.

The standard light microscope at moderately high magnification has a comparatively shallow depth of field. This creates many problems for examining surfaces. If the surface is not extremely flat and perpendicular to the optical axis (for example, a metallographically polished specimen), it cannot all be focused at the same time. Only low magnification light microscopes can be used to examine rough surfaces (e.g., for fractography), and do not give much information about surface geometry. The pattern of light scattered by rough surfaces under diffuse lighting can be used to determine the roughness. It has been shown (Russ, 1994; Pentland, 1984) that a surface with fractal geometry will scatter diffuse light to produce a fractal pattern, and that there is a relationship between the fractal dimension of the surface and that of the light. This has also been reported for scanning electron microscope images of such surfaces. But measuring the overall roughness dimension of the surface is not the same thing as determining the actual coordinates of points on the surface.

On the other hand, the depth of field of the conventional light microscope is too great to measure the important dimensions in the vertical direction on rough surfaces. Paradoxically, the confocal light microscope has a much shallower depth of field (and more importantly rejects stray light from locations away from the plane and point of focus), which allows it to produce true range images from irregular surfaces. In the confocal microscope, the image is built up one point at a time (usually in a raster pattern). Each image corresponds only to points at a particular focal depth, but repeating this operation at many focal depths produces both an extended focus image in which the entire surface is imaged, and a range image in which the elevation at each point is recorded. The resolution in both vertical and lateral directions is much worse than the scanned probe microscopes, but quite useful for many surface measurement applications including metrology of some microelectronic devices.

Because of its very large depth of field, coupled with excellent resolution (typically <10 nm, much better than the light microscope) the SEM is often a tool of choice for the examination of rough surfaces. Furthermore, the appearance of the secondary electron image that is most often recorded from this instrument looks reasonably "familiar" to most observers, who therefore believe they can interpret the image to obtain geometric information. Unfortunately, this is not at all simple. **Figure 8** shows an SEM image of a surface, sintered tungsten carbide particles. This is a relatively simple surface composed of uniform composition

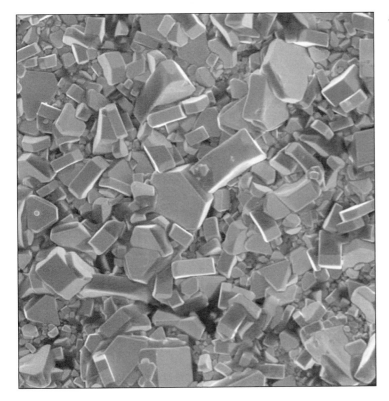

Figure 8. SEM image of the surface of sintered tungsten carbide.

particles with relatively flat facets. But there is no unique or simple relationship between elevation or slope and the local pixel brightness. For relatively smooth surfaces, "shape from shading" methods can convert changes in intensity to changes in slope and thus extract the geometry. The influence of fine-scale roughness, edges, surface contamination or compositional variation, etc., prevents this from being a general purpose approach. Backscattered electron imaging is less sensitive to many of these effects and is used for some metrology applications, but only gives "real" geometric dimensions when comparison to standards is available or extensive modeling of the interactions between electron and sample is performed.

The great frustration in using the SEM to examine surfaces is that while the images look quite natural to human viewers, and seem to represent surface elevation in a familiar way, determining actual dimension values from them is nearly impossible except in very constrained cases. Metrology of integrated circuits is used to determine lateral dimensions, but even in these cases the definition of just what the relationship is between the physical contour of an edge and the voltage profile of the signal is far from certain (and highly dependent upon the voltage used, the material being imaged, the detector type and location, etc.). Metrology is used for quality control in which consistency rather than absolute accuracy is important, and there is no attempt to extract measurements in the Z direction from such images (indeed, even the visibility of points near the bottoms of grooves or contact holes is a problem).

Stereometric imaging in which two (or more) different views of the surface are combined to measure elevation is the same in principle as the generation of topographic contour maps from aerial photographs (Wong, 1980; Wang, 1990). However, this is not an easy technique to automate (Wrobel, 1991; Heipke, 1992; Barnard & Thompson, 1980; Zhou & Dorrer, 1994; Abbasi-Dezfouli & Freeman, 1994), and even with careful control of imaging conditions and measurement of angles, the vertical resolution is typically much worse than the lateral resolution of the individual images. This is because the tilt angle δ between the two views must usually be small (7–10 degrees is typical) to prevent points being hidden in one of the two views, and the angle enters the calculation as $1/\sin(\delta)$. Small uncertainties in δ are magnified and limit the precision of the final result.

Measurement of the elevation difference between individual points is usually quite straightforward using a human to locate the same points in the two images. Then the parallax or offset of the points gives the elevation by straightforward trigonometry. However, to generate an elevation map for an entire surface requires matching a great many points, and requires automation to be practical. The two methods used for this are area-based or feature-based. Area-based matching uses cross-correlation (either in the spatial domain or the frequency domain) to find the location of an area in the second image that most closely matches each area in the first. Any change in the visibility or contrast of the area between the two images, or the presence of repetitive structures, produces problems for this approach. Feature matching detects locations in each image which have some characteristic such as a local maximum value of variance. These points are then matched against the similar list of points in the other image. This is generally more successful, but may match only a few thousand locations in the two images out of perhaps a million pixels, so that the intervening locations can only be interpolated. In all cases, constraints such as preserving the order of points from left to right and knowing the direction of tilt so that searching for matches need only occur in a small fraction of the total image area are important aids to the practical implementation of the methods.

The SEM is also used to generate X-ray maps of surface composition, discussed separately below.

Instead of using electrons, light or other radiation to form an image of the surface, quite a lot of information is available from the scattering or diffraction patterns that are produced. X-ray patterns contain data about the structure of either crystalline or amorphous layers. Electron scattering patterns contain information on the crystallographic arrangement and also on local strains in the material. Scattered patterns of electromagnetic radiation are in effect the Fourier transform of the elevation profiles of the surface and their measurement is therefore a direct way to study the surface elevation in a way that separates the information on the form or figure (the intended large scale geometry of the part), the waviness (medium scale departures from the figure), and the texture or roughness (the fine scale details on the surface). In many cases, the scattering of reflected light may also be directly related to the intended use of the surface, for instance if it is a high-precision mirror. Patterns such as diffraction patterns can be processed and measured using many of the same techniques as more conventional images, but are not discussed here in any detail.

Surface composition imaging

The variety of techniques for probing surfaces is astoundingly broad. Some of the more common ones are the SEM using an X-ray detector, the ion microscope or microprobe using secondary ion mass spectrometry (SIMS), and Fourier transform infrared (FTIR) spectroscopy. There are many other tools used as well particularly for measuring the thickness and composition of coatings. These include the backscattering of particles, which samples the composition and density of the sample at depths up to several micrometers beneath the surface. Also of rather specialized interest is acoustic microscopy, which is sensitive to debonding between the coating layer and substrate. Gigahertz acoustic waves have a wavelength similar to visible light, and can be used to image surface and near-surface structures that are difficult to detect with other signals. Surface waves are strongly reflected by cracks (even closed ones that cannot be seen otherwise) and bulk waves are similarly reflected by the surfaces of pores (although these subsurface waves only propagate at lower frequencies, with correspondingly poorer resolution). The speed of sound in the material can also be measured to determine the modulus of elasticity and other physical properties. Ellipsometry takes advantage of the fact that for many types of thin layer coatings, the plane of polarized light is rotated as it passes through the coating. Measurement of that rotation can provide highly precise coating thickness measurements, and when different wavelengths of light are used (or a spectrometer is used to scan an entire range of wavelengths) can also reveal details about the internal structure of the coating. However, this method is primarily used to measure relatively large spots and not to produce images of the surface. Similarly, another spot-analysis analytical technique uses a laser-beam directed at a selected point on the surface using a light microscope to vaporize material from a pit (typically several μm across and deep) blasted from the surface so that the atomic and molecular fragments can be weighed in a mass spectrometer.

There are several different types of ion microscopes. Many can produce elemental composition maps of the surface, or a series of such images at various depths in the material. An incident beam of ions knocks the uppermost layer of atoms loose from the specimen, either one point at a time (the ion microprobe) or over the entire surface at once. These atoms are ionized and are then accelerated into a mass spectrometer which separates them according to their mass/charge ratio, identifying specific elements and isotopes. A detector or detector array then produces an image. This typically represents the spatial distribution of one selected element at a time across the imaged area, with a lateral resolution of about 1 μm (depending on the diameter of the incident beam in the case of the ion microprobe and the resolution of the ion optics in the case of the ion microscope) but with a depth resolution of one atomic layer. Rapid switching from one element to another as layers are removed produces complete data sets of the structure of the material.

Compositional mapping of surfaces is particularly important for examination of deposited coatings and the identification of contamination. The most common approach to this mapping uses a raster-scanned electron beam to generate characteristic X-rays from the atoms present, which are then detected. The unique energy or wavelength of the X-rays identifies the elements, and calculations based on the physics of X-ray generation can be used to determine their amounts. The lateral and depth resolution is limited to the order of 1 μm by the range of the electrons.

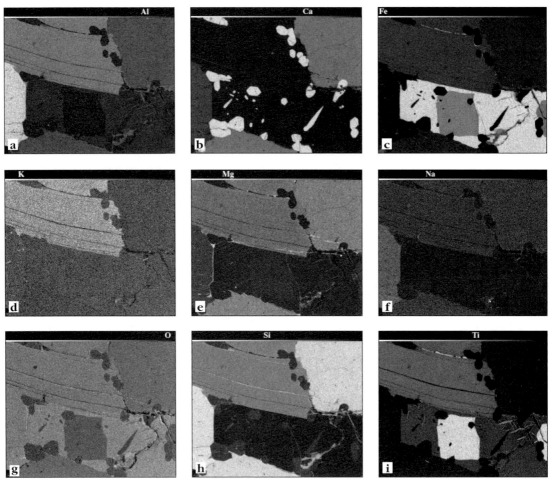

Figure 9. *X-ray maps from a mineral (mica) showing the location of several elements (as labeled on each image). Each dot corresponds to the location of the beam when one X-ray with the proper energy was detected. Some of these X-rays are the Bremsstrahlung background and not characteristic X-rays of the element selected, which produces a finite background level in parts of the image where the specimen may not contain the element. Only in areas of high concentration are the boundaries of phase regions well delineated. (Images courtesy Pia Wahlberg, Danish Technological Institute).*

Several different types of X-ray spectrometers are used; the diffractive or wavelength-dispersive type measures X-rays from one element at a time but with good trace element sensitivity while the more common energy-dispersive type can measure all of the elements present at the same time, but with poorer detectability. These typically produce "dot map" images for several elements at once (**Figure 9**) which only approximately delineate the regions containing the elements and must be processed and combined as discussed below. Other signals, such as Auger electrons, come from a smaller region near the point of entry of the focused electron beam and have better spatial and depth resolution, but because the signal to noise level is poor are not so good at detecting minor and trace elements.

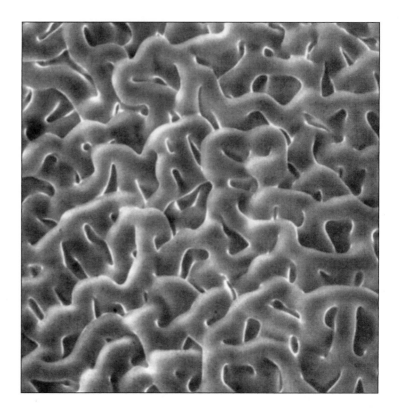

Figure 10. *Scanning electron microscope of the complex surface of a polymer, with undercuts and bridges.*

Molecular identification of coatings and contamination can be made using infrared spectroscopy, in which various vibratory modes of the molecules are excited to produce characteristic spectral peaks. This method is most suitable to the analysis of organic materials and coatings, such as plastics. The spatial resolution of this approach is limited to several micrometers by the light optics used.

Processing of range images

Elevation data from surfaces produced by the various methods discussed above are typically recorded as 8- or 16-bit greyscale images. Each pixel has a value that represents the physical elevation or composition of the corresponding surface location. Since most of the techniques described look vertically down upon the surface, the data are single valued and represent only the uppermost point for surfaces whose irregularity is so great that undercuts and bridges can occur. The SEM is an exception to this, as shown in **Figure 10**, which shows a complex polymer surface with undercuts and bridges which a range image cannot reveal. Integer data stored for each pixel in a range image can be converted to an elevation value in appropriate units (nm, μm, etc.) using scale data that are usually stored in the file header. There is unfortunately no standard format for this data, and not only does each manufacturer have its own (which are not always readily available or well documented) but some have more than one corresponding to different instruments.

Reading in these different file formats and storing the data in some standardized format such as TIFF files may require custom programming. Some image processing and display programs do have the ability to read arrays of data (i.e., images) in a wide variety of data formats provided that the user can specify (or deduce) the necessary format information. This typically includes at least the length of the header and perhaps where specific scaling or other information is stored within it, the dimensions of the array and whether the data are stored in rows or columns, and the data format (byte, integer, long integer, real, etc., and whether the byte order is Intel or Motorola — low word first or high word first).

Once the data are available, the kinds of processing that are required for surface images depend strongly on what kind of instrument was used. Some examples will serve to illustrate the possibilities:

Interference microscopes often have drop-out pixels where the local slope of the surface was too great (more than a few degrees from normal) to return enough light to the optics to permit measurement. These points can be detected by filling the array beforehand with an illegal or impossible value that is replaced by real measurement data. Any pixel that retains the original value is a dropout point and must be filled in, and the most common way to do this is with a median filter. A simple median would suffice for single points, but in many cases regions several pixels across or arranged as a line corresponding to some step or ridge on the surface may be dropped out. In this case a modification of the median approach is necessary. For example, for each dropout pixel, build an array of the neighborhood pixels that are not dropouts. If this is not an empty list, rank them into order and find the median, and place it into the missing location. After this has been done for all of the dropout pixels in the image, see if any remain. If so, repeat the process until every point has been filled in. This will fill in even large areas from their periphery and is generally preferable to linear interpolation between pixels around the dropout, which produces blurred and smoothed edges.

A slight improvement in the basic iterated median can be achieved by using a weighted median in which pixels contribute to the decision on the value to be entered into the central pixel in proportion to how far away they are. For a 3×3 neighborhood, the corner pixels are $\sqrt{2}$ farther away than the ones that share an edge. Placing each corner pixel value into the list of values to be sorted twice and placing the edge pixel values into the list three times gives a ratio of 1.5 which is close to 1.414... and produces the desired weighted median when the list is sorted. For a 5 pixel wide circular neighborhood (**Figure 11**) the pixel distances are 1, $\sqrt{2}$, 2, and $\sqrt{5}$. Weights of 3 for the edge neighbors,

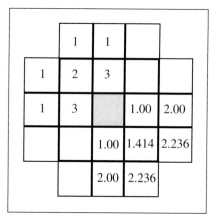

Figure 11. *Weighted median filter duplicates pixel values 2 or 3 times for the closest pixels approximately in inverse proportion to their distance from the center, as shown in the pattern.*

2 for the corner neighbors, and 1 each for the more distant pixels approximate the relative contribution of the neighbors according to their distance. Note that this weighting increases the length of the list of values that must be sorted, which slows the operation significantly and is why larger integer weights which would more closely match the inverse distances are not used. For a single dropout pixel with all 20 neighbors in a 5 pixel wide circle contributing, the sorting list grows from 20 values to 32, approximately doubling the sorting time. If the list of values is even in length rather than odd, the average of the two central values in the sorted list may be used.

Stylus instruments, whether macroscopic ones with diamond tips several micrometers in diameter or atomic force microscopes using Buckytubes to probe much smaller lateral dimensions, share some of the same image analysis problems. The scan rate along each line (the *X*-direction) is typically determined by the dynamics of the stylus itself — the mass of the moving tip and the applied force — which determines the maximum speed at which the tip can move across the surface while remaining in contact with it. Too high a force will result in damage to the surface or the tip, but too low a restoring force will allow the tip to skip over holes or fly from rising slopes. Depending on whether the stylus moves some sensing element (an interferometer, capacitance or inductance gauge for example) or the surface is moved to null the position of the stylus (the typical AFM mode of operation) and the signal to the piezoelectric drivers is recorded, the output signal for the surface elevation is usually an electrical voltage. This must be amplified and then digitized, and in the process suitable filtering can be applied with a time constant appropriate for the scanning speed. This reduces the noise along each scan line, and eliminates the need for subsequent digital filtering to be required to reduce noise. Filtering may be used as discussed below to separate the low frequency signals related to surface form and waviness from the high frequency roughness value, but that is part of the process of measurement rather than image enhancement.

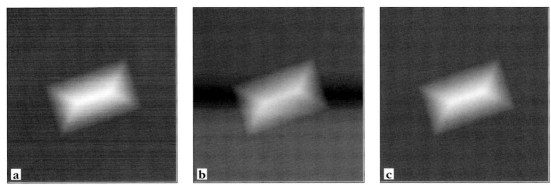

Figure 12. *AFM scan of an etch pit in silicon, showing the line offsets in the raw image* ***(a)***, *the darkening artefact resulting from correction by adjusting the mean value of each line* ***(b)***, *and the improved result using the median value* ***(c)***.

The situation is quite different in the *Y*-direction (from one line to the next). A significant amount of time passes between sequential lines in the raster scan, allowing for changes in the mechanical and electronic components. Most systems scan in one direction only (to minimize hysteresis problems) and have a retrace scan during which the stylus is raised and not in contact with the sample. Repositioning the stylus to the exact same value is very difficult when the resolution of these methods in the vertical direction is of the order of 1 nm. The result is that subsequent scan lines tend to be offset from each other. Since the eye is sensitive to abrupt changes in brightness that extend over large distances, this produces images in which a visible horizontal stripe pattern may be seen. Some AFM manufacturers attempt to alleviate this problem by adjusting each line so that the average value is the same as that of the preceding line. This is rarely a good idea — it means for example that if there is a rising peak somewhere in the image area, the background around the peak will be depressed as the peak rises, producing false data and even an incorrect visual impression of the surface, as shown in **Figure 12**.

There is a better solution than the mean or average value for this line-to-line adjustment, although it requires more computation. The ideal solution would be to align the mode values of sequential lines of data. Under the assumption that the surface consists primarily of a background level with some roughness superimposed on it, plus major features of interest that rise or fall with respect to that plane, the mode is by definition the most probable surface elevation value. For a relatively small collection of data points (most area scans have only a few hundred data points along each line), the mode is not robustly determined. But for any distribution the median is closer to the mode than is the mean. Just as the median value is preferred over the mean for filtering noise from an array of pixels, so the median offers a workable solution for adjusting the scan lines in a raster scan stylus image. **Figure 13** shows this method applied to a typical image of a rough surface.

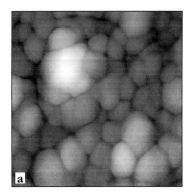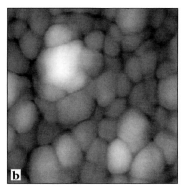

Figure 13. *AFM scan of a chemically deposited surface before (**a**) and after (**b**) the correction of line offsets.*

Another artefact in AFM images that is best avoided by proper attention to the hardware but which seems in principle to be correctable to some extent in software, is the deconvolution of tip shape from the images. As discussed in Chapter 5, if the point spread function of an image can be measured, dividing the Fourier transform of the image by the transform of the point spread function can remove much of the smearing or loss of resolution, so that the inverse transform yields an improved image. Real AFM tips are far from perfect, exhibiting various departures from a ideal symmetrical point. Scanning the tip over a known artefact such as a circular disk (Jarausch et al., 1996; Keller & Franke, 1991, 1993; Markiewicz & Goh, 1994, 1995; Villarrubia, 1994, 1996) allows calculation of the tip shape, and permits this deconvolution. In practice the tips have a short life and no two are identical, so that frequent recalibration is required. However, the correction is only important at the highest magnification and finest resolution levels.

Processing of composition maps

Most surface composition maps that are obtained by ion mass spectroscopy, X-ray energy spectroscopy, or other methods, suffer from low signal levels. As discussed in Chapter 3 this can in principle be rectified by collecting more data, but this is generally not desirable on economic grounds and sometimes is impossible because the analysis alters or consumes the surface. Hence noise reduction methods such as weighted smoothing or median filtering are often applicable. **Figure 14** shows the Potassium X-ray map from **Figure 10** processed with a Gaussian smoothing operator, a conventional median and a hybrid median. Compare the preservation of edges, corners and fine lines by the various methods.

When multiple images are obtained of the same area showing the spatial distribution of different elements or other chemical data, it is very important to find ways to display them in combinations that will communicate the information to the observer, and to find ways to delineate and distinguish the various phases that are present. Combining multiple images as color planes

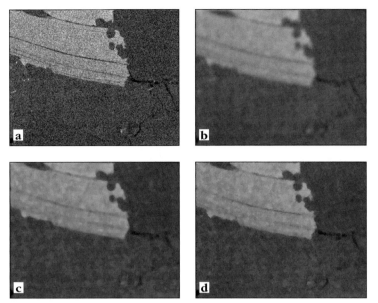

Figure 14. X-ray image for K from Figure 9:

a) *with the random statistical fluctuations in X-ray intensity from point to point reduced by*

b) *a Gaussian blur, σ = 1.5 pixels;*

c) *a conventional median filter (5 pixel wide circular neighborhood); and*

d) *a hybrid median filter of the same size.*

offers one approach to this, as shown in **Figure 15**. However, because of the way that the display hardware (and human vision) works this allows only three planes (R, G, and B) to be assigned and there may be many more individual images available than that. The situation is analogous to the situation for remote sensing images; the Landsat thematic mapper records 7 wavelength bands from the visible into the infrared, and other satellites capture even more. There is no straightforward way to "see" all of this information at one time, and the choice of which planes to show and in which colors can be quite subjective and can reveal (or conceal) quite different aspects of the information.

If the individual elemental maps can be thresholded to correspond to the intensity levels from individual phases, then Boolean combination of the planes using AND and NOT permits forming binary images of each phase, which can then be measured. This process corresponds to setting up threshold ranges in an *N*-dimensional intensity space corresponding to the number of

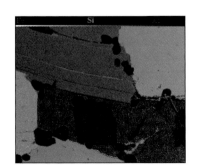
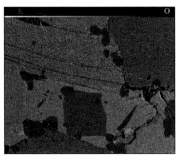
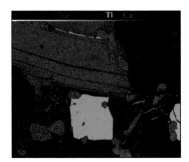

Figure 15. *Color combinations from the nine elemental X-ray maps in Figure 9. Since each of the three planes (R, G, B) can be assigned to any of the nine planes, there are more than 500 different way to display this one data set.*

elements present, in which the ranges are rectangular prisms in shape. This is often adequate to distinguish the phases present in real materials, but a more free-form shape that corresponded to the natural variations in intensity for each phase would be preferred.

There are statistical techniques that plot the intensity of each pixel in each of the image planes as a vector or point in n-space (9 dimensions for the example shown here), and then search for clusters in that space. Once clusters are identified and the boundaries around them defined, the various phases present can be identified (MacQueen, 1968; Anderberg, 1973; Hartigan, 1975). The pixels whose values lie within each cluster are then classified as belonging to the corresponding phase, and a new image can be generated with unique colors for each class so that the phases are delineated (Bright et al., 1988; Mott, 1995; DeMandolx & Davoust, 1997). **Figure 16** shows the results of an unsupervised cluster analysis technique using principal components analysis applied to the raw data from **Figure 9**; seven phases are identified and arbitrarily color coded.

When there is *a priori* information about the composition of the various phases expected to be present, this method works quite well. However, cluster detection without such information suffers from several problems. First, the statistical techniques will always be better able (in a statistical sense) to segment the space by defining more clusters, so unless the number of phase clusters is known the results are suspect. Second, clusters for minor phases representing only a few percent by volume of the structure will be represented by only a few percent of the points. Although these phases may be very important (e.g., for the properties of materials and the economics of mineral ores) they will be poorly defined in the n-space plot and very hard to detect. They are likely to be overlooked amid the background of points from pixels that straddle boundaries between major phases. Principal components methods are more likely to segment single phase regions based on minor gradients in composition or statistical variations in intensity, rather than to identify the presence of important minor phase regions.

Data presentation and visualization

Many types of surface measurement instruments produce data arrays with very large range-to-resolution ratios. In other words the number of bits that encode the elevation or other surface characterization data are very large. Most image processing and display programs cope adequately with 256 grey levels, but even this exceeds the ability of human vision to distinguish them on a computer screen. Resolution of 1 nm over a range of 1 mm, which is quite possible with a high-precision stylus or interferometric instrument, produces a million levels (20 bits). This exceeds the capabilities of displays or of perception. Conse-

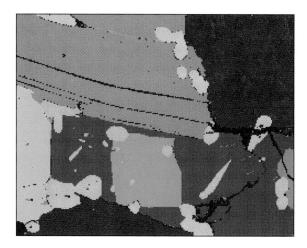

Figure 16. *Color-coding of the seven major phases in the mica sample from Figure 9, as identified by an unsupervised cluster analysis method.*

quently the display routines must either select one part of the entire range to display, or compress the data to show the entire range. Processing can help, for instance by dealing with local slopes or derivatives rather than absolute values, but this also requires some user experience to interpret.

Range images, in which the grey scale value at each pixel represents the elevation (or some other surface parameter) at that point, contain all of the raw information in the data array. Even if the range can be accommodated by the display (for instance by dividing down the resolution with which the data were acquired), the resulting image is an unfamiliar one to human observers, and requires experience to interpret. Using false colors to increase the ability to visually discriminate small changes makes the resulting images even more unfamiliar.

Contour maps draw isoelevation lines, which are exactly the same as topographic maps of the earth's surface. These are familiar to many people and can be more easily interpreted because they make it easy to follow the contour lines to identify the shape of protrusions and valleys, and to identify points at the same elevation. Of course, they also eliminate a great deal of information (the elevation data for all of the other pixels on the surface), but this is part of the simplification that makes interpretation easier. **Figure 17** shows the elevation of a familiar object displayed as a grey scale range image, one that has been color-coded, and one reduced to a small number of contour lines (which have also been color coded to make it easier to distinguish their elevation values).

Contour maps are less successful at communicating visual information when the lateral scale of detail is finer, or when the surface is very anisotropic, as shown in **Figure 18**. In these cases the individual lines are close together and hard to distinguish, and the lines do not tie together different areas of the surface very well. Whenever contour lines become close together because of

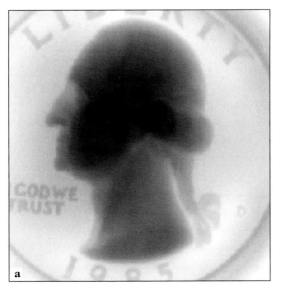

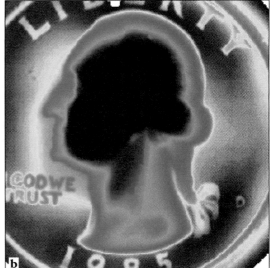

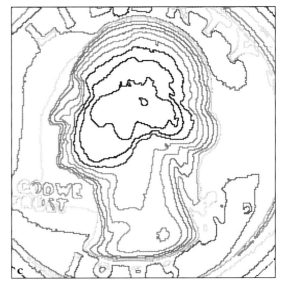

Figure 17. Range image of a coin (from scanning stylus instrument, data courtesy of Paul Scott, Rank Taylor Hobson Ltd.), displayed as:

a) *a greyscale range image;*

b) *a color-coded range image;*

c) *a color-coded contour map with ten isoelevation lines.*

the presence of fine detail or steep slopes, it is necessary to reduce the number of contour lines to help clarify the map.

The visual impression of surface relief can be improved by processing. A directional derivative creates an "embossed" appearance with light and dark contrast along edges and gradients. As discussed in Chapter 4, a kernel of weights of the form

$$
\begin{array}{ccc}
+1 & +1 & 0 \\
+1 & 0 & -1 \\
0 & -1 & -1
\end{array}
$$

produces the effect of lighting the surface from the upper left corner and produces the effect of shadows which the eye interprets as relief. The direction should always be from the top; if bright

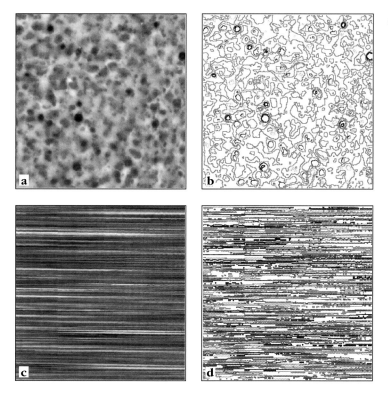

Figure 18. Range images and contour maps (with five isoelevation lines) for an injection molded polymer surface (a,b) and a ground metal surface (c,d).

edges appear on the bottoms of edges the human vision system (which is accustomed to lighting from above) inverts the interpretation of the data and perceives hills as pits and vice versa.

The derivative image shows fine detail but hides the overall elevation changes in the data. This can be alleviated by combining the greyscale range image with the derivative. This may be done by adding the two (simply change the central value in the kernel from 0 to 1), but results that correspond more closely to the way vision perceives texture on surfaces can be obtained by multiplying the two images together. This is shown in **Figure 19**. A particularly attractive version of this display can be constructed by using the information from a color coded range image as well. In **Figure 19d** a hue, saturation, intensity (HSI) model was used with the elevation assigned to the hue for each pixel and the derivative assigned to the intensity (saturation is set to 50%). The shadows create an impression of relief while the color informs the eye about overall elevation values.

These results compare quite favorably to the results of a true rendering of the surface using each triangle of neighboring pixels as a facet and calculating the reflection of light from a light source in a fixed position as shown in **Figure 20**. In this type of calculation the surface can be given various reflectivity characteristics, either more diffuse or more specular. In the examples shown a full ray-tracing and Phong shading was used. The latter method varies the shade across each facet according to the angle varia-

Figure 19. *Enhancement of the image of the coin from Figure 17 using:*

a) *a directional derivative;*

b) *the derivative multiplied by the original grey values;*

c) *the same with the original grey values inverted to place white at the high elevations;*

d) *a color image with the elevation in the hue plane and the derivative in the intensity image.*

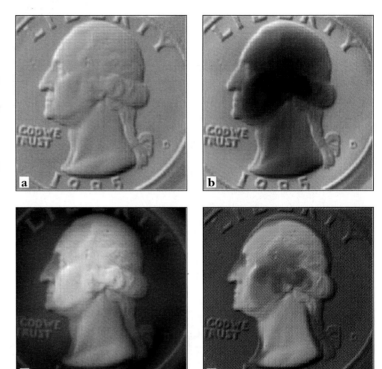

Figure 20. *Rendered surfaces of the coin (from Figure 17) and the polymer (from Figure 18), treating the surface as though it were a diffuse scatterer (plaster of Paris) or a specular one (shiny plastic or metal). The grid pattern visible in the coin image is an artefact of the scanner used to obtain the images, which becomes more visually evident in this display mode.*

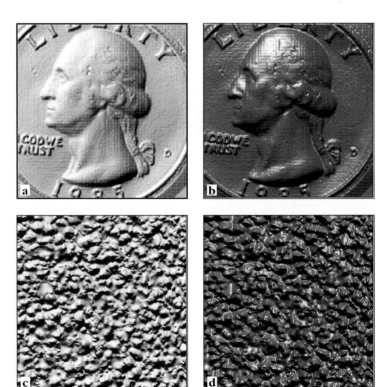

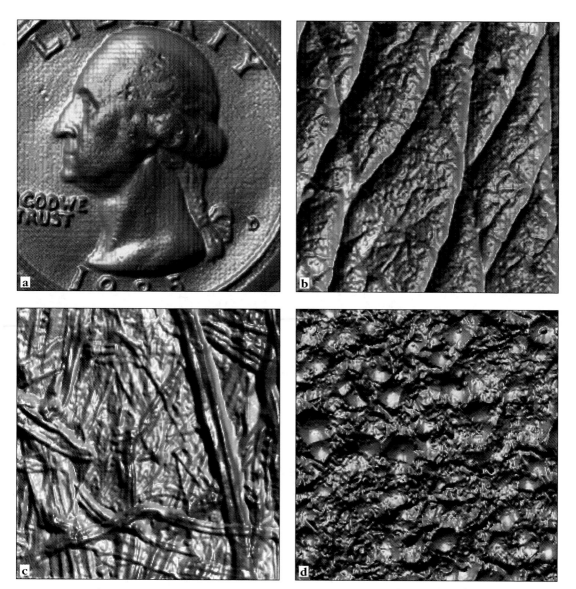

Figure 21. Color coded rendered surfaces using the hue/intensity combination method from Figure 19 with rendering as in Figure 20:
a) coin (from Figure 18);
b) skin (from Figure 7);
c) paper (from Figure 3a);
d) shotblasted metal (from Figure 1d).

tion between neighboring facets, and produces a very smooth and realistic rendered surface as used in computer-assisted drafting (CAD) workstations. The rendered image can also be color-coded, by using the grey scale rendering of reflectivity as the intensity channel and the elevation as the hue channel as discussed above. Examples of this are shown in **Figure 21**.

Rendering and visualization

The views shown above all look onto the surface from directly above. This normal view shows all of the data, but is not the most familiar to a human observer. The use of computer graphics to render the surface from an oblique point of view (which many programs allow to be selected or even interactively

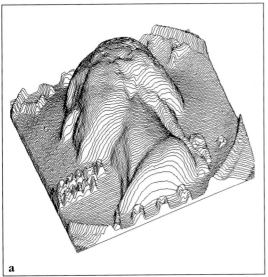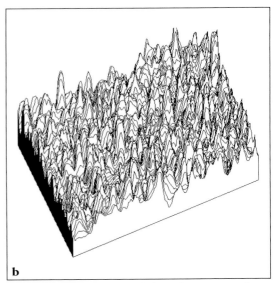

Figure 22. *Isometric line profile displays of the coin image from Figure 17 (**a**) and the polymer image from Figure 18 (**b**).*

rotated) produces an image that makes it easier to visualize the surface morphology, and perhaps to detect the features of interest. The oldest and simplest approach to this is to plot elevation profiles along some of the horizontal rows of pixels, displacing each line vertically and laterally to create the effect of a surface, and skipping some rows so that the lines are adequately spaced apart. **Figure 22** shows two examples of this. In the first, the coin image from **Figure 17**, the lines are well spaced and the surface slopes gradual enough that there are only a few places where lines are hidden (and erased). The result is a fairly easy surface to interpret. In the second example, the polymer image from **Figure 18**, the presentation is harder to interpret because so many lines cross each other and the overall morphology is obscured. Also in these displays the width of each line profile is the same, so that there is no perspective applied to the view. In this type of isometric presentation the human familiarity with the rules of perspective causes this constant width of the data to be misinterpreted as giving the array a wider apparent dimension at the back than at the front.

With the continued advance in computer graphics capabilities, in the form of more processing power and displays with more grey levels and colors, much more realistic presentations can be generated. Adding perspective also makes the data seem more realistic, and adding cross lines that connect together points on successive line profiles breaks the surface up into an array of square or rectangular tiles that improve the interpretability of the surface morphology by showing slopes in the second direction. Increasing the line density provides more information, but still must omit many lines and rows of pixels in order to avoid overwhelming the eye with too many disappearing lines. Coloring in the tiles

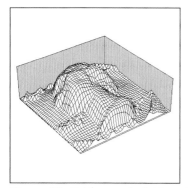 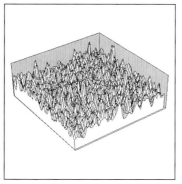 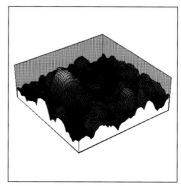

Figure 23. *Grid or mesh displays of the coin (Figure 17), polymer (Figure 18) and deposited surface (Figure 12).*

according to the elevation of the points provides additional cues to depth. The results (shown in **Figure 23**) represented the state of the art for desktop computers only a few years ago.

The most visually realistic presentation uses actual surface rendering to control the brightness of each facet on the surface. Rather than square tiles which must be bent to fit the four corner points (which in general will not lie in a plane), triangular tiles are simpler to deal with. Three corner points define the triangle and the orientation of the facet with respect to the line of sight, and a light source location permits calculation of the intensity to be assigned to the facet. This can be done with complete photorealism given the time and computing power, but there will in general be a very large number of facets to render and faster methods are sought. We can turn again to the technique used in **Figure 19** and shade each facet according to the product of its absolute height and its derivative to produce a very quick and visually realistic rendering.

Figure 24 illustrates this method. In **Figure 22a** the edges of the individual triangular facets are drawn in for clarity. But with this

Figure 24. Deposited surface rendered with triangular facets whose brightness is the product of the elevation and slope:
a) *large facets that are 6 pixels wide;*
b) *facets for each pixel and its immediate neighbors.*

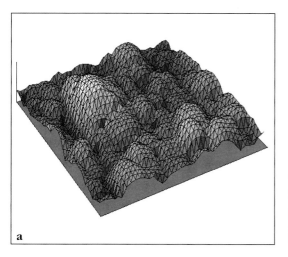 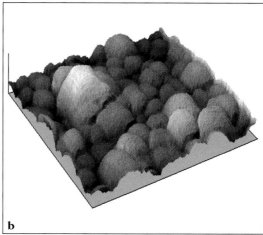

a

b

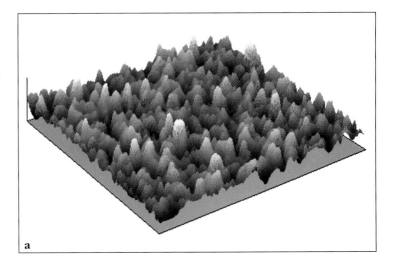

a

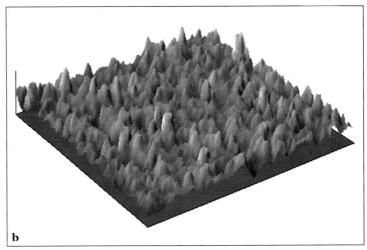

b

method it is practical to create a facet for every pixel and its immediate neighbors, so the full resolution of the data set can be displayed. The result is shown in **Figure 22b**. In computer graphics (as used in CAD programs for example) it is common to apply shading to facets so that they blend in with their neighbors (Gourard or Phong shading) and do not reveal lines where they meet. But while that method is important for the small number of large facets encountered in CAD renderings, it is unnecessary for the tiny facets that correspond to each pixel, because the facets may cover only 1 or 2 points on the display. This also speeds up the process.

It is useful to compare this method against the slightly simpler display procedure of using the elevation to shade the facets, or using false colors to indicate elevation, as shown in **Figure 25**. These methods produce much less realistic results for visualization, and require a more educated eye on the part of the user. It is important to understand that human vision is an important tool for

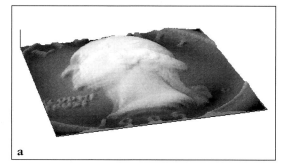

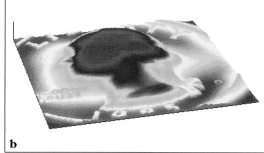

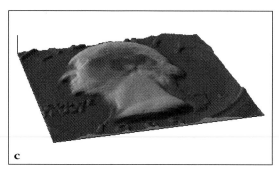

Figure 26. Elevation data from the coin image shown as:

a) *a grey scale representation with each facet shaded according to the product of elevation and slope;*

b) *with each facet assigned a color representing elevation;*

c) *using the hue to represent elevation and the intensity to represent slope.*

examining surface images, since the presence of defects or other features of interest is usually far more readily discerned by an experienced observer than is possible with computer pattern recognition programs.

It is also possible to introduce color to these displays using the same procedure as shown in **Figure 19**, applying the elevation as a color in the hue channel and the slope in the intensity channel, while drawing each facet in its appropriate place on the screen to generate a perspective-corrected visual representation of the surface geometry. This is far more visually interpretable than simply applying false color, as shown in **Figure 26**. Generating such displays requires only seconds on a typical modern desktop computer.

Using this type of presentation communicates a much more effective representation of the surface geometry to most users, even ones with some experience, than does the simple grey-scale range image. **Figure 27** shows this mode of presentation for the same surface images presented in **Figure 1**. Even though the range images contain all of the data, and the perspective-corrected visualizations actually obscure some of it, comparison suggests that the latter are more realistic in appearance and hence more useful.

Modern computer graphics is also capable of rapidly redrawing surface views from different viewpoints. This can be used in several ways. Generating two realistic renderings of a surface from slightly different points of view allows using human stereo vision to interpret the depth of a surface. Creating a series of such images from different viewpoints can be used to display a "movie" showing a fly-over across the surface, and with enough

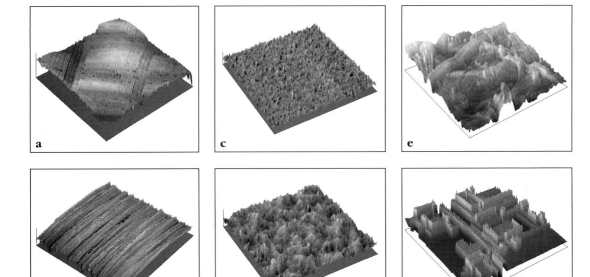

Figure 27. *The surface data from the four surfaces in Figure 1* ***(a-d)*** *and the two surfaces in Figure 3* ***(e,f)*** *rendered to show perspective-corrected visualizations with facets shaded according to the product of slope and elevation. The graphics have been expanded in the vertical (Z) direction to increase the perception of roughness and relief in the data.*

computer horsepower this can be done in real time as an operator manipulates a joystick to interactively control the flight path. Combining this with the stereo display creates a virtual reality world in which the surface can be viewed in detail.

Analysis of surface data

There is no doubt that human visual examination of well-presented visualizations of the surface geometrical and compositional information offers a powerful tool for recognizing defects and other specific characteristics of the surface. But for many purposes there is a need for numerical measures of the surface, which can be used for control purposes and to correlate the surface geometry or compositional variations with the creation and processing history of the surface, and with its performance behavior. For these purposes analytical methods relying on computer processing of the data are needed, and it is far from clear just what should be measured to provide effective parameters for any given requirement.

The traditional measures of surfaces include the thickness of coatings, and the geometric features of the surface geometry. Most of these values, while quite precise, are highly dependent on other factors such as the material composition (and spatial variations of composition), the particular measurement procedure used, and the size of the measured area. Most thickness measuring procedures and some elevation measuring instruments naturally average

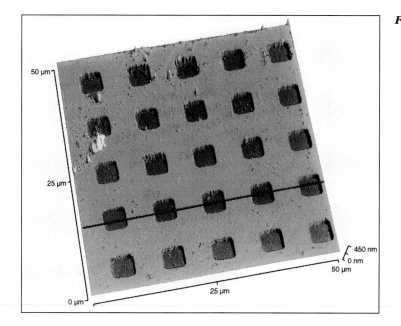

Figure 28. AFM image of a lithographic test pattern used to select the location for a single line scan used for dimensional measurement. When used for this purpose the AFM requires quantitative position sensing such as an interferometer, rather than relying on measuring the signals sent to the piezoelectric positioners.

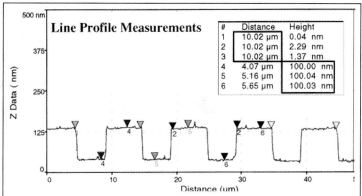

over a lateral distance that is at least several micrometers and often much more. This is much larger than the vertical resolution most techniques are capable of, and may hide important details of the coating. Sampling strategies must be employed to determine spatial uniformity.

Dimensional measurement of surfaces is one application where coordinate measuring machines, stylus instruments and optical interference techniques are all used. In many cases very specific dimensions are specified in the design of the part, and so the measurement does not require an area scan or an image, but simply the proper alignment of the measuring tool with the component. However, as dimensions become small, as in the case of microelectronic devices, it may be necessary to acquire an image to locate the point where measurement is to be performed. **Figure 28** shows an elevation profile taken from one scan line of an AFM, from which highly precise measurements can be taken on the width and height of the steps present.

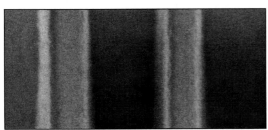 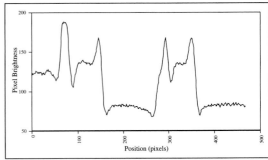

Figure 29. *Position of an SEM image of two parallel lines of photoresist on a silicon wafer and the signal profile across them. The relationship between the physical profile and the signal depends upon the slope and roughness of the sides of the lines, the composition of the material, the electron accelerating voltage used, and the electron detector used.*

Because the AFM is a relatively slow device which has difficulty handling large parts, and because there is always concern about surface damage when a physical contact is made with it, many of the metrology measurements on these devices are presently made by SEM. (The light microscope was used with earlier generations of devices, but the dimensions are now too small for the wavelength of light to resolve them.) **Figure 29** shows an SEM image of two lines of photoresist on a silicon wafer. Unfortunately, the SEM image is only indirectly related to the surface geometry. Consequently the signal profile along a scan line (actually averaged over multiple scan lines to improve the signal to noise ratio) is difficult to interpret to determine the line width. The pitch or spacing of the lines can be determined with fair accuracy under the assumption that the lines have the same shape, and thus generate the same signal profile. Consequently selecting any reproducible characteristic of the signal—the peak, or the maximum slope, etc.—can be used to measure the distance between the lines. But to measure the peak width accurately there must be some absolute determination of where the edge lies (and even what that means given the slightly irregular shape of typical lines).

Computer modeling of the process of generating the SEM image signal can be carried out for various specimen geometries (and as a function of composition, electron beam voltage and detector characteristics and placement). This is a time consuming process but still easier than fabricating physical standards for comparison. Even so, little accurate metrology is done in reality. Most manufacturers who use SEM images for metrology select some arbitrary feature of the signal that can be easily and reproducibly measured, such as the point of maximum slope or halfway between the darkest and lightest signal levels, and use that to monitor changes in dimension but without trying to determine the actual dimension. This is the classic difference between accuracy and precision, and works adequately for production control but is not able to support the development of new geometries and devices.

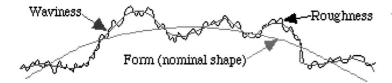

Waviness

Roughness

Form (nominal shape)

Figure 30. *Deviations from intended shape.*

Profile measurements

Unlike the SEM, most instruments considered here do produce actual physical elevation profiles. Surface measurements have historically been assessed from these elevation profiles rather than using full two dimensional images (because the instrumentation is simpler and the time required is much less, and hence because familiarity with the methods became established). By applying filters to the data (either digitally or in the amplifier electronics), different ranges of frequencies in the profiles can be separated which are traditionally described as the figure or form, waviness, and texture or roughness (**Figure 30**). Form is the overall gross geometrical shape, which is generally specified in engineering drawings, controlled by set dimensions, and described by conventional Euclidean geometry. The medium frequencies are called waviness and the high frequencies the texture or roughness. In machining processes, waviness is assumed to result from vibrations or deflections in the machine, while roughness results from more local interactions between the tool and the local microstructure in the material. These divisions are somewhat arbitrary and may differ according to the size of the part. The cutoff frequencies used to define the filters are typically set to wavelengths from about 0.25 mm up to several mm to separate waviness from roughness. International standards specify these as part of the measurement procedure for many mechanical engineering applications.

Filtering to separate roughness from waviness and form data was originally done using analog RC filters in the electronics. In modern systems digital processing is used, with a least-squares line or arc fitted to remove the form and spatial Gaussian filter to separate the waviness and roughness. This generalizes directly to area scans which can also be filtered with an equivalent Gaussian filter, or the Fourier transform of the image can be filtered to select the desired range of frequencies. The form data are most often separated by least squares fitting of a plane, or some other Euclidean shape such as a cylinder or sphere that corresponds to the known intended form, or a generalized polynomial. **Figure 31** shows a simple example of form removal, in which roughness on a ball bearing (spherical) surface is made more evident visually and also becomes easier to measure after the general curvature is subtracted. Deviations are then measured from the nominal form of the ball.

The roughness of surfaces is typically determined from the roughness profile after the low(er) frequency components have

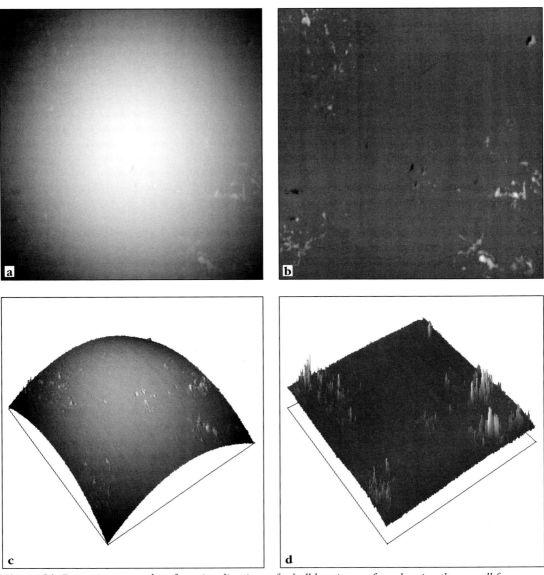

Figure 31. *Range images and surface visualizations of a ball bearing surface showing the overall form* **(a,c)** *and the results of flattening the data by subtracting the spherical shape* **(b,d)** *. Vertical expansion of the data is possible after form removal.*

been removed. A wide variety of measurement parameters are used, some of them codified in various ISO or other international standards, and some of them corresponding to specific industries or equipment manufacturers (Rosen & Crafoord, 1997). A complete review of instrumentation and methods is in Whitehouse (1994). The most widely used perform statistical analysis on the elevation data without regard to its spatial arrangement. Examples include the maximum peak-to-valley range of elevations along the profile, the average absolute value of the deviation from the mean (Ra), or the statistical standard deviation of the elevation data (Rq). Another measure of the magnitude of

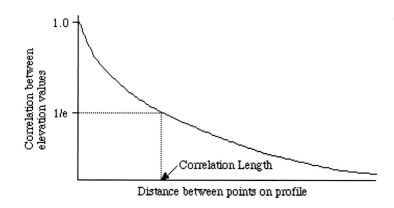

Figure 32. *The correlation plot shows the probability that points will have the same elevation value as a function of their lateral separation. The correlation length is defined as the point at which this plot drops to 1/e or 36.79%.*

the roughness is the difference in elevation between the five highest peaks and five lowest valleys (*Rz*), but this requires defining a peak or a valley. This problem becomes more difficult when applied to area scans or images.

Information on the spatial distribution of the elevation data includes parameters such as the number of peaks along the profile and the correlation length. The latter may be defined as the average distance between successive peaks, or between points at some specific elevation such as the mean elevation line left by removing the form and waviness. A more general definition of the correlation length comes from a plot as shown in **Figure 32**; this is just the magnitude of the autocorrelation function which can be determined from the Fourier transform of the profile. The autocorrelation function (ACF) is also of interest because for surfaces produced by a large number of independent events (shot blasting, grinding, ballistic deposition, etc.) it has the same shape as the ACF of the "average event" that produced the surface.

Functional parameters are also used, which are presumed to correspond to particular usage of the surfaces. The "Abbott curve" is simply the cumulative histogram of the elevation data (**Figure 33**); it gives the area of contact which would be obtained by removal of a portion of the surface, either by in-service wear or by an additional fabrication step such as plateau honing of automotive cylinder liners.

Another approach called "Motif," originally introduced in the French automobile industry and now used throughout Europe (Dietzsch et al., 1997), simplifies the profile to just the peaks which would contact another surface based on the height of the peaks relative to the intervening valleys and the width of the valleys. **Figure 34** shows the principle. Peaks are characterized by their depth (the height above the valley) and their separation distance. Peak and valley patterns are then combined according to their separation distance and depth to eliminate the small peaks on the sides of larger ones, until a minimum is reached which contains just the most important peaks.

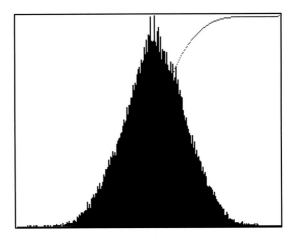

Figure 33. *The histogram (black) of the shotblasted surface range image (Figure 1d) and the same data shown as a cumulative histogram (red). This plots the fraction of points on the surface whose elevation is less than the value on the horizontal axes, and is also called the Abbott-Firestone curve.*

All of these methods have serious limitations. They are highly dependent on the length of the profile scanned and the lateral resolution of the data points. They involve some very arbitrary definitions of what constitutes a peak or valley, ignore the fact that the profile path will not cross the highest or lowest points of most surface peaks and valleys, and do not correlate very well with the real subjects of interest, which are the processes by which surfaces are produced and their behavior for whatever service they are used. They are primarily suitable for specific quality control applications in which the real meaning of the parameters is hidden but consistency of measurement results can be used to keep a working process in control. Furthermore, they are very difficult to generalize to surface images produced by area scans of elevation.

All profile methods suffer from the fact that most real surfaces are not isotropic but have some directionality that results either from the way the surface was generated, the characteristics of the material itself, or the use it has been subjected to. This so-called "lay" of the surface can be simple (e.g. the ground surface in **Figure 1** is highly directional) or very complex and subtle. Measuring a profile perpendicular to the principal lay direction is the recommended approach, but for complicated surfaces this misses much of the actual character of the surface.

Because the history of profile measurements had generated (or accumulated) a rash of parameters, an effort is being made to

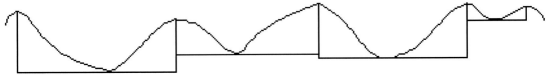

Figure 34. *The basics of Motif combination: each peak and valley motif is measured by the depth (height of the peak above the valley) and width. Motifs which have peaks smaller than the neighbor on either side (a width less than an arbitrary cutoff and a depth less than 60% of the largest depth in the profile) are combined with their neighbors to reduce the number of motifs present.*

rationalize the measurement of area scans. Supported by the ISO committee and spearheaded by researchers at the University of Birmingham (Stout et al., 1993), a set of statistical, spatial and functional parameters have been proposed which will probably evolve to form the basis of future international standards. These still contain some of the same limitations as the profile measures, such as the need to define what constitutes a peak and a strong dependence upon the size of the scan area and the lateral resolution of the points. And they do not include some of the potentially important methods such as topographic analysis, envelope or motif analysis, and fractal geometry. But because they represent an important starting point for surface description, some consideration of them is appropriate.

The Birmingham measurement suite

Four classes of measurement parameters are proposed, ones that deal with the elevation values without regard to their location (called amplitude parameters), ones that deal with lateral distances on the surface (called spatial parameters), ones that combine these together (called hybrid parameters), and ones that are believed to have some direct correlation with surface history and properties (called functional parameters). Within each group only a very few parameters, ones which have the most direct relationship to the more widely accepted profile measurement parameters, are selected. The symbols proposed for these parameters use the same nomenclature as those for profiles except that S (surface) is substituted for the R used in profile standards.

The amplitude parameters are simple extensions to area scans of the statistical measures that are used with profile plots. For instance, Sa is the analog to Ra, the arithmetic mean deviation. For an area scan it is the arithmetic mean of the absolute values of the elevation values from the mean plane (fit as discussed above). Sa is preserved only because Ra is widely used, and that is so in turn because it was comparatively easy in the precomputer days to design instruments to measure it. The root-mean-square deviation of the elevation points is a more robust measure, which is simply the standard deviation of the distribution of the elevation values, Sq. The variance (the square of the standard deviation) is the second moment of the distribution. The third and fourth moments are the skew and kurtosis, respectively, and these are also used as amplitude measurement parameters, called Ssk and Sku respectively. For simple distributions which are not bimodal, these three parameters offer a reasonably compact statistical description of the surface heights.

The histogram of the surface elevation data (examples are shown in **Figure 35**) shows the overall range of surface elevation. The skew in the distribution distinguishes such cases as the narrow and deep grooves that may be important for distributing lubricant on plateau-honed cylinder liners in automobile engines

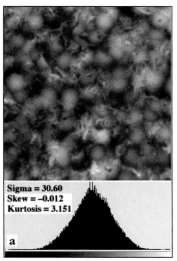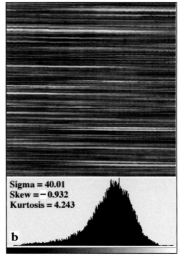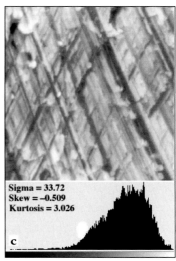

Sigma = 30.60
Skew = –0.012
Kurtosis = 3.151

a

Sigma = 40.01
Skew = – 0.932
Kurtosis = 4.243

b

Sigma = 33.72
Skew = –0.509
Kurtosis = 3.026

c

Figure 35. Histograms of elevation values for a few metal surfaces:
a) shotblasted brass, which has a symmetrical distribution;
b) ground stainless steel, which has a slight negative skew due to the presence of a few deep grooves;
c) a plateau-honed cylinder liner with a negative skew resulting from the deep grooves which distribute lubricant.

(**Figure 35c**). In this case most of the surface has a very narrow range of elevations but the grooves, which cover only a small fraction of the area, reach down to much lower depths. A skew in the opposite direction would correspond to a surface with just a few high peaks or ridges rising up from a relatively smooth surface. But the histogram by itself contains no information on the spatial arrangement of the pits and valleys or the peaks and ridges. The same histogram would result from a surface with all of the high points collected together in one plateau or distributed as thousands of tiny peaks. The properties of these two extreme surfaces would be quite different.

Just as for profiles, these statistical measures of amplitude are sensitive to the size of the sampled area. For most surfaces the standard deviation increases with the number of points measured. In fact for a fractal rough surface the slope of a curve plotting the variance as a function of size on log-log axes is one of the ways used to measure the fractal dimension.

For profiles, the parameter Rz is the difference in elevation between the average of the five highest peaks and five lowest valleys. For an area scan of a surface this is generalized to Sz, the difference between the ten highest peaks and ten lowest valleys. However, this is not purely an amplitude parameter because it depends critically on the definitions of a peak and a valley. They cannot be simply the highest and lowest points on the surface (or pixels in the surface image), since these could be (and often will be) adjacent to each other and would all represent a single peak and valley. For a profile, the presence of a low point separating two high points might be taken to indicate separate peaks. This is a flawed definition because infinitesimal irregularities should not be considered significant, and so some criterion for the depth of the valley between the peaks is required. But on an area scan of a surface even more is needed because the peak (or valley) covers an area and two or more local peaks may connect along intricate paths to be considered part of the same peak (and vice versa for valleys). In tracing this connectivity, it matters whether pixels are considered to touch all 8 of their immediate neighbors or only the four that share edges with them.

There is much more information in the identification of peaks and valleys than just the Sz parameter that is the elevation difference between the average of the ten highest and ten lowest. Different surfaces give rise to very different shapes for peaks and valleys, and their sizes and shapes, orientation and spacing may all contain important characterization information. In **Figure 36** several examples are shown in which peaks are defined as 8-connected (pixels touch 8 neighbors), and are required to be distinct down to 80% of the height of the peak. Valleys are defined in the same way. In this example the 20 highest peaks and lowest valleys are found. The method is similar to the "flood fill" algorithm used in image processing, starting with the highest local maximum (and proceeding down) and including all touching pixels that extend down to the 80% limit, while checking to see if the peak merges into an existing labeled peak. Notice that for the shotblasted surface the valleys are relatively smooth in outline while the peaks are very irregular. Also, for the ground surface the peaks (ridges) tend to be broader than the valleys (crevices), and for the honed surface the peaks are very large while the valleys are much smaller. All of these differences are consistent with our understanding of how such surfaces are produced, and they may give important insights into other surfaces.

Another parameter involving the peaks present in the surface is the number of them per unit area, called Sds. Again, this depends upon the definition of a peak as discussed above. It is likely that secondary information about the peaks will also be important in a variety of applications. For instance, the uniformity of spacing of the peaks may play a role in cases where the surfaces are involved in electrical or thermal contact, friction and wear, or to judge the visual and aesthetic appearance. As discussed under image measurement, the mean nearest neighbor distance can be used to determine the tendency toward uniform spacing or clustering by comparing the value to the mean distance that a Poisson random distribution of the same number of points per unit area would have. **Figure 37** shows the surface of an injection molded polymer in which the peaks are relative evenly spaced (a complex function of the surface finish of the die, the temperature, pressure and viscosity of the polymer, and its molecular weight). This uniformity coupled with a spacing between peaks that is close to the spatial resolution limit of human vision produces an aesthetically pleasing appearance for the product.

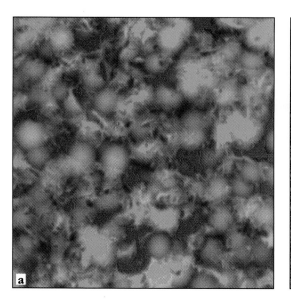

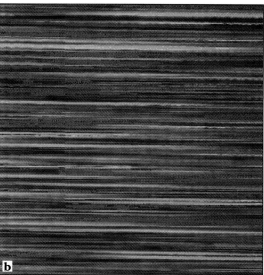

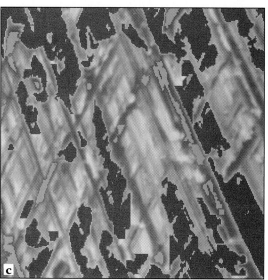

Figure 36. *The twenty highest peaks (red) and lowest valleys (green) on the shotblasted (**a**), ground (**b**) and plateau-honed (**c**) surfaces shown in Figure 35.*

In some other applications the same information about the density and uniformity of pits rather than peaks would be of interest. An example is the surfaces of plates used to retain ink for printing applications.

Surfaces with anisotropy or lay can be characterized by spatial parameters derived from the autocorrelation function. As discussed in the chapter on Fourier space processing, the autocorrelation function (ACF) is obtained by squaring the magnitude of the complex variables in the Fourier transform while setting the phase to zero, which removes all spatial location information. The inverse transform produces the two-dimensional spatial image of the ACF. The parameters defined from this function are the texture aspect ratio *Str*, the texture direction *Std*, and the

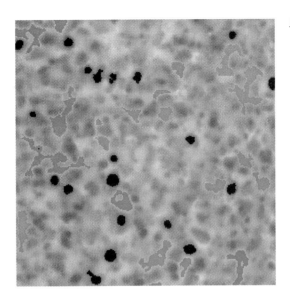

Figure 37. *The highest 20 peaks and lowest 20 valleys in a one-square-millimeter area of the molded polymer surface from Figure 18. The peaks are color coded from purple to red according to height and the valleys from green to cyan. Notice that one valley completely surrounds a small peak, and that the peaks are much more regular in shape than the valleys.*

autocorrelation length *Sal*. Understanding these may be helped by examining the ACF images in **Figure 38**. The autocorrelation length is defined in the Birmingham report as the shortest distance in which the magnitude of the ACF drops to 20%. For the examples shown, this is the minimum radius of the contour line drawn at the 20% intensity level. The texture aspect ratio is the ratio of the minimum radius to the maximum radius, and the texture direction is the orientation of the maximum radius.

For the examples in **Figure 38**, the ACF of the polymer surface (**Figure 18**) is quite isotropic (indicating that the surface is also isotropic), so the aspect ratio is unity and there is no pronounced direction. The ground surface (**Figure 1b**) on the other hand has a strong preferred orientation which is evident in the ACF and can be measured there. For the flycut surface (**Figure 1a**) the texture is more complicated, as is indeed evident in the original image which shows two predominant machining directions. The *Str*, *Std* and *Sal* values as defined can of course be measured from the ACF but it is not clear that they contain all of the information about the surface lay that would be desired for characterization.

The hybrid properties involve both the elevation and lateral data (as indeed do many of the preceding parameters). $S\Delta q$ is the root-mean-square slope of the surface, which can be calculated from the same triangular tiling procedure used to generate the visualizations shown earlier. Formally it is defined as the square root of the mean value of the sum of squares of the derivatives of the image in the vertical and horizontal directions, which can be determined simply as the local difference of elevation values between adjacent pixels. The mean summit curvature *Ssc* is similarly related to the second derivatives of elevation, but calculated only for those pixels located at peaks. This depends, of

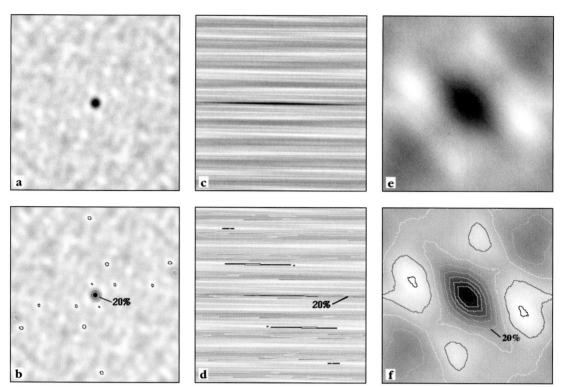

Figure 38. Autocorrelation function calculated for:

a) *the polymer surface from Figure 18;*

c) *the ground surface from Figure 1b;*

e) *the flycut surface from Figure 1a, with superimposed contour lines* ***(b, d, f)*** *indicating the shape of the function and the distance at which it drops to 20%.*

course, on first arriving at a meaningful and accepted definition of which peaks are to be included. The third hybrid property is the ratio of the actual surface area to the projected area *Sdr*. This can be obtained by summing up the areas of the triangles making up the visualization.

None of these hybrid properties is very difficult to compute, but they all depend critically on the sampling interval or spacing of the pixels. Changing lateral resolution will alter the parameter values dramatically so that they are not really functions of the surface but of the measurement technique, and can be used only for comparisons in the most limited way. This is also the case for many of the profile-based measurements, but one of the goals in moving to area-based measurements was to overcome some of the limitations of the older methods. In fact, many engineering surfaces have been shown to have a fractal geometry whose actual surface area is undefined (it increases without limit as the lateral resolution of the measurements improves).

It is a more subtle point, but measurements like these also depend upon whether the elevation data at each pixel are samples of the surface or averages over the pixel area. The mathe-

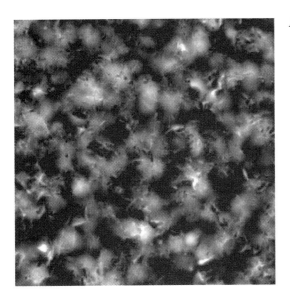

Figure 39. *Thresholding the range image (in this example the shotblasted surface from Figure 1d) at any particular elevation (in this example 31% below the maximum value) shows the surface area that would be in contact with a plane after a corresponding amount of wear (in the absence of any elastic or plastic deformation).*

matics apply for the case of sampling, where the elevation at each pixel is measured at a precise mathematical point and whatever happens between that pixel and the next is not taken into account. In fact, many measurement methods such as conventional stylus instruments and optical interferometers perform some averaging of measurement over the entire area of the pixel, which may either report the maximum value in that area or a weighted average of the elevation values. The mathematics appropriate to these cases has not been worked out and would affect not just the hybrid parameters but all of the parameters described here.

Functional parameters are intended to relate surface geometric data to specific aspects of surface performance, and these are generally related to mechanical engineering applications since the greatest use of surface metrology has thus far been in that field. One typical example is the surface bearing area ratio *Stp*, which is the fraction of the image area that would be in contact with a flat plane parallel to the base if a given height of all peaks was removed by wear (**Figure 39**). This value, of course, can be read directly from the histogram of the elevation data in the image.

Similarly, the amount of volume removed in the process (the material volume ratio *Smr*) can be calculated by integrating the histogram, or using the cumulative histogram. The void volume ratio *Svr* is the volume of empty space within the surface of the specimen, which may be available for retaining or distributing a lubricant. It is measured by integrating the spaces at each elevation level, but this can also be done efficiently using the cumulative histogram. **Figure 40** shows the same data from **Figure 39** but as a surface visualization that reveals the nature of the contact surface and the void volume after some of the

Figure 40. Visualization of the data from Figure 38:

a) *the original shotblasted surface;*

b) *the same surface truncated 31% below the top of the highest peak, showing the contact areas and the void volume.*

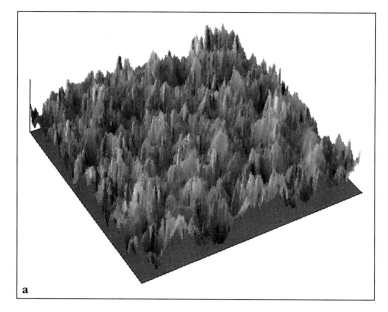

a

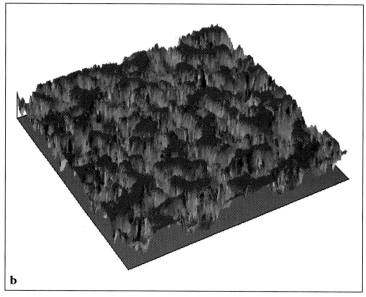

b

peaks have been removed by wear (but assuming that there is no deformation of the remaining surface nor filling in of pits with debris).

There is really more information needed about the contact areas than these parameters provide. The size of the individual contacts is important for heating and deformation, and the void volume may either be completely connected, or consist of isolated pockets, or be a mixture of the two, with very different consequences for lubrication. There are other functional parameters proposed to deal with these and other aspects of surface performance, but these become very specific to each application and will require considerable research to properly define. Many of them are handicapped to a significant degree because the surface elevation data in a range image are single valued. The elevation recorded at each pixel is the maximum height at that point, as detected by a stylus or optical reflection, etc. Undercuts, caves or pores within the surface that do not show up in the range image may become important if wear removes some of the surface overburden.

Image processing and analysis using the tools already developed in preceding chapters can be used to obtain many of the parameters of interest for surfaces from range images. For example, min and max operators can be used to modify the image to form the envelope of the surface which a contact of known form would feel, basically a two-dimensional form of the motif logic mentioned above for profiles. Cross-correlation with the image of a defect (crack, dust particle, etc.) can be used to locate such defects. Measurement of features obtained by thresholding can provide data on the contact areas and their distribution after wear has modified a surface. Skeletonization of the pore volume can be used to determine its connectivity as a pathway to distribute lubricants. Using these tools is straightforward once the significant parameters have been determined so that their relationships to surface behavior and history can be assessed.

New approaches — topographic analysis and fractal dimensions

The limitations and inadequacies of the traditional methods of analysis discussed above prevent them from fully describing real surfaces. They are primarily being used for process control applications in mechanical engineering, where comparison of measurements with prior history provides an indication of change, so long as the measurement technique and instrumentation remains unchanged. Newer methods have become available, but their full meaning and interpretation still remain to be explored. It is hoped that these new approaches may provide more insight into the description and makeup of surfaces.

Human vision uses global topographic information to organize information on surfaces (Scott, 1995). The arrangement of hills and dales, ridges, courses and saddle points, contains quite a bit of information for describing a surface. A landscape or surface can be divided into regions consisting of hills (points from which all uphill paths lead to one particular peak) and dales (points from which all downhill paths lead to a pit). Boundaries between hills are courses and boundaries between dales are ridge lines (**Figure 41**).

A Pfalz graph (Pfalz, 1976) or change tree (**Figure 42**) connecting the peaks and dales through the respective saddle points where ridge and course lines meet summarizes the topological structure. The change tree can represent directly the height difference and

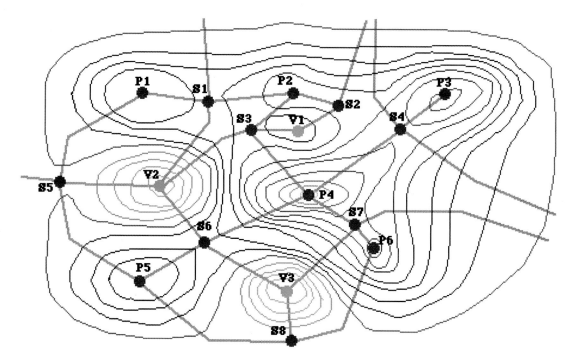

Figure 41. *A contour map representing a surface, with the peaks (red), valleys (green) and saddle points (purple) marked.*

lateral distance between features, which makes decisions straightforward about eliminating features that have either small vertical or lateral extent. This is a direct extension to surfaces of the motif combination used for profiles. Scott (1997) has recently proposed methods for dealing with the finite extent of real

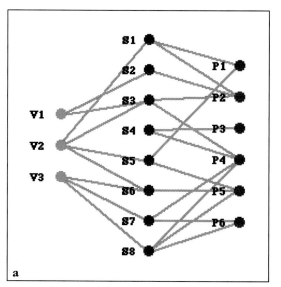

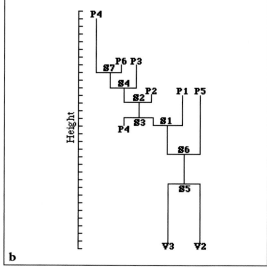

Figure 42. *The Pfalz graph (a) showing which peaks, saddle points and valleys are connected in Figure 41, and the change tree (b) which can be drawn to show the height difference and lateral distance between them.*

images and the corrections necessary for dealing with the intersection of ridges and courses with the edges of the image area. It is not yet clear just how this information will be used for surface measurement, but parameters such as the volume of connected valleys, the spatial distribution of valleys and peaks across the surface, and orientation of watercourses and ridges seem likely to be important for surface characterization.

At quite a different extreme of local roughness, many surfaces (but emphatically not all) are characterized by a self-similarity (more exactly, a self-affinity) that can be described by a fractal dimension. There are several ways to measure this (which do not exactly agree) plus the need to provide an additional parameter that describes the magnitude of the roughness, and perhaps others to describe the directionality of the surface. The appeal of the fractal dimension is that it is not dependent on the measurement scale, and that it summarizes much of the "roughness" of surfaces in a way that seems to correspond to both the way nature works and the way humans perceive roughness. Given a series of surfaces, the "rougher" the surface as it appears to human interpretation (for a variety of basic reasons), the higher the fractal dimension. At the same time it must be noted that the recognition of fractal geometry (even the name) is comparatively new, and there is a "bandwagon" tendency that probably causes it to be applied where it should not be, or with more enthusiasm than critical thinking.

The fractal dimension of a surface is a real number greater than 2 (the topological dimension of the surface) and less than 3 (the topological dimension of the space in which the surface exists). A perfectly smooth surface (dimension 2.0) corresponds to Euclidean geometry, and a plot of the actual area of the measured area as a function of measurement resolution would not change. But for real surfaces an increase in the magnification or resolution with which it is examined will reveal more nooks and crannies and the surface area will increase. For a surprising variety of natural and man-made surfaces, a plot of the area as a function of resolution is linear on a log-log graph, and the slope of this curve gives the dimension D as shown in **Figure 43**.

This description comes directly from the earlier recognition that boundary lines around islands had a length that depended upon the measurement scale. A so-called Richardson plot of the length of the west coast of Britain (Mandelbrot, 1967) as a function of the length of the measurement tool showed this log-log relationship and was one of the triggering ideas that led Mandelbrot to study the mathematics of self-similar structures (ones that appear equally irregular at all scales) and to coin the name fractal for the field. Many other subsequent publications have shown that an extremely broad variety of surfaces also exhibit this kind of geometry, investigated a number of ways to measure the dimension, and begun to study the relationships between the

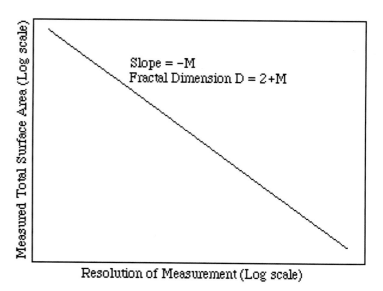

Figure 43. Schematic diagram of fractal dimension measurement: as the measurement resolution becomes smaller the total measured area increases.

dimension and the history and performance characteristics of surfaces.

Measuring the surface area over a range of resolutions is in fact a rather difficult thing to do (one way is by adsorbing molecules of different sizes), and for basic reasons is not actually appropriate for many surfaces because they are not ideally self-similar. For most surfaces, the lateral directions and the normal direction are distinct in dimension and physical properties, which means that the scaling or self-similarity that exists in one direction may not be the same as the others. At a sufficiently large scale most surfaces approach an ideal Euclidean flat surface. For anisotropic surfaces this situation is more severe and even lateral directions are different. This means that the surfaces are mathematically self-affine rather than self-similar. The fact that elevation measurements are single valued and cannot reveal undercuts means that the measured data would be self-affine even for a truly self-similar surface (for instance one produced by diffusion-limited aggregation of particles on a substrate). For self-affine surfaces and data sets there are still a variety of correct and practical measurement techniques. A few of the more practical ones will be summarized here (and a more complete discussion is available in Russ, 1994).

In most cases, the most robust measure of the fractal dimension is the same procedure that can characterize surfaces that are not ideally fractal, nor perfectly isotropic. The Fourier power spectrum can also be used to characterize the instrumental response function, to distinguish it from the surface information. Instead of the usual display mode for the power spectrum, a plot of log (magnitude) vs. log (frequency) reveals a fractal surface as a straight line plot whose slope gives the dimension. The principal drawbacks to using the power spectrum plot to measure the

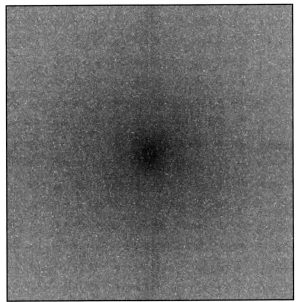

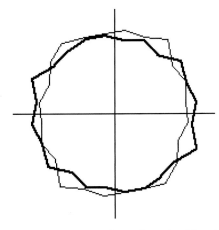

Rose plot of slope : Log(magn.) vs. Log(freq.)

Slope : 1.3671 to 1.7335 Ds(av)=2.2445
Icept : 4.5417 to 5.788 Ave.=5.0692

Log Magnitude : From 6.8024 to 12.0807   Av.slope=-1.4014

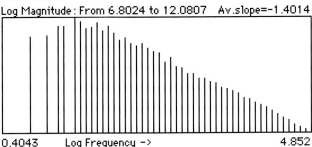

0.4043   Log Frequency ->   4.852

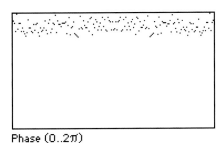

Phase (0..2π)

Figure 44. *The Fourier transform power spectrum (upper left) of the shotblasted metal image (Figure 1d), with its subsequent analysis. The plot of log magnitude vs. log frequency (lower left) averaged over all directions shows a linear relationship which confirms the fractal behavior, whose slope gives the dimension (2.24). A rose plot of the slope as a function of orientation (upper right, bold line) shows that the surface is isotropic and has the same dimension in all directions. The thin line on the same plot shows the intercept of the plot as a function of direction, which is a measure of the amplitude of the roughness and also shows isotropy for this surface. Finally, a plot of the distribution of phases of the terms in the Fourier transform shows them to be uniformly random, which is required for a fractal.*

dimension are that it tends to overestimate the numerical value of the dimension for relatively smooth surfaces (dimensions between 2.0 and about 2.3), and that the numerical precision of the measured value is lower than some of the other methods can provide for images of a given size. **Figure 44** shows an example of a fractal surface and the power spectrum plot giving the fractal dimension.

Generating the two-dimensional Fourier transform of the surface range image reveals any fractal anisotropy (which can be either weak anisotropy in which the dimension is the same in all directions but the magnitude is not, or strong anisotropy in which the dimension also varies). Plotting the slope and inter-

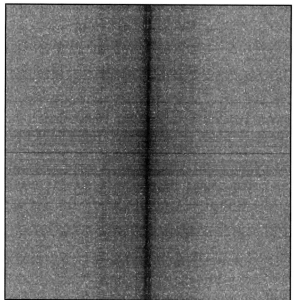
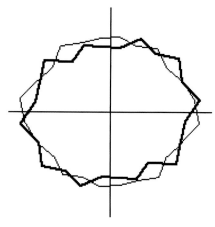

Rose plot of slope : Log(magn.) vs. Log(freq.)

Slope : 0.8218 to 1.1862 Ds(av)=2.509
Icept : 4.966 to 6.5227 Ave.=5.5424

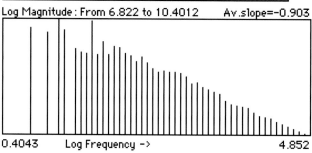

Log Magnitude : From 6.822 to 10.4012   Av.slope=-0.903

0.4043   Log Frequency ->   4.852

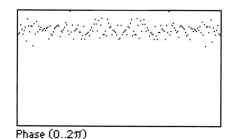

Phase (0..2π)

Figure 45. *The same data presentation as in Figure 44, but for the anisotropic ground surface shown in Figure 1b. Both the slope and intercept of the power spectrum plot are different in the vertical and horizontal directions. The surface is an anisotropic fractal.*

cept of the plot of log (magnitude) vs. log (frequency) as a function of orientation provides a quantitative tool to describe the fractal anisotropy. **Figure 45** shows an example. The separation of the low frequency data that describe the figure and high frequencies that often reveal instrument limitations from the intermediate frequencies can be used to isolate the surface fractal dimension.

By itself, the fractal dimension is only a partial description of surface roughness even for ideally fractal surfaces. Stretching the surface vertically to increase the magnitude of the roughness does not change the slope of the power spectrum or the fractal dimension. An additional measure, which has units of length, is needed to characterize the magnitude. The intercept of the plot of the power spectrum has units of length, and can be used for this purpose. So can the topothesy, which is formally defined as the horizontal distance over which the mean angular change in slope is one radian.

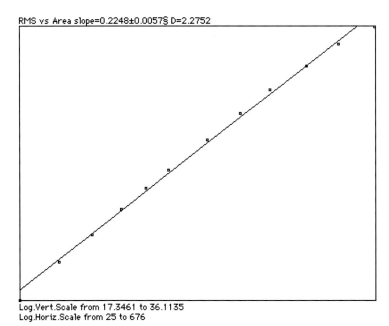

RMS vs Area slope=0.2248±0.0057§ D=2.2752

Log.Vert.Scale from 17.3461 to 36.1135
Log.Horiz.Scale from 25 to 676

Figure 46. *Plot of mean variance vs. neighborhood size to determine the fractal dimension of the shotblasted surface (same image as Figure 44).*

There are a variety of other measurement approaches that can be properly used with self-affine fractal surfaces. Two widely used techniques that deal with the range image of the area directly are the covering blanket and the variogram. Both work correctly for isotropic surfaces but do not reveal anisotropy and can produce nonsense values in those cases rather than an average. The latter is simply a plot of the variance in elevation values as a function of the size of the measured region. Small areas placed systematically or randomly over the surface are averaged, and a single mean value obtained. This process is repeated at many different sizes and a plot (**Figure 46**) made that gives the dimension.

The covering blanket or Minkowski method measures the difference (summed over the entire image) between an upper and lower envelope fitted to the surface as a function of the size of the neighborhood used. The minimum and maximum brightness rank operators discussed under image processing are applied with different diameter neighborhoods, and the total difference between them added up. This produces a plot as shown in **Figure 47** that gives a dimension. Notice that these three methods give only approximate agreement as to the numerical value of the dimension. Part of this is just finite measurement precision, but part of the difference arises from the fact that all of these techniques measure something that is slightly different. These are limits to the actual dimension and in general will not agree, so when comparisons are being made between surfaces it is important to use only one technique for all of the measurements.

It is often attractive to perform measurements in a lower dimension, since a smaller number of data points are involved. His-

Figure 47. *Plot of the Minkowski cover volume as a function of neighborhood size to determine the fractal dimension (same image as Figures 44 and 46).*

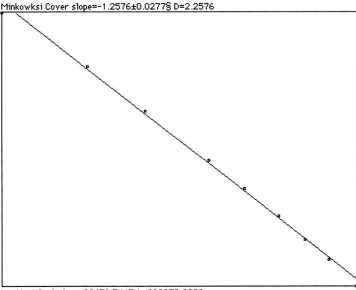

Minkowksi Cover slope=-1.2576±0.0277§ D=2.2576

Log.Vert.Scale from 28458.3447 to 209852.8889
Log.Horiz.Scale from 9 to 293 pixels

torically, much of the work with fractal measurement has been done with boundary lines, whose dimension lies between 1.0 (the Euclidean or topological dimension of a line) and 1.999... (a line whose irregularity is so great that it wanders across an entire plane). There is a way to do this with fractal surfaces, by intersecting the surface with a plane and then measuring the dimension of the line that is the intersection. It is vitally important, however, that this plane be parallel to the nominal surface orientation rather than a vertical cut. The vertical cut would produce the same profile as that obtained with a profilometer, but because the surface is self-affine and not self-similar the proper measurement of this profile is complicated and the common techniques such as the Richardson plot mentioned above do not apply. Also, of course, the profile will be oriented in a particular direction and cannot be used with anisotropic surfaces.

The horizontal cut is called a slit-island method, and it corresponds exactly to the case Richardson was dealing with. The horizontal plane corresponds to sea level and the outlines are the coastlines of the islands produced by the hills that rise above the sea. A plot of the length of these coastlines as a function of measurement scale produces a dimension that is exactly 1 less than the surface dimension (the difference between the topological dimensions of a surface and a line). It is not usually convenient to measure the length of a coastline using a computer in the way Richardson did, by setting a pair of dividers to a particular scale length and "striding" around the coastline so that the boundary length was the divider setting times the number of strides. But there are a variety of other methods that are readily implemented in a computer.

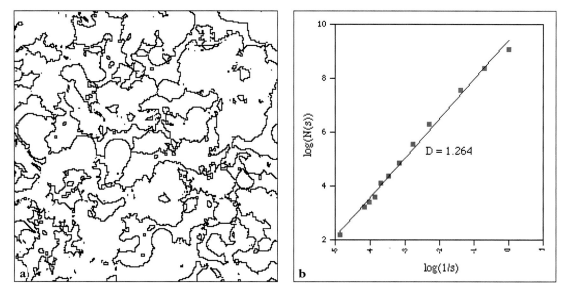

Figure 48. *Contour lines produced by thresholding the image from Figure 1d at 50% of its elevation range, and the plot from a box-counting measurement.*

The analog to the Minkowski blanket for the surface is a Minkowski sausage produced by thickening the boundary line by various amounts and plotting the area covered vs. the width of the stripe or sausage. The Euclidean distance map discussed in the chapter on binary image processing accomplishes this procedure very efficiently and without the directional variation that results from conventional pixel-based dilation. Another method is box-counting (**Figure 48**) in which a grid is placed on the image and the number of squares through which the boundary line passes is counted as a function of the size of the grids. While these methods are quite fast, they are only applicable to isotropic surfaces.

It is beyond the scope of this text to discuss the relationships that have been found between fractal dimensions and various aspects of the history and properties of surfaces. In brief, most processes of surface formation that involve brittle fracture or deposit large amounts of energy in small regions tend to produce fractal surfaces, and the numerical value of the dimension is often a signature of the process that was involved (Russ, 1997). Likewise, many surface contact applications (electrical, thermal, etc.) depend upon the relationship between contact area and pressure and fractal geometry is pertinent to this case. Under some circumstances friction and wear may also be related to the surface dimension. Fractal description of surfaces is a new and somewhat "trendy" approach to surface characterization. While it clearly offers powerful methods that apply to some surfaces, for others such as ductile deformation it is inappropriate.

References

M. Abbasi-Dezfouli, T. G. Freeman (1994). Patch matching in stereo-images based on shape. *ISPRS Int. Arch. Photogramm. Remote Sensing,* 30(3/1):1-8.

M. R. Anderberg (1973). *Cluster Analysis for Applications.* Academic Press, New York.

Agfa Compugraphic Division (1992). *Digital Color Prepress* (Vols. 1 & 2), Agfa Corp., Wilmington, MA.

E. H. Aigeltinger, K. R. Craig, R. T. DeHoff (1972). Experimental determination of the topological properties of three dimensional microstructures. *J. Microsc.* 95:69-81.

J. Astola, P. Haavisto, Y. Neuvo (1990). Vector median filters. *Proc. IEEE* 78:678-689.

N. Baba, M. Naka, Y. Muranaka, S. Nakamura, I. Kino, K. Kanaya (1984). Computer-aided stereographic representation of an object reconstructed from micrographs of serial thin sections. *Micron Microsc. Acta* 15:221-226.

N. Baba, M. Baba, M. Imamura, M. Koga, Y. Ohsumi, M. Osumi, K. Kanaya (1989). Serial section reconstruction using a computer graphics system: application to intracellular structures in yeast cells and to the periodontal structure of dogs' teeth. *J. Electron Microsc. Tech.* 11:16-26.

R. Balasubramanian, C. A. Bouman, J. P. Allebach (1994). Sequential scalar quantization of color images. *J. Electron. Imaging* 3(1):45-59.

A. J. Baddeley, C. V. Howard, A. Boyde, S. Reid (1987). Three-dimensional analysis of the spatial distribution of particles using the tandem-scanning reflected light microscope. *Acta Stereol.* 6 (Suppl. II) 87-100.

D. Ballard (1981). Generalizing the Hough transform to detect arbitrary shapes. *Patt. Recog.*13(2):111-122.

D. H. Ballard, C. M. Brown (1982). *Computer Vision.* Prentice Hall, Englewood Cliffs, NJ.

S. T. Barnard, W. B. Thompson, (1980). Disparity analysis of images. *IEEE Trans. Patt. Anal. Mach. Intell.,* PAMI-2(4): 333-340.

F. L. Barnes, S. G. Azavedo, H. E. Martz, G. P. Roberson, D. J. Schneberk, M. F. Skeate (1990). *Geometric Effects in Tomographic Reconstruction.* Lawrence Livermore National Laboratory Rep. UCRL-ID-105130.

M. F. Barnsley, V. Ervin, D. Hardon, J. Lancaster (1986). Solution of an inverse problem for fractals and other sets. *Proc. Natl. Acad. Sci. U.S.A.* 83:1975-1977.

M. F. Barnsley (1988). *Fractals Everywhere.* Academic Press, San Diego.

M. F. Barnsley, L. P. Hurd (1993). *Fractal Image Compression.* Peters, Wellesley, MA.

H. G. Barth, S-T. Sun (1985). Particle size analysis. *Anal. Chem.* 57:151.

M. A. Bassiouni, N. Tzannes, M. Tzannes (1993). High-fidelity integrated lossless/lossy compression and reconstruction of images. *Opt. Eng.* 32(8):1848-1853.

J. K. Beddow, G. C. Philip, A. F. Vetter (1977). On relating some particle profiles characteristics to the profile Fourier coefficients. *Powder Technol.* 18:15-19.

G. Bertrand, J-C. Everat, M. Couprie (1997). Image segmentation through operators based on topology. *J. Electron. Imaging* 6(4):395-405.

V. Berzins (1984). Accuracy of Laplacian edge detectors. *Comput. Vis. Graph. Image Proc.* 27:1955-2010.

S. Beucher, C. Lantejoul (1979). Use of Watersheds in Contour Detection. Proc. Int. Workshop Image Process., CCETT, Rennes, France.

J. L. Bird, D. T. Eppler, D. M. Checkley, Jr. (1986). Comparisons of herring otoliths using Fourier series shape analysis. *Can. J. Fish. Aquat. Sci.* 43: 1228-1234.

R. A. S. Blackie, R. Bagby, L. Wright, J. Drinkwater, S. Hart (1987). Reconstruction of three-dimensional images of microscopic objects using holography. *Proc. R. Microsc. Soc.* 22:98.

F. R. Boddeke, L. J. van Vliet, H. Netten, I. T. Young (1994). Autofocusing in microscopy based on the OTF and sampling. *Bioimaging* 2:193-203.

A. Boyde (1973). Quantitative photogrammetric analysis and quantitative stereoscopic analysis of SEM images. *J. Microsc.* 98:452.

R. N. Bracewell (1984). The fast Hartley transform. *Proc. IEEE* 72:8.

R. N. Bracewell (1986). *The Hartley Transform.* Oxford Univ. Press.

R. N. Bracewell (June 1989). *The Fourier Transform.* Scientific American.

G. Braudaway (1987). A procedure for optimum choice of a small number of colors from a large color palette for color imaging. Proc. Electronic Imaging '87, San Francisco, CA.

L. G. Briarty, P. H. Jenkins (1984). GRIDSS: an integrated suite of microcomputer programs for three-dimensional graphical reconstruction from serial sections. *J. Microsc.* 134:121-124.

D. S. Bright, D. E. Newbury, R. B. Marinenko (1988). Concentration-concentration histograms: scatter diagrams applied to quantitative compositional maps, in *Microbeam Analysis 1988* (D. E. Newbury, Ed.). San Francisco Press, pp. 18-24.

D. S. Bright, D. E. Newbury, E. B. Steel (1998). Visibility of objects in computer simulations of noisy micrographs. *J. Microsc.* 189(1):25-42.

R. K. Bryan, J. Skilling (1980). Deconvolution by maximum entropy, as illustrated by application to the jet of M87. *Mon. Not. R. Ast. Soc.* 191: 69-79.

J. Canny (1986). A computational approach to edge detection. *IEEE Trans. Patt. Anal. Mach. Intell.* (PAMI) 8(6):679-698.

I. C. Carlsen (1985). Reconstruction of true surface topographies in scanning electron microscopes using backscattered electrons. *Scanning* 7:169-177.

W. A. Carrington (1990). Image restoration in 3D microscopy with limited data, in Bioimaging and Two Dimensional Spectroscopy, *Proc. SPIE,* Vol. 1205 (L. C. Smith, Ed.), 72-83.

K. R. Castleman (1979). *Digital Image Processing.* Prentice Hall, Englewood Cliffs, NJ.

R. L. T. Cederberg (1979). Chain-link coding and segmentation for raster scan devices. *Comput. Graph. Image Proc.* 10:224-234.

P. Chieco, A. Jonker, C. Melchiorri, G. Vanni, C. J. F. van Noorden (1994). A user's guide for avoiding errors in absorbance image cytometry. *Histochem. J.* 26:1-19.

C. K. Chui (1992). *An Introduction to Wavelets.* Academic Press, London.

J. Cookson (1994). Three-Dimensional Reconstruction in Microscopy. *Proc. R. Microsc. Soc.* 29(1) Jan., 1994, pp. 3-10.

J. W. Cooley, J. W. Tukey (1965). An algorithm for the machine calculation of complex Fourier series. *Mathematics of Computation.*

D. M. Coppola, H. R. Purves, A. N. McCoy, D. Purves (1998). The distribution of oriented contours in the real world. *Proc. Natl. Acad. Sci.* 95:4002-4006.

A. M. Cormack (1963). Representation of a function by its line integrals with some radiological applications. *J. Appl. Phys.* 34:2722-2727.

A. M. Cormack (1964). Representation of a function by its line integrals with some radiological applications II. *J. Appl. Phys.* 35:2908-2913.

T. N. Cornsweet (1970). *Visual Perception.* Academic Press, New York.

M. Coster, J-L.Chermant (1985). Précis D'Analse D'Images Éditions du Centre National de la Recherche Scientifique, Paris.

P. E. Danielsson (1980). Euclidean distance mapping. *Comput. Graph. Image Process.* 14:227-248.

D. G. Daut, D. Zhao, J. Wu (1993). Double predictor differential pulse coded modulation algorithm for image data compression. *Opt. Eng.* 32(7):1514-1523.

J. Davidson (1991). Thinning and skeletonization: a tutorial and overview, in *Digital Image Processing: Fundamentals and Applications* (E. Dougherty, Ed.). Marcel Dekker, New York.

E. R. Davies (1988). On the noise suppression and image enhancement characteristics of the median, truncated median and mode filters. *Patt. Recog. Lett.* 7:87-97.

H. W. Deckman, K. L. D'Amico, J. H. Dunsmuir, B. P.Flannery, S. M. Gruner (1989). Microtomography detector design. *Adv. X-ray Anal.* 32:641.

R. T. Dehoff, F. N. Rhines (1968). *Quantitative Microscopy.* McGraw Hill, New York.

D. DeMandolx, J. Davoust (1997). Multicolor analysis and local image correlation in confocal microscopy. *J. Microsc.* 185: 21-36.

G. Diaz, A. Zuccarelli, I. Pelligra, A. Griani (1989). Elliptic Fourier analysis of cell and nuclear shapes. *Comput. Biomed. Res.* 22: 405-414.

G. Diaz, D. Quacci, C. Dell'Orbo (1990). Recognition of cell surface modulation by elliptic Fourier analysis. *Comput. Methods Programs Biomed.* 31: 57-62.

M. Dietzsch, K. Papenfuss, T. Hartmann (1997). The MOTIF method (ISO 12085) — a suitable description for functional manufactural and metrological requirements, in *7th Int. Conf. Metrol. Prop. Eng. Surf.* (B. G. Rosen, R. J. Crafoord, Eds.), Chalmers Univ., Göteborg, Sweden, pp. 231-238.

E. R. Dougherty, J. Astola (1994). *An Introduction to Nonlinear Image Processing.* SPIE, Bellingham, WA.

R. Duda, P. Hart (1972). Use of the Hough transform to detect lines and curves in pictures. *Commun. ACM* 15(1):11-15.

T. R. Edwards (1982). Two-dimensional convolute integers for analytical instrumentation. *Anal. Chem.* 54:1519-1524.

R. Ehrlich, B. Weinberg (1970). An exact method for characterization of grain shape. *J. Sediment. Petrol.* 40:205-212.

R. Ehrlich, S. K. Kennedy, S. J. Crabtree, R. L. Cannon (1984). Petrographic image analysis: 1. Analysis of reservoir pore complexes. *J. Sed. Petrol.* 54:1365-1378.

A. Engel, A. Massalski (1984). 3-D reconstruction from electron micrographs: its potential and practical limitations. *Ultramicroscopy* 13:71-84.

Y. Fahmy, J. C. Russ, C. Koch (1991). Application of fractal geometry measurements to the evaluation of fracture toughness of brittle intermetallics *J. Mater. Res.* 6(9):1856-1861.

J. Feder (1988). *Fractals.* Plenum Press, New York.

L. A. Feldkamp, L. C. Davis, J. W. Kress (1984). Practical cone beam algorithm. *J. Opt. Soc. Am.* 1(6):612.

S. F. Ferson, F. J. Rohlf, R. K. Koehn (1985). Measuring shape variation of two-dimensional outlines. *Syst. Zool.* 34: 59-68.

L. F. Firestone, K. Cook et al. (1991). Comparison of autofocus methods for automated microscopy. *Cytometry* 12: 195-206.

Y. Fisher, E. W. Jacobs, and R. D. Boss (1992). Fractal image compression using iterated transforms, in *Image and Text Compression*, (James A. Storer, Ed.), pp. 35-61. Kluwer Academic Publishers, Boston, MA.

A. G. Flook (1978). Use of dilation logic on the Quantimet to achieve fractal dimension characterization of texture and structured profiles. *Powder Technol.* 21:295-298.

A. G. Flook (1982). Fourier analysis of particle shape, in *Particle Size Analysis* 1981-2 (N. G. Stanley-Wood, T. Allen, Ed.). Wiley Heyden, London.

J. D. Foley, A. Van Dam (1984). *Fundamentals of Interactive Computer Graphics.* Addison Wesley, Reading MA.

J. Frank, (Ed.) (1992). *Electron Tomography*, Plenum Press, NY.

H. Freeman (1961). On the encoding of arbitrary geometric configurations. *IEEE Trans.* EC-10:260-268.

H. Freeman (1974). Computer processing of line-drawing images. *Comput. Surveys* 6:57-97.

W. Frei, C. C. Chen (1977). Fast boundary detection: a generalization and a new algorithm. *IEEE Trans. Comput.* C-26:988-998.

B. R. Frieden (1988). A comparison of maximum entropy, maximum *a postiori* and median window restoration algorithms, in *Scanning Microscopy,* Suppl. 2 (P. Hawkes et al., Eds.), pp. 107-111, Scanning Microscopy International, Chicago.

J. P. Frisby (1980). *Vision: Illusion, Brain and Mind.* Oxford Univ. Press, Oxford U.K.

K. S. Fu, J. K. Mui (1981). A survey on image segmentation. *Patt. Recog.* 13:3-16.

H. Fuchs, S. M. Pizer, L. C. Tsai, S. H. Bloomburg, E. R. Heinz (1982). Adding a true 3-D display to a raster graphics system. *IEEE Comput. Graphics Applic.* 2:73-78.

K. Fukunaga (1990). *Statistical Pattern Recognition, 2nd Edition.* Academic Press, Boston.

R. S. Gentile, J. P. Allebach, E. Walowit (1990). Quantization of color images based on uniform color spaces. *J. Imag. Technol.* 16(1):12-21.

R. C. Gonzalez, P. Wintz (1987). *Digital Image Processing, 2nd Edition.* Addison Wesley, Reading, MA.

R. Gordon (1974). A tutorial on ART (Algebraic Reconstruction Techniques). *IEEE Trans.* NS-21:78-93.

Y. A. Gowayed, J. C. Russ (1991). Geometric characterization of textile composite preforms using image analysis techniques. *J. Comput. Assist. Microsc.* 3(4): 189-200.

C. Gratin, F. Meyer (1992). Morphological three-dimensional analysis. *Scanning Microsc.*, Suppl. 6:129-135.

F. C. A. Green, I. T. Young, G. A. Lighart (1985). A comparison of different focus functions for use in autofocus algorithms. *Cytometry* 6:81-91.

P. Gualtieri, P. Coltelli (1992). An automated system for the analysis of moving images. *J. Comput. Assist. Microsc.* 3(1):15-22.

H. J. G. Gundersen et al. (1988). Some new, simple and efficient stereological methods and their use in pathological research and diagnosis. *Acta Pathol. Microbiol. Immunol. Scand.* 96:857.

K. J. Halford, K. Preston (1984). 3-D skeletonization of elongated solids. *Comput. Vis. Graph. Image Process.* 27:78-91.

Y. S. Ham (1993). Differential Absorption Cone-Beam Microtomography, Ph.D. Thesis, North Carolina State University.

R. M. Haralick (1978). Statistical and structural approaches to texture. Proc. 4th Int. Joint Conf. Patt. Recog., Kyoto, p. 45.

R. Haralick (1979). Statistical and textural approaches to textures. *Proc. IEEE* 67:786-804.

R. M. Haralick, I. Dinstein (1975). A spatial clustering procedure for multi-image data. *Comput. Graph. Image Process.* 12:60-73.

R. M. Haralick, L. G. Shapiro (1988). Segmentation and its place in machine vision. *Scanning Microsc.,* Suppl. 2:39-54.

R. M. Haralick, K. Shanmugam, I. Dinstein (1973). Textural features for image classification. *IEEE Trans.* SMC-3:610-621.

J. A. Hartigan (1975). *Clustering Algorithms.* John Wiley & Sons, New York.

R. V. L. Hartley (1942). A more symmetrical Fourier analysis applied to transmission problems. *Proc. IRE.*

D. Hearn, M. P. Baker (1986). *Computer Graphics.* Prentice Hall, Englewood Cliffs NJ.

P. Heckbert (1982). Color image quantization for frame buffer display. *Comput. Graph.* 16(3):297-307.

R. Hegerl (1989). Three-dimensional reconstruction from projections in electron microscopy. *Eur. J. Cell Biol.* 48 (Suppl. 25):135-138.

H. Heijmans (1991). Theoretical aspects of grey-level morphology. *IEEE Trans. PAMI* 13(6):568-582.

C. Heipke (1992). A global approach for least-squares image matching and surface reconstruction in object space. *Photogramm. Eng. Remote Sens.* 58(3):317-323.

J. Van Helden (1994). CrestPathway algorithm (personal communication).

G. T. Herman (1980). *Image Reconstruction from Projections — The Fundamentals of Computerized Tomography.* Academic Press, New York.

E. C. Hildreth (1983). The detection of intensity changes by computer and biological vision systems. *Comput. Vis. Graph. Image Process.* 22:1-27.

T. J. Holmes, S. Bhattacharyya, J. A. Cooper, D. Hanzel, V. Krishnamurti (1995). Light microscopic images reconstructed by maximum likelihood deconvolution, in *Handbook of Biological Confocal Microscopy* (J. Pawley, Ed.) Plenum Press, New York, 389-402.

B. K. P. Horn (1970). Shape from Shading: A Method for Obtaining the Shape of a Smooth Opaque Object from One View (AI Tech Report 79, Project MAC). Massachusetts Institute of Technology, Cambridge, MA.

P. Hough (1962). Method and means for recognizing complex patterns. U.S. Patent 3,069,654.

J. Huang, S. M. Dunn, S. M. Wiener, P. DeCosta (1994). A method for detecting correspondences in stereo pairs of electron micrographs of networks. *J. Comput. Assist. Microsc.* 6(2):85-102.

T. S. Huang (1979). A fast two-dimensional median filtering algorithm. *IEEE Trans.* ASSP-27:13-18.

D. H. Hubel (1988). *Eye, Brain, and Vision.* Scientific American Library, W. H. Freeman, New York.

H. E. Hurst, R. P. Black, Y. M. Simaika (1965). *Long Term Storage: An Experimental Study.* Constable, London.

C. Hwang, S. Venkatraman, K. R. Rao (1993). Human visual system weighted progressive image transmission using lapped orthogonal transform classified vector quantization. *Opt. Eng.* 32(7):1524-1530.

S. Inoue, K. R. Spring (1997). *Video Microscopy: The Fundamentals.* Plenum Press, New York.

A. K. Jain (1989). *Fundamentals of Digital Image Processing.* Prentice Hall, London.

P. A. Jansson, ed. (1997). *Deconvolution of Images and Spectra.* Academic Press, London.

E. T. Jaynes (1985). Where do we go from here? in *Maximum Entropy and Bayesian Methods in Inverse Problems* (C. R. Smith, W. T. Grandy, Eds.). D. Reidel Publishing Co., Dordrecht, Holland, 21-58.

K. F. Jarausch, T. J. Stark, P. E. Russell (1996). Silicon structures for in-situ characterization of atomic force microscopy probe geometry. *J. Vac. Sci. Technol. B* 14(6):3425.

J. P. Jernot (1982). Thése de Doctorat és Science, Université de Caen, France.

E. M. Johnson, J. J. Capowski (1985). Principles of reconstruction and three-dimensional display of serial sections using a computer, in *The Microcomputer in Cell and Neurobiology Research* (R. R. Mize, Ed.). Elsevier, New York, pp. 249-263.

L. R. Johnson, A. K. Jain (1981). An efficient two-dimensional FFT algorithm. *IEEE Trans.* PAMI-3:698-701.

Q. C. Johnson, J. H. Kinney, U. Bonse, M. C. Nichols, R. Nusshardt, J. M. Brase (1986). Micro-Tomography using Synchrotron Radiation. Lawrence Livermore National Laboratory Preprint UCRL-93538.

S. Joshi, M. I. Miller (1993). Maximum *a posteriori* estimation with good roughness for 3D optical sectioning microscopy. *Opt. Soc. Am. A.* 10:1078-1985.

A. C. Kak, M. Slaney (1988). *Principles of Computerized Tomographic Imaging.* IEEE Pub. PC-02071.

J. N. Kanpur, P. K. Sahoo, A. K. C. Wong (1985). A new method for grey-level picture thresholding using the entropy of the histogram. *Comput. Vis. Graph. Image Process.* 29:273-285.

M. Kass, A. Witkin, D. Terzopoulos (1987). Snakes: active contour models. *Int. J. Comput. Vis.* 1(4):321-331.

A. E. Kayaalp, R. C. Jain (1987). Using SEM stereo to extract semiconductor wafer pattern topography. *Proc. SPIE* 775: 18-26.

B. H. Kaye, J. E. LeBlanc, G. Clark (1983). A study of physical significance of three-dimensional signature waveforms. Proc. Fineparticle Characterization Conference.

B. H. Kaye (1986). Image analysis procedures for characterizing the fractal dimension of fineparticles. Proc. Particle Technol. Conf., Nürnberg.

A. Keating (1993). Duke University, private communication.

D. J. Keller (1991). Reconstruction of STM and AFM images distorted by finite-size tips. *Surf. Sci.* 253:353-364.

D. J. Keller, F. S. Franke (1993). Envelope reconstruction of probe microscope images. *Surf. Sci.* 294:409-419.

S. Kim, J. Lee, J. Kim (1988). A new chain-coding algorithm for binary images using run-length codes. *Comput. Vis. Graph. Image Process.* 41:114-128.

J. H. Kinney, Q. C. Johnson, M. C. Nichols, U. Bonse, R. A. Saroyan, R. Nusshardt, R. Pahl (1989). X-ray microtomography on beamline X at SSRL. *Rev. Sci. Instrum.* 60(7):2471-4.

J. H. Kinney, M. C. Nichols, U. Bonse, S. R. Stock, T. M. Breunig, A. Guvenilir, R. A. Saroyan (1990). Nondestructive imaging of materials microstructures using X-ray tomographic microscopy. Proc. MRS Symp. Tomograph. Imaging, Boston, MA.

R. Kirsch (1971). Computer determination of the constituent structure of biological images. *Comput. Biomed. Res.* 4: 315-328.

J. Kittler, J. Illingworth, J. Foglein (1985). Threshold selection based on a simple image statistic. *Comput. Vis. Graph. Image Process.* 30:125-147.

A. Kriete (Ed.) (1992). *Visualization in Biomedical Microscopies: 3D Imaging and Computer Applications.* VCH Publishers, Weinheim.

F. P. Kuhl, C. R. Giardina (1982). Elliptic Fourier features of a closed contour. *Comput. Graph. Image Process.* 18: 236-258.

K. J. Kurzydlowski, B. Ralph (1995). *The Quantitative Description of the Microstructure of Materials.* CRC Press, Boca Raton, FL.

L. Lam, S. Lee, C. Suen (1992). Thinning methodologies — a comprehensive survey. *IEEE Trans.* PAMI 14:868-885.

C. Lantejoul, S. Beucher (1981). On the use of the geodesic metric in image analysis. *J. Microsc.* 121:39.

D. L. Lee, A. T. Winslow (1993). Performance of three image-quality metrics in ink-jet printing of plain papers. *J. Electron. Imag.* 2(3):174-184.

S. U. Lee, S. Y. Chung, R. H. Park (1990). A comparative performance study of several global thresholding techniques for segmentation. *Comput. Vis. Graph. Image Process.* 52: 171-190.

S. Levialdi (1972) On shrinking binary picture patterns. *Commun. ACM* 15(1):7-10.

H. Li, M. Novak, R. Forchheimer (1993). Fractal-based image sequence compression scheme. *Opt. Eng.* 32(7):1588-1595.

W. Lin, T. J. Holmes, D. H. Szarowski, J. N. Turner (1994). Data corrections for three-dimensional light microscopy stereo pair reconstruction. *J. Comput. Assist. Microsc.* 6(3):113-128.

M. Lineberry (1982). Image segmentation by edge tracing. *Applications of Digital Image Processing IV*, Vol. 359.

S. Lobregt, P. W. Verbeek, F. C. A. Groen (1980). Three-dimensional skeletonization: principle and algorithm. *IEEE Trans.* PAMI-2:75-77.

E. Mach (1906). Über den Einfluss räumlich und zeitlich variierender Lichtreize auf die Gesichtswarhrnehmung. *Sitzungsber. Akad. Wiss. Wien. Math. Naturwiss. Kl.* 115: 633-648.

J. B. MacQueen (1967). Some methods for the classification and analysis of multivariate observations. *Proc. 5th Berkeley Symp. Math. Stat. Probab.* 1: 281-297.

B. B. Mandelbrot (1967). How long is the coast of Britain? Statistical self-similarity and fractional dimension. *Science* 155:636-638.

B. B. Mandelbrot (1982). *The Fractal Geometry of Nature.* W. H. Freeman, San Francisco.

B. B. Mandelbrot, D. E. Passoja, A. J. Paullay (1984). Fractal character of fracture surfaces of metals. *Nature* 308:721.

P. Markiewicz, M. C. Goh (1994). Atomic force microscopy probe tip visualization and improvement of images using a simple deconvolution procedure. *Langmuir* 10:5-7.

P. Markiewicz, M. C. Goh (1995). Atomic force microscope tip deconvolution using calibration arrays. *Rev. Sci. Instrum.* 66:3186-3190.

D. Marr (1982). *Vision.* W. H. Freeman, San Francisco.

D. Marr, E. Hildreth (1980). Theory of edge detection. *Proc. R. Soc. London Ser. B,* 207:187-217.

D. Marr, T. Poggio (1976). Cooperative computation of stereo disparity. *Science* 194:283-287.

G. A. Mastin (1985). Adaptive filters for digital image noise smoothing: an evaluation. *Comput. Vis. Graph. Image Process.* 31:102-121.

A. D. McAulay, J. Wang, J. Li (1993). Optical wavelet transform classifier with positive real Fourier transform wavelets. *Opt. Eng.* 32(6):1333-1339.

J. J. Mecholsky, D. E. Passoja (1985). Fractals and brittle fracture, in *Fractal Aspects of Materials.* Materials Research Society, Pittsburgh, PA.

J. J. Mecholsky, T. J. Mackin, D. E. Passoja (1986). Crack propagation in brittle materials as a fractal process, in *Fractal Aspects of Materials II*. Materials Research Society, Pittsburgh PA.

J. J. Mecholsky, D. E. Passoja, K. S. Feinberg-Ringel (1989). Quantitative analysis of brittle fracture surfaces using fractal geometry. *J. Am. Ceram. Soc.* 72:60.

G. Medioni, R. Nevatia (1985). Segment-based stereo matching. *Comput. Vis. Graph. Image Process.* 31:2-18.

D. L. Milgram (1975). Computer methods for creating photomosaics. *IEEE Trans.* C-24:1113-1119.

D. L. Milgram, M. Herman (1979). Clustering edge values for threshold selection. *Comput. Graph. Image Process.* 10: 272-280.

M. W. Mitchell, D. A. Bonnell (1990). Quantitative topographic analysis of fractal surfaces by scanning tunneling microscopy. *J. Mat. Res.* 5(10):2244-2254.

J. R. Monck, A. F. Oberhauser, T. J. Keating, J. M. Hernandez (1992). Thin-section ratiometric Ca2+ images obtained by optical sectioning of Fura-2 loaded mast cells. *J. Cell Biol.* 116:745-759.

H. P. Moravec (1977). Towards automatic visual obstacle avoidance. *Proc. 5th IJCAI*, 584.

R. B. Mott (1995). Position-tagged spectrometry, a new approach for EDS spectrum imaging. *Proc. Microsc. Microanal.,* p. 595. Jones and Begall, NY.

J. C. Mott-Smith (1970). Medial axis transformations, in *Picture Processing and Psychopictorics* (B. S. Lipkin, A. Rosenfeld, Eds.). Academic Press, New York.

K. S. Nathan, J. C. Curlander (1990). Reducing speckle in one-look SAR images. *NASA Tech. Briefs,* Feb:70.

R. Nevatia, K. Babu (1980). Linear feature extraction and description. *Comput. Graph. Image Process.,* Vol. 13.

W. Niblack (Ed.) (1993). Storage and retrieval for image and video databases. *SPIE Proc.,* Vol. 1908.

A. Nicoulin, M. Mattavelli, W. Li, M. Kunt (1993). Subband image coding using jointly localized filter banks and entropy coding based on vector quantization. *Opt. Eng.* 32(7):1430-1450.

A. Nieminen, P. Heinonen, Y. Nuevo (1987). A new class of detail-preserving filters for image processing. *IEEE Trans. Patt. Anal. Mach. Intell.* PAMI-9:74-90.

J. F. O'Callaghan (1974). Computing the perceptual boundaries of dot patterns. *Comput. Graph. Image Process.* 3(2):141-162.

K. Oistämö, Y. Neuvo (1990). Vector median operations for color image processing. Nonlinear Image Processing (E. J. Delp, Ed.). *SPIE Proc.* 1247:2-12.

C. K. Olsson (1993). Image Processing Methods in Materials Science. Ph. D. Thesis, Technical University of Denmark, Lyngby, Denmark.

N. Otsu (1979). A threshold selection method from gray-level histograms. *IEEE Trans.* SMC-9: 62-69.

D. P. Panda, A. Rosenfeld (1978). Image segmentation by pixel classification in (gray level, edge value) space. *IEEE Trans. Comput.* 27:875-879.

T. Pavlidis (1980). A thinning algorithm for discrete binary images. *Comput. Graph. Image Process.* 13:142-157.

S. Peleg, J. Naor, R. Hartley, D. Avnir (1984). Multiple resolution texture analysis and classification. *IEEE Trans. Patt. Anal. Mach. Intell.* PAMI-6:518.

A. P. Pentland (1983). Fractal-based description of natural scenes. *IEEE Trans.* PAMI-6:661.

A. P. Pentland, (Ed.) (1986). *From Pixels to Predicates*. Ablex, Norwood, NJ.

J. L. Pfalz (1976). Surface networks. *Geogr. Anal.* 8(2):77-93.

M. T. Postek, A. E. Vladar, M. P. Davidson (1998). Image sharpness measurement in scanning electron microscopy. *Scanning* 20:1-9 and 24-34.

W. K. Pratt (1991). *Digital Image Processing*, Second Ed. Wiley, New York.

T. Prettyman, R. Gardner, J. Russ, K. Verghese (1991). On the performance of a combined transmission and scattering approach to industrial computed tomography. *Advances in X-Ray Analysis*, Vol. 35. Plenum Press, New York.

J. M. S. Prewitt, M. L. Mendelsohn (1966). The analysis of cell images. *Ann. N. Y. Acad. Sci.* 128:1035-1053.

L. Quam, M. J. Hannah (1974). *Stanford Automated Photogrammetry Research* AIM-254, Stanford AI Lab.

C. F. Quate (1994). The AFM as a tool for surface imaging. *Surf. Sci.* (Netherlands) 299-300, 980-95.

J. Radon (1917). Über die Bestimmung von Funktionen durch ihre Integralwerte längs gewisser Mannigfaltigkeiten. *Berlin Sächsische Akad. Wiss.* 29:262-279.

M. G. Reed, C. V. Howard, C. G. Shelton (1997). Confocal imaging and second-order stereological analysis of a liquid foam. *J. Microsc.* 185(3):313-320.

M. G. Reed, C. V. Howard (1997). Edge corrected estimates of the nearest neighbor function for three-dimensional point patterns. *J. Microsc.* (in press).

M. G. Reed, C. V. Howard (1998). *Unbiased Stereology*. Bios Scientific Pub., Oxford.

A. A. Reeves, Optimized Fast Hartley Transform with Applications in Image Processing, Thesis, Dartmouth University, March 1990.

R. G. Reeves, (Ed.) (1975). *Manual of Remote Sensing*. American Society of Photogrammetry, Falls Church, CA.

W. H. Richardson (1972). Bayesian-based iterative method of image restoration. *J. Opt. Soc. Am.* 62:55-59.

J. P. Rigaut (1988). Automated image segmentation by mathematical morphology and fractal geometry. *J. Microsc.* 150:21-30.

G. X. Ritter, J. N. Wilson (1996). *Handbook of Computer Vision Algorithms in Image Algebra*. CRC Press, Boca Raton, FL.

B. G. Rosen, R. J. Crafoord, (Eds.) (1997). *Metrology and Properties of Engineering Surfaces*. Chalmers University, Göteborg Sweden.

A. Rosenfeld, A. C. Kak (1982). *Digital Picture Processing*, Vols. 1 and 2. Academic Press, New York.

I. Rock (1984). *Perception*. W. H Freeman, New York.

L. G. Roberts (1965). Machine perception of three-dimensional solids, in *Optical and Electro-Optical Information Processing* (J. T. Tippett, Ed.). MIT Press, Cambridge, MA.

F. J. Rohlf, J.W. Archie (1984). A comparison of Fourier methods for the description of wing shape in mosquitoes (*Diptera: culicidae*). *Syst. Zool.* 33: 302-317.

F. J. Rohlf (1990). Morphometrics. *Annu. Rev. Ecol. Syst.* 21: 299-316.

J. C. Russ (1984). Implementing a new skeletonizing method. *J. Microsc.* 136:RP7.

J. C. Russ (1986). *Practical Stereology*. Plenum Press, New York.

J. C. Russ (1988). Differential absorption three-dimensional microtomography. *Trans Am. Nucl. Soc.* 56(3):14.

J. C. Russ (1990a). *Computer Assisted Microscopy*. Plenum Press, New York.

J. C. Russ (1990b). Surface characterization: fractal dimensions, Hurst coefficients and frequency transforms. *J. Comput. Assist. Microsc.* 2(3):161-184.

J. C. Russ (1990c). Processing images with a local Hurst operator to reveal textural differences. *J. Comput. Assist. Microsc.* 2(4):249-257.

J. C. Russ (1991). Multiband thresholding of images. *J. Comput. Assist. Microsc.* 3(2):77-96.

J. C. Russ (1993). JPEG Image Compression and Image Analysis. *J. Comput. Assist. Microsc.* 5(3):237-244.

J. C. Russ (1993). Method and application for ANDing features in binary images. *J. Comput. Assist. Microsc.* 5(4):265-272.

J. C. Russ (1994). *Fractal Surfaces*. Plenum Press, New York.

J. C. Russ (1995a). Computer-assisted manual stereology. *J. Comput. Assist. Microsc.* 7(1):35-46.

J. C. Russ (1995b). Median filtering in color space. *J. Comput. Assist. Microsc.* 7(2):83-90.

J. C. Russ (1995c). Thresholding images. *J. Comput. Assist. Microsc.* 7(3):41-164.

J. C. Russ (1995d). Designing kernels for image filtering. *J. Comput. Assist. Microsc.* 7(4):179-190.

J. C. Russ (1995e). Optimal greyscale images. *J. Comput. Assist. Microsc.* 7(4):221-234.

J. C. Russ (1995f). Segmenting touching hollow features. *J. Comput. Assist. Microsc.* 7(4):253-261.

J. C. Russ (1997). Fractal dimension measurement of engineering surfaces, in *7th Int. Conf. Metrol. Prop. Eng. Surf.* (B. G. Rosen, R. J. Crafoord, Eds.), Chalmers University, Göteborg, Sweden, 170-174.

J. C. Russ, J. C. Russ (1988a). Automatic discrimination of features in grey scale images. *J. Microsc.* 148:263-277.

J. C. Russ, J. C. Russ (1988b). Improved implementation of a convex segmentation algorithm. *Acta Stereolog.* 7:33-40.

J. C. Russ, J. C. Russ (1989a). Uses of the Euclidean distance map for the measurement of features in images. *J. Comput. Assist. Microsc.* 1(4):343.

J. C. Russ, J. C. Russ (1989b). Topological measurements on skeletonized three-dimensional networks. *J. Comput. Assist. Microsc.* 1:131-150.

J. C. Russ, H. Palmour, III, T. M. Hare (1989). Direct 3-D pore location measurement in alumina. *J. Microsc.* 155(2):RP1-2.

F. F. Sabins, Jr. (1987). *Remote Sensing: Principles and Interpretation (2nd Ed.).* W. H. Freeman, New York.

P. K. Sahoo, S. Soltani, A. C. Wong, Y. C. Chen (1988). A survey of thresholding techniques. *Comput. Vis. Graph. Image Process.* 41:233-260.

A. Santos et al. (1997). Evaluation of autofocus functions in molecular cytogenetic analysis. *J. Microsc.* 188(3):264-272.

A. Savitsky, M. J. E. Golay (1964). Smoothing and differentiation of data by simplified least squares procedures. *Anal. Chem.* 36:1627-1639.

D. J. Schneberk, H. E. Martz, S. G. Azavedo (1991). Multiple energy techniques in industrial computerized tomography, in *Review of Progress in Quantitative Nondestructive Evaluation* (D. O. Thompson, D. E. Chimenti, Eds.). Plenum Press, New York.

H. P. Schwartz, K. C. Shane (1969). Measurement of particle shape by Fourier analysis. *Sedimentology* 13:213-231.

H. Schwarz, H. E. Exner (1980). Implementation of the concept of fractal dimensions on a semi-automatic image analyzer. *Powder Technol.* 27:107.

H. Schwarz, H. E. Exner (1983). The characterization of the arrangement of feature centroids in planes and volumes. *J. Microsc.* 129:155.

P. J. Scott (1995). Recent advances in areal characterization. *IX Int. Oberflächenkolloq,* Technical University of Chemnitz, Zwickau, 151-158.

P. J. Scott (1997). Foundations of topological characterization of surface texture, in *7th Int. Conf. Metrol. Prop. Eng. Surf.* (B. G. Rosen, R. J. Crafoord, Eds.). Chalmers University, Göteborg Sweden, 162-169.

J. Serra (1982). *Image Analysis and Mathematical Morphology.* Academic Press, London.

L. A. Shepp, B. F. Logan (1974). The Fourier reconsruction of a head section. *IEEE Trans.* NS-21:21-43.

J. Skilling (1986). Theory of maximum entropy image reconstruction, in Maximum Entropy and Bayesian Methods in Applied Statistics, *Proc. 4th Max. Entropy Workshop,* University of Calgary, 1984 (J. H. Justice, Ed.), pp. 156-178. Cambridge University Press, Cambridge.

B. D. Smith (1990). Cone-beam tomography: recent advances and a tutorial review. *SPIE Opt. Eng.* 29:5.

D. L. Snyder, T. J. Schutz, J. A. O'Sullivan (1992). Deblurring subject to nonnegative constraints. *IEEE Trans. Signal Process.* 40:1143-1150.

I. Sobel (1970). *Camera Models and Machine Perception*, AIM-21. Stanford Artificial Intelligence Lab, Palo Alto.

S. Srinivasan, J. C. Russ, R. O. Scattergood (1990). Fractal analysis of erosion surfaces. *J. Mat. Res.* 5(11):2616-2619.

J. A. Stark, W. J. Fitzgerald (1996). An alternative algorithm for adaptive histogram equalization. *Comput. Vis. Graph. Image Process.* 56(2):180-185.

D. C. Sterio (1984). The unbiased estimation of number and sizes of arbitrary particles using the disector. *J. Microsc.* 134:127.

P. L. Stewart, R. M. Burnett. Seminars in Virology. Cited in C. J. Mathias, "Visualization Techniques Augment Lab Research into Structure of Adenovirus." *Sci. Comput. Autom.* 7(6):51-56.

J. A. Storer (1992). *Image and Text Compression.* Kluwer Academic Publishers, New York.

K. J. Stout, P. J. Sullivan, W. P. Dong, E. Mainsah, N. Luo, T. Mathia, H. Zahouani (1993). The development of methods for the characterization of roughness in three dimensions. Publication EUR 15178 EN of the Commission of the European Communities, University of Birmingham, Edgbaston, England.

R. E. Swing (1997). *An Introduction to Microdensitometry.* SPIE Press, Bellingham, WA.

M. M. Thompson, (Ed.) (1966). *Manual of Photogrammetry.* American Society of Photogrammetry, Falls Church, VA.

E. E. Underwood (1970). *Quantitative Stereology.* Addison Wesley, Reading, MA.

E. E. Underwood, K. Banerji (1986). Fractals in Fractography. *Mat. Sci. Eng.* 80:1.

G. M. P. Van Kempen, L. J. Van Vliet, P. J. Verveer, H. T. M. Van der Voort (1997). A quantitative comparison of image restoration methods in confocal microscopy. *J. Microsc.* 185(3):354-365.

J. G. Verly, R. L. Delanoy (1993). Some principles and applications of adaptive mathematical morphology for range imagery. *Opt. Eng.* 32(12):3295-3306.

H. Verschueren, B. Houben, J. De Braekeleer, J. De Wit, D. Roggen, P. De Baetselier (1993). Methods for computer assisted analysis of lymphoid cell shape and motility, including Fourier analysis of cell outlines. *J. Immunol. Methods* 163: 99-113.

J. S. Villarrubia (1994). Morphological estimation of tip geometry for scanned probe microscopy. *Surf. Sci.* 321:287-300.

J. S. Villarrubia (1996). Scanned probe microscope tip characterization without calibrated tip characterizers. *J. Vac. Sci. Technol.* B14:1518-1521.

G. Wang, T. H. Lin, P. C. Cheng, D. M. Shinozaki, H. Kim (1991). Scanning cone-beam reconstruction algorithms for X-ray microtomography. *SPIE Scanning Microsc. Instrument.* 1556:99.

R. J. Wall, A. Klinger, K. R. Castleman (1974). Analysis of image histograms, *Proc. 2nd Jt. Int. Conf. Patt. Recog.*, IEEE 74CH-0885-4C:341-344.

E. R. Weibel (1979). *Stereological Methods, Vols. I & II.* Academic Press, London.

A. Wen, C. Lu (1993). Hybrid vector quantization. *Opt. Eng.* 32(7):1496-1502.

J. S. Weszka (1978). A survey of threshold selection techniques. *Comput. Graph. Image Process.* 7:259-265.

J. Weszka, C. Dyer, A. Rosenfeld (1976). A comparative study of texture measures for terrain classification. *IEEE Trans.* SMC-6: 269-285.

J. S. Weszka, A. Rosenfeld (1979). Histogram modification for threshold selection. *IEEE Trans.* SMC-9:38-52.

D. J. Whitehouse (1994). *Precision — The Handbook of Surface Metrology.* Institute of Physics Publishing, Bristol.

H. K. Wickramasinghe (1991). Scanned probes old and new. *AIP Conf. Proc.* (USA), 9-22.

R. Wilson, M. Spann (1988). *Image Segmentation and Uncertainty.* Wiley, New York.

Z. Wang (1990). *Principles of Photogrammetry (with Remote Sensing).* Press of Wuhan Technical University of Surveying and Mapping, Beijing.

G. Wolf (1991). Usage of global information and *a priori* knowledge for object isolation. *Proc. 8th Int. Congr. Stereol.*, Irvine, CA, 56.

K. W. Wong (1980). Basic Mathematics of Photogrammetry, in *Manual of Photogrammetry, 4th Ed.*, American Society of Photogrammetry, Falls Church, VA, 57-58.

S. H. Wong, S. F. Yau (1998). Linear neural network for the solution of limited angle problems in computer-aided tomography. *J. Electron. Imaging* 7(1):70-78.

B. P. Wrobel (1991). Least-squares methods for surface reconstruction from images. *ISPRS J. Photogramm. Remote Sensing*, 46:67-84.

S. Wu, A. Gersho (1993). Lapped vector quantization of images. *Opt. Eng.* 32(7):1489-1495.

G. J. Yang, T. S. Huang (1981). The effect of median filtering on edge location estimation. *Comput. Graph. Image Process.* 15:224-245

Y. Yakimovsky (1976) Boundary and object detection in real world images *J. Assoc. Comput. Mach.* 23:599-618.

R. W. Young, N. G. Kingsbury (1993). Video compression using lapped transforms for motion estimation/compensation and coding. *Opt. Eng.* 32(7):1451-1463.

C. T. Zahn, R. Z. Roskies (1972). Fourier descriptors for plane closed curves. *IEEE Trans. Comput.* C-21: 269-281.

X. Zhou, E. Dorrer (1994). An automatic image matching algorithm based on wavelet decomposition, *ISPRS Int. Arch. Photogramm. Remote Sensing* 30(3/2):951-960.

S. Zucker (1976). Region growing: childhood and adolescence. *Comput. Graph. Image Process.* 5:382-399.

Index

Abbott curve..727
absolute color information 52
accumulator space 525
ACF, see autocorrelation function
acoustic microscopy..662
ADC, see analog-to-digital converter
addressing circuits...228
aerial photography 75, 76, 77, 82, 287
aerial survey 565
AFM, see atomic force microscope
algebraic reconstruction technique (ART)......586, 589,
                                                                    608
aliasing...172, 321
amblyopia..650
Amiga HAM format records....................................126
amplitude parameters 729
analog-to-digital converter (ADC)............................17
ANDing...462
animation, time-based...639
archival storage 119
ART, see algebraic reconstruction technique
artificial intelligence 429
ASCII representation 125
aspect ratio 553
astronomy..25, 163, 299
ATM, see atomic force microscope
atomic force microscope (AFM).................61, 67, 276,
                                                               277, 693, 709
atom probe ion microscope 629
attenuation profiles 580
Auger electrons 705
autocorrelation 367
     function (ACF)...............................727, 732, 733
     image 369
automatic leveling..198, 199
automatic scaling...291, 296
autoradiograph image..186

background image 81, 195, 197
backprojection....................................582, 583, 586, 590
banding..103
Barnsley approach 157
beam hardening 596, 598
Bernoulli drives...118

best fit circles 527
bias, correction for..530
binary image....................................375, 410, 420, 532
     combined..433
     creating...452
     mask 440
     processing 539
binary image processing 431–508
     Boolean logic with features.....................447–451
     Boolean operations 431–434
     boundary lines and thickening................485–489
     coefficient and depth parameters............471–476
     combining Boolean operations 434–438
     custer..481–483
     double thresholding................................456–460
     erosion and dilation 460–461
     Euclidean distance map 489–494
     examples of use 476–481
     extension to grey scale images 469–471
     fractal dimension measurement 501
     from pixels to features............................440–447
     isotropy...465–467
     masks 438–440
     measurements using erosion and dilation ..467–469
     medial axis transform...............................501–508
     opening and closing 461–465
     selecting features by location 451–455
     skeletonization..483–485
     ultimate eroded points............................498–501
     watershed segmentation 494–498
blur vector 362
Boolean logic 68, 384, 438, 449, 454
boundary
     lines...413, 485, 558
     representation 421, 441, 544, 557, 635
bounding-box coordinates 531
brightness 57
     broadcast television 16, 130
     browsing..124
     brute-force correlation methods 73
     Gaussian random 295
     histogram.............................235, 286, 372, 409, 412
     information...83
     level 496

pattern 190
profile 149, 252, 514
range 285
rank operators..743
value 33, 229, 287, 358, 491, 507, 670
variation in 192, 324
Butterworth low-pass filters 339

CAD, see computer-aided design
calibration scale.............................512, 513
caliper dimensions.................................543
camcorders...39
camera specification 21
camouflage...6
Canny filter..268
Cartesian coordinates.............................524
CAT scans, see Computer Assisted Tomography scans
cathode ray tube (CRT).............22, 23, 26, 99, 48,
                                       135, 139, 229
CBED, see convergent beam electron diffraction
CCD, see charged coupled device
CCITT, see International Telegraph and Telephone
Consultative Committee
CD-ROM.......................114, 117, 118, 160
cellophane display.................................682
center-to-center distances.....................505
center of gravity.....................................518
chain code...............................561, 570
charge injection device (CID) 7
charged coupled device (CCD)...........7, 8
    array.................................28, 163
    camera................................164
    chip.......................................37
    detector array 64
chemical etching 486, 690
chord
    encoding.................................420
    table 421
chrominance..............................36, 146
CID, see charge injection device
CIE, see Commission Internationale de L'Éclairage
classification problem 427
Clementine mission.................................80
clusters.....................................428, 504
CMYK, see cyan-magenta-yellow-black
CODEC, see Compressor-decompressor
coding schemes.......................................131
Collage Theorem.....................................157
color
    balancing.................................510
    coding......................568, 573
    composites 34
    correction.................................206
    correction for shift in 208
    displays....................................56
    images 32, 52
    laser printers.............................107
    matching.................................101
    median filter.............................177
    palettes...................................135
    phosphors.................................58
    printing.......................98, 104
    separation.............53, 54, 102
    shading....................................205
    shifts 11
    spaces 47
    subtractive 108
colorimetry 206

Comet Halley 1, 33
Commission Internationale de L'Éclairage (CIE).......47
    color diagram.............................378
    in color management systems.............51
compositional mapping.........................704
compression 151, 154
    effects of...................................344
    methods.................132, 155, 159
    ratios 136, 160
Compressor-decompressor (CODEC) 158
computer
    -aided design (CAD) 210–211, 667, 717, 720
    algorithm 523
    displays.........................58, 74
    drawing programs.........................516
    graphics 210, 615, 675, 718, 721
    memory.....................................38
    modeling...................................724
    processing.......................80, 474
    reconstruction methods 622
    software....................................123
    systems 371
Computer Assisted Tomography (CAT) scans 578, 667
confocal light microscope 364
confocal optics 698
confocal scanning light microscope (CSLM) 30, 61, 70,
                                     299, 418, 624, 626
contours.............................176, 238, 416, 664, 713
contrast expansion.........................191, 348
convergent beam electron diffraction (CBED)...........3
convolution 354
correlation 354, 366
counting
    errors 538
    procedures, special 532
    statistics...........................183, 404
cross-correlation.....................................367
crossing fibers 532
CRT, see cathode ray tube
crystalline silicon..................................327
CSLM, see confocal scanning light microscope
custer 481
cyan-magenta-yellow-black (CMYK) 100, 101, 102
cycloids...447

daisy wheel printer....................................88
data
    3D 649
    management................................113
    presentation...............................712
    set...................636, 661, 673, 680
database
    constructing................................113
    for images.................................120
    management programs.............120, 122, 126, 128
DCT, see discrete cosine transform
Debye-Scherer X-ray...................152, 293
decompression 143
degraded signals 17
delta compression 129
densitometry gels.....................................83
depth
    parameters.................................471
    resolution..................................605
    scale..622
    value..636
derivative calculations.............................265
desktop

color printers......................................98
computers...22
systems 370
detrending...64
Difference of Gaussians (D.O.G.)...........................263
diffraction pattern 3
digital cameras.................................41, 43
digital image processing...............................27
digital movies.....................................158
digital signal processing 337
digital video (DV) 40, 41
digitizers, sonic....................................657
dilation.....................406, 460, 462, 463, 467, 472
2D images, see two-dimensional images
3D images, see three-dimensional images
discrete cosine transform (DCT).....................141–142
display
    cellophane..................................682
    hardware 654
    line profile.................................718
    mesh.......................................719
    methods................................640, 687
    modes......................................670
    volumetric..................................646
distance map 492
distortion...................................219, 621
dithering...96
D.O.G., see Difference of Gaussians
Doppler shift 79
dot-matrix printers 91
dots per inch (dpi)..................................88
    laser writer.................................229
    resolution...................................96
double thresholding.................................456
dpi, see dots per inch
dry inks..105
DV, see digital video
dye sublimation printer 104, 107, 108

edge
    effects.....................................506
    enhancement................................259
    -finding methods.........................262, 266
    following, automatic..........................414
EDM, see Euclidean distance map
electrical signals 305
electrochemistry 694
electromagnetic radiation 78
electron
    diffraction patterns.......................4, 527
    images, secondary...........................535
    microscopist 322
    tomography.................................606
electronic cameras 9
elevation
    contour map................................419
    maps.......................................78
    measurements of.............................702
    profile..................................723, 725
ellipse......................................551, 552
emission tomography 603
empty magnification 18
entropy
    methods................................190, 406
    maximum................................189, 590
erosion...................406, 461, 463, 464, 473
    /dilation procedures 479
    directional.................................475

measurements using 467
methods...492
rate..628
Euclidean boundary 469
Euclidean distance map (EDM)...........251, 342, 489,
                491, 502, 508, 534, 546, 581
    locating...................................251
Euclidean geometry 556, 725

face-centered cubic (FCC) configuration.................634
fan-beam geometry 603
fast Fourier transform 270
fate table...474
fatigue striations 204
fax machines 134, 421
FCC configuration, see face-centered cubic
    configuration
feature(s)
    counting...........................529, 530, 563
    irregular...................................517
    selecting...................................450
    size.......................................536
file server..128
film recorders 110, 111
filtering......................................343, 369
filter shapes......................................594
Fizeau optics......................................65
flood fill algorithm.................................731
floppy disks.......................................45
fluorescence microscopy.................8, 25, 165, 299
formed-character printer.............................88
formfactor..554
Fourier analysis 561
Fourier coefficients 313
Fourier inversion 607
Fourier space reconstruction 582
Fourier transform 140, 306, 307, 311, 314, 333,
            336, 341, 347, 350, 352, 581, 584, 741
Fourier transform infrared (FTIR) spectroscopy......703
fractal(s)
    analysis....................................282
    behavior....................................550
    compression 157
    dimension................501, 555, 557, 558, 737, 739,
                    740, 742, 745
    line, computer-generated 332
    outlines....................................559
    pattern.....................................700
    surface dimension...........................331
    texture and.................................330
frame averaging....................................163
freeze-fractured cell walls...........................205
freeze frame playback 16
Frei and Chen operator 444, 680, 681
frequency transform.....................327, 344, 363, 387
frequency space, processing images in 305–370
    convolution and correlation 354–370
    filtering images...........................334–354
    mathematical preliminaries...............305–320
    measuring images in frequency domain..320–333
FTIR spectroscopy, see Fourier transform infrared
    spectroscopy
functional parameters 729
fuzzy logic 122

gamma ray tomography...............................606
ganglia 248
Gaussian

curves 342
   distribution 168, 191
   filter...725
   function 404
   kernel..204, 407
   random brightness 295
   shape 408
   smoothing kernel 203
GCR, see grey component replacement
geographic information systems (GIS) 641
geometric probability..536
Gestalt theory..6
GIS, see geographic information systems
Global Positioning System (GPS)...........................124
GPS, see Global Positioning System
gradient image...418
graphics design 656
grey component replacement (GCR).....................100
grey scale 54, 94, 97, 258, 417
   dilation..276
   erosion...185, 187, 202
   image.................230, 376, 429, 469, 489, 541, 692
   noise, random 551
   power spectrum...329
   transfer functions 232
   value 193, 235, 439, 533, 547

halftoning 89, 91
hand-held scanners...31
Haralick operator 288, 395
harmonic analysis 559, 560, 562
HCP configuration, see hexagonal close packed
   configuration
HDTV, see high-definition television
heat emission 1
hexagonal close packed (HCP) configuration.........634
high resolution imaging...25
high-definition television (HDTV) ...13, 28, 29, 40, 138
histogram(s)...542, 730
   equalization...233, 236, 239
   examples of...372
   modification of..408
   one-dimensional 377
   peaks 373
   plot of...413
   selective 410
   texture/brightness 400
   three-dimensional 234
   two-dimensional 391
HLS, see hue, lightness, and saturation
holograms...4
homogeneity, measure of...281
horizontal brightness profile 254
Hough transform..524, 527
HSI, see hue, saturation, and intensity
HSV, see hue, saturation, and value
hue, lightness, and saturation (HLS).........................49
hue, saturation, and intensity (HSI)...49, 144, 177, 715
hue, saturation, and value (HSV)...............................49
Huffman code 131, 133
human vision 4, 101, 139, 247, 555, 720
Hurst operator 286, 288
hybrid
   median..181
   parameters...729
   properties 734
hysteresis problems 709

illumination 81, 123, 198, 199, 408
illusion 5
image(s)
   alignment of 214, 216
   ambiguous...423
   analysis 52, 86, 227, 289, 523
   archival storage of...119
   as-acquired 227
   background...195, 197
   blurring of...652
   brightness 249
   browsing through 125
   capture..14, 447
   common type of...536
   compression..128
   databases 124
   derivative 715
   digitized color 515
   enhancement of 84
   fidelity..39
   file sizes 145
   filtering 334
   gradient..418
   halftone 90
   hardcopy representations of 87
   histogram-equalized...237
   inverted..499
   ion microprobe 418
   math..290
   morphing to align 224
   multiband 374, 384
   multiplication 295
   noise-free 191
   out-of-focus 359
   pixel-based 401, 402
   posterizing...181
   processing operations...671
   quality..143, 306, 593
   reconstructed..316
   removal of debris from...465
   representation 420
   restored 139
   segmenting 458
   sensing chip 44
   smoothing of 394
   sparse dot 405
   spatial domain..317
   statistical averages of 127
   subtracting 292
   test 218
   texture..278
   thresholded 565
   types 59
   vertical averaging of 251
   warping 220
image acquisition 575–616,
   see also images, acquiring
   algebraic reconstruction methods 585–590
   basics of reconstruction 578–585
   defects in reconstructed images...............592–603
   device 195
   hardware 86
   high resolution tomography 613–616
   imaging geometries...................................603–605
   maximum entropy......................................590–592
   three-dimensional tomography 605–613
   volume imaging vs. sections....................575–578
image enhancement..................................227–303, 708

contrast manipulation 228–233
derivatives...250–255
fractal analysis 282–288
histogram equalization............................233–242
image math 290–292
implementation notes 288–290
Laplacian..242–250
multiplication and division 295–303
rank operations 268–277
Sobel and Kirsh operators 255–268
subtracting images...................................292–294
texture...278–282
image measurements................................509–574
alignment..523–528
brightness measurements 510–515
caliper dimensions 543–549
counting features....................................529–532
describing shape 553–555
determining location 516–518
ellipse fitting 551–552
feature identification 566–569
feature size 536–543
fractal dimension....................................555–559
harmonic analysis...................................559–562
neighbor relationships 519–522
orientation 518–519
perimeter 549–551
special counting procedures....................532–535
three-dimensional measurements............569–574
topology...562–566
images, acquiring 1–86
color displays 56–59
color imaging 32–41
color spaces 47–55
digital cameras 41–47
high resolution imaging...........................25–32
human reliance on images 1–7
image types 59–61
imaging requirements 80–86
multiple images 68–72
range imaging 61–68
stereoscopy...72–80
using video cameras 7–25
image visualization, three-dimensional...........617–687
arbitrary section planes...........................641–644
3D data sets 633–636
image processing in 3D 679–683
measurements on 3D images 683–686
multiply connected surfaces....................673–679
optical sectioning 624–627
ray tracing..657–662
reflection..662–667
sequential removal 627–629
serial sections 619–624
slicing data set 636–641
sources of 3D data 617–619
special display hardware 654–657
stereo 629–633
stereo viewing 650–654
surfaces..667–673
use of color..645–646
volumetric display 646–649
imaging
astronomical 614
3D 686
infrared 515
metallographic..623
methods...691

modalities 625
requirements 80
sources...35
system characteristics.............................358
stereometric...702
imaging defects, correcting.........................161–225
alignment...216–221
color shading..205–209
contrast expansion 191–194
fitting background function 196–199
geometrical distortion 213–215
maximum entropy 189–191
morphing 222–225
neighborhood averaging..........................166–174
noisy images 162–165
nonplanar views......................................209–213
nonuniform illumination.........................194–196
other neighborhood noise reduction
    methods...182–189
rank leveling...199–205
imaging surfaces..689–745
analysis of surface data...........................722–724
Birmingham measurement suite...............729–737
data presentation and visualization.........712–717
devices imaging surfaces by physical
    contact...692–696
microscopy of surfaces 700–703
noncontacting measurements...................696–700
processing of composition maps 710–712
processing of range images 706–710
producing surfaces 689–692
profile measurements..............................725–729
rendering and visualization 717–722
surface composition imaging...................703–706
topographic analysis and fractal
    dimensions 737–745
immunogold labeling.................................353
indirect interference techniques..................699
infrared imaging..515
inhibition 248
ink-jet printers 91, 105, 106
interactive pointing devices........................413
interference microscopes............................707
interferometric light microscope 63, 64
international standards................................726
International Standards Organization (ISO) 142, 726
International Telegraph and Telephone
    Consultative Committee (CCITT)...........142
interpolation...220, 638
inverse filter..584
ion microprobe image 418
ion microscopy..660, 704
ISO, see International Standards Organization
isoelevation lines.......................................631, 713
isotropy..465, 466, 493

Joint Photographers Expert Group (JPEG).............137,
                                            153, 155, 159, 635
compaction schemes 137
compression 42
standard...140
technique..141
JPEG, see Joint Photographers Expert Group

Kacmarz' method 588
kernel(s)
multiplication 167, 679
operation 166

size...168, 252
    spatial-domain...356
Kirsch operator.......................................255, 257
K value..362

label positioning...294
LaGrange multipliers.......................................591
Landstat thematic mapper (TM).................68, 297, 711
Laplacian
    difference operations...........................267
    enhancement....................................244
    image.....................................244, 257
    operator.........................242, 243, 245, 449
laser printer 87, 104
lattice structure...368
LCD, see liquid crystal display
least-squares fit..284
Lempel-Ziv technique 134
lenslets...13
light
    longer wavelength 626
    microscopy.......................................62, 486
    polarized...303
    sensor 8
    source 511, 625
    staining 192
line profile display 718
linear attenuation coefficient.........................579, 659
liquid crystal display (LCD)......................56, 99, 654
local roughness 739
logic 453
lookup tables (LUTs) 26, 34, 35, 136, 196, 228, 233,
    239, 256, 340, 670
lossless coding 128
lossy compression............................41, 46, 136, 155
luminance.......................................47, 50, 146
LUTs, see lookup tables

Mach bands 246
machining..689
Macintosh PICT format 126, 145
magnetic
    domains...325
    recording 118
    resonance imaging (MRI) 72, 578
    storage 119
magnitude image..319
Marr-Hildreth operator......................................264
mask image 27, 452
MAT, see medial axial transform
mathematical morphology....................................460
matrix multiplication..211
mean summit curvature 733
measurement(s)
    feature-specific 683
    noncontacting....................................696
    parameters.......................................568
    success of 446
mechanical interaction, between parts 689
medial axial transform (MAT)..........501, 503, 546, 547
median filter.................175, 176, 178, 179, 184, 630
medical tomography 578, 600
memory
    addressing 18
    cards 45
    temporary 289
Mercator's projection 209, 213, 224
mesh display 719

Michelson-Morley interferometer 699
micromechanical devices....................................690
microscope slide 122
microstructure 497
mineral identification.......................................297
Minkowski
    fractal dimension................................470
    method 743
    sausages...501
Mirau optics 65
models, non-parametric.....................................569
modulation transfer function (MTF) 66, 359
moment axis 518
monitor design 111
monochrome camera 53
morphing...222
motif combination.........................727, 728, 738
motion blur...362
moving-picture compression methods 159
Moving Pictures Experts Group (MPEG)........138, 143,
    159, 635
MPEG, see Moving Pictures Experts Group
MRI, see magnetic resonance imaging
MTF, see modulation transfer function
mullite structure 323
multiband
    images...374
    thresholding 381
Muybridge, Eadweard.................................639, 640

National Television Systems Committee (NTSC) 35–36,
    51
nearest-neighbor pairs 522
Necker cube 373
neighbor
    patterns.....................................472, 483
    relationships 482, 519, 570
neighborhood
    averaging 166
    operations...................................290, 681
    ranking 174
    region 283
neutron beams 617
noise
    isolated periodic.................................334
    method for removing............................186
    periodic 341
    reduction 163
    variations 171
noisy images.............................162, 170, 185
noncrystalline silicon 327
nonplanar views..209
nonuniform illumination....................................194
notch filter...345
NTSC, see National Television Systems Committee
nucleator...449
Nyquist frequency 308

object motion 294
Olympic filter 182
optical
    axis...700
    disks, read-write.................................117
    sectioning 624
    storage media 114
orientation 518
    determination 261
    preferred...324

paint pigment particles 437
PAL television 15
Parzen window function 337
patterned dots 96
pattern recognition 85
perimeter measurements 550
PET, see positron emission tomography
phantom 580, 600
phosphor dots 56
photographic film 8
photolithography 58
photons..162, 510, 609
piezo scanner movement 695
pixel(s) 7, 15, 95, 133, 180, 188, 192, 200, 217, 227,
                                        268, 299, 379, 400
    accuracy...621
    address...632
    array, reconstruction of 442
    background 490, 513
    blocks 148, 150
    bright 399
    brightness..............62, 88, 149, 190, 193, 512, 515
    color values..55
    corner-touching..549
    counting..............................469, 538, 540, 544, 684
    differences of 459
    dimensions 516
    dropout...707, 708
    edge-straddling...412
    elements 633
    finding 500
    foreground 432
    interpolation 219
    level 282
    limitations 503
    location...301, 355
    missing..462
    noise 24, 44
    ON 448
    patterns..69
    removing 461
    resolution 19, 572
    spacing 21, 401, 699
    square 422
    touching...417
    value 136, 153, 166, 182, 241, 302, 509, 522
planar resectioning..643
plastic replicas 697
point
    distributions..520
    finder 271
    probes..698
Poisson distribution 191, 404, 520, 521
polarization effects..514
polygon perimeter 566
polyhedron..428
position information 403
positron emission tomography (PET) 578
posterization...103, 176
PostScript compatible controllers..........................110
power spectrum 322
pressure waves...612
primary colors...37
printing and storage 87–160
    browsing and thumbnails 124–128
    color palettes...135–136
    color printing..98–104

databases for images..............................120–124
digital movies 158–160
dots on paper 92–97
film recorders 110–112
film storage 113–114
lossless coding..128–135
lossy compression 136–155
magnetic recording 118–120
optical storage media 114–118
other compression methods 155–157
printing 87–91
printing hardware....................................104–110
probability, definition of.............................591
profile-based measurements...........................734
profilometer..63, 65
program fragment 309
progressive scan..28
projection
    data 594
    devices..57
    images..605, 648
    profiles...599
    sets 616
pruning...459
pseudo-color 33, 34, 61, 196, 258, 645
pseudo-resolution 171, 172
pseudo-rotation 651
pseudo-topographic display 668
Pythagorean distance 490, 491, 549

QBIC, see query by image content
quality control 84, 293
query by image content (QBIC)............................121

radar mapping...665, 667
radioactive-labeled drug 185
radioisotope source..592
radio telescope data..2
random
    -access device 115
    dots 96
    intensity variations 183
    sectioning 537
range
    image.......................20, 61, 63, 277, 664, 666, 706
    information..73
    operator 279, 288
    -to-resolution ratios...712
    values..692
rank
    filter...184, 347
    leveling 199
    operations........................202, 268, 269, 278, 679
raster
    pattern 694
    scan...14
ray
    integral equation 579
    paths 612
    tracing..657, 663, 674
real time imaging 24
reconnaissance images 294, 365
reconstruction..338
    basis of 578
    global tomographic...613
    methods, algebraic..585
    technique...574
    tomographic 591, 678

red, green, and blue (RGB)......................................31
    components...52
    pixel values...375
    signals..50
    space..177
reference area...542, 543
region of interest (ROI) 528
relative alignment, of images 216
resolution..379
response curve 408
retina..246
retransformation..351, 361
reverse transformation.....................................583
RGB, see red, green, and blue
Richardson plot...550, 557, 744
ridge-finding algorithm....................................273
ringing..151
RLE, see run-length encoding
RMS, see root-mean-square
Roberts' Cross operator....................................253
ROI, see region of interest
rolling ball
    filter..273
    technique...188
root-mean-square (RMS)....................................280
roughness values...67, 708
routine, automatic...415
rubber-sheeting..220
run-length encoding (RLE) 134, 420

sample preparation 123
SAR, see synthetic aperture radar
satellite images.................114, 207, 225, 280, 281, 294
saturation image...385
scanner 511
scanning
    acoustic microscope image 2
    linear array 46
    tunneling microscope (STM)..............29, 30, 61,
                              67, 333, 693, 695
scanning electron microscope (SEM) 29, 30, 31, 61,
                  68, 74, 75, 194, 217, 535, 629, 701
    chamber...196
    correction of trapezoidal 221
    frustration using 702
    image.................................165, 435, 443, 501, 724
    trapezoidal distortion in 215
    X-ray images from..660
secondary ion mass spectrometer (SIMS)..........70, 71,
                      628, 661, 703
section planes, arbitrary....................................641
segmentation
    methods..423, 425
    process...496
    refining of...427
    watershed 494, 497, 499, 533
segmentation, thresholding and 371–429
    accuracy and reproducibility 400–403
    boundary lines..413–416
    contours...416–420
    general classification problem................427–429
    image representation 420–423
    including position information.............403–410
    multiband images.....................................374–377
    multiband thresholding..........................381–386
    multiple thresholding criteria 391–395
    other segmentation methods 423–427
    selective histograms 410–413

textural orientation.....................................395–400
    thresholding...371–374
    thresholding from texture 386–390
    two-dimensional thresholds 377–381
seismic reflection mapping................................662
seismography..611
self-affine compression.....................................156
SEM, see scanning electron microscope
serial sections 572, 618
shape descriptors 553, 554
shear waves...612
Sierpinski fractal...469
signal-to-noise ratio 24
SIMS, see secondary ion mass spectrometer
skeletonization 446, 456, 457, 483, 484, 487, 683
skiz...507
smoothing..174, 186, 435
Sobel
    derivative..439
    edge..389
    filter...290, 526
    gradient...411
    operator...262, 397
solid-state camera 10, 11, 13, 29
sonar...79
space probes 79
spacing, orientation and 320
spatial domain
    image..............................317, 320, 328, 349, 350
    kernels..356
spectral analysis 560
split-and-merge 424
square pixel array 422
statistical analysis 726
stereo 629
    images...651
    pair images 655
    viewing...650
stereological calculation, classical................537
stereoscopy 72, 73
STM, see scanning tunneling microscope
storage devices, write-once 116
stretching coefficients 212, 214
structural research..84
stylus instruments..693
subpixel accuracy...517
Sunspot technology..108
Super-VHS 36
surface
    data, analysis of 722
    elevation...664
    facets..675
    fractals 331
    geometric data...735
    images...668
    lay of 728
    performance...736
    reconstruction 302
    relief...714
    rendering..677
    science..694
surveillance photos 85, 127, 566
synthetic aperture radar (SAR) 78, 183

tape drives..119
TEM, see transmission electron microscope
template matching....................................365, 474, 679
termination impedance..16

tesselation 223, 274
test
    image 218, 386
    pattern 329, 361
texture
    estimator of 279
    of images 278
    orientation 395
    thresholding from 386
Thermal Infrared Multispectral Mapper 297
thermal wax printer 104, 106
thickness measuring...722
three-dimensional (3D) imaging 85, 520, 575, 577
thresholding, see also segmentation, thresholding
and..424, 425, 488
    brightness values...................................431, 443
    criteria, multiple................................391
    logical extension of..374
    mask obtained by 439
    of original image 464
TIFF files...126, 707
TM, see Landstat thematic mapper
tomography 611, 617
    high resolution 613
    medical 600
    three-dimensional 605
top hat filter.......................................271, 272, 273
topographic analysis 737
topological properties.........................563, 564
topothesy...742
touching particles, counting 534
training classes 567
transfer function 229, 230, 231
transform power spectrum 315
transistors 12, 37
transmission electron microscope (TEM) 32, 59, 60,
86, 284, 631
    deposits 81
    image 200, 205, 326, 351, 535, 623
    lattice 349
    replica 203, 204
    specimens...627
tube cameras 11
tumor 121
two dimensional (2D) images 575, 577
typesetter 93

UCR, see undercolor removal
UEPs, see ultimate eroded points
ultimate eroded points (UEPs) 495, 498, 683
undercolor removal (UCR) 100
unsharp masking...272

vacuum tube 8

Van Cittert filter 653
variance operator 265, 392, 399, 458, 459
Venn diagrams....................................433
video camera.......................................7, 15, 191, 334
vidicon camera 10
viewfinder...44
virtual reality..112
vision defects 1
visual
    classification 564
    discrimination....................................193
    inhibition 247
    switching 656
    system......................................6
visualization
    3D 658
    programs 384
    task 576
volume imaging 575, 617
Voronoi tesselation.......................................223
voting system, proportional...............................526
voxel(s)......................................70, 587, 618, 642
    arrays 647
    counting....................................570
    cubic 569
    images 71
    patterns 571
    reconstructed....................................615
    values......................................658
    weights 590

watershed segmentation...................494, 497, 499, 533
wax-based inks 106
weather satellite 214, 224
WORM drives 116, 117

X-ray
    absorption 578, 601, 602
    dot maps.................................405, 477
    energy....................................32, 710
    films 83
    images 33, 231, 451
    incidence.....................................604
    intensity......................................435
    mapping 23
    maps....................................436, 476, 646
    photons....................................592
    scattering....................................596
    spectrometers....................................705
    tomography.................................72, 455, 457, 609
    tubes 596, 610, 614

zone of inhibition.....................................248